Dynamic Nutrition for
MAXIMUM PERFORMANCE

A COMPLETE NUTRITIONAL GUIDE FOR PEAK SPORTS PERFORMANCE

DANIEL GASTELU
Dr. FRED HATFIELD

Avery Publishing Group

Garden City Park, New York

The information and procedures contained in this book are based upon the research and the personal and professional experiences of the authors. They are not intended to be a substitute for consulting with your physician or other health-care provider. The publisher and the authors are not responsible for any adverse effects or consequences resulting from the use of any of the suggestions, preparations, or procedures discussed in this book. All matters pertaining to your physical health should be supervised by a health-care professional.

Cover designers: William Gonzalez, Rudy Shur, and Ken Rajman
In-house editor: Elaine Will Sparber
Typesetter: Elaine V. McCaw

Avery Publishing Group
120 Old Broadway
Garden City Park, NY 11040
1–800–548–5757

Permission Credits

The table on page 29 is used with the permission of the American Diabetes Association. It is from adapted *Diabetes Care*, Vol. 5 (1982).

The definition on page 33 is reprinted with the permission of Chapman & Hall, New York, NY. It is from *The Nutrition and Health Encyclopedia*, Second Edition, by David F. Tver and Percy Russell, Ph.D.

The material on herbs on pages 107 to 114 is used with the permission of Avery Publishing Group, Garden City Park, NY. It is adapted from *Prescription for Nutritional Healing*, Second Edition, by James F. Balch, M.D., and Phyllis A. Balch, C.N.C.

The food-count listings on pages 347 to 372 are used with the permission of Avery Publishing Group, Garden City Park, NY. They are adapted from *The NutriBase Complete Book of Food Counts*, by Dr. Art Ulene.

The photos on the front cover and pages 201, 205, 216, 219, 244, 253, 257, 260, 264, 268, 272, 279, 283, 287, 296, 302, 311, 315, 327, 331, and 335 are used courtesy of PhotoDisc.

The photos on the front cover and page 238 are used courtesy of the United States Field Hockey Association/Steve Parker.

The photo on page 208 is used courtesy of Jason Mathas.

The photo on page 212 is used courtesy of the Professional Bowlers Association.

The photo on page 226 is used courtesy of Dana McCaw.

The photo on the back cover and page 232 is used courtesy of the National Equestrian Federation of the United States and Ed Lawrence, photographer, Video and Stills.

The photo on page 276 is used courtesy of Fred C. Hatfield, Ph.D.

The photo on page 324 is used courtesy of Tony Svensson, Trimarket.

Library of Congress Cataloging-in-Publication Data

Gastelu, Daniel.
    Dynamic nutrition for maximum performance : a complete nutritional
guide for peak sports performance / Daniel Gastelu, Fred Hatfield.
        p.   cm.
    Includes bibliographical references and index.
    ISBN 0-89529-756-6
    1. Athletes—Nutrition. I. Hatfield, Frederick C. II. Title.
TX361.A8.G37 1997
613.2' 024796—dc21   97-23443
                                                       CIP

Printed in the United States of America

10 9 8 7 6 5 4 3 2 1

CONTENTS

Appendix

Dynamic Nutrition for Maximum Performance
is dedicated to all the athletes and fitness exercisers
who train hard to be their very best,
and to those who nurture, teach, and coach them.

It is also dedicated to the memory
of my grandparents, Isidro and Rose Gastelu
and Gustav and Margaret Walther.

Daniel Gastelu, Jr.

ACKNOWLEDGMENTS

Special thanks to the following people, who encouraged me through this several-year endeavor—my wife, Gail Gastelu; my parents, Daniel and Joan Gastelu, Sr.; my brothers, Christopher and Gary Gastelu; managing editor, Rudy Shur; editor, Elaine Will Sparber; typesetter, Elaine V. McCaw; proofreaders Dara Stewart, Jennifer L. Santo, and Lisa James; and co-author, Dr. Fred Hatfield. Additionally, thanks to my friends, colleagues, and mentors, whose influence along my career path was an important part in my attaining this goal—Richard Vartan, Robert Mizerek, Dr. John H. Crow, Dr. Mark Kraus, Bob Fritz, Dr. Shari Lieberman, Ed Frankel, and Keith Frankel.

Daniel Gastelu, Jr.

The names of the people I owe gratitude could fill volumes. I have learned from scientists and athletes. I have learned from family and friends. My greatest debt of thanks I offer to my son Fred, who performed some of the background research that made this effort possible.

Fred C. Hatfield, Ph.D

PREFACE

The creation of this book has been a project taking several years and forming a story in itself.

We, the authors, recognized the need for a new, comprehensive sports-nutrition book a number of years ago. To try to meet this need, we first drew up an outline that included chapters presenting background information on the various aspects of sports nutrition. We then expanded our original idea to include a section featuring a variety of sports and fitness activities on an individual basis. Finally, we decided to present all this information in a user-friendly manner so that everyone in sports and fitness, regardless of age, experience, and educational background, could make immediate use of the book.

The need for such a practical educational tool is constantly being underscored by dietary surveys conducted among not only Americans in general but athletes, coaches, and trainers. These surveys reveal that most people, athletes included, do not follow an optimum-performance diet. Even more alarmingly, they indicate that many personal trainers, coaches, and professional nutritionists need to learn more about the special nutritional requirements of optimum performance. With these surveys in mind, we determined to create a book that would not only be a valuable, useful tool for all readers but that would also provide background information on various topics related to sports nutrition for the benefit of both fitness exercisers and sports professionals.

After several years of research and writing, we have produced *Dynamic Nutrition for Maximum Performance*, an encyclopedic resource on sports nutrition that athletes and fitness exercisers, as well as the specialists who guide them, can put to immediate use. In this book, we present information on basic performance-nutrition factors, dietary supplements, and energy production, plus provide guidelines for designing a personalized training program. In writing the book, we relied both on nutritional principles that are established in the scientific literature and on those that evolved from our personal-practice experiences, the experiences of the elite athletes with whom we

work, and the research of the International Sports Sciences Association. The performance-nutrition information that we present bridges the gap between theoretical research and practice. We never meant for this book to be a critical scientific overview, so we limited ourselves to presenting useful facts, not theoretical debate. For technical and professional readers, we include an extensive bibliography of reference sources for further study.

Most often, the athletes who are led astray nutritionally are enticed into choosing their diet or dietary-supplement program by marketing slogans or similar forms of misinformation. Sidetracked by this Madison Avenue hype, these athletes are blinded to the new scientific advances being made in performance nutrition. In this book, we present and discuss proven scientific performance-nutrition techniques and will help you reach your peak physical-performance level by explaining how to apply them.

Although this book focuses primarily on performance nutrition, it also includes tips for designing a personalized, sport-appropriate training program. Every physical activity creates its own specific nutritional demands, and in order for athletes to achieve their performance potential, they must both eat and train correctly for their particular activity.

The book begins with an introduction to nutrition that presents important guidelines from which you can benefit from your very first hour of reading. For immediate help, you can also turn to your sport-specific plan in Part Four.

Part One covers the A-to-Z's of nutrition as they apply to increasing athletic performance and maintaining fitness and good health. You will learn about the macronutrients—carbohydrates, protein, lipids, water, and oxygen—and the micronutrients—vitamins, minerals, metabolites, and herbs. A discussion of food and dietary supplements is also presented, as is information on ergogenic aids (any substances or procedures that enhance athletic performance).

Part Two includes such topics as basic anatomy to give you a foundation on which to base the rest of the material in the book. A discussion of body composition will show you how to determine the amounts of muscle and fat that make up your body and what your body should contain for peak performance. Additional topics include digestion, absorption, and metabolism.

Part Three is a special-nutrition section that offers straightforward information on fat loss, muscle building, and carbohydrate loading. It ends with a discussion of additional factors important to performance improvement and stresses how these factors combine to create a successful formula.

Part Four is the heart and soul of the book. It presents an easy-to-use nutrition plan for each individual sport and fitness activity. If, for example, you are a football player, you can simply turn to the football plan for all the nutrition information that you in particular need. If you enjoy aerobic exercise, you can turn to the plan for fitness activities for nutrition information individualized for your needs. If you cannot find your athletic or fitness activity in Part Four, turn to the list of additional activities presented on pages 198 to 200 for the covered activity that most closely resembles yours.

Rounding out the book are a complete explana-tion of how to put together the best diet for your athletic or fitness efforts and eight sample daily menus to use as guides. An hourly caloric breakdown chart will also help you create your perfect diet, and a personal inventory form will help you stay on top of your changing body composition and nutritional requirements. We include a daily nutrition log to help you keep track of your food intake and assess which foods and diet plans do and do not work for you. And for reference purposes, we offer the most recent listings of the Reference Daily Intakes and Daily Reference Values, as well as a detailed three-part diagram of the muscles of the human body. Finally, an extensive glossary, bibliography, and index will help you get the most out of all the information presented in the book.

Dynamic Nutrition for Maximum Performance is your comprehensive resource for nutrition success. With its easy-to-use format and library of information, it will become an important part of your life. Use it to design a personalized nutrition and supplement program that will lead you to maximum performance and health.

Good luck in your athletic and fitness endeavors.

HOW TO USE THIS BOOK

Dynamic Nutrition for Maximum Performance is a comprehensive guide intended to help you achieve and maintain the highest level of fitness and performance through proper dietary intake and nutritional supplementation. Even if you are a good athlete, you will benefit from this book because it will help you achieve optimum health and performance, and increase your energy, power, and endurance. Written by a certified specialist in performance nutrition and certified master of fitness science along with the head of the International Sports Sciences Association and world-class powerlifting champion, this book blends the latest scientific research with traditional locker-room treatments. It provides all the information you need to design your own individualized performance-nutrition program. In addition, it explains such key nutritional techniques as carbohydrate loading and taking megadoses of selected supplements, discusses how to modify your diet for fat loss and/or muscle gain, and presents training tips and advice on how to construct a state-of-the-art training program—all in easy-to-understand language.

Dynamic Nutrition for Maximum Performance is divided into four parts. Parts One and Two present the basic principles of nutrition and health. Part One reviews the macronutrients (carbohydrates, protein, and lipids), the micronutrients (vitamins, minerals, metabolites, and herbs), and the forgotten nutrients (water and oxygen). It also explains how to obtain the macro- and micronutrients from food and supplement sources and describes the variety of popular sports supplements found in grocery stores, health-food stores, and pharmacies. Part Two explains how and why the body uses the nutrients discussed in Part One. It looks at the cells, tissues, and systems of the body, discusses digestion and absorption, and presents the latest information on metabolism and body composition.

Part Three takes an in-depth look at several key sports-nutrition techniques. Proven methods for successful fat loss and muscle building are fully described, with tables and insets included to make your calculations easier. Three methods for effective carbohydrate loading are also presented, as is an overview of the non-nutritional elements that are included in any top-notch nutrition and training program.

Part Four is the heart and soul of the book. It presents sport-specific performance-nutrition plans for activities from baseball to wrestling. Use the guide on page 198 to help you find the plan that you in particular should follow. Each plan takes the information from Parts One, Two, and Three and presents it in a format that is both user-friendly and concise. After a brief introduction to the activity, the energy demands of the activity are fully described, with a table showing how much energy each of the body's major energy systems contributes for different aspects of the activity. The table is then translated into concrete guidelines on how to structure your diet for maximum energy, power, and endurance, and two tables list exactly which nutritional supplements to take to augment your diet and in what amounts. Either read Parts One, Two, and Three for a solid foundation in sports nutrition and then turn to your sport-specific plan for the guidelines pertinent for you, or turn to your sport-specific plan first, dipping into Parts One, Two, and Three as necessary for explanations and background information.

Rounding out the book are a personal inventory form to help you keep track of your body composition, daily caloric requirements, and protein requirement; a chart to help you determine your caloric requirements; detailed instructions and sample daily diets to help you eat appropriately for your performance goals; and a daily nutrition log to help you keep track of your food intake. For reference, the current Reference Daily Intakes of the vitamins and minerals and Daily Reference Values of the macronutrients are also provided, as is a three-part diagram of the muscles of the human body. A glossary of terms used in the book will help if you come upon a word whose definition you have forgotten, and an extensive bibliography will point you to additional reference sources to expand your knowledge of sports nutrition even further.

The supplementation programs recommended in this book are dynamic and depend upon your individual body composition and needs; your sport or fitness activity; and the recommendations of your health-care provider. Incorporate the recommended supplements into your regimen one at a time. Before you begin taking them on a regular basis, test them out to make sure you do not experience any negative reactions. When taking your supplements, always wash them down with a full glass of water. Some nutritional supplements are concentrated and can overburden the liver and other bodily systems if they are not accompanied by enough liquid. Additionally, water enhances absorption and is needed to help carry the nutrients to the cells.

Learn to listen to your body and keep an accurate training log. Over time, you will notice changes in your body and will be able to identify their causes. After a supplementation period is completed, decrease your supplement dosages gradually so that your body has a chance to adjust.

It is important to stress that the suggestions offered in this book are not intended to replace appropriate medical or nutritional consultation or treatment. The supplements recommended for a particular purpose should be approved and monitored by your doctor or a trained health-care professional.

AN INTRODUCTION TO NUTRITION
THE VITAL LINK TO SUPER PERFORMANCE AND ENERGY

Looking back through history, we can see clear evidence that humans have been searching for performance-enhancing foods since before they even began banding together to form the earliest civilizations. Anthropologists believe that in primitive times, early humans searched for foods that would increase their strength and performance and help them become better hunters and warriors. History is filled with tales about men who ate and drank certain foods to boost their combat prowess. There are even gruesome accounts of victors eating the hearts of their opponents to capture the spirit of the opponents' strength.

What these early hunters and warriors realized was that nutrition is an important factor in physical performance. Just as most cultures have traditional potions to boost sexual performance, many also have customary foods and rituals for increasing athletic performance. The Greeks are credited with the first documented attempt to improve sports performance through special nutritional practices. According to historians, around 450 B.C., Dromeus of Stymphalus advocated such dietary habits as the consumption of large amounts of meat to improve muscular strength. Many athletes in various sports still eat high-protein diets for increased performance.

Today, we know much more about how nutrition affects performance. Furthermore, we know that athletes, to be successful, must eat sufficient amounts of all the nutrients, not just protein, and we reserve high-protein diets for special times and for certain athletes. We understand that no one food or nutrient can increase athletic performance. The myth of the "magic food solution" is the reason there are so many misconceptions concerning nutrition and such tremendous controversy within the field of sports nutrition. Nutrition for peak performance is an involved science, and many factors must be considered to help any one athlete achieve maximum results.

THE NEW AGE OF SPORTS NUTRITION

When you think of the high-tech society in which we live today, you may find it hard to believe that we first began practicing carbohydrate loading and consumption of carbohydrates during athletic events in the 1970s. Many readers probably still remember the days when marathon runners experienced the phenomenon called "hitting the wall." Marathoners felt this sensation when they depleted their body's glycogen (carbohydrate) stores and began running primarily on stored body fat. Today, long-distance athletes know that they can increase their times and avoid hitting the wall simply by practicing carbohydrate loading and ingesting carbohydrate drinks immediately before and during the race. This physical phenomenon and its simple dietary solution exemplify perfectly why a scientific approach toward nutrition is necessary.

We know so much more today about how to improve athletic performance through nutrition than our predecessors ever imagined, even just twenty years ago. Thousands of studies on how nutrients and nutritional practices can improve performance have been conducted during the past two decades. Still, however, most people succumb to the misinformation that is spread around locker rooms and published in magazines. Surprisingly, recent scientific surveys have revealed that the majority of athletes, as well as the coaches, trainers, and other professionals who tend to them, do not have a working knowledge of what constitutes a good sports-nutrition program. This is why many athletes continue to resort to ridiculous nutritional practices and then turn to snake oils or even drugs in an attempt to compensate for their poor habits. These practices are not only dangerous but counterproductive.

The performance-nutrition information presented in this book will help you reach your athletic peak quicker and achieve optimum health in the process. You will learn new ways to keep your energy level up

1

on a consistent basis. You will also find new information on special nutrition topics such as weight loss, muscle building, and macronutrient modulation for the achievement of maximum output.

Everyone has experienced, directly or indirectly, the need to lose weight for a sport such as wrestling, football, or gymnastics. Losing weight, in fact, is a multi-billion-dollar-a-year industry. However, do you think that the common methods for losing weight—for example, starving, taking laxatives, sweating, or following gimmick diets—are healthy or effective? Of course they are not! And what about building muscle? Athletes will try almost anything to put an extra inch on their biceps or to gain extra strength to lift a few additional pounds. This is true for the athletes of every sport. Athletes want to be leaner and more muscular.

If you are involved in athletics or fitness, or just want to improve yourself, it is now time for you to leave the dark ages of nutrition and join the renaissance age of scientifically based high-tech performance nutrition. This text is intended to guide you. It is written for all athletes—professionals and amateurs—as well as for coaches, trainers, and fitness exercisers, and is intended to be both informative and easy to use. Proper nutrition is the key to getting the competitive edge that all athletes need to win in sports and that all people need to win in life.

WHAT IS NUTRITION?

Nutrition is the process of eating and converting food into structural and functional body tissues such as skin, muscle, and hair. It is required for growth, maintenance of bodily functions, repair of tissues, performance, and health. Different parts of the body need different nutrients to function properly. As an example, the nervous system has different nutritional needs than the muscles do. These differences must be taken into consideration when attempting to make the whole body perform at its best.

On the surface, getting the nutrition you need seems to be easy enough. After all, you eat something every day. But recent government reports show that the vast majority of Americans eat too much of the wrong things—fat, sodium, and sugar—and not enough of the good stuff—complex carbohydrates, lean meats, and fresh fruits and vegetables. It is astounding how many athletes, especially teen athletes, frequent fast-food restaurants and munch down large amounts of snack foods but still believe they are consuming high-protein, low-fat diets. In truth, these people are eating high-fat, high-sodium diets that are low in the essential nutrients.

The problem of poor nutrition is highly complex but originates in the simple fact that most of us learned about nutrition way back in grade school. What was taught then, and even what is taught today in grade schools, has nothing to do with nutrition for athletes and barely provides a good foundation for nonathletes.

The basic guidelines that you probably remember are based on the food-group approach to nutrition. This approach says that a diet is balanced if it consists of foods from the fruit and vegetable group; the meat, poultry, and fish group; the dairy group; and the bread and cereal group.

In theory, this food-group approach should work. In practice, however, we are a nation suffering from fatal diseases due to poor nutrition. Qualitative approaches to nutrition do not address exactly how much of each nutrient every individual needs, nor do they deal with the special requirements of athletes. All they do is recommend the consumption of several servings from certain food categories on a daily basis.

Additionally, you cannot be certain that the food you eat provides reliable nutrition. Scientists have determined that the nutritional content of food can vary greatly according to where the food was grown. This means that potatoes from Maine and potatoes from Idaho may vary tremendously in the amounts of the vitamins and minerals they have. Many studies have shown that athletes are deficient in important minerals and vitamins. Athletes are just not eating correctly.

Nutrition, especially sports nutrition, is a quantitative science. While nonathletes can survive day to day by following general do's and don'ts, athletes need more sophisticated and precise guidelines to achieve performance excellence. Therefore, a 120-pound female swimmer needs to eat a different diet from a 250-pound male shot-putter.

Billions of people eat and live on the planet Earth. The food supply is quite different on every continent, and so is health. Most of us associate being well fed with being healthy. However, millions of people each year die from diseases that are caused by such dietary bloopers as eating too much fat. Athletes must do more than just eat and live. They must operate at a heightened level. For this reason, they must follow special high-performance nutrition programs. The average athlete consumes two, three, or more times the number of calories than a nonathlete. Typically, athletes consume over 3,000 calories per day. At these high levels of food intake, athletes had better make sure that they are eating the correct foods.

Understanding exactly what constitutes a healthy diet is therefore of primary importance. With the basics down, we can then move on to the scientific intricacies of performance nutrition.

THE THREE E'S OF NUTRITION

By now, you have probably come to believe that no one really knows which nutrition plan is correct. In one sense, you are right. Scientific advances and new research are constantly changing the way we believe we should eat for good health.

The nutrition philosophies that are followed today fall into three main categories:

1. Essential nutrition for survival.
2. Essential nutrition for optimum health.
3. Essential nutrition for maximum athletic performance.

In the following pages, we will discuss these different levels of nutrition and attempt to shed new light on why your nutrition program may be incomplete.

Essential Nutrition for Survival

The diets that are eaten by most of the general population can be classified as providing essential nutrition for survival. This category is based on the nutrition standard that you have heard so much about—the Recommended Dietary Allowances (RDAs). The RDAs were first established in 1943 by the National Research Council (NRC) of the U.S. Department of Health and Human Services as a goal for good nutrition. Experts at that time recognized that nutritional goals needed to be set to help propagate good health on a national basis. Every several years, the NRC has published updated RDAs to reflect the best current scientific judgment on nutrient allowances for good health. In addition, the NRC established the Estimated Safe and Adequate Daily Dietary Intakes (ESADDIs), a group of nutrient values that represent safe and adequate intake levels for a number of essential nutrients for which the data were sufficient to estimate a range of requirements but not sufficient enough to assign RDAs. The RDAs have

also served as the baseline against which the diets of certain specialized groups of people can be compared for adequacy. In this way, the RDAs have been a particularly useful reference point for health-care practitioners. However, in 1985, the scientists involved in updating the RDAs disagreed so widely on the recommended allowances that the tenth edition of the guidelines was not published until 1989. Nutritionists from the NRC and Health Canada (the Canadian equivalent of the U.S. Department of Health and Human Services) are currently working together to compile a new database, the Dietary Reference Intakes. (For a discussion of the Dietary Reference Intakes, see "The Nutritional Alphabet Soup" on page 4.) This new database is expected to replace the RDAs within the next ten years.

As a member of the general public, though, you have probably only rarely come face-to-face with the RDAs and ESADDIs. What you actually see, on food and supplement nutrition labels, are the Reference Daily Intakes (RDIs)—or, rather, the Daily Values (DVs), which are used by manufacturers to present a product's RDI information to the public. Before the RDIs, you probably encountered the U.S. Recommended Daily Allowances (USRDAs). The USRDAs were a group of nutrient values created by the Food and Drug Administration (FDA) to help the manufacturers of processed foods and supplements meet its nutrition-labeling criteria. The USRDA values were based on the RDAs. The FDA took the RDAs, which are the recommended nutrient intakes for health reasons, and created the USRDAs, which were the nutrient values applied to food and supplement regulations. In an effort to make the system more user-friendly, the FDA replaced the USRDAs with the more general RDIs after the passage of the Nutrition Labeling and Education Act in 1993, and the USRDA nomenclature has not been used since January 1997. RDIs have been given to twenty-seven vitamins and minerals. (For the list, see Appendix E on page 377.) These values are represented on the new nutrition labels as percent Daily Values.

Along with the RDIs, the FDA has also created a group of food- and supplement-label nutrient values called the Daily Reference Values (DRVs). The DRVs describe the macronutrients that are present in a food or supplement and are based on a reference diet of 2,000 calories. The same as the RDIs, they are represented on the new nutrition labels in terms of percent DVs. The terms *Reference Daily Intakes*,

Daily Reference Values, *RDI*, and *DRV* never actually appear on food and supplement labels.

Now that the FDA has made its successful switch from the USRDA system to the RDI and DRV systems, nutritionists are anxiously awaiting the NRC's switch to its new database, the Dietary Reference Intakes. Many progressive health-care practitioners claim that the RDAs are not adequate for good health. New and evolving research is demonstrating that eating more of certain nutrients can help improve and protect health. For example, research has shown that taking more vitamin E than the RDA for that nutrient can reduce the risk for certain diseases.

This shift away from the RDA approach to nutrition is founded on the health-driven philosophy of achieving optimum nutrition. The RDAs, as well as similar governmental nutritional standards around the world, are concerned primarily with preventing diseases that result from deficiencies of essential nutrients, such as scurvy, which is caused by the lack of vitamin C. The goal of the RDAs is not optimum health. In fact, most of the RDA values are based on the average intakes of those nutrients by the entire American population. For this approach to result in optimum health, everyone in the population must already be eating a healthy diet and everyone must have the same nutritional requirements. As mentioned earlier, though, the reality is that the majority of Americans are eating poor diets. The 1988 Surgeon General's *Report on Nutrition and Health* even named the typical American diet as responsible for causing disease or death in millions of people annually.

The goal of the RDAs has never been optimum health. In fact, when the RDAs were first established in 1943, values were listed for just nine nutrients—protein, vitamin A, vitamin B_1 (thiamine), vitamin B_2 (riboflavin), vitamin B_3 (niacin), vitamin C, vitamin D, calcium, and iron. Today, RDA values have been set for nineteen nutrients—protein, vitamin A, vitamin B_1, vitamin B_2, vitamin B_3, vitamin B_6 (pyridoxine), vitamin B_{12} (cobalamin), folate, vitamin C, vitamin D, vitamin E, vitamin K, calcium, iodine, iron, magnesium, phosphorus, selenium, and zinc. In addition, ESADDIs have been set for seven vitamins and minerals—vitamin B_5 (pantothenic acid), biotin, chromium, copper, fluoride, manganese, and molybdenum. (For a discussion of any of these nutrients, see the appropriate chapter in Part One.)

It is enlightening that just thirty years ago, Americans based their nutritional needs on only nine essential nutrients, and today, on twenty-six. Many experts recognize that even more essential nutrients exist and look to the RDAs only as a guideline for maintaining survival and avoiding deficiencies. Additionally, they acknowledge that the RDAs are based on population averages and are intended to maintain the average national health, not individual health. To underscore this point, the tenth edition of the book *Recommended Dietary Allowances* warns, on page 1, that "individuals with special nutrition needs are not covered by the RDA's." This warning certainly applies to athletes. And athletes should keep this warning in mind as they try to break away from erroneous beliefs and wives' tales and forge ahead to discover, with a clear mind, what performance nutrition is all about.

Even if you are not an athlete, you need to understand the limitations of the RDA system so that you can upgrade your nutrition without feeling hesitant or doubtful. The RDA system is useful as a baseline and reference point for nutrient intake. The current RDAs, as just mentioned, provide values for twenty-six nutrients, but most nutrition experts identify forty-five as essential for life. (For the list, see "The Essential Nutrients" on page 6.) As time goes on, researchers will discover even more essential nutrients, as well as more uses for those currently recognized.

The Nutritional Alphabet Soup

Unless you are a student majoring in nutrition or a recent graduate, you probably do not understand the differences between the various nutrient values in popular use today. You may not even realize that there are any differences. In fact, some professional nutritionists have trouble defining the systems with a fair degree of accuracy.

To aid you in your quest to improve your nutritional acumen, or at least to help you figure out how much vitamin C you are *really* getting, we have compiled the following list of brief definitions of the nutritional alphabet soup:

☐ *Recommended Dietary Allowances (RDAs).* A database originally compiled by the National Research Council that has become the accepted source of nutrient allowances for healthy people. The RDAs served as the basis for the U.S. Recommended Daily Allowances (USRDAs), which were the Food and Drug Administration's standards for nutrition labeling on foods and supplements until January 1997, and now serve as the basis for the Reference Daily Intakes (RDIs), which have replaced the USRDAs. The RDAs are presented in a book entitled *Recommended Dietary Allowances,* first published in 1943; the tenth edition was published in 1989. The RDAs are to be replaced by the Dietary Reference Intakes (DRIs), a new database being compiled jointly by the United States, Canada, and possibly Mexico.

☐ *Estimated Safe and Adequate Daily Dietary Intakes (ESADDIs).* A group of nutrient values compiled by the National Research Council that represents safe and adequate intake levels for a number of essential nutrients for which the data were sufficient to estimate a range of requirements but not sufficient enough to assign RDAs.

☐ *Dietary Reference Intakes (DRIs).* An umbrella term referring to a new three-tier database being compiled to take the place of the Recommended Dietary Allowances (RDAs). It is being compiled jointly by the National Research Council of the U.S. Department of Health and Human Services and Health Canada (the Canadian equivalent of the U.S. Department of Health and Human Services). It is hoped that Mexico will also join the effort, so that one standard database can be compiled for the entire North American continent.

While the names of the tiers are tentative, the three tiers will include:

• *Estimated Average Requirements (EARs).* The mean requirement of each nutrient in a number of age-gender categories.

• *Recommended Dietary Allowances (RDAs) for an individual.* The mean requirement plus two deviations for a reference individual of each nutrient. The combination of these three values will meet the biological needs of 97.5 percent of the population.

• *Maximum upper levels.* The upper limit of intake for each nutrient that is known or predicted to be associated with a low risk of adverse effects in almost all the people of the reference group.

According to current plans, DRIs will be set for non-essential nutrients in addition to the essential nutrients. Furthermore, the goal of the DRIs is optimum health, not just survival.

☐ *U.S. Recommended Daily Allowances (USRDAs).* A group of nutrient values created by the Food and Drug Administration to help the manufacturers of processed foods and supplements meet its nutrition-labeling criteria. The values were based on the National Research Council's Recommended Dietary Allowances (RDAs). The FDA took the RDAs, which are the recommended nutrient intakes for health reasons, and created the USRDAs, which are the nutrient values applied to food and supplement regulations. The USRDAs were completely phased out and replaced with the FDA's Reference Daily Intakes (RDIs) by January 1997.

☐ *Reference Daily Intakes (RDIs).* Food- and supplement-label nutrient values created by the Food and Drug Administration to replace its U.S. Recommended Daily Allowances (USRDAs) but still based on the National Research Council's Recommended Dietary Allowances (RDAs). The original mandate, which grew out of a number of proposals, was published in January 1994; and the RDIs completely took the place of the USRDAs by January 1997. RDIs have been assigned to twenty-seven vitamins and minerals—vitamin A, vitamin B_1 (thiamine), vitamin B_2 (riboflavin), vitamin B_3 (niacin), vitamin B_5 (pantothenic acid), vitamin B_6 (pyridoxine), vitamin B_{12} (cobalamin), biotin, folate, vitamin C, vitamin D, vitamin E, vitamin K, calcium, chloride, chromium, copper, iodine, iron, magnesium, manganese, molybdenum, phosphorus, potassium, selenium, sodium, and zinc. These values are represented on the new nutrition labels as percent Daily Values (DVs).

☐ *Daily Reference Values (DRVs).* Food- and supplement-label nutrient values created by the Food and Drug Administration for the macronutrients and two electrolytes. DRVs, based on a reference diet of 2,000 calories, have been assigned to fat, saturated fat, cholesterol, total carbohydrate, fiber, protein, sodium, and potassium. These values, the same as the Reference Daily Intakes (RDIs), are presented on the new nutrition labels as percent Daily Values (DVs).

☐ *Daily Values (DVs).* A system created by the Food and Drug Administration to help manufacturers present their Reference Daily Intake (RDI) and Daily Reference Value (DRV) information on food and supplement labels. The RDI and DRV values are presented as percent Daily Values—that is, the amount of the nutrient in the product is described as a percentage, with 100 percent being equivalent to the total amount of the nutrient required by a reference individual consuming a 2,000-calorie-per-day diet. The terms *Reference Daily Intakes, Daily Reference Values, RDI,* and *DRV* never actually appear on the nutrition labels.

For more information on the above terms, visit your local library or contact the Center for Food Safety and Applied Nutrition, Food and Drug Administration, 200 C Street, Southwest, Washington, DC 20204; or the Food and Nutrition Board, Institute of Medicine, National Academy of Sciences, 2101 Constitution Avenue, Northwest, Washington, DC 20418.

The Essential Nutrients

The following nutrients are substances vital for good health that the body cannot produce itself or that it cannot produce in sufficient amounts:

☐ *Amino acids*—Cystine, histidine, isoleucine, leucine, lysine, methionine, phenylalanine, threonine, tryptophan, tyrosine, and valine.

☐ *Carbohydrates*—Fiber and glucose.

☐ *Lipids*—Alpha-linolenic acid, arachidonic acid, and linoleic acid.

☐ *Metabolites*—Choline and inositol.

☐ *Minerals*—Calcium, chloride, chromium, cobalt, copper, fluoride, iodide, iron, magnesium, manganese, molybdenum, phosphorus, potassium, selenium, sodium, sulfur, and zinc.

☐ *Vitamins*—Vitamin A, vitamin B_1 (thiamine), vitamin B_2 (riboflavin), vitamin B_3 (niacin), vitamin B_5 (pantothenic acid), vitamin B_6 (pyridoxine), vitamin B_{12} (cobalamin), biotin, folate, vitamin C (ascorbic acid), vitamin D, vitamin E, and vitamin K.

☐ *Water and oxygen.*

In addition to these known nutrients, there are nutrients that have not yet been determined to be essential but that are vital for good health and performance.

Essential Nutrition for Optimum Health

As just discussed, the focus of the government and of the many nutrition professionals who follow the government's RDA standards is nutrition that provides just enough of the essential nutrients to prevent dietary deficiencies. The focus is not optimum nutrition. Furthermore, the government and these nutrition professionals do not put any emphasis on the so-called nonessential nutrients. (For a discussion of the term *nonessential*, see *"Nonessential* Does Not Mean Unimportant" on page 7.) Thanks to the developing health industry, however, these past few decades have witnessed a nutrition revolution promoting a diet rich in all nutrients, in amounts greater than those previously recommended. At long last, we are looking at a total nutrition approach.

Progressive nutritionists such as Shari Lieberman, Ph.D, a coauthor of *The Real Vitamin and Mineral Book* (Garden City Park, New York: Avery Publishing Group, 1997), now tell us that for optimum health, our bodies need more nutrients and in higher amounts than the RDAs recommend. Dr. Lieberman is one of the nutritional pioneers who coined the term *Optimum Daily Intake* for the higher amounts of vitamins and minerals that we require and for the nonessential nutrients and herbal factors that offer us so many benefits.

There are many reasons why our nutritional requirements are so high. Our bodies face, on a daily basis, a host of environmental stresses, such as air pollution, poor or contaminated drinking water, pesticides, and non-nutritive food additives, some of which are even toxic. The foods that we eat do not supply the proper amounts of the nutrients for optimum health. Moreover, most people do not eat proper diets to begin with. On top of this, researchers are continually finding new uses for all the nutrients besides their roles in basic survival. For example, a group of vitamins and minerals called antioxidants has been found to protect the body against free radicals. Free radicals are byproducts of normal chemical reactions in the body that involve oxygen. They are known to injure cell membranes and cause defects in the deoxyribonucleic acid (DNA), the genetic material of the cells, plus are believed to contribute to the aging process and to degenerative illnesses such as cancer, arthritis, atherosclerosis (hardening of the arteries), and cataracts. Increased activity, sunlight, and chemicals all cause the body to produce higher amounts of free radicals, which means that it is especially important for athletes to take nutrients with antioxidant capabilities. Antioxidants seek out and neutralize free radicals in the body and stimulate the body to recover more quickly from free-radical damage. (For a discussion of free radicals and antioxidants, see Chapter 5.)

The Optimum Daily Intakes (ODIs) form the framework of the sports-nutrition program presented in the chapters that follow. The program includes eating a diet that contains the essential and many nonessential nutrients in amounts that are two or more times greater than the RDAs.

Essential Nutrition for Maximum Athletic Performance

Essential nutrition for maximum athletic performance is the most recent advancement in the field of nutrition. Sports scientists have been making new discoveries almost daily, uncovering the intimate connection between nutrition and performance. Eating for maximum athletic performance includes consuming food for the maintenance of optimum health as well as for extra nutrients to achieve maximum performance.

Macronutrient modulation is also part of an athlete's performance-nutrition program. Macronutrient modulation is the practice of eating specific percentages of protein, fat, and carbohydrates to enhance performance. In addition, meal timing and frequency are important. While nonathletes can achieve optimum health by eating three or four moderately sized, balanced meals, athletes must consume a diet that is much more complex. Athletes need to vary their intake of carbohydrates, protein, and fat, and to consume a precise amount of dietary supplements, such as vitamins and minerals, at each meal and in conjunction with their specific training schedules. Some athletes must implement a special nutrition plan, such as carbohydrate loading, several days before competition. Still others must concentrate on attaining a certain body weight for competition while still maintaining peak performance.

To help athletes meet their special needs, the nutrition program presented in this book is individualized for twenty-eight major sports and fitness activities using a new set of standards called the Performance Daily Intakes (PDIs). The PDIs, like the RDIs and ODIs, are guidelines for the intake of nutrients based on the findings of researchers and, in this case, sports researchers. They were developed using research results as well as the vast library of reference publications on nutrition. The PDI guidelines are for both men and women. They compensate for the higher nutritional requirements that athletes have over nonathletes and are customized according to athletic or fitness specialty. They are dynamic, taking into consideration a wide range of needs, activity levels, and body sizes. They offer, for the first time, guidance in the purchase of dietary supplements by providing examples of the ingredients to look for when shopping.

General PDI values are presented in Table 1 on page 8. These general values are for physically active, healthy adults. For the supplement amounts that you in particular need, turn to your sport-specific plan in Part Four. Note that all the nutrition plans utilize supplement sources in addition to food sources. In most cases, the lower limit of a nutrient's recommended range of intake is equal to or higher than its RDA value, so food sources alone probably will not suffice, or will just barely do so. The intake recommendations are given in ranges because individuals' needs vary according to size and activity level. Smaller or less active individuals need less of each nutrient than do larger or more active individuals. No matter how active or large you are, however, do not take more than the highest amount recommended, except under a doctor's supervision. (For

Nonessential Does Not Mean Unimportant

An essential nutrient is a nutrient that the body cannot make or that it cannot make in sufficient amounts to maintain good health. Scientists have discovered over forty nutrients that fit this description. These nutrients include the carbohydrate glucose, certain amino acids from protein, certain fatty acids such as alpha-linolenic acid, thirteen vitamins, and seventeen minerals.

The label *nonessential* is terribly misleading. The nonessential nutrients are all the nutrients that are not considered essential—that is, the nutrients that the body does make in sufficient amounts to maintain good health. However, when you eat for maximum performance and optimum health, getting the nonessentials from your diet can be just as important as getting the essentials. For example, by eating a full-profile protein, which contains all the nonessential as well as essential amino acids, you give your body the amino acids that it needs in a much quicker fashion, as it will not have to spend time making the nonessentials from the essentials. For maximum performance and health, you also need to eat the right proportions and amounts of both the essential and nonessential nutrients. In addition, there are other performance factors—such as herbs, metabolites (substances created by or necessary for metabolism), and phytochemicals (chemical substances from plants)—that are not essential for survival but that are essential for improved performance.

Table 1.   General PDIs for Physically Active, Healthy Adults

Nutrient	Forms Used in Supplements	PDI
VITAMINS		
Vitamin A	Vitamin A acetate, vitamin A palmitate	5,000–25,000 IU
Beta-carotene	Beta-carotene	15,000–80,000 IU
Vitamin B_1	Thiamine hydrochloride, thiamine mononitrate	30–300 mg
Vitamin B_2	Riboflavin	30–300 mg
Vitamin B_3	Nicotinic acid, niacinamide	20–100 mg
Vitamin B_5	D-calcium pantothenate	25–200 mg
Vitamin B_6	Pyridoxine hydrochloride	20–100 mg
Vitamin B_{12}	Cyanocobalamin	12–200 mcg
Biotin	Biotin	125–300 mcg
Folate	Folic acid	400–1,200 mcg
Vitamin C	Ascorbic acid, buffered vitamin C, mineral ascorbates, rose hips, ester C polyascorbate	800–3,000 mg
Vitamin D	Ergocalciferol (vitamin D_2), cholecalciferol (vitamin D_3)	400–1,000 IU
Vitamin E	D-alpha-tocopherol succinate, d-alpha-tocopherol acetate, dl-alpha-tocopherol, dl-alpha-tocopherol acetate, mixed tocopherols	200–1,000 IU
Vitamin K	Phylloquinone (vitamin K_1), menadione (vitamin K_3)	80–180 mcg
MINERALS		
Boron	Boron tri chelate, boron glycinate, boron citrate	6–12 mg
Calcium	Calcium carbonate, calcium citrate, calcium malate, calcium glycinate	1,200–2,600 mg

Nutrient	Forms Used in Supplements	PDI
Chloride	Sodium chloride*	1,500–4,500 mg
Chromium	Chromium dinicotinate glycinate, chromium picolinate, chromium polynicotinate	200–600 mcg
Copper	Copper lysinate, copper gluconate	3–6 mg
Iodine	Iodine from kelp concentrate	200–400 mcg
Iron	Ferrous fumarate, iron glycinate	25–60 mg
Magnesium	Magnesium oxide, magnesium glycinate, magnesium carbonate	400–800 mg
Manganese	Manganese arginate, manganese glycinate, manganese gluconate	15–45 mg
Molybdenum	Molybdenum chelate, sodium molybdate	100–300 mcg
Phosphorus	Phosphorus	800–1,600 mg
Potassium	Potassium chloride, potassium ascorbate, potassium–amino acid complexes	2,500–4,000 mg
Selenium	Selenomethionine	100–300 mcg
Sodium	Sodium chloride*	1,500–4,500 mg
Zinc	Zinc citrate, zinc arginate	15–60 mg
METABOLITES		
Bioflavonoids	Rutin, hesperidin, citrus, quercetin, flavone, the flavonols	200–2,000 mg
Choline	Choline bitartrate, choline dihydrogen citrate, phosphatidyl-choline	600–1,200 mg
Inositol	Myo-inositol	800–1,200 mg

Note: Refer to the appropriate chapters in Part One for details on and special considerations regarding these nutrients. Guidelines for the nutrients not included in this table—such as the amino acids, carbohydrates, lipids, herbs, and metabolites—can also be found in Part One.

IU = international units, mcg = micrograms, mg = milligrams.
* Sodium and chloride are derived mainly from food sources.

comprehensive guidelines on each nutrient, consult the appropriate chapter in Part One.)

When you study the advancements made in nutritional research and see how the field of nutrition has evolved over the years, you can easily understand why people who wish to improve their performance need to use an updated, comprehensive approach. This is the approach we take in *Dynamic Nutrition for Maximum Performance*—scientifically based performance nutrition that is individualized according to your physical and metabolic needs as well as the special needs of your sport or fitness activity. In the following chapters, we will further elaborate on this dynamic approach.

PART ONE

THE NUTRIENTS

1. Nutrients and Athletic Performance

From Amino Acids to Zinc

Every day, the body requires many nutrients for energy, growth, and performance. The nutrients needed for athletic performance are grouped into several categories. Most, however, fall into two main categories—macronutrients and micronutrients. In this chapter, we will provide an overview of the primary nutrients that athletes need and, at the same time, will introduce the basic terminology that scientists, nutritionists, and health professionals use to categorize and represent the many nutritional concepts covered in this book. In the remaining chapters of Part One, we will explore the individual nutrients in more detail and will focus on their relationships to improving athletic performance and health.

MACRONUTRIENTS—MEETING ENERGY AND GROWTH REQUIREMENTS

Macronutrients are nutrients that are required daily in large amounts and that are thought of in quantities of ounces and grams. They include carbohydrates, protein, lipids, and water. Macronutrients are important because they supply the body with energy and serve as the building blocks for growth and repair. They are found in all foods, but they occur in each food in a different proportion. For example, meat is high in protein and fat but has almost no carbohydrates. Pasta, on the other hand, is very high in carbohydrates but has just a moderate amount of protein and a very small amount of fat.

Carbohydrates and lipids are the chief macronutrients that supply the body with energy. Different people have different energy requirements, since the requirements vary with age, activity, and diet. Energy needs can range from a low of 1,700 calories per day to more than 6,000 calories per day. The caloric contents of the macronutrients and of alcohol are listed in Table 1.1, right.

As shown in Table 1.1, on a per-weight basis, fat has the most calories, followed by alcohol and then by carbohydrates and protein. In the past, scientists assumed that the body metabolized all the calories supplied by

nutrients in the same way and used them all for energy in an equal fashion. In recent years, however, scientists have determined that the energy contents of the different macronutrients vary, depending on the macronutrient being measured, the ratio of all the macronutrients in the diet, the vitamins and minerals in the diet, the level of hydration of the body, and the physical condition of the body. For example, protein is considered a protected nutrient because the body reserves it for the synthesis (formation) of tissues and molecules instead of using it all for energy. The body prefers to use its fat and glycogen (stored glucose) supplies for energy over ingested protein or the protein that makes up muscle tissue. In fact, scientists have detected a thermogenic response in individuals eating diets high in protein. (For an explanation of thermogenesis, see "What Is Thermogenesis?" on page 14.) This indicates that the body uses more energy to metabolize protein than to metabolize the other macronutrients.

Carbohydrates affect energy and performance according to when they are eaten and what kind they are. The two kinds of carbohydrates are the complex carbohydrates, or starches, and the simple carbohydrates, such as glucose and fructose. Starch provides the body with a slow, steady supply of glucose because it is composed of chains of glucose that must first be broken down during digestion. Glucose itself does not need to be broken down and therefore enters the bloodstream immediately, providing a quick supply of energy. Fructose gets into the bloodstream at a rate

Table 1.1. Caloric Contents of the Macronutrients and Alcohol

	Calories per Gram	Calories per Ounce
Fat	9	255.6
Alcohol	7	198.8
Carbohydrates	4	113.6
Protein	4	113.6
Water	0	0.0

What Is Thermogenesis?

Thermogenesis is the process by which the body generates heat, or energy, by increasing the metabolic rate above normal. This rise in metabolic rate is referred to as the thermogenic effect, thermogenic response, or specific dynamic action (SDA).

Thermogenesis is activated by a few different mechanisms, including nutrition, exercise, and exposure to cold. Among the nutritional activators, the various macronutrients have different effects on the thermogenic response. When you ingest food, your metabolic rate increases above the fasting level. In the case of protein, this is thought to occur because the body must use energy to process the protein, which is then used for tissue growth and repair. On the other hand, carbohydrates and fat function primarily as fuel and are used more efficiently as such by the body. Carbohydrates and fat therefore have a much lower thermogenic effect than protein.

that is somewhere between starch and glucose.

Lipids are fats, oils, and other plant and animal nutrients that are insoluble in water. Triglycerides, the fatty acids that make up fat, contain the most energy of any macronutrient on a per-weight basis. Other lipids, such as cholesterol, are not important energy sources but are major components of some hormones and bile acids.

The body always uses a mixture of carbohydrates and fat, plus a little protein, for energy. This energy mixture varies depending upon the intensity and duration of the physical activity and the composition of the food from which the energy is derived. Endurance sports, such as marathon running, tend to cause the body to burn a higher proportion of fat for energy, while power sports, such as powerlifting, tend to cause the body to burn a greater amount of carbohydrates. The physical demand therefore dictates the proportion of macronutrients needed in the diet. A marathon runner generally needs a diet high in carbohydrates and moderate in fat and protein, while a sprinter needs a diet high in carbohydrates and protein and low in fat.

The way the body uses protein during and after exercise is more complicated than the way it uses carbohydrates or fat for energy. Protein supplies the body with building blocks in the form of amino acids. The body therefore tends to avoid using protein or amino acids for energy. However, during exercise, the body does use certain amino acids for energy and other metabolic functions. This cannot be prevented, but it can be counterbalanced by ingesting proteins with higher amounts of the amino acids used during exercise, such as the branched-chain amino acids. (For a discussion of these special amino acids, see "The Branched-Chain Amino Acids" on page 40.) Research has shown that even while athletes rest, their highly trained muscles still use certain amino acids for energy, despite the presence of carbohydrates and fat. Athletes can use special dietary supplements that are designed to boost the efficiency and utilization of dietary protein plus supply certain vitamin and mineral cofactors that help prevent muscle breakdown and encourage muscle repair. A cofactor is a substance that must be present for another substance to perform a certain function.

Water and Electrolytes

Water is the macronutrient that is most essential to life, but it provides no calories or nutrition. Water is the universal solvent that all life on Earth depends upon and the medium that transports the food materials used in the body. A person can survive for several weeks without food but for only several days without water.

Scientists have always recognized the importance of water, but recently, additional research has shown that sustaining the optimum level of hydration is important for maintaining peak performance and for achieving adequate recovery. In a sport such as soccer or basketball, an athlete can lose several pounds of water weight during just one game. This can adversely affect performance and, in the long run, can cause peaks and valleys in the athlete's performance curve.

In addition to remaining hydrated, the body also needs to maintain its electrolyte balance. The major electrolytes found in the bodily fluids are chloride, magnesium, potassium, and sodium. Water is a part of every cell. How much water a cell contains depends on the function of the cell. Likewise, specific quantities of the electrolytes are found in intracellular and extracellular fluid. These water and electrolyte concentrations are closely controlled, even under extreme temperature conditions. The same as water, the electrolytes are lost through sweat. Replenishing water and electrolyte stores during exercise and throughout the day has become an increasingly complex task for the athlete, as scientists are continually discovering new roles that these nutrients play in the body.

Macronutrient Modulation

The body needs a constant intake of protein and the other macronutrients all day long. However, the ratio of the macronutrients that is needed by the body changes during the day and should be planned around the training and resting periods. This variation in macronutrient intake is called macronutrient modulation, or macronutrient manipulation.

Macronutrient modulation refers simply to the practice of varying the intake of the macronutrients to meet specific metabolic needs. For example, consuming water, some amino acids, and simple carbohydrates just before and during exercise will help the body maintain energy and spare its glycogen stores and muscle tissue. Avoiding fat and large amounts of protein directly before and during training helps because these macronutrients take longer to break down and slow the digestive process.

Macronutrient modulation is not a complex undertaking. Even such practices as carbohydrate loading and water loading are relatively simple. For instructions on how to manipulate your daily diet to maximize your athletic performance, see your sport-specific plan in Part Four, which will give you the best macronutrient ratio to follow during your season, preseason, and off-season, and guidelines on how to adjust your diet to improve your performance in your particular sport. Instructions for water loading and carbohydrate loading can be found on pages 59 and 184, respectively.

MICRONUTRIENTS—METABOLIC COFACTORS

Even more diverse as a group than the macronutrients are the micronutrients. As the name implies, micronutrients are nutrients that are present in the diet and the body in small amounts. They are measured in milligrams and micrograms. They do not provide significant amounts of calories to the body but act as cofactors in making molecules, play various structural roles, and function as electrolytes and enzymes. Broadly speaking, the essential and nonessential vita-

mins and minerals, vitaminlike substances, and other dietary substances that are important to performance and health fall into the micronutrient category.

Vitamins are organic compounds that the body needs for the maintenance of good health and for growth. By convention, the name *vitamin* is reserved for certain nutrients that the body cannot manufacture and therefore must get from food. Vitamins are further classified as fat soluble or water soluble. The fat-soluble vitamins include vitamins A, D, E, and K. Because they are soluble in fat (lipids), these vitamins tend to become stored in the body's fat tissues, fat deposits, and liver. This storage capability makes the fat-soluble vitamins potentially toxic. Care should be exercised when taking the fat-soluble vitamins. For guidelines on the safe consumption of the fat-soluble vitamins, see Chapter 6.

The water-soluble vitamins include the B vitamins and vitamin C. In contrast to the fat-soluble vitamins, the water-soluble vitamins are not easily stored by the body. They are often lost from foods during cooking or are eliminated from the body.

Vitamins are not usually metabolized for energy, but some are essential for the production of energy from the macronutrients and act as cofactors. As with the macronutrients, vitamin research has only begun to illuminate how these nutrients benefit performance and health beyond the prevention of nutritional deficiencies. However, current findings give us a good picture of how vitamins are important to health and performance.

Minerals are inorganic nutrients or inorganic-organic complexes that are essential structural components in the body and necessary for many vital metabolic processes, even though they make up only about 4 percent of the body's weight. Every day, the body needs minerals such as calcium in large amounts, about 1,200 milligrams or more, while it needs other minerals, such as chromium, in smaller amounts, measured in micrograms. A microgram is one-thousandth of a milligram. Although the minerals are needed on a daily basis in a wide range of amounts, their relative importance is equal. Some minerals are found in the body in an inorganic form; examples are calcium salts in the bones and sodium chloride in the blood. Other minerals are present in organic combinations; examples are iron in hemoglobin (the oxygen carrier in red blood cells) and iodine in thyroxine (a thyroid hormone). How well the body absorbs each mineral varies greatly. Researchers are discovering that just because a mineral, or a vitamin, is present in a food does not mean that all of it will be absorbed into the body. This is another reason that dietary supplements are recommended. Supplements ensure that the body receives exact amounts of the nutrients. Additionally, the nutrients in supplements are of a high quality, unaccompanied by the fat, salt, pesticides, and other junk that is found in many foods.

In addition to the essential vitamins and minerals, a host of micronutrients exist that are manufactured in the body but that can still be provided through foods or supplements for additional benefits. These substances, called metabolites, are also sometimes known as accessory nutrients or nonessential nutrients. (For a discussion of metabolites, see Chapter 8.) For athletes, many of these accessory nutrients actually improve performance. Sodium bicarbonate can boost performance in the power sports. Carnitine, an amine that is essential for the oxidation of long-chain fatty acids into energy, has been shown to benefit fat metabolism and to increase endurance when taken in supplemental amounts. And inosine, which is taken by many athletes, is touted for its energy-enhancing effects and usefulness in power sports.

In addition to the vitamins, minerals, and accessory nutrients, substances found in plants and animals can also helps improve health and performance. A group of naturally occurring plant compounds, the bioflavonoids, helps maintain the artery walls of the circulatory system. Herbs such as ginseng, yellow dock, kava kava, burdock, yerba maté, garlic, and sarsaparilla are taken for a variety of purposes including stress reduction, digestion, energy, muscle growth, fat loss, and sleep. Enzymes, both those that are nutritionally derived and those that are bodily manufactured, are important in areas such as recovery, fat loss, and muscle building. Furthermore, vitamins, minerals, and nutrients such as the amino sugar glucosamine and the herb turmeric are important for healing.

NUTRIENT DENSITY

Foods contain macronutrients and micronutrients in many different combinations and amounts. A potato is high in complex carbohydrates; is a good source of vitamin C; contains some protein, B vitamins, and minerals, especially potassium and phosphorus; and has a trace amount of fat. Meat—steak, for example—is high in protein and fat but has no carbohydrates. Steak

is also a good source of vitamin A and has some B vitamins, phosphorus, potassium, iron, and magnesium. These two foods additionally demonstrate that while most foods contain some of the essential nutrients, they lack others. The nutritional content of a food also varies according to when and where it was grown.

In these modern times, a vast proportion of food is processed, and most processed foods are very low in the micronutrients. For example, white pasta, which is a good source of carbohydrates, is made of flour that was stripped of most of its micronutrient content during the bleaching process. In fact, most pastas are vitamin fortified to compensate for this. Canned vegetables are low in vitamins and enzymes, which are lost during the cooking and preparation processes.

Eating whole foods and taking supplements is necessary for ensuring high-quality nutrition. For instance, even though sugar is a carbohydrate, it does not supply the essential vitamin cofactors in the proper amounts to enable the body to get the most efficient and highest level of energy out of the carbohydrates. Consuming foods that are high in quality nutrients is important for reaching top performance. For athletes, attaining a nutrient-dense diet necessitates combining certain foods with supplements.

BIOAVAILABILITY OF NUTRIENTS

Scientists once assumed that if a nutrient was present in a particular food, the body would make full use of it. However, we now know that this is not true for many nutrients.

Bioavailability refers to the ability of an ingested nutrient to cross from the digestive tract into the bloodstream and then from the bloodstream into the cells in which it will be utilized. A nutrient's bioavailability is affected in many ways. Some nutrients compete with each other over which one will be absorbed through the intestines. Certain methods of food preparation affect some nutrients' bioavailability. Digestive problems can interfere with nutrient absorption. And some nutrients are absorbed better in the presence of other nutrients; for example, vitamin D improves the intestinal absorption of phosphorus.

When constructing a nutrition program for maximum athletic performance, you must select foods and supplements that contain bioavailable nutrients. Even the nutrients used in supplements vary in degree of bioavailability. Therefore, you must be careful to choose supplements that contain highly bioavailable nutrients. (For guidelines on choosing supplements, see Chapter 9.)

LIMITING NUTRIENTS

While the nutrients in food are usually absorbed into the body, the absence of even one nutrient can limit the utilization of other nutrients or the functioning of the body. For example, the mineral chromium is an essential cofactor for the proper functioning of the hormone insulin. When you eat a meal, your pancreas secretes insulin, which helps glucose and amino acids pass from the bloodstream into the cells. Even if your body makes enough insulin, a shortage of chromium can prevent the complete passage of these substances into the cells. Researchers have determined that chromium is not present in optimal amounts in most diets, especially in the diets of athletes. When chromium is not present in an optimum amount, the dietary glucose and amino acids in the bloodstream that cannot get into the cells will circulate back to the liver and may end up being converted to fat. Additionally, the muscle cells will be deprived of the amino acids necessary for proper growth and recovery and of the glucose needed for the replenishment of the glycogen stores. In this example, chromium is a limiting nutrient because it limits the cellular uptake of other nutrients.

Some of the amino acids that build proteins can also become limiting nutrients. As mentioned earlier, during exercise, some amino acids are used for energy. The amino acid leucine is an example. Leucine is an essential amino acid. It is used to make other amino acids and is important in metabolic functioning. For athletes, leucine can become a limiting nutrient and can affect the utilization of the other amino acids if it is used selectively for energy and the other amino acids are not. The body uses amino acids to build proteins, which are chains of amino acids. When one amino acid runs out, the rate of protein synthesis is inhibited and reduced, and the growth and repair of the body is slowed. One way to compensate for the disproportionate use of leucine for energy is to consume supplemental amounts of it. Ingesting the correct amounts of the nonessential amino acids and of the other nonessential nutrients is equally important for keeping the body from having to waste time and energy making those nutrients.

You can probably now see how eating for maximum athletic performance is different from eating just for survival or for optimum health. First, you must determine what nutrients, both essential and nonessential, your body uses, and how and when it uses them. Then, you must learn how to supply them through your diet. Planning a diet for maximum performance is like formulating a supercharged fuel for a high-performance engine. The engine in this case, however, is the human body, which is a dynamic engine. For help in designing a diet that is appropriate for your individual needs, see your sport-specific plan in Part Four. Your sport-specific plan offers dietary and supplementation guidelines as well as lists of nutrients and intake ranges.

OTHER USES OF NUTRIENTS

In addition to taking nutrients because of their primary dietary roles, athletes should also take certain nutrients in large amounts for their other desirable effects. When taking nutrients at high levels, however, both the pharmacological actions and the toxic effects must be taken into account. For example, some people have used vitamin A and related retinoids in high amounts to heal skin disorders and to improve night vision. Athletes, too, have recognized the benefits of vitamin A. However, taking large amounts of this fat-soluble vitamin may cause acute or chronic side effects. Signs of toxicity usually appear only with sustained daily intakes exceeding 50,000 international units, which is ten times the RDA. One way to reap the benefits of vitamin A without risking the side effects is to eat foods and take supplements that contain beta-carotene. Beta-carotene is water soluble and converts to vitamin A in the body when needed. It is also a powerful antioxidant, which helps protect the body from oxidative stress. (For a complete discussion of vitamin A and beta-carotene, see page 74.)

People have been increasingly consuming isolated amino acids for specific therapeutic purposes. For example, research has shown that the concentrations of some of the neurotransmitters in the brain are influenced by diet. These neurotransmitters are important for alertness, memory, and sleep. Certain amino acids are precursors of these neurotransmitters—that is, the amino acids are intermediate compounds in the body's production of the neurotransmitters. The amino acid tryptophan was popular as a supplement because of its role in synthesizing serotonin, which improves sleep and combats depression.

Tyrosine, phenylalanine, and gamma-aminobutyric acid (GABA) also have histories as dietary supplements. However, just as with the vitamins and minerals, taking too much of an isolated amino acid can have negative side effects. You must always exercise caution when self-administering these nutrients at high dosages.

Enhancing immunity has become popular of late. The immune system fights off diseases that try to invade the body. During periods of increased stress, the immune system is challenged and the body is more likely to catch a disease, such as the flu or a cold. Using nutrients and herbs to boost the immune system has become a very important way to protect against disease and to get rid of an illness faster.

The recognition of the pharmacological effects of nutrients further demonstrates the dynamic nature of nutrition for athletes. According to numerous personal interviews, most athletes take nutrients mainly for their muscle-building and energy roles. The athletes questioned never even considered the intricacies of nourishing the nervous system, promoting healing, or protecting against metabolic damage. Use of nutrients for these purposes makes for some interesting possibilities, and the sum total of applying all these scientific nutritional principles will make a better athlete.

SAFETY OF NUTRIENTS

How do you know if the food you are eating is safe? This is not an easy task these days. Most people assume that if a food can be purchased in a store, it is safe to eat. The NRC has published reports linking diseases such as cancer, hypertension, and heart disease to food. Too much fat can cause a diversity of problems. Excessive amounts of saturated fat are even a suspect cause of certain cancers. Fat is also indirectly responsible for weight problems—when too much fat is consumed, the excess is converted to body fat.

The list of non-nutrients that are either suspected or proven to be carcinogenic (cancer causing) to humans or laboratory animals is growing. These non-nutrients include naturally occurring carcinogens and mutagens in foods as well as chemical food additives and contaminants. Examples are saccharin, tannins, polychlorinated biphenyls, aflatoxins, mycotoxins, and alcohol. It should be underscored here that even some natural foods and substances may be harmful to health and can ultimately hinder performance.

How do scientists determine if a food or food constituent is harmful? There are two ways. The first uses epidemiological evidence. Epidemiological evidence is gathered by studying groups of people in different areas of the world. For example, newspapers occasionally run articles about a group of people living in a particular region who develop fewer cases of certain cancers because their diet is low in fat and high in fiber. Epidemiological evidence can also be gathered on the same population or group of people over a period of years. In this way, researchers can see if there are increases or decreases in diseases on an annual basis that can be correlated to changes in the diet.

The second way to determine whether a food will cause a disease is through direct experimentation. Since it is unethical to experiment on people with potentially harmful substances, researchers use laboratory animals. The laboratory animals are fed different amounts of the suspected food substance to see what happens. In the case of cancer, the researchers might have observed epidemiological evidence indicating that a certain food component may be a cause of a certain type of cancer. The researchers then isolate the suspected compound, test different concentrations of the compound on laboratory animals, and observe the incidence of cancer formation.

It is interesting to note that even when a substance has been proven to be harmful to health, it may still be available for human consumption. The artificial sweeteners cyclamate, saccharin, and dulcin have all been shown to cause cancer in laboratory animals, but they are still available in foods. The same is true for saturated fats and cholesterol. Research has clearly shown that a diet in which more than 30 percent of the total daily calories comes from fat increases the chances of developing heart disease and cancer. Because of this, you would think that the Food and Drug Administration (FDA) would require warnings on the labels of foods that are high in fat. It does not, however. The reality is that eating a healthy diet is in your own hands. The dietary guidelines in this book were designed to help you minimize the use of unhealthy foods and foods containing additives that can be harmful to health and performance.

Table 1.2 on page 19 lists many of the food additives commonly used in the sports-nutrition industry that are on the FDA's Generally Recognized as Safe (GRAS) list or that are otherwise allowed in foods. The FDA feels that, based on prior and current use, these nutrients and substances are safe. However, the

Table 1.2.   Common Additives and Their Status in Relation to Performance Nutrition

While the following additives are found in many foods and supplements, some are better—that is, healthier—than others. Therefore, choose foods that contain additives with an "acceptable" status rating, and avoid or minimize consumption of those with additives that are "not acceptable."

Additive	Status
Acetic acid	Acceptable
Aerosol sprays other than nitrogen or carbon dioxide	Not acceptable
Algin	Acceptable
Alpha-tocopherol	Acceptable
Alpha-tocopherol acetate	Acceptable
Ammonium bicarbonate	Acceptable
Ammonium compounds	Acceptable
Ammonium phosphate	Acceptable
Ammonium sulfate	Acceptable
Annato	Acceptable
Artificial colors	Not acceptable
Ascorbic acid	Acceptable
Ascorbyl palmitate	Acceptable
Aspartame	Acceptable but not preferred
Benzoyl peroxide	Not acceptable
Beta-carotene	Acceptable
Biotin	Acceptable
Bleached flour	Acceptable but not preferred
Brominated vegetable oil	Not acceptable
Butylated hydroxyanisole (BHA)	Not acceptable
Butylated hydroxytoluene (BHT)	Not acceptable
Calcium carbonate	Acceptable
Calcium chloride	Acceptable
Calcium citrate	Acceptable
Calcium disodium ethylene-diaminetetraacetic acid (EDTA)	Not acceptable
Calcium pantothenate	Acceptable
Calcium peroxide	Not acceptable
Calcium phosphate	Acceptable
Calcium propionate	Not acceptable
Calcium stearoyl-2-lactylate	Not acceptable
Calcium sulfate	Acceptable
Canthaxanthine	Not acceptable
Caramel color	Acceptable
Carmine	Not acceptable
Carob bean gum	Acceptable

Additive	Status
Carrageenan	Acceptable
Casein	Acceptable
Caustic soda	Not acceptable
Cellulose	Acceptable
Certified colors	Not acceptable
Cholecalciferol	Acceptable
Choline bitartrate	Acceptable
Choline chloride	Acceptable
Citrates	Acceptable
Citric acid	Acceptable
Cobalamin	Acceptable
Cochineal	Not acceptable
Coconut oil	Acceptable but not preferred
Corn syrup	Acceptable
Cream of tartar	Acceptable
Cyanocobalamin	Acceptable
Cyclamates	Not acceptable
Dextrose	Acceptable
Diglycerides	Acceptable
Dioctyl sodium sulfosuccinate	Not acceptable
Disodium guanylate	Not acceptable
Disodium inosinate	Not acceptable
Egg albumin	Acceptable
Equal	Not acceptable
Ergocalciferol	Acceptable
Ethylenediaminetetraacetic acid (EDTA)	Not acceptable
Ferrous gluconate	Acceptable
Fructose	Acceptable
Glucono delta-lactone	Acceptable
Guanosine monophosphate (GMP)	Not acceptable
Guar gum	Acceptable
Gum acacia	Acceptable
Gum arabic	Acceptable
Gum tragacanth	Acceptable
High-fructose corn syrup	Acceptable
Hydrogen peroxide in foods	Not acceptable
Hydrogenated oil	Acceptable but not preferred

Additive	Status
Hydrolyzed protein	Acceptable
Inositol	Acceptable
Karaya gum	Acceptable
Lactalbumin	Acceptable
Lecithin	Acceptable
Locust-bean gum	Acceptable
Lye	Not acceptable
Magnesium carbonate	Acceptable
Malic acid	Acceptable
Maltodextrin	Acceptable
Mannitol	Acceptable but not preferred
Methyl silicone	Not acceptable
Methylene chloride	Not acceptable
Methylparaben	Not acceptable
Modified food starch	Not acceptable
Monoglycerides	Acceptable
Monosodium glutamate (MSG)	Not acceptable
Niacin	Acceptable
Niacinamide	Acceptable
Nitrates	Not acceptable
Nitrites	Not acceptable
NutraSweet	Not acceptable
Olestra	Not acceptable
Oxystearin	Not acceptable
Palm kernel oil	Acceptable but not preferred
Palm oil	Acceptable but not preferred
Papain	Acceptable
Partially hydrogenated oil	Acceptable but not preferred
Pectin	Acceptable
Polysorbates	Not acceptable
Potassium acid tartrate	Acceptable
Potassium bicarbonate	Acceptable
Potassium bisulfite	Not acceptable
Potassium bromate	Not acceptable
Potassium chloride	Acceptable
Potassium iodide	Acceptable
Potassium sorbate	Not acceptable
Propyl gallate	Not acceptable

Additive	Status
Propylene glycol	Not acceptable
Propylparaben	Not acceptable
Pyridoxine hydrochloride	Acceptable
Quinine	Not acceptable
Riboflavin	Acceptable
Saccharin	Not acceptable
Simplesse	Not acceptable
Sodium aluminum phosphate	Not acceptable
Sodium benzoate	Not acceptable
Sodium bicarbonate	Acceptable
Sodium bisulfite	Not acceptable
Sodium caseinate	Acceptable
Sodium ferrocyanide	Not acceptable
Sodium hydroxide	Not acceptable
Sodium nitrate	Not acceptable
Sodium nitrite	Not acceptable
Sodium pyrophosphate	Not acceptable
Sodium stearoyl-2-lactylate	Not acceptable
Sorbic acid	Not acceptable
Sorbitol	Acceptable but not preferred
Soy protein isolates	Acceptable
Stannous chloride	Not acceptable
Sulfites	Not acceptable
Sulfur dioxide	Not acceptable
Sweet'n Low	Not acceptable
Tartaric acid	Acceptable
Textured vegetable protein (TVP)	Acceptable
Thiamine hydrochloride	Acceptable
Thiamine mononitrate	Acceptable
Tocopherols	Acceptable
Turmeric	Acceptable
Vanillin	Acceptable
Vegetable gums	Acceptable
Vitamin A acetate	Acceptable
Vitamin A palmitate	Acceptable
Whey	Acceptable
Xanthan gum	Acceptable
Xylitol	Acceptable but not preferred
Yellow prussiate of soda	Not acceptable
Zinc compounds	Acceptable

amounts eaten of these nutrients and substances also determine their safety. Table 1.2 gives the status of each additive as it pertains to the interests of athletes, fitness exercisers, and other health-minded individuals. Notice that hydrogen peroxide is on the list. In large amounts, this substance is harmful to life.

RESEARCH ON NUTRIENTS

Historically, most of the research on nutrition has been focused on nutrient deficiencies, nutritional care for metabolic disorders such as diabetes, and clinical nutrition. Research on using nutrition to improve physical performance and optimum health has been scanty. However, since the late 1970s, more and more research has been conducted on the ways in which nutrition affects performance and health. Researchers have been breaking the confines of traditional dogma, delving into unexplored areas of nutrition, and looking at the relationships between human performance and nutrition.

A lot has yet to be discovered about nutrition and performance; this area of research is wide open and growing. The good news is that many fundamental and even some quite sophisticated discoveries have been made concerning the effects that nutrition has on athletic performance. Many of these important scientific findings will be discussed in the chapters on the nutrients.

ERGOGENIC AIDS

Ergogenic is a catchall term that describes anything that can be used to enhance athletic performance. Ergogenic aids can be either dietary or nondietary and include special training techniques, blood doping, mental strategies, and drugs. Dietary ergogenic aids range from water to large dosages of vitamins. In the most fundamental sense of the definition, a dietary ergogenic aid can cause an immediate, observable benefit involving athletic performance. Some, however, provide long-term benefits that are not immediately observable.

As far as we are concerned in this book, the entire nutrition and training program is an ergogenic aid. While we employ certain short-term performance-enhancing methods, such as macronutrient modulation and carbohydrate loading, we believe that you must focus on perfecting your total nutrition and training program to increase and maximize your performance. If your baseline nutrition is not optimum, you will not derive the maximum benefits from any dietary ergogenic aids. For example, if you consume large amounts of vitamin B_{12} for energy but do not eat the proper amounts of carbohydrates, you will not see any of the performance-enhancing benefits of the B_{12}. As you review the nutrients one by one in the following chapters, remember that the total nutrition approach will far exceed any of its individual parts.

2. CARBOHYDRATES
THE ULTIMATE PERFORMANCE FUEL

In the United States, the average daily intake of carbohydrates is 287 grams for adult males and 177 grams for adult females. Approximately half of the carbohydrates that normal American adults consume are simple carbohydrates, with the other half being complex carbohydrates. This is off-balance. The National Research Council and the Surgeon General have determined that the typical American diet is too high in fat, sodium, and sugar (simple carbohydrates), and too low in complex carbohydrates and fiber.

Most athletes eating for top performance should get at least 55 percent of their total daily calories from carbohydrates. For some kinds of athletes, the percentage should be even higher. In addition, research has shown that the type of carbohydrate eaten can affect performance.

Take the simple carbohydrate glucose as an example. Studies have shown that consuming a high-glucose food or drink approximately thirty minutes to two hours before exercising stimulates a rise in the insulin level. This rise in insulin in turn promotes the uptake of glucose by cells throughout the body and may cause hypoglycemia (low blood sugar). The net result is decreased performance and early onset of fatigue. In contrast, a glucose drink taken just prior to—that is, about five minutes before—and during exercise maintains the blood sugar, spares glycogen, and increases the time it takes the body to become exhausted. In other words, it increases performance and capacity. Complex carbohydrates eaten two to three hours before exercise also increase performance and delay fatigue in endurance activities because they enter the bloodstream at a slow, steady rate.

The most recent studies show that carbohydrates are the body's primary high-energy fuel source for all activities. Early researchers studied the effects of nutrient intake on work performance. By putting their subjects on a variety of nutritional regimens—from outright starvation to diets consisting of different proportions of fat, protein, and carbohydrates—they found a few interesting dynamics. First, when the body runs out of its stored glycogen and must turn to fatty acids as its primary source of energy, physical performance declines dramatically. The body must push much harder to keep up the work pace. Endurance athletes call this "hitting the wall." They commonly encountered this phenomenon before the importance of carbohydrate loading and ingesting carbohydrate drinks during exercise were discovered. Carbohydrate loading is a supercompensation in glycogen storage. Studies have revealed that it can be initiated by depleting the body's glycogen stores and then replenishing them using a diet high in carbohydrates. (For a complete discussion of carbohydrate loading, see Chapter 15.)

Since all this early research, even more light has been shed on the importance of carbohydrates to performance. As well as consuming an adequate supply of carbohydrates by means of a mixed diet, athletes must consider the type of carbohydrates they eat, the time of day they eat them, and their intake of cofactors. All these elements together help increase the glycogen stores and enhance energy production during exercise.

In this chapter, we will discuss the basic types of carbohydrates that are found in food and dietary supplements. We will then examine the ways in which these basic types of carbohydrates can be used to enhance athletic performance.

TYPES OF CARBOHYDRATES

There are several types of carbohydrates, some of which are better than others. Starch, sugar, and dextrose are examples. The different types of carbohydrates can be divided into three general categories. Monosaccharides are carbohydrates that have one sugar molecule. Disaccharides are carbohydrates that have two sugar molecules. And polysaccharides are carbohydrates that have three or more sugar molecules. Monosaccharides and disaccharides are commonly called sugars, while polysaccharides are called complex carbohydrates or glucose polymers. Some of the more commonly encountered carbohydrates in these three categories include the following:

☐ *Monosaccharides*—Glucose, fructose, sorbitol, galactose, mannitol, and mannose.

☐ *Disaccharides*—Sucrose, which is made of one molecule each of glucose and fructose; maltose, made of two molecules of glucose; and lactose, made of one molecule each of glucose and galactose.

☐ *Polysaccharides*—Starch, dextrin, cellulose, and glycogen, which are all made of chains of glucose and are called glucose polymers or maltodextrins; and inulin, a unique carbohydrate made of multiple molecules of fructose.

Another kind of carbohydrate is fiber, which is composed mainly of the indigestible polysaccharides that make up a plant's cell walls. These polysaccharides include cellulose, hemicellulose, pectin, and a variety of gums, mucilages, and algal polysaccharides.

SIMPLE CARBOHYDRATES

The principal monosaccharides in food are glucose and fructose. Glucose, which is also called dextrose or grape sugar, is found commonly in fruit, sweet corn, corn syrup, certain roots, and honey. Fructose, which is also called levulose or fruit sugar, is found together with glucose and sucrose in honey and fruit. (For a discussion of the different names used for sugar, see "Sugar By Any Other Name . . . ," below.)

While glucose has traditionally been a frequently encountered dietary sugar, fructose is becoming more popular due to the discovery that it does not cause the rapid rise and fall in the blood-sugar level that glucose does. Researchers realized this in 1984 when they undertook the first extensive comparisons of the different sweeteners available at the time. (For a discussion of the different types of sweeteners available, see "The Many Faces of Sweeteners" on page 25.) They found that the main reason fructose is easier on the blood-sugar level is that the body absorbs and utilizes fructose much slower than it does glucose. In fact, they discovered, the body starts absorbing glucose in the stomach. Fructose allows people to enjoy sweets without suffering a roller-coaster ride in the blood-sugar level and has therefore become a main ingredient in health foods.

As a result of all the recent attention, fructose is now used in a variety of drinks and foods in place of glucose and sucrose. It is pitched as the "healthy sugar." But while fructose may have some benefits over the other sugars, it is still a sugar and supplies raw energy without much other nutrition. Furthermore, the exact athletic benefits of fructose, other than the help it provides in controlling the appetite by maintaining the blood-sugar level, are not very apparent. In addition, remember that eating too much of any sugar

Sugar By Any Other Name . . .

There are many different types of sugar, and some have names that disguise their true nature. Despite the fact that several have been touted as healthy alternatives to common sugar, all of them are essentially the same.

White table sugar is also called sucrose and is basically the same as brown sugar, confectioners' sugar, invert sugar, raw sugar, and turbinado. Glucose masquerades under the name *dextrose* and is also found in corn syrup and corn sweeteners. High-fructose corn syrup is not the same as pure fructose, which is usually labeled as *fructose*. Honey is a natural syrup made of glucose and fructose. Sorbitol, mannitol, and xylitol are naturally occurring sugar alcohols.

All of the foregoing sugars provide few essential nutrients and are usually referred to as empty calories. In an attempt to give their products sweetness but not extra calories, manufacturers commonly use several artificial sweeteners, including aspartame (NutraSweet and Equal), acesulfame K (Sunette and Sweet One), and saccharin (Sweet'n Low, Sprinkle Sweet, and Sweet 10).

Once you get into the habit of examining food labels, you will be surprised at how many hidden sources of sugar you discover. The average American consumes over 100 pounds of sugar a year. In fact, most Americans get 25 percent of their total daily calories from sucrose.

Food labels rarely announce the amount of sugar that a product contains, but you can get a rough idea from where it appears within the list of ingredients. Manufacturers are required to list ingredients in descending order according to weight. Therefore, you should stay away from products that list sugar or any of its cousins high on the list.

The Many Faces of Sweeteners

While white table sugar has long had a reputation as an enemy of the thighs and waistline, some other sweeteners have acquired reputations as health foods. For example, many people would never consider adding white table sugar to a recipe but do not hesitate to add scoopfuls of brown sugar.

Sugar does not need to be totally avoided. But brown sugar, like many other types of sugar, is essentially the same as common table sugar. Strictly speaking, the problem with sugar is not the calories. As with other carbohydrates, sugar has just 4 calories per gram. (However, some sweets, such as chocolate, are high in both sugar and fat.) The problem with sugar is that it can cause fluctuations in the blood-sugar level, and these fluctuations can ultimately increase the appetite and cause a craving for more sugar.

One crafty way around the ill effects of sugar has been the development of artificial sweeteners. Aspartame is a popular artificial sweetener made from two naturally occurring amino acids—phenylalanine and aspartic acid. While aspartame was not designed for use in cooking, it does provide an alternative means of enjoying a sweet taste without interfering with fat loss or weight maintenance. One word of advice on artificially sweetened diet beverages: Although these beverages are low in calories, drinking a lot of them every day sharpens the sweet tooth and provokes sugar cravings. Stick to drinking water and reserve the diet sodas for treats.

Commonly encountered dietary disaccharides, or double sugars, include sucrose (white table sugar, cane sugar, and beet sugar), maltose (malt sugar), and lactose (milk sugar). Disaccharides are broken down into their monosaccharide subunits during digestion, before they are absorbed into the body. When sucrose is commercially hydrolyzed, a one-to-one mixture of glucose and fructose is formed. This mixture is called invert sugar and is seen as such on food labels.

---

can lead to tooth decay. Concern over cavities is not just for children. Adult athletes with tooth decay may end up with disrupted seasons due to root-canal surgery or tooth extractions.

Fructose does have its place, though, and is a wise choice in beverages. In addition to its less damaging effects on the blood-sugar level, it has also been found to replenish the glycogen stores in the liver over the glycogen stores in the muscles. This is important because the brain derives most of its energy supply from the liver, which is especially low in glycogen in the morning. Perhaps the desire to drink juices high in fructose in the morning is more than coincidence, since these juices provide the mental surge of energy that so many people need to start the day.

Note, however, that once fructose is mixed with food, its effects on the bood-sugar level becomes less clear.

COMPLEX CARBOHYDRATES

The two polysaccharides that are the most important energy contributors to the body are starch and glycogen. Processed forms of polysaccharides are maltodextrin and glucose polymers, which are shorter polymers of glucose than starch and are commonly used in sports drinks because they are more soluble in water than starch is. Starch occurs in various parts of plants and consists of long chains of glucose units. It is found in grains, roots, vegetables, pasta, bread, and legumes. Starch and other polysaccharides are called complex carbohydrates.

When starch is eaten, it is digested slowly in the body, releasing glucose molecules from the intestines into the bloodstream at a slow, steady rate. This is unlike most simple sugars, which are absorbed quickly from the digestive system into the bloodstream. Quick absorption leads to a high blood-sugar level and conversion of the food to fat by the liver. This is one reason why individuals on fat-reduction diets should minimize their intake of simple sugars as well as their consumption of fat. (For a discussion of starch's impact on the diet, see "Is Starch Fattening?" on page 26.) Additionally, individuals who participate in power sports should minimize their intake of simple carbohydrates and fat because their bodies obtain energy by burning primarily muscle glycogen, not the large amounts of fatty acids that endurance athletes burn. (For a list of the best complex carbohydrates for athletes, see "Top Twenty Grains and Legumes for Athletes" on page 27.)

FIBER

Fiber is another type of polysaccharide, but one that cannot be digested in the human gut and that does not provide any energy of which to speak. It does,

Is Starch Fattening?

Many people think that starchy foods such as bread and pasta are fattening. Not so. Most of the fat calories connected with starchy foods come from the spreads and sauces that are put on them, such as sour cream, butter, margarine, gravy, jelly, and jam. The starchy foods themselves are not fattening, unless, of course, they are overeaten. What the body does not need for immediate energy it converts to fat. Starches provide only 4 calories per gram, while fat provides 9 calories per gram. Fat is therefore more than twice as caloric as starch. If you, like most people, eat a diet that is high in fat, you can cut your total caloric intake at least in half just by replacing the fat with carbohydrates—while still keeping your total food intake the same! A pound of lean ground beef contains 1,252 calories, 90 grams of fat, 106 grams of protein, and 2 grams of carbohydrates. Compare this with a pound of pasta, which contains only about 665 calories, 3 grams of fat, 25 grams of protein, and 136 grams of carbohydrates.

Is it surprising that athletes who eat large amounts of meat chronically suffer from poor performance and struggle with body fat? Just by eating more complex carbohydrates and less fat, you can increase your athletic performance.

Recent research has proven that the body prefers to convert to body fat the calories from fat over the calories from carbohydrates. All carbohydrates have only 4 calories per gram, which the body prefers to use directly for energy. If the body has to convert glucose molecules to fat, it must expend energy to complete the biochemical process. This, obviously, is not as efficient as just storing fat from fat.

Researchers have also found that when comparing people who eat the same amount of calories per day, the ones who eat more fat have a greater tendency to gain body fat. So, eating starchy foods is a good way to fill up with fewer calories, as long as you go easy on the condiments and do not overeat.

however, play an important role as the main contributor to the roughage content of the diet. Among its protective qualities, roughage, which is also known as dietary fiber, helps promote efficient intestinal functioning and aids the absorption of sugars into the bloodstream.

Fiber is found along with simple and complex carbohydrates in various plant foods, such as fruits, leaves, stalks, and the outer coverings of grains, nuts, seeds, and legumes. Dietary fiber helps soften the stool and encourages normal elimination. Fiber-rich diets also promote satiety. In addition, research has shown that people who eat high-fiber diets experience reduced rates of cardiovascular disease, colon cancer, and diabetes. A high-fiber diet works best when it includes plenty of fluids.

How much dietary fiber do adults need to get these benefits? The NRC estimates that the average intake of fiber in the United States is 12 grams per day. This is much lower than what has been observed in other cultures, some of which boast fiber-intake levels as high as 150 grams per day. Health-care practitioners recommend that the average adult consume at least 40 to 60 grams per day. You can achieve this intake goal by eating foods high in fiber and by adding a fiber supplement to your diet. (For a list of foods high in fiber, see "Fiber 10 Foods for Athletes" on page 28.)

Some experts fear that diets high in fiber interfere with mineral absorption. This interference, however, can be offset by a daily dietary supplement or even by the minerals already present in the high-fiber foods themselves.

DIGESTION OF CARBOHYDRATES

The chemical digestion of carbohydrates begins immediately in the mouth via enzymes that are present in the saliva. In the stomach, the digestive juices further break down the long chains of glucose that make up starch. The stomach has some capacity to allow glucose to enter the bloodstream, which helps endurance athletes who drink glucose drinks during exercise in an effort to promote glycogen sparing (the saving of glycogen for other functions). Once they reach the intestines, glucose and fructose are absorbed at their respective rates, with glucose taken up more quickly than fructose. When complex carbohydrates are eaten, either alone or with sugars, their short chains of glucose polymers slowly release glucose in the intestines for an hour or two. This slow release provides both a prolonged supply of glucose to the bloodstream and a supply of nutritional energy that further spares and replenishes muscle glycogen.

Carbohydrates are more quickly released from the stomach to the intestines than either protein or fat. The more protein and fat that you eat, the longer your stomach will take to empty. Logically, therefore, you should eat and drink foods that are very high in carbohydrates before and during exercise to take advantage of this process. Again, this is why special sports-nutrition drinks can help increase performance.

CARBOHYDRATES IN THE BODY—GLUCOSE AND GLYCOGEN

Glycogen is similar to the starch that is found in plants in that it consists of chains of glucose units. However, glycogen and starch differ in structure. In addition, while starch occurs only in plants, glycogen occurs only in animals. Very little glycogen is found in food, however. This is mainly because meat contains only small amounts of glycogen. Due to the human body's small storage capacity for glycogen, it needs a relatively constant supply of carbohydrates throughout the day. The body converts a portion of all ingested complex carbohydrates into glycogen, thereby replenishing its limited glycogen supply.

In the human body, glycogen is found in all the cells. However, it is present in greater percentages in the muscle fibers and liver cells. In this way, the liver and muscles act as reservoirs for glucose. The liver's glycogen supply is used to regulate the blood-sugar level. Furthermore, the glucose that is fed into the bloodstream from the liver's glycogen supply is the main source of energy for the brain. The brain can use over 400 calories per day of glucose from the liver's glycogen. Athletes and other physically active individuals sometimes have a feeling of being bogged down. Many

times, this feeling is due to a low level of liver glycogen. Eating a good amount of complex carbohydrates, especially at night, will replenish the glycogen supply and restore mental alertness and physical energy. High-fructose drinks also replenish the liver glycogen. (For a discussion of how foods affect the blood-sugar level, see "The Glycemic Index" on page 29.)

Glycogen is not stored by itself in the liver. Rather, it is stored together with water. In fact, every 1 ounce of glycogen is stored with about 3 ounces of water. This means that when glycogen is used, water is also removed from the body. Many fad diets take advantage of this phenomenon by requiring a low caloric intake coupled with a high protein consumption, which causes liver and muscle glycogen to be depleted in twenty-four to forty-eight hours. This glycogen depletion can result in a loss of several pounds of water, which many dieters mistake for a loss of body fat. Moreover, because most weight-loss diets are low in calories, the body eliminates a few pounds of gastrointestinal bulk within a few days. Dieters usually mistake this, too, for a loss of body fat. So, a week or two of fad dieting may result in a loss of several pounds of water weight and gastrointestinal bulk but perhaps only a mere pound or two of body fat. This is one reason why fad dieters quickly, almost overnight, gain back the weight they lost. Understanding this is especially important for weight-conscious athletes, who typically deplete their glycogen supplies on low-calorie diets, blow up when they return to a normal diet, and then have to lose several pounds again a few days later. By keeping their caloric and carbohydrate intakes at normal levels, athletes can help their bodies work better and can maintain their glyco-

---

Top Twenty Grains and Legumes for Athletes

The following foods are top protein sources, consisting of more than 20-percent protein and less than 20-percent fat:

☐ Soybeans	☐ Lima beans
☐ Split peas	☐ Black-eyed peas
☐ Kidney beans	☐ Lentils
☐ Dried whole peas	☐ Black beans
☐ Wheat germ	☐ Navy beans

The following foods are top carbohydrate sources, consisting of less than 5-percent fat and more than 70-percent carbohydrate:

☐ Brown rice	☐ Wild rice
☐ Whole barley	☐ Whole corn
☐ Whole buckwheat	☐ Pearl millet
☐ Whole rye	☐ Whole wheat
☐ Foxtail mullet	☐ Rolled oats

Including these grains and legumes in your daily diet will help ensure that you get a good supply of low-fat, nutritious complex carbohydrates.

Fiber 10 Foods for Athletes

While fiber does not supply much in the form of energy, it does serve the vital function of promoting digestive efficiency. Diets high in fiber also make you feel full, which helps to control caloric intake, and they aid in the fight against cardiovascular disease, colon cancer, and diabetes.

The average adult should consume about 40 to 60 grams of fiber a day. Each of the following foods contains approximately 10 grams of dietary fiber:

☐ **Grains**
- 1/2 cup All Bran cereal
- 1 cup rolled oats
- 1 cup whole-grain cereal
- 2 ears sweet corn
- 3 slices whole-rye bread
- 3 cups Puffed Wheat cereal
- 4 slices whole-wheat bread
- 4 squares Shredded Wheat cereal
- 4 ounces popcorn

☐ **Vegetables**
- 1/2 cup mixed beans
- 1/2 cup peas
- 1/2 cup lentils
- 1 cup peanuts
- 2 cups soybeans
- 3 cups steamed vegetables
- 4 large carrots
- 4 cups sunflower seeds
- 5 cups raw cauliflower

☐ **Fruits**
- 3 pears
- 3 bananas
- 4 peaches
- 4 ounces blackberries
- 5 apples
- 6 oranges
- 6 dried pear halves
- 10 dried figs
- 20 prunes

To check the fiber content of other foods, see *The NutriBase Complete Book of Food Counts*, by Art Ulene (Garden City Park, New York: Avery Publishing Group, 1996).

---

gen supplies for better overall performance.

Glycogen is also stored along with potassium. Therefore, when dietary conditions encourage the depletion of the body's glycogen stores, potassium is also lost. The loss of potassium, which is an important electrolyte, can result in impaired performance. So, if you go through periods of glycogen depletion, make sure that you maintain an adequate intake of potassium, as well as of the other essential vitamins and minerals. (For a discussion of potassium, see page 99.)

Glycogen depletion followed by glycogen replenishment, which is also known as carbohydrate loading, causes the muscles to increase their water content considerably. When glycogen replenishment is complete, the increased body weight may induce the muscles to feel heavy and stiff. This can interfere with physical performance in certain athletic events, particularly in connection with sports that rely on repeated short bursts of all-out effort, such as sprinting, football, and basketball. Bodybuilders can take advantage of this phenomenon, however, and experienced bodybuilders know how to add size and hardness to their physiques on contest days for an added competitive edge.

Understanding glycogen storage and dynamics is a cornerstone of improving athletic performance nutritionally. Knowledgeable athletes recognize that they must keep their muscle and liver glycogen stores filled up. They comprehend that they must follow a daily nutrition program that encourages glycogen replenishment and spares glycogen utilization. And they know how to use carbohydrate loading to maximize their glycogen stores for endurance sports and tournaments.

CARBOHYDRATES FOR INCREASED ATHLETIC PERFORMANCE

To maintain their glycogen stores, athletes must focus on their carbohydrate intake on a twenty-four-hour basis and on a pre-event basis. This means that they must devote attention to the following important factors:

☐ Maintenance of carbohydrate balance at each meal.

☐ Increase in carbohydrate intake before athletic events or exercise sessions.

☐ Ingestion of selected types of carbohydrates during exercise.

☐ Ingestion of carbohydrates after exercise.

☐ Methodical buildup of muscle and liver glycogen stores before events.

☐ Carbohydrate loading for events lasting more than one and a half hours and for tournaments. (For a complete discussion of carbohydrate loading, see Chapter 15.)

☐ Ingestion of high amounts of complex carbohydrates, with intake of increased amounts of simple carbohydrates at breakfast, during exercise, and directly after exercise to quickly replace depleted glycogen stores.

You can easily maintain carbohydrate balance by eating several servings of carbohydrates per day. In general, you should eat a plentiful amount of complex carbohydrates with each meal and reserve simple car-

bohydrates for special parts of the day. This means that you must make sure that you eat carbohydrates with every meal and with snacks.

Carbohydrates Before, During, and After Exercise

When consuming carbohydrates before, during, or after exercise, you also need to take in fluids and the electrolytes. Before exercise, your meal should be high in carbohydrates, moderate in protein, and low in fat. You should eat this meal about three hours before

The Glycemic Index

The glycemic index is a measurement of the way the blood sugar responds two hours after a certain food is ingested in comparison to the way it responds two hours after an equivalent amount of pure glucose is ingested. The lower a food's glycemic index is, the less is the body's glycemic response to that food. By eating foods with lower glycemic indexes, you can maintain a more stable blood-sugar level. For the glycemic indexes of some common foods, see the table to the right.

The glycemic index is important for two primary reasons—it indicates the metabolic consequences that different foods can have, and it helps when foods with certain glycemic indexes need to be consumed at specific times. For example, it is better to consume foods with low glycemic indexes for meals and snacks, since these foods help maintain the proper blood-sugar level and ensure a sustained energy supply. Conversely, during workouts and competitions, it is better to eat foods with high glycemic indexes because these foods help spare glycogen in the body and supply quick energy to exercising muscles. For more guidelines on when you should eat foods with high or low glycemic indexes, see your sport-specific plan in Part Four.

Glycemic Indexes of Selected Common Foods

Glycemic Index	Food
Rapid Inducers of Insulin Secretion	
100 percent	Glucose
80–90 percent	Corn flakes, carrots*, parsnips*, potatoes (instant mashed), maltose, honey
70–79 percent	Bread (whole-grain), millet, rice (white), Weetabix cereal, broad beans (fresh)*, potatoes (new), swede*
Moderate Inducers of Insulin Secretion	
60–69 percent	Bread (white), rice (brown), muesli, Shredded Wheat cereal, Ryvita crispbreads, water biscuits, beetroot*, bananas, raisins, Mars Bars
50–59 percent	Buckwheat, spaghetti (bleached), sweet corn, All Bran cereal, digestive biscuits, oatmeal biscuits, Rich Tea biscuits, peas (frozen), yams, sucrose, potato chips
40–49 percent	Spaghetti (whole-wheat), oatmeal, potatoes (sweet), beans (canned navy), peas (dried), oranges, orange juice
Slow Inducers of Insulin Secretion	
30–39 percent	Butter beans, haricot beans, black-eyed peas, chickpeas, apples (Golden Delicious), ice cream, milk (skim), milk (whole), yogurt, tomato soup
20–29 percent	Kidney beans, lentils, fructose
10–19 percent	Soybeans, soybeans (canned), peanuts

*This food item was tested in portions containing 25 grams of carbohydrates.
The above table is adapted from *Diabetes Care*, vol. 5 (1982). It is used with the permission of the American Diabetes Association.

beginning the exercise. This is important because it will take this long for your stomach to empty and for the glucose to enter your bloodstream. If you eat too much protein or fat before exercising, you will lengthen the time it will take for your stomach to empty. You should also drink several glasses of water after finishing your pre-exercise meal and again thirty minutes before beginning the exercise session. Studies have shown that drinking fluids with glucose and some electrolytes several minutes before beginning to exercise is the best way to spare the body's supply of glycogen.

During exercise, you should drink water or a sports beverage containing water plus 70 to 100 calories of carbohydrates per serving and a supply of the electrolytes. However, if the carbohydrate or electrolyte content of the sports drink is too high, your stomach will take longer to empty. For practice sessions and events lasting more than two hours, you must consume a drink containing adequate amounts of carbohydrates and the electrolytes. Preferably, the drink should consist of glucose or sucrose mixed with a complex carbohydrate such as maltodextrin. For events less than two hours long, you should still try to drink at least water to rehydrate your body. The benefits of drinking beverages containing carbohydrates and the electrolytes are less clear for exercise sessions lasting less than two hours. But while sports drinks might not supply immediate benefits, they could help preserve glycogen stores and prevent glycogen depletion on a day-to-day basis. Research indicates that many athletes suffer from chronic glycogen depletion, with decreased performance and increased recovery time.

After exercise—any exercise—you must replenish your body with water, carbohydrates, the B-complex vitamins, vitamin C, and protein. You can do this by consuming a supplement drink designed especially for this purpose followed by a full meal. If you trained after your last evening meal, you should consume a high-carbohydrate, multinutrient supplement drink containing 300 to 600 calories about one to two hours after finishing the session. In addition, you should drink two or more glasses of water.

The practice of drinking carbohydrate beverages before, during, and after exercise may be new to you. Give it a try and see how your system responds. If you find that your stomach cannot tolerate a carbohydrate beverage before or during exercise, eat extra amounts of carbohydates before and directly after exercise instead. In addition, drink plain water while exercising. Before giving up on the practice completely, however, experiment with different brands of beverages and different caloric totals. Your problem may not be with carbohydrate beverages in general but just with a certain brand or formula. Generally, carbohydrate solutions that are pure glucose and contain about 50 calories in every 8 ounces are the easiest to stomach. As the amount of carbohydrates goes up and more electrolytes and other nutrients are added in, the rate at which the stomach empties slows down and the feeling of being bloated may become more pronounced.

FOOD AND SUPPLEMENT SOURCES OF CARBOHYDRATES

Carbohydrates tend to be the least expensive of the macronutrients. You can buy several pounds of potatoes for only a few dollars and have a week's supply of high-quality complex carbohydrates. Other foods that are high in carbohydrates—that is, over 60 percent of their calories come from carbohydrates—are ready-to-serve and cooked cereals, whole-grain bread, crackers, popcorn, rice, pasta, corn, winter squash, and yams.

Supplement sources of carbohydrates include sports drinks, which vary in caloric content and carbohydrate type. The caloric content of sports drinks generally runs from 90 to 400 calories per 8-ounce serving. Many different types of sports drinks are available, but most are based either on a simple-carbohydrate source or on a complex formulation that contains a mixture of simple carbohydrates, glucose polymers, and micronutrients. Some research has indicated that while foods alone can be used for glycogen sparing and carbohydrate loading, these special supplement products are slightly better for improving performance. However, they are also more expensive. Most athletes on tight budgets use these special products just during the season or during the week preceding an important competition.

It is interesting that carbohydrates, such a seemingly simple group of macronutrients, are utilized by the body in such a diversity of ways. It is equally fascinating that they have such profound effects on performance. Keeping close track of your carbohydrate intake, however, is just one ingredient in your performance-nutrition formula.

3. PROTEIN AND AMINO ACIDS
MUSCLE BUILDERS AND MORE

The relationship between protein and the athlete has become legendary. As already mentioned, one of the earliest recorded athletic nutritional practices was that of consuming large amounts of protein to improve strength and performance. The most recent research confirms protein's role as a vital component of health and performance. However, studies have also established that diets that are too high in protein can be as counterproductive as diets that are too low in protein. One thing is certain—athletes require at least twice as much protein as nonathletes do.

Protein is an essential part of the diet and plays many roles in the body. Protein's roles are primarily structural, but it is also sacrificed by the body for energy during intensive exercise or when nutrition is inadequate. In these situations, to meet its metabolic needs, the body breaks down precious muscle tissue, which is a setback for an athlete who has been training hard to make gains. In addition, athletes need to eat just the right amount of protein to minimize the formation of metabolic waste products. When too much protein is consumed, the body converts the excess to fat and increases the blood levels of ammonia and uric acid. Ammonia and uric acid are toxic metabolic waste products. The athlete's goal therefore is to maintain proper protein intake.

In this chapter, we will discuss protein and its special relationship with the athlete. We will learn about the various methods used to rate the quality of proteins and how to estimate individual daily requirements. We will also look in detail at the amino acids, which are the building blocks of protein.

WHAT IS PROTEIN?

Protein is a large molecule called a macromolecule or supermolecule. It is a polypeptide, a compound containing from ten to one hundred amino-acid molecules. The amino acids are linked together by a chemical bond called a peptide bond.

When we talk about protein, we are really discussing these amino-acid subunits. There are about twenty-two amino acids that are considered biologically important, but many more exist in nature, including in the body. Amino acids are important not only for being the building blocks of protein, however, but also for the individual roles that they play in the body. For example, some amino acids are used by the body in metabolic processes such as the urea cycle. Others act as neurotransmitters, the chemical substances that help transmit nerve impulses.

Protein is needed for the growth, maintenance, and repair of cells, including muscle cells, and for the production of enzymes, hormones, and DNA. It occurs in various sizes and shapes and is divided into two main categories—simple proteins and conjugated proteins. Simple proteins consist only of amino acids, while conjugated proteins also have nonprotein molecules as part of their structures. Some simple proteins are serum albumin, which is present in blood; lactalbumin, which is present in milk; ovalbumin, which is present in eggs; myosin, present in muscle; collagen, present in connective tissue; and keratin, present in hair. Examples of conjugated proteins are nucleic acid, found in chromosomes; lipoprotein, found in cell membranes; glycoprotein, chromoprotein, and metaloprotein, all found in blood; and phosphoprotein, found in casein (milk protein). Protein constitutes about 74 percent of the dry weight of most body cells.

PROTEIN AND ENERGY

In addition to the functions discussed above, protein—the same as fat and carbohydrates—can also be used for energy. Under conditions of both outright and training-induced starvation, the body releases amino acids from muscle tissue for use as energy or in energy cycles. This catabolism (breakdown) of protein occurs during exercise—especially during intensive workouts, in particular power exercises and prolonged endurance activities—or when the body runs out of carbohydrates from the diet or glycogen from its muscle and liver stores. Even though the body can depend on the fat that it has stored, it still uses muscle protein, unless it is fed protein as food. When dietary circumstances cause the body to use amino acids as a source of energy, it cannot also use these amino acids for building muscle tissue or for performing their other metabolic functions. This is why a proper protein intake is essential every hour of the day.

Even if you do consume a proper diet, your body will still use certain amino acids as fuel during grueling exercise bouts. The muscles use the branched-chain amino acids (BCAAs)—isoleucine, leucine, and valine—to supply a limited amount of energy during strenuous exercise. (For a discussion of these special amino acids, see "The Branched-Chain Amino Acids" on page 40.) However, research has shown that although the body can utilize all three BCAAs for energy during exercise, it uses leucine the most. As demonstrated by studies, a trained person's muscles use leucine even while that person is at rest. This disproportionate use of leucine, as well as of the other BCAAs, affects the body's overall use of amino acids for growth. Here, the BCAAs, especially leucine, are limiting nutrients.

For optimum muscle growth, cellular growth, metabolism, and recovery, the body needs to receive the amino acids in the proper proportions. Merely eating amino-acid sources, such as meat and eggs, does not ensure that the amino acids they supply will be available for muscle growth or for the formation of other proteins. For example, suppose you consume a total of 100 grams of protein, with all the essential amino acids present in equal amounts. How will your body use these amino acids? To begin, it will utilize a considerable percentage of the leucine for energy for exercising muscles. This means that only a small amount of leucine will be available for growth and repair purposes. When your leucine supply runs out, your protein formation will be negatively affected because leucine is an essential amino acid—that is, your body cannot manufacture it. The result is that perhaps only 15 grams of the original 100 grams of protein will be available for growth and repair.

On a similar note, a trend in some circles of athletes—bodybuilders in particular—has been to ingest pure-protein meals or supplements. This practice is counterproductive because the body also needs carbohydrates to rebuild its glycogen stores. When it does not receive carbohydrates, it must break down some of the protein and convert it to glucose and fatty acids in the liver. Therefore, you should always consume at least some carbohydrates, and even a modicum of fat, to prevent the undesirable destruction of ingested protein for energy.

RATING PROTEINS

Just as there are differences among the carbohydrates, the various proteins are not created equal. Some proteins have more-complete amino-acid contents than others and are therefore better suited for growth purposes. Scientists are currently using a number of methods to rate proteins. Most of these rating methods do not take into account the extra protein and the specific amino acids that are required by athletes. However, as more research is conducted using athletes, methods for rating proteins for athletic purposes will hopefully result.

Complete Versus Incomplete Proteins

Due to the fact that an adequate protein intake is essential for optimum growth in children, the World Health Organization (WHO) has conducted significant research on protein requirements. What the WHO researchers determined was that not all proteins supply the proper amounts and proportions of the amino acids necessary for adequate growth and development. Complete proteins are proteins that contain the essential amino acids in amounts that are sufficient for the maintenance of normal growth rate and body weight. Complete proteins are therefore said to have a high biological value. Most animal products have complete proteins.

Incomplete proteins are usually deficient in one or more of the essential amino acids. This amino-acid deficiency creates a limiting-amino-acid condition, which adversely affects growth and development rates. Most plant proteins are incomplete. However, considering the dynamics of amino acids in the body, even high-quality proteins can be incomplete for athletes' needs. Furthermore, research indicates that the proper proportions of both the essential and nonessential amino acids are required for optimum growth and recovery. This means that athletes should consume protein supplements as well as high-quality food protein sources. Their dietary goals should be to eat a diet fortified with the amino acids that are used for energy and nongrowth functions and to ensure an adequate intake of the amino acids that are necessary for growth and recovery—but not to eat so much protein that there will be an excess that is converted to fat.

Protein Efficiency Ratio

Another method of determining the quality of protein is the protein efficiency ratio (PER). The PER is calculated using laboratory animals. It refers to the amount of weight gained versus the amount of protein ingested. For example, casein has a PER of 2.86, which means that 2.86 grams of body weight are gained for every 1 gram of casein eaten. Table 3.1, below, provides a sampling of foods and their PER values.

One criticism of the PER system as a method for determining the quality of proteins for human consumption is that the values were derived through testing on animals, mostly rats. Does a rat's growth rate correlate to a human's? Perhaps not. Additionally, rats and other laboratory animals have a large amount of fur all over their bodies. This places an extra demand on amino acids such as methionine, which is used in fur growth and which is a common limiting amino acid in plant protein sources. Moreover, we now realize that athletes need higher amounts of certain amino acids, such as the BCAAs. Therefore, the PER and other similar data should be used only as guidelines for determining minimum intakes of protein for nonathletes. Additionally, different proteins can be combined to improve the quality of the individual proteins. This is commonly done to increase the PER of plant proteins. Many powder supplements now include a mixture of two or more of the less-expensive lesser-quality proteins, such as soy and casein, which boost each other's PERs when used together, instead of using one of the more-expensive high-quality protein sources, such as egg white.

An interesting note is that WHO suggests that newborns need complete dietary proteins containing about 37 percent of the protein's weight in essential amino acids. Adults, on the other hand, require complete dietary proteins containing just 15 percent of the protein's weight in essential amino acids. This demonstrates that the proportion of essential to nonessential amino acids is an important factor in growth and development. Athletes training to develop stronger and bigger muscles should try to maintain higher proportions of the essential amino acids in their diets.

Net Protein Utilization

Net protein utilization (NPU) is a way of determining the digestibility of a protein. It does this by measuring the percentage of nitrogen that is absorbed from a protein's amino acids. Generally, the more nitrogen that is absorbed from a protein, the more digestible the protein is.

The NPU of a protein is calculated by measuring an individual's intake of nitrogen from amino acids, comparing that amount to the amount of nitrogen that the individual excretes, and determining how much of the protein in question is needed to balance out the two amounts. If a protein has a low NPU, more of it is needed to achieve nitrogen balance. (For a more complete discussion of this, see "Nitrogen Balance" on page 34) Therefore, proteins with high NPU values, such as egg and milk proteins, are more desirable for athletes.

Biological Value

While the methods used to determine a protein's biological value (BV) are not entirely standardized, the one that most scientists prefer is described as "the efficiency with which that protein furnishes the proper proportions and amounts of the essential or indispensable amino acids needed for the synthesis of body proteins in humans or animals."

The general formula for determining BV is as follows:

$$BV = \text{nitrogen retained} \div \text{nitrogen absorbed} \times 100$$

When applying mathematical data, the breakdown of the above equation is as follows:

$$\text{Nitrogen retained} = (\text{dietary } N) - (F - Fm) + (U - Ue)$$

$$\text{Nitrogen absorbed} = (\text{dietary } N) + (F - Fm)$$

In the above breakdown, dietary N represents dietary nitrogen, F equals the fecal nitrogen excreted during the testing of a protein, Fm equals the fecal nitrogen excreted on a protein-free diet (endogenous fecal

Table 3.1. Selected Foods and Their Protein Efficiency Ratios

FOOD	PER
Eggs	3.92
Whey	3.6–3.9
Fish	3.55
Lactalbumin	3.43
Whole milk	3.09
Casein	2.86
Soy flour	2.30
Beef	2.30
Oatmeal	2.25
Rice	2.18

Nitrogen Balance

Nitrogen balance is a topic that is frequently encountered when reading articles about athletes' protein and amino-acid requirements. In addition to carbon and hydrogen, amino acids also contain nitrogen as part of their molecular structure. This is a unique characteristic, one that we can use to our advantage, since it allows us to determine if our protein intake is adequate. Specifically, nitrogen balance refers to the condition in which the amount of dietary nitrogen taken in is equal to the amount of nitrogen excreted. A nitrogen balance that is positive indicates a possible net growth in body tissues. A nitrogen balance that is negative indicates an inadequate protein intake and the possibility that the body is cannibalizing its muscle tissue. During the season, athletes who want to maintain their body weight should strive to equalize their nitrogen intake and excretion. Athletes who want to increase their muscle mass should aim for a positive nitrogen balance.

Determining nitrogen balance is not an easy task, however. Because nitrogen from broken-down amino acids can be excreted in both the urine and the feces, and because some is lost as sweat, all these excretions must be collected and analyzed. In addition, all the nitrogen ingested from protein must be accurately measured. This is impractical for most individuals. However, some companies have now developed methods that enable athletes to get a rough idea of their nitrogen balance by taking measurements using just their urine and measuring their nitrogen ingested as protein. This approach makes assumptions about the relative amount of nitrogen lost in feces and sweat. Although you would have to spend time making calculations every day, you would probably find it interesting to learn what your nitrogen balance is to give you an approximate guideline for what your daily protein intake should be. You could then experiment with combining different food and supplement protein sources to tailor-make an efficient protein-intake program for yourself.

nitrogen), U equals the urinary nitrogen excreted during the testing of a protein, and Ue equals the urinary nitrogen excreted on a protein-free diet (endogenous urinary nitrogen). The highest BV that can be obtained using this method is 100. By substituting your mathematical readings for these factors listed in the general formula, you can determine the BV of a food.

No matter what method is used to determine BV, the score does not indicate the ultimate fate of the amino acids in the body—that is, it does not show whether they will be used for muscle growth or enzyme synthesis. In addition, BV measurements vary for the same protein according to the animal species tested. For example, chickens have different amino-acid needs than do rats due to, among other things, the fact that chickens have feathers and rats have fur. Because feathers require different amino acids than fur does, the two animals need different proportions of the amino acids. Therefore, unless the BV for a particular type or brand of protein was determined specifically for humans, that protein may not offer any advantages to humans, even though it may have a high BV according to the testing done with animals.

Amino-Acid Score

The amino-acid score is one additional method of determining the quality of proteins that is worth mentioning, since sports-nutrition advertisers are using more and more scientific jargon to sell their products. The amino-acid score of a food protein is determined by comparing its content of essential amino acids with a reference pattern. This is a crude method, however, because the reference pattern does not relate to athletes' needs. It does not account for the digestibility of the protein, the availability of the amino acids, or the utilization of the amino acids by the body.

Ideally, more research needs to be conducted on athletes to determine protein scores for athletic purposes. In 1990, a group of inventors led by Robert Fritz developed the first effective home testing tool for measuring urinary nitrogen. Called NitroStix, these diagnostic sticks are available commercially and give athletes, as well as nonathletes, a tool for monitoring their nitrogen balance on a daily basis to determine if their protein intake is sufficient. Use of these diagnostic sticks can also help athletes determine how other factors, such as training and nutrient intake, affect their nitrogen balance.

THE FUTURE FOR PROTEIN PRODUCTS

The future for protein and amino-acid sports science lies in designing an amino-acid source that brings about nitrogen balance using a minimum amount of protein.

This goal can be reached in several ways, and manufacturers have already developed pioneering ingredients and products that accomplish it. Creating an amino-acid profile that has all the essential amino acids with extra BCAAs and the nonessential amino acids is a start. Products with a variety of amino-acid combinations are available. Among their benefits are growth-hormone (GH) stimulation, blood-ammonia detoxification, increased mental alertness, and mental relaxation.

Absorption is also an important factor. Some protein manufacturers are inventing better ways to purify the protein from milk and other sources. One manufacturer even combined medium-chain triglycerides with high-quality protein to increase utilization; the resulting product is marketed under the brand name SuperProtein. Adding nonprotein ingredients can further improve utilization, as well as supply other growth factors, such as glucosamine for connective tissue. (For a discussion of glucosamine, see page 105.)

The diversity of amino-acid combinations possible and the benefits that they offer make protein and amino acids a very interesting field of research and a very important part of the athlete's nutrition program.

FREE-FORM AND PEPTIDE-BONDED AMINO ACIDS

When referring to the amino-acid content of food or supplements, the terms *free form* and *peptide bonded* are used. In fact, the debate seems to be constant over which supplement form is better. Free-form amino acids are amino acids that are in their free state, or single. When protein is digested, some of its amino acids are eventually broken down into their free forms for transport and use in the body. Peptide-bonded amino acids are amino acids that are linked together. Di-peptides are two amino acids linked together, tri-peptides are three amino acids linked together, and polypeptides are four or more amino acids linked together. Interestingly, the intestines can absorb free-form, di-peptide, and tri-peptide amino acids but not polypeptides.

Because the body has the capacity to digest protein, it can make use of whole-protein supplement sources. However, many supplements now contain free-form amino acids or combinations of free-form and peptide-bonded amino acids. Some also contain hydrolyzed proteins. Hydrolyzed proteins are already broken down, usually by enzymes, and are a mixture of free-form, di-peptide, and tri-peptide amino acids. Many people consider them better than nonhy-drolyzed proteins because their partial digestion possibly makes them more easily absorbed by the body. Preliminary research, however, is unclear regarding the benefits of hydrolyzed proteins in healthy individuals.

The benefits of using a multi-amino-acid supplement that is composed of just free-form amino acids are even less clear. The trend apparently got its start in early nutrition studies that attempted to chemically create a balanced protein by using free-form amino acids, along with other nutrients. In the United States, the use of free-form L-tryptophan was banned a number of years ago. (For a discussion of the FDA's action, see "The Ban on Tryptophan" on page 45.) Any multi-amino-acid supplement that consists of free-form essential amino acids minus L-tryptophan is basically useless. Make sure that your multi-amino-acid formulation is full spectrum—that is, has all the essential amino acids in addition to nonessential amino acids.

The use of free-form amino acids is still common in clinical applications when intravenous solutions are used to supply amino acids directly into the bloodstream. Free-form amino acids can also be used to fortify food proteins. Taking the BCAAs with meals can be useful for compensating for the amino acids already used for energy. Additionally, when you just want to take extra amounts of one or several amino acids, a free-form amino-acid formulation makes perfect sense. Concerning multi-amino-acid and powder supplements, however, whole-protein or hydrolyzed-protein sources are the best.

Another reason why a mixture of free-form and peptide-bonded amino acids is better than free-form amino acids alone is that the intestines can better absorb mixtures for transport into the bloodstream. While it might seem logical that free-form amino acids could be absorbed more quickly, the upper part of the small intestine is better able to absorb amino acids in twos and threes. Furthermore, free-form amino acids are manufactured, and ingestion of large amounts of these synthetics for long periods of time can cause problems in the stomach and intestines. If you choose to up your protein intake, you should use whole proteins or hydrolyzed proteins from foods and supplements as your primary sources of protein. Limit your use of free-form amino acids to supplementing your meals with the BCAAs, ammonia-detoxifying agents, or single amino acids for precursor therapy, as is done with L-tyrosine.

D-, L-, AND DL-FORMS OF AMINO ACIDS

Most amino acids come in two forms. The two forms are isomers, mirror images of each other, and are denoted by the letter "D" or "L" placed in front of the name of the amino acid. Scientists can identify which isomer an amino acid is by the direction of the rotation of the spiral that is the chemical structure of the molecule—L-form amino acids rotate to the left and D-form amino acids rotate to the right. "L" stands for *levo*, which is Latin for "left," and "D" stands for *dextro*, which is Latin for "right." In general, the L-form is more compatible with human biochemistry and the only form that should be ingested. Never use a supplement that contains only the D-form.

A third form in which some amino acids can be found is the DL-form, a mixture of the D- and L-forms. However, the only two amino acids whose DL-forms have been observed to have metabolic advantages are phenylalanine and methionine. The D-forms of these two amino acids can apparently be converted to the L-forms in the liver. This seems to produce a positive effect in some cases.

THE COMMONLY ENCOUNTERED AMINO ACIDS

The following amino acids are the major ones that are important to the body and commonly encountered in supplements. (For a quick listing of these essential and nonessential amino acids, see Table 3.2, above right.) In addition to being a part of proteins, many amino acids have specific metabolic functions. For example, arginine stimulates the release of GH. However, please note that while the following information is comprehensive, many of the amino acids have uses that are not included. These uses are mainly in the treatment of clinical and metabolic disorders, which are beyond the scope of this book.

A word of caution: Although amino acids have been used for years by the medical profession and have been taken as supplements by all types of individuals, our intention in this book is not to recommend the use of isolated amino acids or free-form amino-acid combinations. While many studies have used amino acids safely, some reports have documented side effects. If you wish to use any amino-acid supplements, seek the guidance of your health-care practitioner and make sure that you exercise caution.

If you do choose to take an amino-acid supplement, the best way is on an empty stomach or as directed on the label. This allows the amino acid to enter the body

Table 3.2. Important Amino Acids Commonly Used in Supplements

Essential	Nonessential
L-valine	Glycine
L-lysine	L-alanine
L-threonine	L-serine
L-leucine	L-cystine
L-isoleucine	L-tyrosine
L-tryptophan	L-aspartic acid
L- or DL-phenylalanine plus L-tyrosine[1]	L-proline
	L-hydroxyproline
L- or DL-methionine plus L-cystine[1]	L-citrulline
	L-arginine
L-histidine[2]	L-ornithine
	L-glutamic acid[3]

[1] Because tyrosine can replace about 50 percent of the phenylalanine that is required and cystine can replace about 30 percent of the methionine that is required, these amino acids must also be considered in association with the traditional essential amino acids.
[2] Essential for infants and athletes only.
[3] Conditionally essential, particularly during intensive weight training, when it is useful in combating the catabolic effects of cortisol.

in a pure form and prevents competition with other amino acids and nutrients. For specific dosing recommendations, see the individual amino acids.

Alanine

Alanine is found in high concentrations in most muscle tissue and is grouped with the nonessential amino acids because it can be manufactured by the body. Alanine is involved in an important biochemical process that occurs during exercise—the glucose-alanine cycle. In the muscles, glycogen stores are broken down to glucose and then to a three-carbon-atom molecule called pyruvate. Some of the pyruvate is used directly for energy by the muscles. Some of it, however, is converted to alanine, which is transported through the bloodstream to the liver, where it is converted once again into glucose. The glucose is then transported back to a muscle and again used for energy.

The glucose-alanine cycle serves to conserve energy in the form of glycogen. Sports physiologists believe that this helps maintain the glucose level during prolonged exercise. In this way, supplementing with L-alanine can be useful in the same way that supplementing with the BCAAs is—the supplemental L-alanine helps to spare muscle tissue, as well as liver glycogen.

Arginine

Arginine is another nonessential amino acid that influences several metabolic factors that are important to athletes. Arginine is most famous for its role in stimulating the release of human GH (somatotropin). Several studies have measured the ability of supplemental L-arginine, both alone and in combination with other amino acids, to increase the GH level in a resting individual. Potential benefits of an increased GH level include reduction in body fat, improved healing and recovery, and increased muscle mass. The exact benefits, though, are still in question and awaiting more research.

Research has also been conducted on supplementation with different forms of L-arginine, such as L-arginine-pyroglutamate combined with L-lysine hydrochloride. One study used 1,200 milligrams of each and reported significant elevations of GH levels over what were achieved using either compound alone. However, this particular study has been criticized by other scientists, who have been unable to replicate its findings, so the safety of these particular combinations has not yet been clearly determined. The exact benefits for athletes have not been determined either.

A second important function of arginine is its role as a precursor in creatine production. Creatine combines with phosphate and is an important energy source during power activities, such as weightlifting and sprinting. (For a discussion of creatine, see page 104.) Daily ingestion of 4,000 milligrams each of L-arginine and L-glycine has been shown to cause a small increase in body creatine stores. This can help improve performance for power athletes.

A third function of arginine that may benefit athletes is its role in ammonia detoxification. Arginine is an intermediary in the urea cycle. It converts ammonia to the waste product urea, which can then be excreted from the body. Ammonia is toxic, and its level increases with exercise. Any ammonia-lowering effects of supplemental L-arginine would therefore be beneficial to athletes.

Even though more studies are needed to determine its specific effectiveness, supplemental L-arginine can benefit athletes because of its ability to reduce ammonia, increase GH, and increase creatine. L-arginine supplementation can especially help athletes involved in strenuous sports or training. Furthermore, L-arginine has been found to improve wound healing and to play a role in the immune sys-

tem. More studies are also needed to determine L-arginine's exact safety and dosage levels, but 1,000 to about 3,000 milligrams per day have been successfully used in research to date.

Asparagine

Asparagine is a nonessential amino acid that is manufactured in the body from aspartic acid. Asparagine appears to be involved in the proper functioning of the central nervous system because it helps prevent both extreme nervousness and extreme calmness. L-asparagine supplementation by athletes has not yet been evaluated.

Aspartic Acid

Aspartic acid is a nonessential amino acid that has been shown to help reduce the blood-ammonia level after exercise. Aspartic acid is metabolized from glutamic acid in the body. It is involved in the urea cycle and in the Krebs cycle. In the Krebs cycle, energy is released from glucose, fatty-acid, or protein molecules and used to form adenosine-triphosphate (ATP) molecules, which are the form of energy that the body can utilize.

Researchers have studied potassium and magnesium-L-aspartates for their possible effects on athletic performance, which include reducing blood ammonia, sparing glycogen, and increasing free fatty acids. A total of 8,400 milligrams per day of potassium and magnesium-L-aspartates ingested in two to three dosages during the twenty-four-hour period before exercise has been shown to increase capacity in unconditioned individuals (recreational athletes). The exact benefits for conditioned individuals in active training have not been proven at this time.

Aspartic acid is an excitatory neurotransmitter in the brain. Long-term supplemental use is not recommended. Doses of 4,000 to 8,000 milligrams before an event can benefit performance in unconditioned individuals and may benefit conditioned athletes if taken before competitions and tournaments.

Citrulline

Citrulline is a nonessential amino acid and one of the two amino acids that do not occur in proteins. Both citrulline and ornithine, the other amino acid that does not occur in proteins, are important in the urea cycle for the removal of ammonia from the blood. Citrulline is made from the essential amino acid lysine. The benefits of L-citrulline supplementaion have not been established at this time.

Cysteine

Cysteine is a sulfur-bearing nonessential amino acid. The body manufactures it from methionine. Cysteine is important in the formation of hair and insulin. Besides its major role as a component of proteins, it functions as an antioxidant and detoxifying agent, helping rid the body of carcinogens and dangerous chemicals. (For a complete discussion of antioxidants, see page 69.) In addition, it helps form glutathione, which is another important antioxidant and detoxifying agent. Cysteine also plays a role in energy production. Like other amino acids, it can be converted to glucose and either used for energy or stored as glycogen.

Dosages of L-cysteine of around 250 to 500 milligrams, taken once or twice a day, have been used as part of an antioxidant regimen. Higher dosages taken without medical supervision are not recommended. Some reports indicate that L-cysteine works better when taken along with vitamin B_6, vitamin C, vitamin E, calcium, and selenium. Individuals with the metabolic disorder cystinuria should not take supplemental L-cysteine due to an increased risk of cysteine-gallstone formation.

Cystine

Cystine is another sulfur-bearing nonessential amino acid. It is made from two molecules of cysteine.

Cystine plays a vital role in helping many protein molecules hold their shape as they are carried around the body. It is generally poorly absorbed when taken in supplemental form and is more effectively derived by formation from cysteine. The same as cysteine, cystine is important in the formation of hair and skin. It is also a detoxifying agent. The athletic benefits of supplementation with free-form L-cystine have not yet been clearly defined.

Gamma-Aminobutyric Acid

Gamma-aminobutyric acid (GABA) is a nonessential amino acid that functions primarily as an inhibitory neurotransmitter in the central nervous system. In other words, GABA is calming to the brain. This calming effect can be beneficial for athletes who require concentration or steadiness. It can also help athletes who are affected by stress. GABA works by decreasing neuron activity.

GABA is generally taken in one of two ways—either by holding about 40 to 100 milligrams under the tongue and letting it be absorbed by the tiny capillaries in the mouth or by swallowing from 500 to 2,000 milligrams. GABA may also play a role in appetite control, so athletes taking it should make sure that they eat their prescribed amount of food each day. Supplemental vitamin B_6, manganese, L-taurine, and L-lysine can increase GABA synthesis in the body. Supplemental L-aspartic acid and L-glutamic acid may inhibit the action of GABA.

A word of caution: Some individuals who have taken GABA on an empty stomach have noted a nervous-system reaction beginning about fifteen minutes after ingestion. Among the symptoms are anxiety, increased rate of breathing, headache, and nausea. These individuals also noted that the effects lasted for up to two hours.

Glutamic Acid

Glutamic acid, also known as glutamate, is a nonessential amino acid occurring in proteins. It acts as an intermediary in the Krebs cycle and is therefore important for the proper metabolism of carbohydrates. It is also involved in the removal of ammonia from the muscles. It does this by combining with the ammonia to form glutamine, which is then removed. Glutamic acid is also needed for the production of energy from the BCAAs. In fact, some research has indicated that the amount of energy produced from the BCAAs depends upon the supply of glutamic acid that is available. The same as glucose, glutamic acid can pass readily through the blood-brain barrier, a semipermeable membrane that keeps the blood that is circulating in the brain away from the tissue fluids surrounding the brain cells.

Free-form L-glutamic acid can be used to supplement food proteins and can also be taken along with the BCAAs during exercise in dosages ranging from 500 to 2,000 milligrams per day. Ideally, L-glutamic acid (as well as vitamin B_6) should be part of all BCAA formulations and should be included in high amounts in all full-spectrum amino-acid formulations.

Glutamine

Glutamine is a nonessential amino acid found in proteins. It is formed from glutamic acid by the addition of ammonia and vitamin B_6. Glutamine is a neurotransmitter in the brain, where it can be converted back to glutamic acid. It is essential for the proper functioning of the brain. It is an energy source in the brain and a mediator of glutamic-acid and GABA activity. Glutamine is also vital to immune functioning. New studies show that glutamine is required for cellular replication in the immune system. However, the majority of glutamine is made in the muscles, so the muscles have to supply a large amount of glutamine to the immune system.

Oversupplementation with L-glutamine can contribute to the ammonia load; the use of glutamine alphaketoglutarate is recommended as an alternative. Use of supplemental free-form L-glutamine by athletes is known to produce a strong anticatabolic effect, which neutralizes the cortisol that accompanies strenuous exercise. Cortisol is a steroid hormone and highly catabolic. L-glutamine's anticatabolic action allows more efficient anabolism. Glutamine is also active in recovery and healing.

Supplemental glutamine has reportedly been taken in dosages ranging from 500 to over 20,000 milligrams per day during periods of high stress. Glutamine is now also commonly added to protein drinks.

Glutathione

Glutathione is a tri-peptide that as a supplement is commonly thought of as a free-form amino acid. It is a sulfur-bearing tri-peptide consisting of glutamic acid, cysteine, and glycine. Glutathione occurs in plant and animal tissues and is a vital component of the body's defense mechanism against the effects of oxygen and free radicals. (For a complete discussion of free radicals and antioxidants, see Chapter 5.) It also acts as a detoxifying agent, aids immune functioning, helps protect the integrity of red blood cells, and functions as a neurotransmitter.

Glutathione tends to decrease with age, making supplementation particularly important for adult athletes. In addition, supplemental L-cysteine raises the level of glutathione in the body, as do supplemental L- and DL-methionine. Supplemental intake of L-glutathione along with L-cysteine can be effective in reducing free-radical damage. Exercise can reduce the glutathione level.

Glycine

Glycine is a nonessential amino acid that is synthesized from serine, with folate acting as a coenzyme (enzyme cofactor). Glycine gets its name from the Greek word meaning "sweet." It is a sweet-tasting substance.

Glycine is an important precursor of many substances, including protein, DNA, phospholipids, collagen, and creatine. It is also a precursor in the release of energy. Glycine is used by the liver in the elimination of phenols, which are toxic, and in the formation of bile salts. It is necessary for the proper functioning of the central nervous system and is an inhibitory neurotransmitter. Too much supplemental glycine can displace glucose in the metabolic-energy chain and cause fatigue, but just enough can help produce more energy. During rapid growth, the body's demand for glycine increases.

Studies have shown that the use of 7,000 milligrams of glycine per day causes an increase in the GH level. Some studies have also noted that glycine ingestion causes an increase in strength, possibly due in part to its elevation of the GH level. Supplemental glycine has additionally been shown to increase the creatine level.

The long-term effects of glycine supplementation are not known, although headaches have been reported. The use of supplemental glycine is still in the experimental stage. However, 3,000 to 6,000 milligrams per day may be beneficial for power athletes, and glycine should be part of all full-spectrum amino-acid supplements. Use free-form glycine supplements with caution.

Histidine

Histidine is recognized as an essential amino acid for infants but not for adults. It is extremely important in the growth and repair of human tissue. Because of this, however, histidine is an essential amino acid for athletes, who experience high rates of growth and repair. Histidine is also important in the formation of white and red blood cells. In addition, it has a history of use as a free-form amino acid in the management of arthritis due to its anti-inflammatory properties.

L-histidine has been used as a supplement in dosages of 1,000 to 5,000 milligrams per day. It should be included in multi-amino-acid formulations. The benefits of prolonged use of supplemental free-form L-histidine by athletes are not yet clear.

However, benefits may be derived in the preseason and during injury recovery.

Isoleucine

Isoleucine is an essential amino acid that, along with leucine and valine, is one of the BCAAs. Isoleucine is found in proteins and is needed for the formation of hemoglobin. It is involved in the regulation of blood sugar and is metabolized for energy in muscle tissue during exercise.

Supplemental intake of L–isoleucine, along with the other BCAAs, has been shown to help spare muscle tis-

sue, maintain nitrogen balance, and promote muscle growth and healing. For dosage recommendations, see "The Branched–Chain Amino Acids," below.

Leucine

Leucine is an essential amino acid found in proteins that is, like the other BCAAs, important in energy production during exercise. For many years, the three BCAAs were assumed to contribute equally to energy. Recent studies, however, have shown that both exercising and resting muscle tissue uses far more leucine for energy than either of the other two BCAAs.

The Branched-Chain Amino Acids

The branched-chain amino acids (BCAAs) are the essential amino acids isoleucine, leucine, and valine. Together, these three amino acids make up about 35 percent of the amino-acid content of muscle tissue. Each of these amino acids is also used by the body for energy. Studies confirm that under conditions of stress, injury, or exercise, the body uses a disproportionately high amount of the BCAAs to maintain nitrogen balance. (For a discussion of nitrogen balance, see page 34.) Studies also indicate that leucine is used at a rate two or more times greater than those of isoleucine and valine. Many amino-acid formulations on the market therefore have about twice as much L-leucine as the other two BCAAs.

The BCAAs have a history of use in hospital situations for patients in stressed states, such as burn victims, surgical and trauma patients, and starvation cases. These patients are fed intravenously to stimulate their protein synthesis and nitrogen balance. During the 1980s, sports-nutrition companies picked up on these clinical practices and sponsored research using animals and athletes that revealed that the BCAAs are used for energy. The researchers hypothesized that taking supplemental BCAAs would compensate for the BCAAs used for energy, promote muscle growth, and restore nitrogen balance. Additionally, leucine was found to have other growth-related metabolic effects including releasing GH and insulin.

The amounts of the BCAAs supplied vary with the different products available. Some products contain just the BCAAs, others have the BCAAs as well as a few additional ingredients, and still others contain the full spectrum of eighteen amino acids with extra amounts of the BCAAs plus cofactors. Athletes, especially bodybuilders, report muscle growth and strength benefits from *effective* BCAA formulations. However, the

BCAAs are not just for power athletes. Endurance athletes can also benefit from BCAA supplementation. Research has determined that endurance athletes use as much as 90 percent of their total daily leucine for energy purposes. This means that endurance athletes might need to eat several times the normally recommended amount of protein to maintain nitrogen balance. An alternative method these athletes can use is to fortify their base diet of food proteins with a BCAA-type supplement.

HOW MUCH OF THE BCAAs IS NEEDED?

Exactly how much of each of the BCAAs is needed by the body has not yet been determined, but we have developed the following guidelines from available research and experience. If you wish to take a BCAA supplement, you can take either a combination formulation consisting of just the BCAAs and a few cofactors, a full-spectrum amino-acid formulation that includes the BCAAs, or a full-spectrum amino-acid supplement that contains extra BCAAs. Formulations that have the BCAAs, vitamin B_6, and L-glutamic acid are the best. Supplemental amounts of the BCAAs should range from 1,500 to 6,000 milligrams for L-leucine and 800 to 3,000 milligrams each for L-isoleucine and L-valine. Divide the dosage between two servings a day. Take the two servings thirty to sixty minutes before exercising and directly after exercising on training days, or along with meals on nontraining days, to fortify the base proteins.

The BCAAs compete for absorption with other amino acids, such as L-tyrosine, L- and DL-phenylalanine, and L- and DL-methionine. If you take supplemental amounts of these other amino acids, do so in the evening or morning, at least three hours after taking your BCAA supplement.

According to estimates, up to 90 percent of dietary leucine may be used for energy in exercising muscles. This makes leucine a very limiting amino acid if supplemental amounts are not taken to compensate for the loss. Leucine may also stimulate the release of insulin, which increases protein synthesis and inhibits protein breakdown.

For supplemental L-leucine dosage recommendations, see "The Branched-Chain Amino Acids" on page 40.

Lysine

Lysine is an essential amino acid that is found in large quantities in muscle tissue. It is needed for proper growth and bone development, and it aids in calcium absorption. Lysine has the ability to fight cold sores and herpes viruses. It is required for the formation of collagen, enzymes, antibodies, and other compounds. Together with methionine, iron, and vitamins B_1, B_6, and C, it helps form carnitine, a compound that the body needs in the production of energy from fatty acids. Lysine deficiency can limit protein synthesis and the growth and repair of tissues, in particular the connective tissues. It can become depleted in the brain by excess intake of L-arginine and L-ornithine.

L-lysine should be part of all full-spectrum amino-acid supplements. The effects of the use of supplemental free-form L-lysine by athletes have not yet been determined.

Methionine

Methionine is an essential sulfur-bearing amino acid. It is involved in transmethylation, a metabolic process that is vital to the manufacture of several compounds and important in muscle performance. In transmethylation, an amino acid donates a methyl group to another compound. These methyl donors often function as intermediaries in many biochemical processes. Methionine is the major methyl donor in the body.

Methionine is a limiting amino acid in many proteins, especially in plant proteins. It functions in the removal of metabolic waste products from the liver and assists in the breakdown of fat and the prevention of fatty buildup in the liver and arteries. It is used to make choline, which makes taking supplemental choline a mandatory practice for athletes to spare methionine for its other functions.

DL-methionine is commonly added to meal-replacement drinks and other nutrient beverages con- taining soy protein because it increases the quality of the protein. L-methionine, in supplemental dosages ranging from 500 to 2,000 milligrams per day, may be of benefit to athletes, especially those looking to reduce body fat.

Ornithine

Ornithine is a nonessential amino acid that does not occur in proteins. Ornithine's primary role in the body is in the urea cycle, which makes it important in the removal of ammonia. It is formed from arginine in the urea cycle. Like arginine, ornithine has been proven to be an effective GH releaser. It is this role that has brought it widespread recognition among athletes in recent years.

Supplementation with L-ornithine in various dosages, ranging from 2,000 to 4,000 milligrams per day, has been studied. Research using L-ornithine with other amino acids has also been conducted. Recently, a study using 1,000 milligrams of L-ornithine and 1,000 milligrams of L-arginine per day along with five weeks of weight training showed a decrease in body fat and an increase in muscle mass. However, indications are that the effective dose of L-ornithine may be as high as 5,000 to 15,000 milligrams per day. More research needs to be conducted to determine the exact dosage, as well as the specific benefits. L-ornithine may be particularly beneficial for bodybuilders, power lifters, and sprinters.

Ornithine is also an important component of ornithine alphaketoglutarate, a compound that is gaining popularity among bodybuilders and power athletes. For a discussion of this compound, see "Ornithine Alphaketoglutarate" on page 42.

Phenylalanine

Phenylalanine is an essential amino acid and a precursor of the nonessential amino acid tyrosine. Ingestion of supplemental L-tyrosine therefore spares phenylalanine for its other duties.

Phenylalanine has many functions in the body and is a precursor of several important metabolites, such as the skin pigment melanin, and several catecholamine neurotransmitters, such as epinephrine and norepinephrine. The catecholamines are important in memory and learning, locomotion, sex drive, tissue growth and repair, immune-system functioning, and appetite control. Phenylalanine inhibits appetite by increasing the brain's production of nor-

Ornithine Alphaketoglutarate

OKG, which is short for *ornithine alphaketoglutarate*, is the new buzzword being thrown around in American athletic and bodybuilding circles. The supplement's popularity is due to the marvelous features it offers the athlete. OKG has been used in Europe for a number of years, as far back as the early 1970s, mainly to treat the victims of burns, trauma, or severe malnutrition and to aid postsurgical healing.

OKG consists of two ornithine molecules and one alphaketoglutarate molecule. It seems to be a stimulus for a variety of metabolic functions. It acts as an ammonia scavenger; increases the glutamine pool in muscle tissue, thereby reducing catabolism; elevates the GH level; increases protein synthesis; increases insulin secretion; and aids glutamine and arginine synthesis. While studies still need to be conducted using athletes, clinical use has shown that dosages of 2,000 to 4,000 milligrams taken once or twice a day with meals are of potential benefit for bodybuilders and power athletes.

Before jumping on the OKG bandwagon, however, note that there are other substances that are much more effective for recovery and tissue repair and that have many more studies supporting their use by athletes. Among them are L-glutamine, glucosamine, the herb turmeric, and antioxidant mixtures.

---

epinephrine and cholecystokinin (CCK). CCK is the hormone that is thought to be responsible for sending out the "I am full" message. These functions of phenylalanine can be of tremendous value to athletes, especially those who need to stimulate mental alertness or who need to lose weight or maintain low levels of body fat.

Dosages of supplemental L-phenylalanine ranging from 100 to 500 milligrams, taken once or twice a day, have been reported to produce no side effects. Take L-phenylalanine on an empty stomach in the morning and in the evening. However, note that dosages of over 4,000 milligrams have been shown to cause headaches. Cofactors that appear to be necessary in phenylalanine metabolism include vitamin B_3, vitamin B_6, vitamin C, copper, and iron.

DL-phenylalanine (DLPA) has been shown to be useful in combating pain. This can be beneficial for athletes who suffer from acute or chronic pain from injury. Dosages of 500 to 1,500 milligrams of DLPA per day have been reported to be effective for this purpose. The theorized mechanism is that DLPA "protects" the endorphins in the body from destruction, thereby allowing them to distribute their morphinelike pain relief. Endorphins are a thousand times more powerful than morphine. Remember, however, that more is not always better. If you experience just partial pain relief, contact your healthcare practitioner to evaluate your condition. Do not take megadoses of DLPA, especially without medical supervision.

A word of caution: The artificial sweetener aspartame is a di-peptide made up of phenylalanine and aspartic acid. Soft drinks containing aspartame carry warnings that are aimed at people with phenylketonuria (PKU), a disease in which phenylalanine is not properly metabolized and can be very damaging. People with phenylketonuria should not take any supplemental L- or DL-phenylalanine.

On the other hand, people who drink a lot of caffeine-containing beverages or take energy supplements with caffeine-containing herbs, such as guarana, may need more phenylalanine. Caffeine tends to cause some of the neurotransmitters that are made with phenylalanine to become depleted in the central nervous system. This is why people sometimes feel mentally fuzzy after drinking a lot of coffee. Taking supplemental L- or DL-phenylalanine can help offset the depletion. Better yet, cut down on your caffeine consumption.

Proline

Proline is a nonessential amino acid. It occurs in high amounts in collagen tissue. It can be synthesized from ornithine or glutamic acid. Hydroproline, which is also abundant in collagen, is synthesized in the body from proline. Proline may be important in the maintenance and healing of collagen tissues such as the skin, tendons, and cartilage.

Current knowledge of L-proline and hydroproline supplementation is limited. Therefore, no reliable recommendations are possible at this time.

(For a discussion of hydroxyproline and its effects on the muscles, see "Delayed-Onset Muscle Soreness" on page 43.)

Delayed-Onset Muscle Soreness

Hydroxyproline is one of the amino acids that spills into the interstitial spaces following microtrauma, which involves small but widespread tears in the muscle cells from training stress. The interstitial spaces are the tiny spaces between tissues or organ parts. Over a period of twenty-four to forty-eight hours, the hydroxyproline reaches enough nerve endings to cause a deep, sometimes near-crippling pain called delayed-onset muscle soreness (DOMS) or postexercise muscle soreness (PEMS). Hydroxyproline is highly caustic to nerve endings. Until recently, the cause of DOMS was believed to be lactic acid. Lactic acid, though, is now known to be dispersed and cleared from the body within two hours after intensive exercise.

Serine

Serine is a nonessential amino acid found in proteins and derived from glycine. Its metabolism leads to the formation of many important substances, such as choline and phospholipids, which are essential in the formation of some neurotransmitters and are used to stabilize membranes. Serine is important in the metabolism of fat and the preservation of a healthy immune system. However, dosage guidelines for L-serine supplementation still need to be established.

Taurine

The nonessential amino acid taurine is one of the sulfur-bearing amino acids and occurs in the body only in its free form because it is not a component of proteins. Taurine plays a major role in brain tissue and in nervous-system functioning. It is involved in blood-pressure regulation and in the transportation of the electrolytes across cell membranes. It is found in the heart, muscles, central nervous system, and brain. It is also an inhibitory neurotransmitter—that is, calming to the brain—just like GABA. Taurine is also found in the eye and may be important for maintaining good vision and eye functioning.

Taurine is made from cysteine, with vitamin B_6 as a cofactor. The use of supplemental amounts of L-taurine ranging from 500 to 5,000 milligrams per day have been reported, but no research has yet been done to determine exactly how L-taurine can be used as part of an athlete's nutrition program.

Threonine

Threonine is an essential amino acid found in proteins. It is an important component of collagen, tooth enamel, protein, and elastic tissue. It can also function as a lipotropic agent, a substance that prevents fatty buildup in the liver. Supplemental L-threonine has a reported use in the treatment of depression in patients with low threonine levels. Generally, dosages of 1,000 milligrams per day are used in these depression cases. Studies still need to be undertaken to determine the exact benefits of L-threonine supplementation for athletes.

Tryptophan

Tryptophan is an essential amino acid that has recently been shrouded in controversy due to its suspected link to a rare blood disorder. (For a discussion of the controversy, see "The Ban on Tryptophan" on page 45.) Tryptophan is necessary for the production of vitamin B_3. Therefore, taking supplemental vitamin B_3 can help conserve tryptophan for its other functions. Supplemental L-tryptophan has been taken for years by millions of people for its pronounced calming effects, which include the promotion of sleep and the treatment of depression. Tryptophan is the precursor of the neurotransmitter serotonin. Serotonin helps control the sleep cycle, causing a feeling of drowsiness. L-tryptophan taken in dosages of 500 to 2,000 milligrams has been reported to correct sleep disorders.

L-tryptophan has also been reported to increase the GH level. One interesting study examined the effect of taking 1,200 milligrams of L-tryptophan twenty-four hours before exercising. The researchers found that treadmill performance (total exercise capacity and total exercise time) was greatly increased. However, due to the ban on L-tryptophan, use of this amino acid by athletes is not currently possible.

Tryptophan is one of the least abundant amino acids in food, which makes it one of the limiting essential amino acids. Some foods that are high in tryptophan are cottage cheese, pork, wild game, duck, and avocado. Eating these foods along with vitamin B_3 and the cofactors vitamin B_6 and magnesium may help athletes derive some of the benefits that tryptophan offers.

Tyrosine

Tyrosine is a nonessential amino acid that is made from the essential amino acid phenylalanine. Supplementation with L-tyrosine can have a sparing effect on phenylalanine, leaving phenylalanine available for functions not associated with tyrosine formation.

Tyrosine plays many roles in the body. It is a precursor of the catecholamines dopamine and norepinephrine, regulates appetite, and aids in melanin production. These functions are similar to the ones with which phenylalanine is associated as a precursor of tyrosine. However, tyrosine is believed to be better at stimulating these effects because it is one step closer as a precursor. An antidepressant effect and an increased sex drive in men have also been observed with tyrosine supplementation.

Supplemental L-tyrosine may be useful for athletes who are undergoing stress, who need to lose body fat, or who wish to maintain peak alertness. Dosages ranging from 100 milligrams to several thousand milligrams per day have been reported. *A word of caution*: L-tyrosine may trigger migraine headaches when it is broken down into a product called tyramine.

Valine

Valine is an essential amino acid and a member of the branched-chain amino acids. The same as the other BCAAs, isoleucine and leucine, valine is an integral part of muscle tissue and may be used for energy by exercising muscles. It is involved in tissue repair, nitrogen balance, and muscle metabolism. For supplemental L-valine dosage recommendations, see "The Branched-Chain Amino Acids" on page 40.

DIGESTION OF PROTEIN AND AMINO ACIDS

The mechanical digestion of protein begins in the mouth during chewing. In the stomach, the enzyme pepsin joins in, breaking down the protein into shorter peptides. The partially digested protein then passes into the intestines, where the free-form, di-peptide, and tri-peptide amino acids are absorbed, begin-

ning immediately. Enzymes continue to digest any polypeptides as they travel down the intestines.

Once the free-form, di-peptide, and tri-peptide amino acids enter the bloodstream, they are transported to the liver, where a few things may happen to them. They may be converted into other amino acids; they may be used to make other proteins; they may be further broken down and either used for energy or excreted; or they may be placed into circulation and continue on to the rest of the body.

Proteins empty from the stomach in two to three hours, depending on how much fat is present. This means that you should keep the protein content of precompetition meals low to enable your stomach to pass food into your bloodstream and cells before you begin exercising. (For a further discussion of digestion and absorption, see Chapter 11.)

SPECIAL PROTEIN AND AMINO-ACID NEEDS OF THE ATHLETE

In Chapter 2, we credited carbohydrates with having a protein-sparing effect. This protein-sparing effect is a function of carbohydrates providing enough energy to minimize the body's use of amino acids for energy. Calories, however, are not the only factor involved in the sparing of muscle tissue, which is extremely important to the athlete who has been working hard to build up or maintain muscle mass. For example, if you ate a whopping 10,000 calories a day from only carbohydrate and fat sources, your body still would have to break down muscle tissue to get the supply of amino acids it needed to carry on metabolism. Looking at it this way, you can see that an adequate supply of protein (amino acids) is essential to the maintenance of existing muscle tissue.

To derive optimum protein, you must achieve the proper protein-to-calorie ratio. You can accomplish this by eating enough carbohydrates and fat to meet your energy requirements and enough protein to get the amino acids your body needs for growth, energy, and other metabolic demands. But, as is evident from the material discussed so far in this chapter, adequate amount is not the only requirement for optimum protein intake. What type the protein is affects how it is used by the body, and fortification with certain amino acids and other cofactors influences how efficiently food-source proteins are used. At the very least, protein intake, especially by athletes, is a sophisticated science. Just how much protein an athlete requires depends on body weight, the quality of the protein, and the intensity and duration of the exercise.

The RDA guidelines for protein can provide a baseline for athletes' protein requirements. However, the protein allowances were determined according to body weight, plus they assume normal body weight. Therefore, if you have more than the average amount of body fat, you may end up overcalculating your protein need.

According to the RDAs, an adult male between the ages of twenty-five and fifty requires 63 grams of protein per day, which can be obtained by eating about 6 ounces of chicken. However, research has shown that athletes engaged in daily exercise have difficulty maintaining nitrogen balance when their dietary-protein intake is less than 1.5 grams for each 1 kilogram (2.2 pounds) of body weight. This is about 50-percent higher than the RDA. In fact, researchers estimate that, depending on the type of sport, the requirement for protein is about 1.5 to 2.5 grams per 1 kilogram of ideal body weight. Furthermore, in some special instances—for example, if you are a bodybuilder preparing for a contest—the requirement may exceed 3 grams for every 1 kilogram of body weight. How much food does this translate into? For an athlete weighing 174 pounds, protein intake should be between 118 to 198 grams per day. This is two to three times the RDA and a lot of protein to eat (about 14 to 22 ounces of chicken per day). Remember that

excess protein is not converted to muscle. Rather, it is either broken down and used as energy in the liver or converted to fat. Because protein is also one of the most expensive nutrients, you should take special care to eat just the right amount for your sport, lean body mass, and activity level.

Another consideration in protein consumption is efficiency. You can make the proteins you eat more efficient by fortifying them with a multi-amino-acid supplement that includes the BCAAs. By providing your body with potentially limiting amino acids from supplement sources, you may be able to maintain nitrogen balance with a lower protein intake. While we offer protein-supplement guidelines in this book, the only way you can determine your nitrogen balance for sure is to monitor how it varies with different levels of protein intake and supplement use.

Additionally, protein cofactors are required for the proper metabolism of the amino acids. Vitamin B_6 is the most important cofactor because it is necessary in the functioning of the enzymes that aid this metabolism. Vitamin B_3 is an important vitamin because it spares tryptophan, which is converted to vitamin B_3 in the body. However, do not take large amounts of vitamin B_3 during exercise, as studies have shown that a large intake of vitamin B_3 can increase glycogen use, which results in early onset of fatigue. (For a complete discussion of vitamin B_3, see page 80.) Researchers have also determined that increased pro-

The Ban on Tryptophan

L-tryptophan has been commercially used as a free-form amino acid for many years. It has been self-prescribed as well as recommended by health-care practitioners for the treatment of depression, the management of pain, and help with sleep. In 1989, a sudden outbreak of eosinophilia myalgia, a rare blood disorder, was observed in the United States. The Centers for Disease Control and the FDA quickly linked the development of the disorder to the use of certain L-tryptophan supplements. As a result, the FDA banned the use of L-tryptophan on its own and currently allows it only for the fortification of protein and in other limited applications. The vast majority of supplement users, however, were surprised about the L-tryptophan ban because, during decades of use, the amino acid had never been linked to the rare blood disease. Almost immediately during the investigation, health officials found that the L-tryptophan supplements that had been

used by the people who developed the blood disease came from one particular manufacturer in Japan. Upon further inquiry, the investigators discovered that just several batches of that manufacturer's L-tryptophan were contaminated and that the contaminant—not the L-tryptophan—was responsible for causing the blood disease. Despite this finding, however, synthetic free-form L-tryptophan supplements continue to be prohibited in the United States.

Tryptophan, though, is still included among the amino acids that are profiled on the labels of many protein and amino-acid products. This is okay because tryptophan, the same as other amino acids, is a naturally occurring essential amino acid that is found in all dietary proteins. In fact, humans cannot live without it. As a result, many manufacturers of supplements containing L-typtophan indicate on the label that the amino acid is from natural sources, not a synthetic form.

Estimating Your Daily Protein Requirement

Too often, athletes eat either too much or too little protein. The following method was developed by Dr. Hatfield as an easy way to estimate your daily protein requirement. It will help you determine approximately how much protein you should consume from food and supplement sources on a daily basis.

  Your estimated protein requirement is determined using your lean body mass and activity factor. Your lean body mass is all of your body's bones, muscles, organs, blood, and water—all of your bodily tissues apart from your body fat. Your activity factor is the average intensity of a normal day's activities. If you are more active on a particular day, or during your athletic season, you will need to up your protein intake to meet your increased requirement. If you are less active, you should lower it, since your demand is reduced.

To estimate your daily protein requirement:

1. Calculate your lean body mass (in pounds) using the Quick Method for Determining Body Composition on page 145.

2. Determine your activity factor using the Activity Factors Table, below.

3. Determine your daily protein requirement (in grams) using the Daily Protein Requirement Table, right. First, find the lean body mass closest to your own from step 1 in the Lean Body Mass column. Then, read across the row until you find your activity factor from step 2. The answer is the grams of protein you should consume from food and supplement sources on an average day. For example, if your lean body mass is 173 pounds and you train with heavy weights every day, you would find the 170-pound row and read across to the .9 column. Your daily protein requirement would be 153 grams.

Activity Factors Table

Activity Factor	General Daily Activity	Activity Factor	General Daily Activity
.5	Sedentary; no sports participation or fitness exercising.	.8	Moderate weight training or aerobic training daily.
.6	Jogging or light fitness exercising.	.9	Heavy weight training daily.
.7	Sports participation or moderate fitness exercising three times a week.	1.0	Heavy weight training plus sports training daily ("two-a-day" training).

tein intake leads to an increase in calcium excretion. Increasing phosphorus intake seems to minimize this effect, however, as does increasing calcium intake by individuals on high-protein diets. All the essential vitamins and minerals are important in some way in the body's optimum use of the amino acids.

For a quick and relatively accurate method of estimating your daily protein requirement, see above. This method was developed by Dr. Hatfield and takes into account lean body mass as well as activity level. You need to know your protein requirement as part of your sports-nutrition program and to construct a customized nutrition plan, as explained in Chapter 13. Therefore, once you have calculated your protein requirement, transfer it to the Personal Inventory form provided in Appendix A.

FOOD AND SUPPLEMENT SOURCES OF PROTEIN

Protein is found in animals, in plants, and in supplement form. Animal proteins tend to be of higher quality than plant proteins because they contain the proper proportions of the essential amino acids. Most plant protein sources, such as beans and peas, are incomplete in their essential-amino-acid contents. Therefore, it is necessary to combine different plant proteins to get an adequate balance of the amino acids. Two popular combinations are peas with corn and kidney beans with brown rice. If you are a vegetarian, you need to know how to combine legumes with grains to formulate complete proteins. Check your local library or bookstore for a book that explains how to do this.

Protein is ususally found together with fat in foods, especially in animal products. Some good low-fat sources of protein are low-fat milk, skim milk, and other low-fat dairy products; most fishes, including cod, sole, halibut, tuna, sardines, and salmon; most shellfishes, including scallops, lobster, crab, shrimp, and mussels; lean red meat from which the fat has been trimmed; and skinless poultry.

As supplements, protein and amino acids are avail-

Daily Protein Requirement Table

Lean Body Mass	Activity Factor					
	.5	.6	.7	.8	.9	1.0
IN POUNDS	COLUMNS REPRESENT DAILY PROTEIN REQUIREMENTS IN GRAMS					
90	45	54	63	72	81	90
100	50	60	70	80	90	100
110	55	66	77	88	99	110
120	60	72	84	96	108	120
130	65	78	91	104	117	130
140	70	84	98	112	126	140
150	75	90	105	120	135	150
160	80	96	112	128	144	160
170	85	102	119	136	153	170
180	90	108	126	144	162	180
190	95	114	133	152	171	190
200	100	120	140	160	180	200
210	105	126	147	168	189	210
220	110	132	154	176	198	220
230	115	138	161	184	207	230
240	120	144	168	192	216	240

able in tablet, capsule, liquid, and powder forms. In tablet form, they are generally used to fortify meals or to get extra amino acids before or during exercise or before going to bed. One or several amino acids can be delivered by tablets and capsules. Liquid and powder protein supplements can be eaten between meals or with meals. The ingredients range from just a few amino acids, such as the BCAAs, to the full spectrum of eighteen amino acids with extra amounts of the BCAAs as well as cofactors. If you shop carefully, you should be able to find economical sources of protein in supplement form. The best are high in both protein and carbohydrates. Protein drinks should have whey or whey and egg as the primary sources of protein.

DECIPHERING LABELS

Proteins and amino acids come not only in several forms but also in many combinations. When purchasing a supplement formulation that supplies one or several amino acids, you must know how to determine how much of the actual amino acids you are getting. For example, the ingredient list of a supplement containing L-arginine and L-ornithine may read:

Each capsule supplies:

L-arginine .... 500 milligrams
L-ornithine .... 500 milligrams

This label is reporting the molecular amounts of L-arginine and L-ornithine.

Some products contain amino acids combined with other molecules. The ingredient list of this type of supplement may read:

Each capsule supplies:

L-arginine hydrochloride ..... 500 milligrams
L-ornithine hydrochloride .... 500 milligrams

This label is reporting that each capsule has 500 milligrams of the entire molecule of L-arginine hydrochloride, of which L-arginine may make up only 60 percent, or 300 milligrams; and 500 milligrams of the entire molecule of L-ornithine hydrochloride, of which L-ornithine may make up only 60 percent, or 300 milligrams. Since the capsules in the first example actually have 500 milligrams each of L-arginine and L-ornithine, they are a better choice.

Another product may have a label that reads:

Each capsule supplies:

    L-arginine (hydrochloride) ..... 500 milligrams
    L-ornithine (hydrochloride) .... 500 milligrams

The parentheses around the *hydrochloride*, which is sometimes abbreviated as *HCl*, indicate that this product supplies, per capsule, 500 milligrams each of L-arginine and L-ornithine in the form of hydrochloride. This is the same amount as the product in the first example.

Always be wary of products that do not give the amounts of the amino acids they supply. Some products list only the names of the amino acids, not the quantities. This limited information is worthless, since there is no way you can figure out how much of the product to consume.

The importance of proper protein intake to maximum performance is obvious. Choosing high-quality food protein sources and properly using protein and amino-acid supplements is essential. Ingesting the correct amount of protein for your body size and activity level can help maintain your desirable body weight and improve your healing and recovery abilities.

4. LIPIDS

UNDERESTIMATED ENERGY AND GROWTH FACTORS

The third major macronutrient category, along with carbohydrates and protein, is lipids. The same as carbohydrates, lipids are composed of carbon, hydrogen, and oxygen. Lipids are necessary in the human body for numerous reasons. They contain the fat-soluble vitamins A, D, E, and K. They are a source of the essential fatty acids, which play many vital roles in maintaining the functioning and integrity of cell membranes. They serve as concentrated sources of energy. They add palatability to meals. And they are important in biochemical and biophysical functions such as steroid-hormone synthesis.

The most prevalent type of lipid is the triglyceride. As an energy source, the triglyceride varies in importance according to the type of exercise performed. For endurance sports, such as marathon running, triglycerides are the primary source of energy. For power sports, such as sprinting, glycogen is the primary fuel, but some triglycerides are also used. It is important to understand that the body is constantly metabolizing triglycerides for energy; the only thing that changes is the degree to which it does this.

Power athletes are prone to becoming fat because of this differential use of energy sources—that is, because their bodies use mostly glycogen for energy and just a minor portion of body fat. These athletes must therefore follow nutrition programs that are low in fat and high in fat-metabolizing nutrients. But even though endurance athletes, such as marathon runners, can get away with eating high-fat diets, they will definitely find their performance impeded and health negatively affected if their diets are *too* high in fat.

In this chapter, we will take a look at the different kinds of lipids that exist. We will also discuss ways of cutting down on the bad lipids in the diet without reducing our intake of the beneficial nutrients such as protein.

LIPIDS—THE MOST MISUNDERSTOOD MACRONUTRIENT

In recent years, dietary lipids have gained a bad repu-

tation. Medical research has linked a diet high in lipids to many diseases. Certain lipids are essential to health, however. Rather than cut lipids out of your diet completely, you should learn how to balance the good lipids with the bad lipids in your diet and how to trim total lipid intake.

Lipids serve many essential functions in the body. Their main functions are:

☐ To provide fuel.

☐ To provide insulation.

☐ To aid in the absorption of the fat-soluble vitamins.

☐ To act as energy storehouses.

☐ To supply the essential fatty acids.

☐ To provide protective padding for body structures and organs.

☐ To serve as components of all cell membranes and other cellular structures.

☐ To supply building blocks for other molecules.

The main problem with lipids in the diet is simple—we consume too much total lipid, too much of the wrong lipids, and not enough of the good lipids. While lipids are necessary for health, too much of the wrong kinds of lipids can have negative effects on the body and can lead to certain cancers and cardiovascular diseases. The common culprits are saturated fats and cholesterol. Of course, too much of any lipid can cause obesity. Most experts recommend a total dietary-lipid intake of less than 30 percent of total daily calories; some recommend keeping lipids under 20 percent. Because athletes generally consume over 4,000 calories a day, they can easily get an overdose of lipids in their diets. Keeping total lipid intake down, maximizing the good lipids, and minimizing the bad lipids are therefore the major focus of sports nutrition.

THE MAJOR LIPIDS

Lipids occur in both plants and animals, but plant lipids vary slightly in chemical composition from animal lipids. By definition, lipids are compounds that are soluble in organic solvents but not in water. Mammal fats tend to be more saturated than fish oils or plant oils. Beef tends to be more saturated than pork or poultry. The degree of hardness that a fat displays at room temperature is an indication of how saturated it is. Compare hard beef fat, soft fish fat, and vegetable oil. Vegetable oil has a low amount of saturated fat and a high amount of polyunsaturated fat.

The major lipids found in the diet and body are triglycerides and fatty acids, phospholipids, and cholesterol.

Triglycerides and Fatty Acids

Triglycerides are the major class of lipids in the diet and body. They are the lipids that make up the fats and oils in the diet and the fat that is stored by the body. They include about 98 percent of all the dietary fats.

The difference between fat and oil is simple—fat is solid at room temperature and oil is liquid. This difference in solidity gives an indication of composition. Triglycerides are composed of three fatty acids attached to a three-carbon-atom glycerol molecule. There are hundreds of different fatty acids, and they come in various lengths, from four to twenty-four carbon atoms long. A short-chain fatty acid has four to five carbon atoms; a medium-chain fatty acid has six to twelve carbon atoms; a long-chain fatty acid has thirteen to nineteen carbon atoms; and a very long chain fatty acid has twenty or more carbon atoms.

Fatty acids are also rated according to the hydrogen atoms that are attached to their carbon chains. Saturated fatty acids have the maximum number of hydrogen atoms that they can hold, with no unsaturated carbon molecules. This is why saturated fatty acids are more solid. Hydrogenation is the process of taking unsaturated fatty acids and saturating them with hydrogen atoms to make them more solid. An example is margarine, which is made of vegetable oil, a liquid fatty acid. Monounsaturated fatty acids have one unsaturated carbon molecule, and polyunsaturated fatty acids have more than one unsaturated carbon molecule.

Saturated fatty acids tend to be solid at room temperature. Therefore, fats are high in saturated fatty acids. Polyunsaturated fatty acids tend to be liquid at room temperature. Oils are high in polyunsaturated fatty acids. Saturated fatty acids are always either used for energy or stored as body fat, as are fatty acids containing sixteen or fewer carbon atoms. The fewer carbon atoms a fatty acid has, the easier it is to use that fatty acid for energy. The longer fatty acids can also be used for energy or stored as body fat, but they have other functions as well. For example, they serve as components in the structure of cell membranes, which is important for growth.

Among the fatty acids, the most important ones are the essential fatty acids, the omega-3 fatty acids, gamma linolenic acid, and medium-chain triglycerides.

The Essential Fatty Acids

Of the many fatty acids that exist, only two are essential and only one is conditionally essential. Linoleic acid is a primary essential fatty acid. It is necessary for normal growth and health. Therefore, since the body cannot manufacture it, it must be obtained from the diet. Another fatty acid, arachidonic acid, is made in the body from linoleic acid. Arachidonic acid only becomes essential when a linoleic-acid deficiency exists. However, because arachidonic acid has to be made from linoleic acid and because it is a polyunsaturated fatty acid, arachidonic acid has a linoleic-sparing effect when it is present in the diet. This may be beneficial to athletes because arachidonic acid is also an important structural fatty acid that is present in cell membranes.

Alpha-linolenic acid is the other essential fatty acid. Alpha-linolenic acid is similar to linoleic acid in structure. Among its functions, it is important in growth and is the precursor of two other important fatty acids, eicosapentaenoic acid (EPA) and docosahexaenoic acid (DHA). As with protein and the amino acids, the body would rather use the essential fatty acids for growth and functional needs than for fuel needs. A diet that is high in the essential fatty acids and low in the nonessential fatty acids therefore increases metabolism and discourages increased body-fat formation, assuming that overeating is not a factor. Remember, excess carbohydrates and amino acids can be converted to body fat.

The essential fatty acids are important to existence and performance. Some of their specific functions are:

☐ Presence in phospholipids, which are important in maintaining the structure and the functioning of cellular and subcellular membranes.

☐ Service as precursors of eicosanoids, which are important in regulating a wide diversity of physiological processes.

☐ Involvement in the transfer of oxygen from the lungs to the bloodstream.

☐ Formation of a structural part of all cells.

☐ Reduction of the time required for recovery by fatigued muscles after exercise by helping clear away lactic acid.

☐ Maintenance of proper brain and nervous-system functioning.

☐ Production of prostaglandins, a group of hormones important in metabolism.

☐ Formation of healthy skin and hair.

☐ Assistance in wound healing.

☐ Growth enhancement.

Linoleic acid and alpha-linolenic acid are both unsaturated fatty acids and eighteen carbon atoms long. While scientists recognize that the body requires these two fatty acids for health, they have not yet established RDAs for them for adults because deficiencies in the essential fatty acids are rare.

The Omega-3 Fatty Acids

During the 1980s, there was a resurgence of attention focused on two fatty acids belonging to the omega-3 family—eicosapentaenoic acid (EPA) and docosahexaenoic acid (DHA). Researchers in the 1950s had documented the cholesterol-lowering effects of EPA and DHA. However, it was not until the 1970s, when the low rates of cardiovascular diseases were documented among the fish-eating Greenland Eskimos, that conclusive results were proven.

EPA and DHA can be made in the body from linoleic acid, also a fatty acid, and are found in human tissue as normal components. Despite this, when they are obtained from food sources that are part of a diet that is low in saturated fatty acids, they have beneficial effects. They have the tendency to disperse fatty acids and cholesterol in the bloodstream, which seems to be how their presence helps prevent arteries from clogging. They have a blood-thinning effect and discourage excessive blood clotting. They lower the blood-triglyceride level and raise the level of high-density lipoproteins (HDLs), the good lipoproteins that help prevent cholesterol buildup in the arteries. In addition, EPA and DHA have an anti-inflammatory effect and work by competing with arachidonic acid, which forms pro-inflammatory compounds.

Besides all their known health benefits, EPA and DHA have also been documented to improve athletic performance. Recent studies using 2,000 to 4,000 milligrams per day of EPA and DHA from supplements and fish have reported significant increases in strength and aerobic (with oxygen) performance. The improvements included increased bench-press repetitions, faster running times, reduced muscular inflammation, and longer jumping distances. Scientists believe that these improvements were due to the combined effects that EPA and DHA have on the body, including improved GH production, anti-inflammatory action, enhanced oxygen metabolism, lowered blood viscosity (thickness) leading to better oxygen and nutrient delivery to the muscles, and improved recovery.

EPA and DHA are found in high amounts in cold-water fishes such as cod, salmon, sardines, trout, and mackerel, and in lower amounts in tuna. They are also available in supplemental form, specifically as gelatin capsules and liquid supplements. Aim for a combined intake of 2,000 to 4,000 milligrams of EPA and DHA per day from supplement and food sources.

Gamma Linolenic Acid

Gamma linolenic acid (GLA) is another important fatty acid that can be made in the body from the main essential fatty acid, linoleic acid. GLA is an important precursor of the series-1 prostaglandins, a group of hormones that regulate many cellular activities. The series-1 prostaglandins keep blood platelets from sticking together, control cholesterol formation, reduce inflammation, make insulin work better, improve nerve functioning, regulate calcium metabolism, and function in the immune system. While studies on athletes have not confirmed any performance-enhancing effects, the ingestion of foods and supplements high in GLA does benefit overall health.

Foods containing GLA are not that easy to find, however. GLA is not present in many foods. In fact, the major sources are evening primrose oil, borage oil, and black currant oil, which are also high in linoleic acid. GLA taken in dosages of 100 to 400 milligrams per day, in association with the essential fatty acids and omega-3 fatty acids, may benefit physical performance and health, especially during the season.

Medium-Chain Triglycerides

Medium-chain triglyceride (MCT) formulations were first made in the 1950s using coconut oil. MCTs contain saturated fatty acids with chains of six to twelve carbon atoms. They occur in milk fat and especially in coconut oil and palm oil. MCT formulations are high in caprylic acid and capric acid, which are saturated fatty acids. They are just now coming to the attention of athletes because they are relatively new on the market.

MCT formulations were originally developed as calorie sources for individuals who have certain pathologic conditions that do not allow normal digestion and utilization of long-chain fatty acids. MCTs tend to behave differently in the body than long-chain triglycerides (LCTs) do. They are more soluble in water, and they can pass from the intestines directly into the bloodstream. Fatty acids usually pass from the intestines first into the lymphatic system, then into the bloodstream. Because MCTs get into the bloodstream quicker than LCTs do, they are more easily and quickly digested. In addition, it has been reported in the medical literature that although MCTs can be converted to body fat, they are not readily stored in fat deposits and are quickly used for energy in the liver. They can also pass freely, without the aid of carnitine, into the mitochondria of cells. (For a discussion of carnitine, see page 102.) MCTs are therefore a potentially quick source of high energy for the body. MCTs reportedly also have a thermogenic effect, estimated to be 10- to 15-percent higher than their caloric value, but only when the MCTs in the diet exceed 30 percent of the total calories.

These features of MCTs have recently attracted the attention of athletes, especially bodybuilders. Bodybuilders feel that these features benefit their restricted contest-preparation diets, which are aimed at reducing body fat and sparing muscle tissue. The implications of the use of large amounts of MCTs by athletes on restricted diets are not clearly evident, though. Some bodybuilders report that they are able to get "super lean" when they eat about 400 calories per day of MCTs as part of a 2,000-calorie-a-day contest-preparation diet. Remember, though, that bodybuilders are not concerned with physical performance. In bodybuilding contests, physique is judged.

MCTs may also have a place in the diets of endurance athletes, as part of the precompetition meal. Scientists hypothesize that this quick fuel source may be a better fuel than body stores of fatty acids and can perhaps spare muscle glycogen. Studies on athletes need to be performed to verify this. A major drawback of MCTs is their conversion to ketones during their metabolism by the body. Ketones are produced during the incomplete metabolism of fatty acids. They are acidic and can upset an individual's physiology. Although trained endurance athletes have developed the metabolic pathways (sequences of reactions) to better utilize ketones than untrained individuals, athletes experimenting with MCTs should do so several weeks before a major event to avoid an impaired performance due to an elevated blood-ketone level.

Do MCTs have a place in every athlete's diet? More research is needed to determine the exact benefits of MCTs for athletes in general. While bodybuilders appear to derive certain benefits, some people can suffer side effects from eating too much MCT. The most common complaints are abdominal cramping and diarrhea. Prolonged use may also be harmful. MCTs are saturated fatty acids, and consuming more than 10 percent of total daily calories from saturated fatty acids is not recommended because of the link to various diseases. Additionally, in recent research, individuals who ingested only moderate amounts of MCTs developed elevated triglyceride and cholesterol blood levels. If you plan to experiment with MCTs, you should use formulations that also contain the essential fatty acids and the omega-3 fatty acids.

Phospholipids

Phospholipids are a second major class of lipids. Phospholipids are manufactured by the body. They are a major structural lipid in all organisms, a part of every living cell. In combination with proteins, they are constituents of cell membranes and the membranes of subcellular particles.

Phospholipids consist of two fatty acids attached to a three-carbon-atom glycerol molecule, with a phosphate-containing compound attached to the third carbon atom. Their main function is maintaining the structural integrity of cell membranes. They also act as emulsifiers in the body—that is, during digestion, they help disperse fats in water mediums. They are important structural components of brain and nervous-system tissue and of lipoproteins, the conjugated proteins that transport cholesterol and fats in the blood.

Phospholipids are generally contained in the "invisible" fat of plants and animals, not in the visible fat. Lecithin is the most well known phospholipid. Studies have also been conducted on the inositol-containing phospholipids, the phosphoinositides. The phosphoinositides' primary role is as a precursor of messenger molecules. In this capacity, they have a profound effect on cellular functioning and on metabolism, particularly the metabolism of fats. The research into the phosphoinositides was prompted by observations made about choline- and inositol-deficient diets. Choline and inositol are nutrients that are important in fatty-acid metabolism and are said to help defat the liver. Nutrients that have this defatting action on the liver are called lipotropic agents. Choline also functions in memory, with diets deficient in choline associated with memory impairment. For the athlete, all of these important structural, metabolic, memory, and lipotropic roles of phospholipids are vital for peak performance. (For discussions of choline and inositol, see Chapter 8.)

Of the many phospholipids that exist, lecithin and phosphatidylserine are currently sharing the spotlight regarding supplemental use.

Lecithin

Lecithin (phosphatidylcholine) is a type of phospholipid that has choline attached to the phosphate molecule. Lecithin supplies the body with choline, which is essential for liver and brain functioning. Lecithin is also high in linoleic acid. Egg yolks, liver, and soybeans are rich in lecithin. In addition, lecithin is manufactured by the body.

The use of lecithin supplements came into vogue when researchers made the connection between choline and memory functioning. Lecithin's emulsifying properties are also thought to help keep the blood system clean of fatty deposits. Researchers have documented reduced choline levels in athletes running in the Boston Marathon and have speculated that a low choline level may adversely affect performance as well as have detrimental long-term effects on the nervous system. Choline is important in creatine synthesis and is therefore suspected of playing a role as a strength builder. Studies on athletes using dosages of 20,000 to 30,000 milligrams of lecithin have produced mixed results; some have reported beneficial effects on muscular power, performance, and endurance.

Phosphatidylserine

Recently, attention has turned to another phospholipid, phosphatidylserine (PS). In PS, serine is attached to the phosphate molecule. Serine is a nonessential amino acid whose metabolism leads to the synthesis of PS. Serine functions in fat metabolism and is vital to the health of the immune system. Intake of 200 to 300 milligrams of PS has been associated with improved memory and learning. Intake of 800 milligrams has been linked to a reduced level of cortisol, which is a catabolic hormone, as well as improved muscle growth and recovery after exercise.

Cholesterol

Cholesterol is a member of a group of fats called sterols. It is made by the body and occurs naturally in foods only of animal origin. The highest concentrations of cholesterol are found in liver and egg yolks, although high levels are also present in red meat, poultry (especially the skin), whole milk, and cheese.

Cholesterol has many important functions in the body. It is a component of every cell; a precursor of bile acids, various sex and adrenal hormones, and vitamin D; and an important aid in brain and nervous-system tissues. The body needs a constant supply of cholesterol for proper health and performance. However, a high cholesterol level has been linked to a variety of cardiovascular diseases.

For good health, doctors recommend keeping cholesterol intake to under 300 milligrams per day. Since most meats contain about 90 milligrams of cholesterol in every 3 ounces, this is an almost impossible task for athletes, who generally need to consume high levels of protein. To meet both these needs, athletes must take special care to include plant protein sources, egg whites, and other high-protein, low-fat, low-cholesterol foods and supplements in their diets.

DIGESTION OF LIPIDS

Lipids take the most time and effort to be digested by the human body because of their insolubility in water and their complex structures. As lipids pass through the mouth and stomach, they are treated mechanically and chemically in preparation for the main digestive processes, which take place in the intestines. Lipids take longer than the other macronutrients to empty from the stomach, about three to four hours or more, depending on the size of the meal. Their digestion takes place chiefly in the small intestine, where bile from the liver helps to bring them into contact with fat-splitting enzymes from the pancreas and the intestinal wall. In the intestines, the fatty acids are separated from the glycerol molecules; these components are then reassembled after they pass through the intestinal walls. Along the way, they are coated with protein. They then pass into the lymphatic system. Under normal conditions, about 60 to 70 percent of ingested fat is absorbed into the portal circulation via the lymphatic system. Medium- and short-chain fatty acids are absorbed directly from the intestines.

Once in the bloodstream, fats and cholesterol are transported to the liver in conjunction with lipoproteins. The liver is the main processing center for lipids. In the liver, lipids may be converted for energy use or they may be modified—for example, the carbon chains of fatty acids may be shortened or lengthened or the degree of saturation may be increased or decreased. Any lipids that are not immediately needed by the body are converted into fat stores. The liver also synthesizes triglycerides, lipoproteins, cholesterol, and phospholipids.

Lipids are constantly being broken down, resynthesized, and used for energy in the body. They are in equilibrium when caloric intake is in balance with energy needs. However, when caloric intake from lipids, proteins, and carbohydrates exceeds energy needs, body-fat stores are increased.

YOU ARE WHAT YOU EAT

The type of lipid that you eat actually affects your body's fatty-acid composition. All cell membranes contain fatty acids. However, comparisons between vegetarians and meat eaters have revealed that a vegetarian's body is composed of more unsaturated fatty acids and a meat eater's body is composed of more saturated fatty acids. Also revealed was that people who consume diets high in saturated fat have bodies composed of more saturated than unsaturated fatty acids.

Saturated fatty acids tend to be less stable than unsaturated fatty acids and are therefore more susceptible to damage from free radicals and toxic metabolic waste products. This means that a body made of more unsaturated than saturated fatty acids may be more resistant to certain cellular damage. Since athletes are subject to high amounts of free radicals and metabolic toxins, they may be able to reduce muscle

damage and increase recovery rates by consuming diets that have more unsaturated than saturated fats.

SPECIAL LIPID NEEDS OF THE ATHLETE

The NRC recommends that people of average health keep their total lipid intake below 30 percent of their total daily caloric intake and their saturated fat intake below 10 percent of their total daily caloric intake. This assumes that these people eat only the recommended total daily calories for their age and body size. Combined intake of linoleic and alpha-linolenic acids should be kept to 1 to 2 percent of total daily calories, which works out roughly to 3,000 to 6,000 milligrams. However, some health professionals estimate that males require three times this amount of these two essential fatty acids because of hormonal differences from females.

As far as athletes are concerned, the total amount of fat that should be consumed varies with the sport. In general, endurance athletes need to maintain higher levels of fat intake than do power athletes. The specific level is directly related to the energetics of the sport. Additionally, since the number of calories consumed daily by athletes is two to three times greater than the "average" total daily calories used by the NRC to determine its RDA values, using a rule of thumb can result in overestimation of fat intake.

Most athletes should concentrate on reducing their total lipid intake as well as their saturated-fat intake while at the same time increasing their essential fatty acid intake. Because athletes maintain such a high total intake of calories, they should not obtain over 25 percent of their total daily calories from lipids. In fact, most athletes should maintain a total fat intake of under 20 percent. Weight-conscious athletes should try to maintain a fat intake of about 15 percent. Furthermore, an athlete's essential fatty acid intake should be at least 9,000 or more milligrams per day of linoleic and alpha-linolenic acids. (For a discussion of lipids in the diet, see "Too Much Lipid in Our Diets" on page 55.)

FOOD SOURCES OF LIPIDS

Lipids from plant sources tend to be healthier than lipids from animal sources. At the same time, though, most plant proteins are incomplete and low in quality, while animal proteins are complete and high in quality. When planning your meals and snacks, you

Too Much Lipid in Our Diets

Most of us consume too much lipid in our diets. Typical Americans get 45 percent of their total daily calories from lipids. When you consider that each gram of lipid contains more than twice the number of calories contained by a gram of carbohydrates or protein, you can easily see why fats and oils are such villains.

Furthermore, the very latest scientific studies reveal that fats and oils may be even more villainous than their caloric value suggests. In direct comparisons of high-fat and low-fat diets, even when the number of calories in each diet was identical, the high-fat diet caused much more fat to be stored.

So how much lipid should you consume in your diet? The American Heart Association recommends 30 percent of your total daily calories as the absolute maximum. But the closer you can get to 20 percent, or the more you can go below it, the easier it will be for you to attain your fat-loss or weight-maintenance goals. See the following table for what this means in calories.

Fat Calories Consumed on Different Diets

Total Daily Calories	Total Daily Fat Calories	
	20%-Fat Diet	30%-Fat Diet
2,400 calories	480 calories < 4 tablespoons fat	720 calories < 6 tablespoons fat
3,000 calories	600 calories < 5 tablespoons fat	900 calories < 8 tablespoons fat

The symbol < means "less than."

When calculating your own fat intake, keep in mind that 1 teaspoon of fat equals 5 grams, which equals 45 calories; and 1 tablespoon of fat equals 15 grams, which equals 135 calories.

---

must try to strike a balance between these foods to minimize your intake of saturated fats and cholesterol but still benefit from complete proteins.

As a general rule, the foods you should avoid or eat infrequently include kidney, liver, egg yolks, custard, coconut oil, butter, palm oil, cream cheese, whole-milk products, and fatty meats, especially bacon, pork sausage, hot dogs, bologna, and hamburgers. These foods are high in saturated fatty acids and cholesterol. Instead, eat lean meats such as fish, chicken, and turkey; egg whites; skim-milk products; a combination of plant proteins that form a complete protein; and protein formulations. It is especially important for bodybuilders following a high-protein diet to monitor their lipid intake. Supplement formulations of pure proteins and amino acids can be extremely helpful.

Regarding sources of pure fat, such as oils, food sources high in polyunsaturated fats should be substituted for food sources high in saturated fats. Some fat sources that are low in saturated fats and cholesterol are margarine, corn oil, olive oil, peanut oil, cottonseed oil, safflower oil, sunflower oil, and most nuts. Nuts also supply protein. Fat sources to avoid include butter, bacon fat, cream, mayonnaise, and mayonnaise-based salad dressings.

As this chapter has made evident, you must always be on the lookout for fat, which so easily sneaks into the diet. Choose foods such as low-fat salad oil, then spoon it on rather than pour it on.

As you strive to reduce your fat intake, keep the following good news in mind: Each gram of fat that you replace with a gram of either protein or carbohydrate cuts your calories by more than half. As a result, you may be able to eat more food and lose body fat at the same time.

Why do our bodies store fat so readily when this can be so harmful to our health? The answer is that it was not always harmful. Before food became as plentiful as it is today, the body was able to pack away fat as an energy reserve for lean times. However, now that supermarkets and refrigerators make food plentiful all year long, our fat-storage capability has outlived its usefulness. Rather than serve as energy reserves, fat stores are now energy and health drains.

5. WATER AND OXYGEN
THE NEGLECTED NUTRIENTS

Water and oxygen are two of the most important nutrients for health and performance. Studies have verified that even minute fluctuations in the body's water balance can, and often do, adversely affect performance. Similarly, the availability of oxygen is vital for top performance, and new research has determined that oxygen utilization can be maximized by physical and nutritional means. In spite of this, many people take water and oxygen for granted or neglect them. This is equally true for athletes and nonathletes.

In this chapter, we will take an in-depth look at water and oxygen. We will review their functions and discuss how to optimize water intake and oxygen utilization for maximum performance.

WATER AND THE ATHLETE

Water, whimsically called H_2O by many people, consists of two hydrogen atoms and one oxygen atom. It is the aqueous medium used for transporting the body's food materials and the place where the body's biochemical reactions occur. Water is found throughout the body, and depending on an individual's body fat, it can vary in content from about 45 percent in very obese individuals to 70 percent in very lean individuals. The different parts of the body also vary in water content. For example, blood normally has the highest water content, at about 83 percent; muscle tissue has a water content of about 75 percent; bone is about 22-percent water; and fat tissue is only about 10-percent water.

A body's degree of hydration is affected by the person's rate of water intake in relationship to his or her rate of water loss. Water loss is less under resting conditions than under conditions of high-intensity exercising. Water is obtained from fluids that are ingested as liquids, from fluids that are present in more solid foods, and as a result of metabolic activity within the body. It is estimated that the average-sized man, weighing about 170 pounds and performing moderate nonathletic activities, requires about 80 ounces of water per day to match his water loss.

The major sources of water for the human body are the following:

☐ *Liquids.* Liquids are by far the most abundant source of water for the body, accounting for about two-thirds of a person's water intake per day. Liquids can be readily taken in by the body without much digestive effort. Pure water is taken in the fastest. As the carbohydrate and electrolyte contents of a liquid increase, the length of time that it takes the liquid to empty from the stomach increases. The exact concentration of carbohydrates and electrolytes that an athlete needs depends upon the sport and the level of physical activity.

☐ *Food.* All foods consist of water and solids. The amount of water that a food contains depends on what the food is. For example, fruits, vegetables, cooked cereals, and milk are 80- to 95-percent water. Meat cooked rare is about 75-percent water, while meat cooked well done is about 45-percent or less water. Ready-to-serve cereals are about 3- to 5-percent water. Generally, approximately one-third of daily water intake is from food.

☐ *Metabolic water.* Metabolic water is the water that is produced in the body as a result of energy production. Often overlooked, it totals approximately 10 ounces per day, depending on how many calories are burned. Metabolic water is produced from oxygen and hydrogen atoms. The oxygen atoms are obtained from the atmosphere and brought into the body via the lungs during breathing. The hydrogen atoms are obtained from carbohydrates, fatty acids, and other carbon molecules that are broken down in the body for energy.

☐ *Glycogen-bound water.* Glycogen-bound water is stored in the muscles along with glycogen. About 3 ounces of water are stored along with every 1 ounce of glycogen. Glycogen-bound water becomes important when the glycogen supply is in the process of being depleted for energy use. This occurs during training and endurance events lasting more than one hour and during periods of calorie restriction. During intensive endurance activities, about 16 fluid ounces of water may be released per hour. However, this water will be released only for as long as the glycogen to which it is bound remains stored in the body. Glycogen-bound water must be replenished when it is used. Altogether, approximately 3 to 4 pints of glycogen-bound water can be stored. For endurance athletes and athletes performing in day-long tournaments, glycogen-bound water is an important source of hydration during physical activity. It can be maximized through carbohydrate loading.

The major ways in which water is output by the body are the following:

☐ *Urination.* Urination is the process by which water is filtered out through the kidneys and excreted as urine. Urine output under normal circumstances is roughly 1½ to 2 quarts per day. Interestingly enough, water loss from the kidneys is minimized during exercise. During exercise, fluid loss from the kidneys is slowed down to only ounces per hour. This is due to certain hormones, in particular antidiuretic hormone (ADH), also known as vasopressin. The ADH level increases during exercise, which increases the amount of water that is reabsorbed by the kidneys, thereby decreasing water loss. Note that alcohol (ethyl alcohol) and caffeine have diuretic effects because they inhibit ADH and therefore increase water output from the kidneys. Alcoholic and caffeinated beverages should be avoided during the season and especially during the last seven days prior to a major athletic event.

Food intake can also affect the rate of water loss from the kidneys. It takes about 16 fluid ounces of water to remove 1 ounce of solids from the bloodstream through the kidneys. Therefore, foods that leave higher amounts of waste products, such as protein, can speed up the body's dehydration process and should be minimized twenty-four hours before major competitions in sports where dehydration is a concern.

☐ *Defecation.* Under normal conditions, water loss through defecation is relatively small, about 4 to 8 ounces per day. However, a person with gastrointestinal upset, such as diarrhea or vomiting, can lose 32 to 160 fluid ounces of water in a day. It is therefore important for athletes with gastrointestinal problems to consume more than the normal amount of liquid to compensate for this extra water loss.

☐ *Sweating.* Water is lost through the skin when the body sweats. The body always sweats to some degree, but sweating becomes evident when conditions such as humidity or increased activity cause water to accumulate on the skin. Sweating is the body's cooling mechanism. It removes excess heat to keep the body's core temperature within a limited range and to prevent the body from overheating. If a body overheats from dehydration, the possible results include heat stroke, fainting, and even death. Sweat must evaporate from the skin to have a cooling effect. The production of sweat is just the first step in the process.

Sweating is a major mode of water loss during exercise. Over 1 quart of water can be lost per hour via sweating during prolonged exercise, such as long-distance running. Sweating is also significant in sports such as basketball, football, soccer, and swimming.

☐ *Breathing.* A small amount of water is lost during the process of breathing in the form of water droplets in the air that is exhaled. These water droplets amount to about 10 to 12 fluid ounces per day. This amount is increased during exercise, since breathing is accelerated.

Water intake varies with the size of the individual, the duration and intensity of the activity, and the weather. Water loss is affected by factors such as the weather, the ability to acclimate to the temperature, the duration and intensity of the activity, the rate of sweating, the weight of the clothing worn, health, gastrointestinal problems, alcohol and caffeine consumption, the use of diuretics and other medications, and body fat.

Effects of Dehydration on Performance

Dehydration can and does affect athletic performance. As the body loses water, its core temperature rises. This affects all the metabolic pathways, interferes with cardiovascular functioning, and reduces total exercise capacity. When the water losses reach 1 to 4 percent of the body weight, athletic performance is reduced. During a race, marathon runners can lose several quarts of water, representing 6 to 10 percent of their body weight. If they do not properly rehydrate during the race, they will find that this amount of water loss can significantly impair their performance and possibly even put their well-being at risk. Nonendurance sports such as football, basketball, hockey, and soccer can cause similar water losses. During tournaments, no matter what the sport is, athletes must make sure they increase their water intake to compensate for the prolonged exercise over the one or two days of competition.

Sports in which participants must meet weight-class requirements—boxing and wrestling, for example—are also associated with dehydration. Wrestlers typically dehydrate themselves to make a lower weight class. This type of chronic dehydration decreases performance and adversely affects health.

Chronic dehydration will develop in any athlete who does not make an effort to remain adequately hydrated. The thirst response in humans is not as finely tuned as it should be. This means that the body can enter a state of dehydration and the person may not feel the sensation of thirst for several hours. Therefore, you should not rely solely on your thirst response but should, instead, make a point to keep rehydrating your body all day long.

Special Water Needs of the Athlete

The amount of water you need varies greatly according to your initial level of hydration, the climate, and the duration and intensity of your activity. As a general rule, measure your water intake by your water loss—namely, your frequency of urination. If you are well hydrated, you should be urinating about once every one and a half to two hours. If you urinate only a few times per day, you probably need to increase your water intake. Because thirst is not a good indicator of hydration level, you should get in the habit of drinking water or other fluids frequently through the day.

Daily hydration guidelines are important for all athletes to follow. Studies have shown that endurance athletes who compete for periods longer than thirty minutes improve their performance by drinking fluids during the activity. Athletes competing in shorter events need to be properly hydrated from the start to achieve peak performance.

Daily Hydration Guidelines

Daily hydration is vital for everyone—endurance athletes, power athletes, and even nonathletes. Table 5.1, above right, presents water-intake guidelines for healthy, active individuals who exercise on a regular basis. Researchers have found that the best way to determine the recommended daily water intake is to look at daily energy expenditure. (To determine your

Table 5.1. Daily Hydration Guidelines

Daily Energy Expenditure	Minimum Daily Water Intake
2,000 calories	64–80 ounces
3,000 calories	102–118 ounces
4,000 calories	138–154 ounces
5,000 calories	170–186 ounces
6,000 calories	204–220 ounces

own energy expenditure, see page 150.) Table 5.1 provides a minimum daily water-intake range to accommodate individual differences as well as climatic differences. As the temperature climbs above 70° Fahrenheit (F) and the humidity above 70 percent, water loss will be increased due to increased sweating, especially during exercise.

Hydration Guidelines for Optimum Athletic Performance

Attaining and maintaining a peak hydration level starts by following the daily hydration guidelines discussed above. For athletes competing in endurance events lasting more than thirty minutes, hydration supercompensation (water loading) before an event as well as hydration maintenance during the event have been shown to increase athletic performance. (For a description of hydration supercompensation, see "Pre-event," below.) Other athletes should make sure that they properly maintain their hydration levels leading up to the event, but they do not necessarily need to concern themselves with drinking water during their events. One exception is athletes competing in tournaments that require participation in several events per day or several events over several days.

Specific guidelines for optimum athletic performance to be observed every day plus before, during, and after athletic events are as follows:

☐ *Every day.* During your athletic season, keep track of your water intake on a daily basis. In addition, weigh yourself in the morning and after practice to keep track of your daily body-weight fluctuations. In general, the human body can lose only a maximum of a half pound of fat per day, so if you find yourself losing several pounds of body weight on a particular day, it is most likely from water loss. If you frequently perspire profusely, you should also take a multi-vitamin-and-mineral supplement every day.

☐ *Pre-event.* Whether you are participating in an

endurance or nonendurance event, you should load up on water about two hours before your competition. Depending on your body weight, you should consume between 18 and 24 ounces of water. This will allow you to "top off" your body with water and still give yourself enough time to urinate the excess before your event. Fifteen to twenty minutes before your event, drink another 12 to 20 ounces of water. Do not drink any alcohol, coffee, or other beverages that tend to act as diuretics. Also avoid taking any dehydrating medications.

☐ *During endurance events.* Remember that the main reason for drinking water during endurance events is to replace sweat. Sweating is essential for cooling the body. If your body temperature increases too much during your event, your performance will suffer. To prevent this, you need to encourage sweating and make sure that the sweat evaporates from your body. Take special care on hot, humid days, which are the worst for athletic activities because they cause the most sweating with the least amount of evaporation. Ideally, during your event, drink 6 to 9 ounces of cool water every fifteen to twenty minutes.

☐ *Postevent.* Give your body a chance to cool down and your heart rate a chance to normalize, then start drinking a sports rehydration drink. (For a discussion of sports rehydration drinks, see "Food and Supplement Sources of Water," below.) Make sure to eat a meal within one to two hours after your event and consume the appropriate supplements for your sport. (For the supplements appropriate for you, see your sport-specific plan in Part Four.)

Please note that if you follow these hydration guidelines during events, you should also follow them during practice. This way, your body will have a chance to adjust to ingesting the recommended amounts of water before the day of competition.

In addition, athletes participating in ultra-endurance events—that is, events lasting more than two hours—should consume fluids that contain glucose and the electrolytes. The solution should be hypotonic (diluted) because the more hypertonic (concentrated) a beverage is, the longer it takes to empty from the stomach.

Food and Supplement Sources of Water

Since water is the most abundant and most important nutrient in the body, we cannot live without it. For an athlete who trains regularly, water is even more important. Athletes who participate in endurance events must make sure to drink extra fluids. Some power athletes also perspire a lot and need fluids to replace those lost as sweat.

In recent years, however, the quality of water and other beverages has become a major concern for many people. Reports abound about the harmful effects of contaminants in drinking water and of chemicals in beverages. Because athletes consume far greater amounts of beverages than nonathletes do, their exposure to impurities in these products is greater. Try drinking pure water instead of soft drinks, juices, and other calorie-containing beverages.

Some time ago, scientists discovered that not just water is lost through sweating. Valuable minerals are lost, too. This discovery led to the development of sports rehydration drinks. The solutions that make up these drinks replace not only water but also the electrolytes—and they throw in some sugar for energy.

If you are an endurance athlete, you may find that drinking plain water for fluid replacement results in a low blood-sugar level. Low blood sugar produces early onset of fatigue and reduces endurance. Because the small intestine absorbs fluids from glucose-sodium solutions quite rapidly, sports rehydration drinks containing these two minerals are the best choice. Glucose stimulates sodium uptake in the small intestine, which markedly increases fluid absorption.

There are many different kinds of sports rehydration drinks available. In general, they fall into two broad categories—carbohydrate drinks and carbohydrate-protein drinks. Most of the drinks in both these categories are laced with minerals and/or vitamins. Calorie-wise, carbohydrate drinks range from 90 calories to over 400 calories per 16 fluid ounces of beverage, while carbohydrate-protein drinks have from 200 calories to over 500 calories per 16 fluid ounces. Carbohydrate-protein drinks also have up to 150 grams of carbohydrate and 32 grams of protein per 16 fluid ounces of beverage.

The lower-calorie carbohydrate drinks designed to rehydrate plus replenish the energy supply definitely improve performance for endurance athletes in events lasting more than one and a half hours. The performance benefits of carbohydrate drinks are less clear in athletic events and practice sessions of shorter duration. However, studies indicate that carbohydrate drinks containing a mid-range number of calories do help preserve the glycogen level during workouts lasting less than one and a half hours. Most of the research has shown that carbohydrate drinks work best when they are consumed just before and during exercise.

Carbohydrate-protein drinks can be consumed as a pretraining or precompetition meal about two to three hours before the start of an activity. They also make a convenient meal one hour after the completion of training or competition, plus they replace the protein and carbohydrates that were lost during the activity. They may also offer other benefits during workouts. Some research has indicated that consuming carbohydrate-protein drinks during weight-training sessions helps promote an overall increase in the GH level. GH is an important hormone involved in the mobilization of fatty acids, sparing of muscle glycogen, and promotion of positive nitrogen balance. Increasing the GH level is particularly important for athletes who train intensively, such as power athletes.

No matter what you choose to drink or when, remember that liquids intended to rehydrate the body work best when they are chilled. Both plain water and sports drinks are most effective when consumed at around 40°F. Remember, too, that if you plan to drink water or a sports drink during competition, you should also do so during training. The same way that your body needs to become accustomed to the physical demands of your activity, it also needs to adjust to the ingestion of liquids. The fewer surprises your body has to deal with during competition, the better your performance will be and the fewer gastrointestinal problems you will be rewarded with.

OXYGEN AND THE ATHLETE

The great Green Bay Packers coach Vince Lombardi said it the best: "Fatigue makes cowards of us all." More precisely, postexercise fatigue can devastate an athlete's recovery capabilities. It limits the ability to bounce back and train harder and more often for better gains. Sports scientists learned years ago that postexercise fatigue is caused by three major factors—tissue hypoxia (lack of oxygen to the working muscles); accumulation of waste products, such as lactic acid, in both the liver and the muscles; and microtrauma. Waste-product accumulation and microtrauma are discussed elsewhere in this book. In the remainder of this chapter, we will discuss oxygen and how it is used in the body, especially during athletic and fitness

activities. We will examine methods for improving the body's assimilation and utilization of oxygen. In addition, we will look at how oxygen affects aging and free radicals and how antioxidants can be used to combat their adverse effects.

Oxygen, the Body, and the Training Effect

Oxygen, like water, is something that most people do not consider a nutrient but that the body cannot survive without. It is basic to human life. Oxygen not only keeps the lungs breathing and the heart pumping but feeds every cell of the body. Knowing the dynamics of oxygen uptake and utilization can help you plan a scientific and sound performance-enhancement program. The best training program not only builds muscles and increases stamina but also improves the body's ability to take in and properly utilize oxygen, which builds bigger muscles and increases stamina even further.

Oxygen takes a circuitous route through the body. It enters by the lungs, then travels via the bloodstream through the heart to the cells of the muscles, brain, and other tissues. The lungs are also the last stop for the waste products of oxygen metabolism, which are carried away from the cells through the blood vessels and eventually exhaled into the air.

The Lungs

The lungs are the first step in the operation that brings oxygen into the body system. The lungs are a pair of organs that sit in the chest on either side of the heart. They process the air that is breathed in, removing the oxygen and transferring it to the bloodstream for distribution throughout the body. The amount of air that the lungs can process varies with the condition of the person—a conditioned person can process more air than a deconditioned person can. The amount of air that the lungs can process is therefore a limiting factor.

To use an analogy, the lungs are like a dairy that processes milk. When bulk milk comes in, the cream is separated from it and then bottled and sent off for distribution. When the empty bottles come back, they are flushed out, filled with more cream, and sent out once again. The air that we breathe is like the bulk milk, and oxygen is like the cream. When bulk air comes into the lungs, the oxygen is extracted from it, "bottled" in red blood cells, and sent off in the bloodstream for distribution. When the "bottles" reach the tissues that they are to feed, they exchange their oxygen for carbon dioxide and water, waste products that they then carry back to the lungs to be flushed out of the body. Once emptied of these waste products, the "bottles" are again filled with oxygen and sent out once more for distribution.

The air that we breathe is approximately 21-percent oxygen and 78-percent nitrogen, with negligible traces of other gasses. This ratio never varies. What does vary is the amount of air that can be processed. If the lungs cannot process enough air, they cannot extract enough oxygen to produce enough energy. Two factors limit the lungs' ability to process air.

First, the lungs have no muscles of their own. To expand and contract, they must depend completely upon the muscles of the rib cage and diaphragm. Upon inhalation, the muscles surrounding the lungs increase the available space within the lung cavity. When they do this, they cause a partial vacuum, which helps to suck air into the lungs. Upon exhalation, assisted somewhat by the natural elasticity of the lungs and the chest wall, the muscles contract to create greater atmospheric pressure inside the lungs than outside the body. This causes the air to be pushed out.

This normal breathing is done by the body at rest. As already mentioned, all resting bodies consume basically the same amount of oxygen and consequently inhale and exhale about the same amount of air. When the body is in action, however, the amount of air that the lungs can inhale and exhale becomes limited by the size of the vacuum the muscles can create for the lungs to expand into and the size of the area the lungs can squeeze back down into. A conditioned person in action obviously has the capability to inhale more air and for longer periods of time than a deconditioned person has. A conditioned person is also capable of exhaling more waste products because the muscles around the lungs have been trained to do more work.

The second factor that limits how much air the lungs can process is the condition inside the lungs. Lungs vary in size. A larger person naturally has proportionately larger lungs than a smaller person does. So, in fitness and sports, we are less concerned with the size of the lungs, or total lung capacity, than with how much of that capacity is usable. The usable portion of the lungs is called the vital lung capacity, and it is measured in the laboratory by the amount of air that can be exhaled in one deep breath. Numerous

tests have shown that a conditioned person's vital lung capacity is about 75 percent of total lung capacity. Often, however, an otherwise deconditioned person can match this, so we look at one more factor—the maximum minute volume. This is the amount of air that a person can process during one minute of vigorous exercise, and it usually separates the fit from the unfit. Conditioned persons can force as much as twenty times their vital capacity through the lungs in one minute, while deconditioned persons are often hard-pressed to force even ten times through. Deconditioned persons simply lack the muscle and strength endurance to perform at a higher level.

The remainder of the lungs—or, more specifically, the remainder of the air in the lungs—is called the residual volume. The residual volume is fixed, and even a conditioned person cannot breathe this remaining air in or out. Since residual volume is inversely related to vital lung capacity, too much residual volume is unhealthy. If your body deteriorates from inactivity or disease, the unusable portion of your lungs increases, blocking off more and more space and allowing less space for normal breathing, let alone vigorous exercise. Ultimately, you will find yourself short of breath from even light activity, such as climbing a flight of stairs.

So, if you allow your body to deteriorate, you will live your life with two handicaps in your lungs alone. When you need more oxygen in a hurry, you may have trouble getting it because the muscles controlling your lungs will not be in a good enough condition to force large volumes of air through the lungs. In addition, the usable space within your lungs may be seriously reduced.

Training can reverse both these trends. Exercising the muscles surrounding the lungs can increase the muscles' strength and efficiency, allowing them to open more usable lung space. Opening more usable lung space has the net effect of increasing the vital lung capacity and reducing the residual volume. In each instance, the lungs become more efficient at processing air and extracting oxygen.

The oxygen supply to the blood is only about 1 cup per minute in a resting body. In a trained athlete, this can be stepped up to 1 gallon per minute during intensive exercise. In a resting body, only about 12 percent of the stagnant air in the lungs is renewed during each breath.

A good way to test the breathing condition of your lungs is to take a deep breath and see how long you can hold it. Most adults in moderately good physical condition and with healthy lungs are able to hold their breath for sixty seconds or longer.

The Blood

From the lungs, the oxygen extracted from the bulk air goes directly into the bloodstream, the body's "assembly line." This is accomplished because the lungs contain millions of tiny air sacs, called alveoli, around which the blood flows. The alveoli are like tiny balloons that are filled with air and dangle in the liquid of the bloodstream. The air was originally forced into the alveoli by atmospheric pressure, and now, obeying the Law of Gaseous Diffusion, the oxygen transfers from the air in the sacs, in which the pressure is higher, to the red blood cells, or "empty bottles," in which the pressure is lower. The limiting factors here are the number of red blood cells that exist and the amount of hemoglobin they can carry. Even if the lungs could process more oxygen, the tissue cells would not receive more unless additional "bottles" existed to deliver it.

Training helps here, too. Training produces more hemoglobin to carry oxygen, more red blood cells to carry the hemoglobin, more blood plasma to carry the red blood cells, and, consequently, more total blood volume. Laboratory tests have repeatedly shown that individuals in good physical condition have a larger blood supply than deconditioned individuals of comparable size. An average-sized man can increase his blood volume by nearly a quart in response to aerobic conditioning. The red blood cell count increases proportionately.

The additional "bottles" produced by training not only deliver more oxygen to the tissue cells but carry away more waste products. The removal of carbon dioxide and other waste products is just as important in reducing fatigue and increasing endurance as is the production of energy. Think of your home. Even if you keep your refrigerator stocked with good food, you cannot continue to live in your house unless you also regularly clean out the garbage.

The process by which the "bottles" unload their oxygen into the tissue cells and pick up waste products is called osmosis. The oxygen and food particles, now in liquid form, pass through the cell membranes into the cells in one direction, while the waste products exit the cells through the cell membranes in the opposite direction. This is the life cycle—materials for

nourishment and energy go in and waste products come out. The carbon dioxide and other waste products are then carried away in the bloodstream via the veins, and when they reach the lungs, they follow the Law of Gaseous Diffusion in reverse. The pressure of the carbon dioxide in the veins is greater than the pressure in the empty alveoli, so the carbon dioxide passes freely into the alveoli and is exhaled with the expired air.

The efficiency and capacity of this cycle are both functions of the effects of training. If you increase the system's capacity, you help to increase its efficiency. If you do nothing, the system deteriorates.

The Blood Vessels

In a resting body, blood travels through the large arteries at about 55 feet per minute. By boosting the circulation to two or three times this speed, the same amount of blood can do two or three times the work of feeding the tissue cells and removing waste products.

Muscular activity speeds up the rate of a normal heart, forcing it to pump more blood per minute and increasing the amount of blood returning to the heart. This increases the circulation. As the volume of blood increases, so does the blood supply to the muscles. This improved blood flow, resulting from tissue vascularization (creation of new blood vessels), is probably the most remarkable training effect. To carry on our analogy, it is similar to a dairy expanding its regular delivery routes by opening up new routes into many small neighborhoods that up until now were neglected.

In addition to helping create new blood vessels, training also improves the condition of the existing blood vessels, which has a beneficial effect on the blood pressure. When a blood-pressure reading is taken, two figures are noted. A common reading is 120 over 80, written as "120/80." The top figure is the systolic pressure, the pressure of the blood against the walls of the arteries when the heart is in the process of ejecting blood into the system. The lower figure is the diastolic pressure, the pressure during the relaxed phase of the pumping cycle. In other words, the two figures represent the maximum and minimum pressures inside the blood vessels. In a conditioned person, these figures are usually lower because the blood vessels are more pliable and the resistance to blood flow is at a minimum. In a deconditioned person, the figures are higher because the arteries tend to lose elasticity with disuse (inactivity) and the resistance to blood flow is increased.

When physical activity or emotional stress are added, trouble can result. The heart rate is increased, which raises the blood pressure because the heart is pumping more blood into the system at a faster rate. In a treadmill test, a conditioned man might start with a diastolic pressure of 70 and experience only a slight increase during his run. After the test, his blood pressure returns to normal within a few minutes. A deconditioned man, however, and especially an overweight deconditioned man, might start with a diastolic pressure of 90, have it shoot up to 105 during the test, and then take ten minutes or more to recover.

Almost everyone, especially persons with clinical conditions, can reduce their blood pressure significantly by adhering to an exercise program for even just a few weeks. First, blood vessels tend to make compensatory adjustments to handle increased exercise capacity, something that almost all body systems do in response to increased stress. Once again, this is an effect of training. Second, conditioning the blood vessels causes the creation of an augmented blood supply, the new routes that are opened up into the small "neighborhoods," as discussed above.

One of the most famous, and amusing, tests done in this area was reported by a researcher who lifted a weight with a finger. The researcher set the weight on the floor, tied a rope to it, ran the rope over a pulley fastened to the edge of a table, then sat on the other side of the table and looped the end of the rope over the middle finger of his right hand. In time to a metronome, he repeatedly lifted the weight with his finger. The first time, and for many weeks thereafter, the best he could do was 25 lifts before his finger became fatigued. To expand the experiment, he occasionally had a mechanic in his building lift the weight with a finger. The mechanic always beat him. Then one day, about two months into the test, the researcher did his usual routine but found that his finger was not tired at 25 lifts. He kept going and ultimately reached 100 lifts. He suspected what had happened and brought the experiment to a rather unorthodox conclusion. He invited the mechanic in again and made a small bet that he could beat the man. The mechanic accepted the bet and lost.

What the researcher had suspected was that his finger muscles had undergone vascularization in response to the stress of the lifting exercise. More blood vessels had opened up, creating new routes for delivering more oxygen. However, the new blood vessels apparently did not open up one at a time but a whole network at a time. Other evidence supports this conclusion. Many people practicing conditioning programs recount how they agonized for months, then boom! Almost overnight, the exercise became relatively effortless. Athletes report similar "plateaus of progress," improving not only day by day but in quantum leaps.

Vascularization is the most essential factor in building endurance and reducing fatigue in the skeletal muscles, in saturating the tissues with oxygen, and in carrying away more waste products. It is also an extremely vital factor in the health of the heart, the most important muscle of all. More and larger blood vessels supplying the cardiac (heart) tissue with energy-producing oxygen considerably reduce the chances of cardiac failure. Even if a heart attack does occur, the improved blood supply helps keep the surrounding tissues healthy and improves the chances for a speedy recovery.

There is one final problem involving the blood vessels—fat metabolism. "Metabolism" is a big word with a reasonably simple meaning. It means "change." We have already discussed one kind of metabolism—energy production, also known as energy metabolism. Foodstuffs, burned by oxygen, are changed into energy. Tissue metabolism is another kind. This kind of metabolism is the process by which foodstuffs are changed to make new tissues.

Fat, of course, is one of the foodstuffs. Protein and carbohydrates are the others. Fat is important because it is one of the major factors in the development of arteriosclerosis (hardening of the arteries). The crust found on the inner walls of arteries in arteriosclerosis contains large amounts of cholesterol, the "cousin" of the fat family. The body can tolerate and easily metabolize a moderate amount of fat. However, high-fat diets strain the body's metabolic capabilities. With a high-fat diet, fat circulates in the bloodstream for prolonged periods of time following fatty meals. The length of time it takes an individual to get rid of this circulating fat depends on the person's condition. Healthy fat metabolism results from the combination of a low-fat diet and aerobic exercise.

Training, then, basically does three things for the blood vessels—it enlarges them and makes them more pliable under pressure; it increases their number for saturation coverage; and it helps keep their linings clear of corrosive materials.

The Tissues

The tissues are the end of the assembly line. They are where the oxygen is turned over to the consumer and the waste products are picked up for carting away. The body contains all kinds of tissues. All these tissues are composed of cells, the smallest units in the body. The cells are the ultimate consumers.

Cells are like small factories. Each has its own receiving and shipping facilities, storeroom, and power plant for creating energy, heat, and new protoplasm—the stuff of which all cells, as well as all living things, are made. As complicated as the body is, it is also that simple. All the food you eat and all the oxygen you breathe are meant to serve this tiny factory.

Whether this tiny factory is serviced well or poorly depends to a large extent upon the proportion of food and oxygen it is sent. Unhappily, the ratio is usually too much food and not enough oxygen, so the food just stacks up unused in the storeroom. Even if it is needed, it cannot be burned in the power plant without oxygen. Exercise helps pump oxygen around the body to fuel all the tiny power plants and to burn all the stored food to keep all the little factories in business.

Moving up in size from the microscopic cell, a group of specialized cells together form tissue, such as bone, muscle, and nerve tissue. Various tissues combine to form organs, such as the heart, lungs, and stomach. Several organs and assorted parts combine to form systems, such as the pulmonary, cardiovascular, and muscular systems.

The Muscular System

There are three types of muscles in the body. Voluntary muscles respond to an act of the will. The arm muscles, which are usually moved by decision, are voluntary muscles. Involuntary muscles act independently of the will. These include the muscles lining the blood vessels and digestive tract. The cardiac muscle (heart) is a little of both, beating independently of the will, but still responsive to the will, especially in moments of emotional stress.

The involuntary muscles are affected by training and conditioning, as we discussed in connection with the blood vessels, but not to the same extent that the cardiac and voluntary muscles are. In an aerobic-type weight-training program, tissues tend to grow longer and leaner, causing more of this area to be close to

supply routes—the tiny blood-carrying capillaries—at all times. In addition, a conditioning program itself creates more supply routes. In a person in good condition—good cardiovascular and muscular condition—hardly any part of the muscular system is not well supplied by blood vessels.

This good supply of blood vessels is probably the main reason conditioned people fatigue less easily, even when they spend their workdays at desk jobs. Their assembly lines are in excellent condition, servicing more "factories" and fueling more "power plants."

The Heart

The heart is the magnificent engine that keeps the whole assembly line going. It takes the oxygen-laden blood from the lungs and pumps it throughout the body. At the same time, it takes the carbon dioxide–laden blood back from the body and pumps it into the lungs for eventual disposal. It begins its work before birth and continues until death.

Ironically, the heart works faster and less efficiently when it is given little to do than when it has demands made on it. Studies have shown that both aerobically conditioned men and anaerobically conditioned men (power athletes) who exercise regularly have resting heart rates of about 60 beats or less per minute. Deconditioned men who do not exercise may have resting heart rates of about 80 beats or more per minute. Therefore, even at complete rest, deconditioned men who do not exercise force their hearts to beat nearly 30,000 times more per day every day of their lives:

Conditioned men:

60 beats per minute x 60 minutes = 3,600 beats per hour
3,600 beats per hour x 24 hours = 86,400 beats per day
86,400 beats per day x 365 days = 31,536,000 beats
per year

Deconditioned men:

80 beats per minute x 60 minutes = 4,800 beats per hour
4,800 beats per hour x 24 hours = 115,200 beats per day
115,200 beats per day x 365 days = 42,048,000 beats
per year

Most people, however, are not at complete rest for twenty-four hours a day; and for ordinary activities, such as getting up from a chair or climbing a flight of stairs, the deconditioned heart would beat proportionately faster than a conditioned heart. Obesity, stress, and many other factors can also speed up the heart rate considerably, even though the individual may appear to be in great condition. Women tend to have slightly lower heart rates than men do, as do children.

There are two factors that we look at when considering how healthy a heart is—the cardiac tissue and the heart rate.

Cardiac Tissue. The heart is all muscle tissue. Therefore, unlike the lungs, the heart does its own work, which is unquestionably the most important work in the body. The health of the cardiac tissue depends on the heart's size and how well it is supplied with blood vessels.

Basically, hearts exist in three sizes. A normal but deconditioned heart is relatively weak and small. This is because, the same as any muscle that is not exercised properly, it has wasted away somewhat. An unhealthy deconditioned heart is weak and enlarged. It became enlarged probably to compensate for some deficiency in the cardiovascular system, hypertension, or a vascular deformity. An enlarged heart such as this, however, is not as efficient as a heart that grew large through training. An unhealthy heart's interior volume, despite its exterior size, is not large, so it cannot pump as much blood with each stroke as a healthy heart can. An "athlete's heart," on the other hand, is strong and healthy, relatively large, and highly efficient, pumping more blood with each stroke and with less effort. It is resilient and, if it were visible, would be beautiful to watch. Like a great athlete, it does wonderful things with ease.

Vascularization plays a large role in the heart, the same as it does in the muscles. The heart, for its own energy requirements, needs the same oxygen that it pumps around the body, and a healthy heart is characterized by a conspicuously favorable blood supply. In short, a healthy heart's tissue is saturated with healthy blood vessels. Some sedentary individuals not only lack enlarged arteries, but the small ones they do have are clogged with debris, reducing the openings even further.

The health of a heart depends on the health of its tissue, and the health of cardiac tissue depends on its saturation with large, healthy supply routes. This saturation coverage, or vascularization, is one of the most important benefits of training and is nowhere more evident or more important than in the heart.

Heart Rate. Conditioned hearts, as they grow larger and stronger, are able to beat more slowly because they pump more blood with each stroke. Nearly all of the great long-distance runners have low heart rates. In fact, some reportedly have resting rates of 32 beats per minute. Even highly conditioned anaerobic athletes, such as football players and weight lifters, have resting heart rates far lower than the average person. The average young office worker has a resting rate of about 75 or 80 beats per minute.

Training also reduces the maximum heart rate, which is just as important. Healthy hearts peak out, without strain, at 190 beats or less per minute; while poorly conditioned hearts, during exhausting activity, may go as high as 220 beats or more, which is dangerously high. What a lower heart rate really means, then, is that at rest, the heart conserves energy (saving at least 15,000 beats per day), and during activity, it has built-in protection against beating too fast and suffering strain or failure.

Training can condition the heart not only to reduce its maximum rate but also to increase its ejection fraction, the percentage of blood that is forced out of the heart with each beat; to increase its stroke volume, the total volume of blood that is forced out of the heart with each beat; and to strengthen the heart itself, so that it can hold near-maximum rates for longer periods of time before becoming fatigued. Some of the Gemini astronauts ran heart rates of around 170 during their exhausting extravehicular activity. And Norwegian cross-country skiers are known to hold heart rates of up to 170 for as much as two and a half hours at a clip!

There is also a third heart rate, one that has nothing to do with physical exercise. It is called the anticipatory rate, or tension rate. It could also be called the emotional heart rate. The telephone rings unexpectedly in the middle of the night and you can almost hear your heart pound as you rush to grab the receiver. You are due for a promotion that does not come, and you become worked up just thinking about it. Many of life's little crises touch the heart, but training can reduce these effects, too.

It is the way the heart responds to mental and physical stimuli that makes it such a unique muscle. Two systems in your body prepare you for the fight-or-flight reaction, a series of physiological changes intended to mobilize the body in response to stress. In periods of acute emotional stress, the sympathetic nervous system, an automatic system that speeds up most of the body's activities, works with the adrenal glands to release into the bloodstream a high level of hormones that cause the heart to increase in rate and strength of contraction. Ordinarily, this reaction can be good, helping the heart to pump enough blood to do whatever work the emergency calls for. It is one reason athletes can put that extra effort into a performance, reaching down to "do or die." Ordinarily, a companion system, the parasympathetic nervous system, acts as a damper to keep this hormonal effect down to a safe level. While the sympathetic system urges the heart to "go, man, go," the parasympathetic system tells it to "take it easy, pal!"

However, deconditioned individuals sometimes do not experience the dampening response, their hearts just taking off and beating at excessively fast rates, possibly even suffering heart attacks. In conditioned individuals, the balance is better, and the heart can "go, man, go," but can still remain under enough control to avoid going too far. A high, potentially damaging level of hormones is simply never reached by a conditioned person.

This, too, is a training effect. A conditioned body is less affected by these hormones, possibly due to more efficient utilization of them or to decreased production. Add to this the fact that a conditioned person's heart is already trained to level off at a relatively low maximum rate, and the person has built-in protection against uncontrollable emotional crises. A deconditioned person does not have this protection. And if the deconditioned person is also hyper-reactive, becoming overly excited even in minor emergencies, two strikes exist—too much emotion and too little built-in physical protection.

So training, intimately tied in with the use of oxygen, benefits the entire body in a number of ways. It has remarkable effects on how the body takes up and utilizes oxygen, which helps the body develop into a strong, healthy machine that works more effortlessly during moments of both relaxation and peak physical exertion. By working more efficiently, the body also maintains larger reserves of power to handle whatever physical or emotional stresses are imposed upon it. In short, a healthy cardiovascular system maximizes not only daily functioning but also athletic performance.

The Need for Oxygen

Even before you began reading this chapter, you knew that the human body needs oxygen to survive.

You also knew that breathing is the only way to get that oxygen into the body. All the billions of cells that make up the body must also "breathe." They must "breathe" to produce the energy that fuels the body and makes you able to work and play. Oxygen is the fuel that gives energy to the cells.

One of the principal jobs of the tissues is to produce adenosine triphosphate (ATP). They do this as part of the metabolic process called glycolysis, in which glucose is converted to lactic acid. ATP is the compound that, when broken down, produces the energy that enables the muscles and other organs to function. In essence, without ATP, there is no energy and no life.

According to Dr. Sheldon Henler, author of *The Oxygen Breakthrough,* "When ATP output slows or is interrupted, you have personal energy outages that can result in anything from mild fatigue, to a life threatening disease and disorder." Dr. Henler also states that the body and breathing are extremely sensitive to even very small reductions in ATP production. This sensitivity is expressed in aches and pains, confusion, fatigue, great susceptibility to infection, and, finally, a chronic state of fatigue and persistent illness. Imagine what reduced ATP production could do to a body if it were allowed to persist over a lifetime!

By maximizing your oxygen intake and utilization—and therefore your ATP production—you can boost the functional efficiency of both your muscles and your internal organs. The ability to take in and properly use oxygen is the single most important factor in doing this. Not only must you develop the ability to get a maximum flow of oxygen to the energy-producing centers of the cells, but you must also create conditions that allow the cell membranes to take in the oxygen for utilization. Difficulty doing this seems to be the main problem in many immune-system disorders, such as chronic fatigue syndrome and acquired immune deficiency syndrome (AIDS). Certain nutritional and drug therapies play major roles in treating these problems because they create the necessary fluidity around the cells to allow oxygen to get in and do its work.

Hundreds of diets and other nutrition programs have been created for weight loss, but very few have been designed to promote the maximum amount of biological energy. Diets of this type use a variety of foods and supplements to boost the body's ATP-production capabilities. These foods and supplements play a major role in creating the conditions that allow the body to properly utilize oxygen. Included are above-average intakes of specific vitamins, minerals, herbs, and other substances.

Let us look for a moment inside a single cell—a muscle cell—where oxygen is working to produce ATP-giving energy. Among the tiny components inside the muscle cell is a mitochondrion. Mitochondria are the "furnaces," or "power plants," of the cells because they are where oxygen is used and ATP is produced. When the mitochondrion membrane is fluid, the flow of electrons and electrical currents intimately linked with energy production is smooth and highly efficient and the cell's energy level is great. However, when the membrane loses fluidity, energy diminishes, and with it, immunity and all the other functions of the body. Hardening of the mitochondrion membrane is virtually synonymous with degeneration and aging. (For a discussion of mitochondria and other cellular components, see Chapter 10.)

As we will discuss later in this chapter, age-related maladies are many, and most are directly linked to free-radical damage inside the cells—and inside the mitochondria—over a period of years. Factors that improve mitochondrion-membrane fluidity include decreased cholesterol, increased lecithin, decreased peroxidation (formation of a peroxide), increased unsaturation of fatty acids, optimum breathing, and proper aerobic exercise.

When oxygen cannot get to the cells as needed, free radicals develop. Free radicals in turn cause the cell membranes to become rigid or to become rancid and oxidize (combine with the oxygen). This makes the cell membranes even more rigid, which hampers the flow of oxygen even further. It is a vicious cycle that can be combated only with free-radical scavengers—antioxidants.

The body's need for oxygen can also be examined in regard to some of the more prominent diseases. For example, according to Dr. Henler, recent research has shown that "many viruses including EBV [Epstein-Barr virus], CMV [cytomegalovirus] and others in the Herpes family, as well as the retrovirus involved in AIDS, all have membranes high in cholesterol and are thus relatively rigid." These viral membranes, says Dr. Henler, can be disrupted by a number of medications and nutritional substances. But diet, and especially a high-oxygen diet, can help make life difficult for these viruses. A high-oxygen diet yields maximum amounts of biological energy

(ATP) with minimum production of toxic waste products and free radicals.

Oxygen and Premature Aging

Everyone ages and dies. This is a fact. There is no magic bullet, no cure-all, no Fountain of Youth. There is no alternative to sound health and fitness practices applied over a lifetime. There is no substitute for scientific, state-of-the-art medical care in times of disease.

There is, however, an immense step that you can take in the right direction. That step is fighting free radicals. You cannot win the war against old age, but you can enjoy—and profit from—winning many of the battles. This approach to life makes common sense. Living a fitness lifestyle is the only way the war can be fought. In the process, you will enhance the quality of your life and probably prolong it as well.

Ponce de León sought the Fountain of Youth out of ignorance. Today, we must seek it out of necessity. In the face of massive environmental compromise, brought on by all manner of human misbehavior blithely referred to as progress, scientists are obliged to solve nagging health problems ranging from premature aging to cancer. Perhaps there is no Fountain of Youth in the fabled tradition of the term, but the study of free radicals has expanded our knowledge of many of the ills that befall modern man. A serendipitous outcome of this relatively new research interest is a greater knowledge of the effects of free radicals on premature aging.

Free Radicals

Free radicals are highly reactive molecules that attack the protein bonds in tissues, the DNA in cell nuclei, and the important polyunsaturated fatty acids in cell membranes. A chain reaction, once initiated in a cell, results in the total destruction of that cell. Scientists have determined that more than sixty age-related maladies are a direct result of long-term damage from free-radical activity. So far, scientists have identified seven different "species" of free radicals. (For the seven species of free radicals, see Table 5.2 on page 69.)

Exposure to radiation, ozone, carcinogens, and other environmental toxins, as well as exercise and even normal metabolism, can cause oxygen molecules inside the body to break down. Losing one of its electrons to another molecule during such a breakdown causes an oxygen molecule to become highly reac-

Table 5.2.   Species of Free Radicals and the Scavengers That Can Be Used Against Them

Species of Free Radicals	Free-Radical Scavengers
Hydrogen peroxide	L-glutathione, ginkgo, milk thistle
Hydroxyl radical	Vitamin C, L-methionine, ginkgo, green tea
Organic or fatty-acid hydroperoxide	L-glutathione, ginkgo, milk thistle
Oxidized protein	L-glutathione, ginkgo, milk thistle
Polyunsaturated fatty-acid radical	Beta-carotene, vitamin E, selenium and bilberry, milk thistle
Singlet oxygen	Vitamin A, beta-carotene, vitamin E, selenium and bilberry, L-histidine, ginkgo, milk thistle
Superoxide anion radical	Vitamin C, L-glutathione, ginkgo, milk thistle, green tea

tive, capable of combining with other molecules in its quest for an electron to take the place of the one it lost. In this volatile state, the oxygen molecule is known as a free radical.

When the free radical finds an electron mate, it bonds with it. This additional electron makes the free radical even more reactive, and a vicious, self-perpetuating cycle begins. The molecule destroys cell membranes, compromises the integrity of the immune system, and alters or destroys DNA.

During the 1990s, scientific understanding of the aging process and the many sicknesses associated with it has virtually exploded. The research literature is chock full of articles on how free radicals can cause cancer, atherosclerosis, emphysema, cataracts, glaucoma, high blood pressure, immune-system deficiencies, heart disease, arthritis, stroke, Parkinson's disease, various skin disorders, and wrinkled skin. The big question for everyone living on planet Earth is what to do about these devilish little free radicals.

By far the most important prophylaxis against the ravages of free radicals is prevention. Some preventive measures are abstinence from smoking; strict adher-

ence to a carefully constructed, integrated training program (including diet); avoidance of pollutants and other toxic substances that are known to cause free-radical formation; and avoidance of sun exposure. These practices impact positively on both life span and life quality.

Antioxidants

Other prophylaxes against free radicals are the "scavengers" that are collectively called antioxidants. Some of the more well known antioxidants are beta-carotene, vitamin C, vitamin E, the bioflavonoids, manganese, selenium, zinc, and the amino acids cysteine and glutathione. Antioxidants work both directly and indirectly against the known free-radical species. They either combat these free radicals directly, inhibit the formation of free radicals, potentiate other antioxidants, prevent the depletion of other antioxidants, or prevent the depletion of other substances that potentiate the activity of other antioxidants. The secret to successful antioxidant therapy is an integrated approach, which allows the antioxidants to work synergistically to restore normal functioning to the bodily tissues.

Over the past few years, scientists have proven that antioxidants do make a difference. For example, Dr. William Pryor, professor of biochemistry at Louisiana State University, has studied the effects of smoking on free-radical formation. Aside from the obvious advice of quitting smoking, he advocates a strong antioxidant-supplementation regimen, and he believes he is on solid scientific ground in doing so. "There's been a renaissance in free radical biology in the past decade," he says. "Within the next ten or so years, [our greater knowledge of how best to fight free-radical damage] will promote a modest extension in life span—perhaps five to eight years."

Professor Pryor is not alone in this belief. Working at the Institute for Toxicology at the University of Southern California, Drs. Paul Hochstein and Kelvin Davies, together with their colleagues, have dedicated their time and resources to understanding free radicals, the damage they cause, and the ways in which to combat them or prevent their formation. According to their research, the body's built-in repair mechanisms—certain enzymatic free-radical scavenging and salvage systems—are not capable of handling the onslaught. "The cumulative effect of [free-radical] damage over time may diminish the cell's ability to make these repairs," explains Dr. Davies. "This may be what causes some of the physical degeneration of aging."

The use of antioxidant supplements to protect the body against free-radical damage has become an important nutrition factor for athletes. Free radicals and free-radical damage are increased in exercising bodies. Recent studies using all types of athletes have shown promising results, however. Athletes who took various combinations of antioxidant supplements displayed reductions in free-radical damage. Improved immune-system functioning was also reported. As research continues in this area, newer and better ways of protecting the body against free-radical damage will undoubtedly be discovered. (For recommended dosages of the antioxidant supplements, see your sport-specific plan in Part Four.)

Antioxidants and Wrinkles

A quick glance at the scientific literature on age-related skin conditions reveals that researchers are focusing on at least four important factors. These factors that are believed to contribute to wrinkled skin are:

☐ *Photodamage from the sun's ultraviolet (UV) rays.* There are two types of UV rays, known as UVA and UVB rays, and both cause thermal (heat) damage, immune-system disorders, and chemical reactions through the formation of free radicals.

☐ *Cigarette smoking.* The peripherally restricted blood flow caused by the nicotine and other chemicals in tobacco results in nutritional deficiencies, oxygen starvation, and impeded waste-product elimination.

☐ *Various nutritional deficiencies.* Depending on the deficiency, the resulting problems may include immune-response interference and metabolism-related skin disorders.

☐ *Normal deterioration associated with aging.* This includes loss of muscle tone and formation of cross-links in the supporting tissues of the skin. Cross-links are undesirable bondings between molecules. Induced by free radicals, they result in deformed molecules that cannot function properly.

Scientists seem to agree that a large percentage of the wrinkling of skin with age is the result of photodamage. They also seem to concur that the best prevention is to limit exposure to the sun and to use a good-quality sunscreen.

The skin is the first line of defense against invading free radicals and is therefore equipped with several antioxidants that neutralize both free radicals as well as the penetrating UV rays from the sun. Recent evidence suggests that this built-in protective system can be enhanced by both ingested and topically applied antioxidants.

After about age forty, a person's skin-pigment cells, called melanocytes, begin to decrease in number. One of the most important functions of the melanocytes is to eradicate the free radicals responsible for inducing malignancies and the cross-linking of the skin's connective (supporting) tissue. It therefore makes sense to prevent the melanocytes from decreasing as much as possible and to provide the antioxidants that they once provided.

Are these feats possible? Research indicates that when antioxidants such as vitamins C and E, beta-carotene, and selenium are topically applied, they benefit the skin by immediately supplying their antioxidant-protection factors to the uppermost layers. Orally administered antioxidants, which work system-wide, also look promising in combating photodamage. Vitamins A, C, and E are known to be effective antioxidants in the diet. So, too, are the bioflavonoids, selenium, L-glutathione, and a growing list of phytochemicals.

The verdict is clearly in favor of antioxidants being an important part of your daily supplementation schedule. The benefits, according to compelling and mounting research, are many. For the skin in particular, Drs. Ebhard and Phyllis Kronhausen offer some sound advice in their excellent book *Formula for Life*. They feel that minimum sun exposure over the years, the use of a good-quality sunscreen when you do expose yourself to the sun, and a healthy antioxidant program can protect your skin to a measurable degree. At the very least, they believe that this regimen can help prevent some costly trips to the family doctor or a plastic surgeon.

Everyone—adults, teenagers, and children alike—should take a broad-spectrum antioxidant supplement two or three times a day. Free radicals are caused by air pollution and other environmental toxins, exercise, smoking, sun exposure, and even conditions of normal human metabolism. According to mounting research evidence, the use of an effective antioxidant supplement—one that combats a broad array of the many types of free radicals we are exposed to over our lifetimes—can prolong life by as much as five to ten years.

Table 5.3.   Factors Involved in Improved Recovery and How to Boost Them

Factor	Boosters	Factor	Boosters
Improved blood circulation during and after intensive training for the removal of catabolic waste products and the delivery of nutrients and oxygen.	Vasodilator (blood-vessel expander), such as cayenne or ginkgo; viscosity reducer (blood thinner), such as aspirin; therapeutic modality, such as heat, ice, sauna, or whirlpool.	Improved compensation processes, including: ☐ Improved stress tolerance in the connective tissues. ☐ Improved strength in the muscle tissues. ☐ Improved circulation (vascularization).	Protein drink with twenty-four amino acids and all the cofactors (for the muscle tissues); glucosamine; GH releaser; mucopolysaccharides (for the connective tissues), such as chondroitin sulfate.
Improved protein repair involving: ☐ Sloughing off of destroyed muscle cells. ☐ Bringing in of amino acids, especially the BCAAs, to facilitate the anabolic processes of new growth and to allow for stress adaptation. ☐ Fighting of the unnecessary destruction of cells through the use of anticatabolic agents.	Vitamin B complex, especially vitamins B_6 and B_{12}; BCAAs and L-glutamine; immune-system booster, such as echinacea.	Improved postexercise clearance of adhesions stemming from damaged cells and tissues.	Protease; therapeutic modality, such as stretching, deep-fiber massage, or ultrasound.
		Improved free-radical scavenging.	Vitamins A, C, and E; selenium; L-glutathione; ginkgo; milk thistle; green tea.
		Improved adaptogenic ability (ability to increase the body's resistance to adverse influences) to maintain homeostasis.	Ginseng (Chinese, American, or Siberian); gotu kola.
Improved energy replacement before anabolic processes begin.	Short-, medium-, or long-chain glucose polymers; creatine monohydrate; inosine.	Improved quality of sleep.	Serotonin activator, such as L-tryptophan; tranquilizer or calming agent, such as kava kava or melatonin.
Improved immune-system competence.	Vitamin E; echinacea; astragalus.		

More important to some people, antioxidants can prevent many of the diseases associated with aging.

Oxygen and Recovery

In sports, only one question matters. It is the question asked by all athletes and fitness exercisers: How can I improve my performance capabilities? According to the Russians, the answer lies in the ability to recover fully and quickly from intensive training. In fact, the Russians felt so strongly that recovery is the key that they spent most of their research efforts and sports budget on learning what it is and how to boost it. Improved recovery is why anabolic steroids were so popular until a few years ago. The sole function in sports of these now-banned substances was to improve recovery. Improved recovery ability allows an athlete to train harder amd more often.

The research into recovery and how to improve it

is today being continued by the Russians, as well as by the Americans and others. A number of important factors have so far been isolated. These factors are listed in Table 5.3, above. All of these factors are in large part dependent upon the body's ability to acquire and utilize oxygen efficiently. Oxygen is, after all, the basis of all human life. The next logical question therefore is: Which of the factors can be improved and how? The answer is that all of the factors can be improved, and Table 5.3 shows how.

If you wish to improve your athletic performance, there are a number of things that you can do. Your sport-specific plan in Part Four will show you what you in particular should do. The approach that we use in Part Four, and in this book as a whole, is an integrated approach. An integrated approach involves isolating and addressing all the factors involved in an issue. Improving recovery ability is one of the key factors to address in a program to improve performance. An integrated approach is also the best way to improve the individual factors. If you ignore one factor, and that one factor happens to be a serious problem, your improvement will be hindered. Improvement is only as good as its weakest factor, to paraphrase a popular saying. Therefore, to improve performance, you need to improve your recovery ability. To improve your recovery ability, you need to improve the factors listed in Table 5.3. Pick the combination of methods that works best for you. If one method does not work, find a substitute. Experiment. You may find yourself with an improved recovery ability, improved performance, improved health, and improved self-image. After all, your athletic or fitness involvement is a factor of your life as a whole.

6. VITAMINS
MICRONUTRIENTS FOR MEGAPERFORMANCE

Vitamins are a group of naturally occurring nutrients found in food that are required in the diet for the maintenance of health, metabolic functioning, growth, recovery, and athletic performance. They are organic compounds, which means that they are biologically produced and contain carbon atoms as part of their chemical structures. By definition, vitamins are necessary for health in trace amounts (micrograms to milligrams) and are essential in the diet because the human body either does not make them or does not make them in adequate amounts. If one or more are lacking in the diet, metabolism is affected and symptoms may arise.

There are also hundreds of organic substances essential to health that the body does make in good quantities. Despite this, scientists have determined that supplemental amounts can be beneficial under certain circumstances. These metabolic intermediaries, or metabolites, are sometimes referred to as pseudovitamins or vitaminlike molecules. Examples are choline and inositol. For a full discussion of metabolites, see Chapter 8.

Vitamins are divided into two groups based on their solubility characteristics. The two groups are the fat-soluble vitamins and the water-soluble vitamins. These categories were devised back when researchers first began working on isolating the dietary factors that could prevent nutritional diseases. Scientists called the fat-soluble factors fraction A and the water-soluble factors fraction B. Vitamin A was the first vitamin identified in the fat-soluble fraction, thus the name. Similarly, the B vitamins were the first vitamins identified in the water-soluble fraction. Over time, researchers have found other vitamins in each fraction and have continued using the letter system to name them.

In this chapter, we will review the vitamins on an individual basis. We will discuss the functions of each vitamin, how the vitamin improves athletic performance, its food and supplement sources, the problems induced by deficiency, and the potential side effects caused by excess intake. For each vitamin, we will also present the published safe range of intake and the Performance Daily Intake (PDI). (For the Reference Daily Intakes of the vitamins, see Appendix E.) How to buy vitamins is also briefly discussed (see below).

THE FAT-SOLUBLE VITAMINS

The fat-soluble vitamins are vitamins A, D, E, and K. They are soluble in lipid and organic solvents. Their lipid solubility allows these vitamins to be stored in large amounts in the liver along with fat. The water-soluble vitamins can also be stored in the body, but they usually accumulate in much smaller amounts because of their tendency to be easily flushed out of the system.

The fat-soluble vitamins, especially vitamin A, should be consumed with care because of their storage capabilities. They have the potential of building

How to Buy Vitamins

Hundreds of different kinds of vitamins are stacked on the shelves of health-food stores, pharmacies, and grocery stores, and listed in the catalogs sent out by mail-order companies and wholesale distributors. They range from simple single-nutrient formulations to complex formulations containing an array of vitamins along with minerals, herbs, and other nutrients.

What seems to work best for most individuals is finding a multi-vitamin-and-mineral supplement that provides the vitamins they need in the amounts recommended for their specific body size and sport, then adding single-nutrient formulations for additional nutrients or amounts. (For more guidelines, see Chapter 9.)

up to harmful levels. Even though very few cases of vitamin toxicity have been reported, concern has grown during recent years as the practice of taking megadoses has become popular. If you consume large doses of the fat-soluble vitamins, you may not develop a clear case of vitamin toxicity, but you may find your performance impaired. When it comes to nutrition, more is not always better.

On the other hand, also a concern with the fat-soluble vitamins is deficiency. This is because the proper digestion and absorption of vitamins A, D, E, and K require the presence of lipids in the diet. A low-fat, low-calorie diet can result in malabsorption of these nutrients. Supplements of these vitamins should be oil based or taken with a meal.

Vitamin A

Vitamin A's function in vision makes it one of the most widely known vitamins. As children, we were all forced to eat carrots so that our vision would be at its best and we would not need glasses. In ancient Egypt, the cure for night blindness was to squeeze the liquid from cooked liver onto the eyes. Later, other civilizations combated night blindness by including liver in the diet. We know today that both carrots and liver are very high in vitamin A.

Vitamin A is actually a group of compounds that display vitamin-A activity. The principal vitamin-A compound is retinol, which belongs to a class of chemicals called the retinoids. The retinoids have varying degrees of vitamin-A activity, with retinol the standard against which the other compounds are rated. The retinoids occur in animals.

The carotenoids are another class of chemicals that display vitamin-A activity. They are made by plants but can also be stored in animal fat. They can be converted to vitamin A, mostly retinol, in the body.

The carotenoids, like the retinoids, can build up in the body, but they do not appear to cause toxicity. Persons who wish to maintain a high vitamin-A intake therefore generally combine a moderate amount of vitamin A with a higher amount of beta-carotene. Beta-carotene is the most popular type of carotenoid and has about one-sixth the biological vitamin activity of retinol.

The carotenoids are yellow-red plant pigments that, when taken in high amounts, may give a person's skin a yellow or orange tint due to their accumulation in the subcutaneous fat. The condition, which is reported to

be harmless, is called carotenemia. The coloration disappears when the high dosages are cut back.

Vitamin A plays many roles in the body. It is essential for vision and for cellular growth and development. It is necessary for reproduction, since it is involved in testicular and ovarian functioning. It is needed for the integrity of the immune system; for the formation and maintenance of healthy skin, hair, and mucous membranes; and for bone growth and tooth development. Vitamin A also has anticancer functions. Low intake of the carotenoids, particularly of beta-carotene, is associated with increased risk of lung cancer. This suggests that maintaining a proper intake of the carotenoids may help reduce the risk of lung cancer. Other studies have indicated that vegetables and fruits that are high in vitamin A may reduce the risk of cancer in the mouth, pharynx, larynx, esophagus, stomach, colon, rectum, bladder, and cervix. Scientists speculate that this anticancer activity is due partially to vitamin A's role in promoting normal epithelial cells. Epithelial cells compose such structures as the linings of the lungs and digestive system.

In addition to all of vitamin A's functions, beta-carotene is an antioxidant, able to quench free radicals, particularly singlet oxygen. This helps reduce cellular, molecular, and tissue damage by free radicals, whose numbers are greatly boosted by exercise and increased oxygen uptake. (For a complete discussion of free radicals and antioxidants, see Chapter 5.)

Deficiency

The symptoms of vitamin-A deficiency include night blindness, glare blindness, loss of appetite, increased susceptibility to infections, slowed growth, and rough, dry skin. Deficiency is found mostly in children under the age of five and is usually due to insufficient dietary intake. Deficiency also results from chronic fat malabsorption.

The primary symptoms of beta-carotene deficiency are night blindness and other eye problems, skin disorders, growth disorders, and reproductive-system failure.

Excessive Intake

Excessive intake of vitamin A may lead to toxicity, which can be acute or chronic. The symptoms of toxicity include headaches, vomiting, dry mucous membranes, bone abnormalities, and liver damage. Toxicity seems to occur after prolonged daily retinol intake of

50,000 international units in adults and 20,000 international units in children and infants. These dosages are about ten times the RDA and are difficult to obtain unless large amounts of liver are eaten every day for a long period of time or supplements are taken in enormous quantities. In women, the ingestion of high therapeutic doses of vitamin A has been reported to cause spontaneous abortion and birth defects. Therefore, women who are pregnant or who are planning on becoming pregnant should consult a health-care practitioner concerning supplementation.

Excessive intake of beta-carotene does not appear to produce toxic side effects. Therefore, beta-carotene is recommended over retinol when higher dosages are desired. Note, however, that carotenemia may occur at dosages of over 25,000 international units.

Food and Supplement Sources

The forms of vitamin A that are the most commonly used in supplements are vitamin A acetate and vitamin A palmitate. These are effective and economical synthetic forms of retinol. Natural vitamin A retinol forms are also available, but they are more expensive because they are extracted from natural animal sources, such as fish-liver oil, and are then concentrated.

Beta-carotene, while of plant origin, comes in a synthetic form, too. This synthetic form is used mostly in supplements. Beta-carotene, whether natural or synthetic, is more expensive than vitamin A, both natural and synthetic.

Both vitamin A and beta-carotene are available in tablets, capsules, and gelatin capsules. The dry forms tend to be more stable. The best way to get vitamin A is from a combination of vitamin-A supplements, beta-carotene supplements, and a diet that is rich in vegetables that are high in beta-carotene.

The food sources of vitamin A include liver, fish-liver oil, egg yolks, crab, halibut, whole-milk products, butter, cream, and margarine. The food sources of beta-carotene include carrots, green leafy vegetables, spinach, broccoli, squash, apricots, sweet potatoes, and cantaloupe.

Estimated Safe Range of Intake

The estimated safe range of intake for vitamin A for average adults is 5,000 to 50,000 international units per day. The estimated safe range of intake for vitamin A for large, healthy, active adults is 25,000 to 50,000 international units per day.

Performance Daily Intake

The PDI of vitamin A for men and women who are healthy and actively training is 5,000 to 25,000 international units.

The PDI of beta-carotene for men and women who are healthy and actively training is 15,000 to 60,000 international units. For endurance athletes, the PDI of beta-carotene is 20,000 to 80,000 international units.

Athletic Performance Goals

Studies support the adequate intake of vitamin A and beta-carotene for the maintenance of overall health and athletic performance. However, current research does not support the practice of taking megadoses of vitamin A for the improvement of athletic performance. Keep your daily vitamin-A intake from food and supplement sources to within the PDI guidelines. Increase your beta-carotene intake as you increase your activity level to make sure you get adequate antioxidant benefits, especially if you are an endurance athlete.

Vitamin D

Vitamin D was originally isolated when researchers were seeking the active nutrient in cod-liver oil, which was the treatment of choice for rickets and similar disorders. Rickets is a childhood disease marked by bones that are soft and malformed. Later, researchers determined that UV rays from both sunlight and lamps can also cure rickets. We now know that vitamin D occurs in high amounts in cod-liver oil and that the body manufactures vitamin D when exposed to UV light.

Four compounds exhibit vitamin-D activity. The two most commonly found in food are cholecalciferol and ergocalciferol. Cholecalciferol, also known as vitamin D_3, is the major form of vitamin D that is manufactured in the body. When UV light hits the skin, it induces the conversion of 7-dehydrocholesterol, a sterol widely distributed in the skin, into cholecalciferol. Ergocalciferol, also known as vitamin D_2 or calciferol, is produced in plants when UV light hits and converts the sterol ergosterol. The body can utilize both these forms of vitamin D by converting them to the biologically active form, 25-hydroxycholecalciferol. Vitamin D_1 and vitamin D_4 (dihydroergocalciferol) are not commonly found in food.

Vitamin D has several important functions. It is essential for growth, especially the normal growth and development of bones and teeth in children. Its main function is assisting in many aspects of calcium and phosphorus metabolism, including their intestinal absorption and utilization. In this way, vitamin D supports the normal mineralization (hardening) of the bone, making it an important tool in the fight against both rickets and osteoporosis. In osteoporosis, the bones become extremely porous and break very easily. There is also some evidence that vitamin D functions to improve muscular strength, prevent hypocalcemia (a low blood-calcium level), and enhance immunity. Taking megadoses, however, does not appear to increase benefits.

Deficiency

Vitamin-D deficiency is characterized by inadequate mineralization of the bones and associated abnormalities such as soft bones, bowlegs, poor teeth, and skeletal deformity. In children, deficiency can result in rickets. In adults, bone loss and increased susceptibility to fractures can ensue. Although the fortification of milk and other foods has greatly reduced the incidence of vitamin-D deficiency, certain individuals are still at increased risk. Infants who are breastfed, not given supplemental vitamin D, and not adequately exposed to sunlight are susceptible. So are the elderly and persons who spend most of their time indoors. The characteristic biochemical changes include lowered blood levels of calcium and phosphorus. Housebound individuals should make an effort to get at least the RDA of vitamin D from food and supplement sources.

Excessive Intake

Excessive intake of vitamin D may lead to toxicity, which is potentially harmful, especially in young children. It may also lead to calcium buildup in the soft tissues and irreversible kidney and cardiovascular damage. Harmful levels of vitamin-D intake have not been clearly established, but consumption of as little as 1,800 international units of cholecalciferol per day has caused hypervitaminosis (overdose toxicity) in children. Because exposure to the sun causes vitamin D to be manufactured in the body, supplemental intake should be closely monitored. In some cases, doses of only five times the RDA produced side effects. While intake greater than the RDA may be

beneficial for athletes, taking megadoses of vitamin D should be avoided, unless it is done under medical supervision.

Food and Supplement Sources

The forms of vitamin D that are generally used in supplements are ergocalciferol (vitamin D_2) and cholecalciferol (vitamin D_3). Look for supplements that contain both.

The food sources of vitamin D include fish-liver oil, eggs, butter, cream, halibut, herring, liver, mackerel, salmon, sardines, and shrimp. In the United States, foods fortified with vitamin D, especially milk, are major food sources.

Individuals who are not frequently exposed to sunlight need more vitamin D from food sources than do persons who are frequently exposed.

Estimated Safe Range of Intake

The estimated safe range of intake for vitamin D (as cholecalciferol) for adults is 400 to 2,000 international units per day.

Performance Daily Intake

The PDI of vitamin D for men and women who are healthy and actively training is 400 to 1,000 international units.

Athletic Performance Goals

Studies support the adequate intake of vitamin D for the maintenance of overall health and athletic performance. However, current research does not support the practice of taking megadoses of vitamin D for the improvement of athletic performance. Keep your daily vitamin-D intake from food and supplement sources to within the PDI guidelines.

Vitamin E

Vitamin E's role in reproduction is widely recognized. In fact, its supplemental use has become extremely popular among persons hoping to enhance their sexual performance. Research has now also disclosed other potential benefits of vitamin-E supplementation.

There are two major groups of compounds found in food that display vitamin-E activity. They are the tocopherols and the tocotrienols. The tocopherols are the primary sources of vitamin E, since they display much higher activity levels than the tocotrienols. Among the tocopherols, alpha-tocopherol is the most active form.

Vitamin E has a host of functions. It assists in red blood cell formation, acts as an antioxidant, and aids in the regulation of prostanoid synthesis. Prostanoids are compounds that are important in the reproductive process, blood-platelet aggregation (clustering), energy production, synthesis of deoxyribonucleic acid (DNA) and ribonucleic acid (RNA), and retardation of aging, cancer, and heart disease. Vitamin E, therefore, protects cell membranes against oxidation, prevents blood clots, retards oxidation of the other fat-soluble vitamins, helps cells breathe, and treats or prevents vitamin deficiency in premature or low-birth-weight infants. Of interest to athletes, vitamin E has also been shown to lower the blood-lactate level, decrease the formation of certain waste products during exercise, reduce oxidative cellular damage, maintain muscle tissue, and possibly help testosterone production.

A recent study showed that adults taking 100 international units of vitamin E per day have a reduced risk of cardiovascular disease. In other studies, high experimental intakes (between 200 and 1,200 international units) have been found to benefit athletes by improving energy production, reducing cellular damage, and stabilizing membranes. Supplementation has also been shown to noticeably benefit physical performance and tissue protection at high altitudes.

Deficiency

While symptoms of vitamin-E deficiency have been observed in animals, they are less clear in humans. Furthermore, the diagnosis of vitamin-E deficiency in humans is complicated by the mineral selenium playing a role in vitamin E's metabolism. Symptoms in animals have disappeared when selenium or the sulfur-bearing amino acids were supplied. (For a complete discussion of selenium, see page 96.) Among the suspected symptoms of vitamin-E deficiency are muscle weakness, increased destruction of cell membranes, abnormal disposition of fat in the muscles, and rupture of red blood cells. However, even though its deficiency is difficult to clearly diagnose, vitamin E is known to be an important essential nutrient that should be ingested in amounts higher than the RDA.

Excessive Intake

Compared to the other fat-soluble vitamins, vitamin E is relatively nontoxic when orally ingested. This is fortunate, since taking megadoses of the vitamin has become so popular in recent years. Adults have been observed to ingest 100 to 800 international units per day without signs of toxicity. However, a high level of vitamin E may interfere with the activity of vitamin K, leading to problems with blood clotting. (For a complete discussion of vitamin K, see page 78.)

Food and Supplement Sources

Both the natural and synthetic forms of vitamin E are found in supplements. The natural forms, d-alpha-tocopherol succinate and d-alpha-tocopherol acetate, are generally recommended by experts due to their higher rates of absorption. The synthetic forms, dl-alpha-tocopherol and dl-alpha-tocopherol acetate, appear to be less bioactive. Also recommended is a combination form known as mixed tocopherols.

Vitamin E is available in tablets and gelatin capsules. Both are satisfactory, but the tablets tend to be more stable.

The food sources of vitamin E vary greatly in quality according to their storage and preparation. The richest sources are vegetable oils, such as soy, corn, cottonseed, peanut, and safflower oils. Products made from or containing these oils include margarine, wheat germ, and nuts. Meat, fish, animal fat, and fruit are generally low in vitamin E.

Estimated Safe Range of Intake

The estimated safe range of intake for vitamin E for adults is 20 to 1,200 international units per day.

Performance Daily Intake

The PDI of vitamin E for men and women who are healthy and actively training is 200 to 1,000 international units.

The PDI of vitamin E for men and women recovering from injuries or competing at high altitudes is 600 to 1,200 international units. Note, however, that this is recommended only for short periods of time, several weeks at the most.

Athletic Performance Goals

Studies support the adequate intake of vitamin E for the maintenance of overall health and a higher-than-average intake of vitamin E for the maintenance of athletic performance. However, keep your daily vitamin-E intake from food and supplement sources to within the PDI guidelines for men and women who are healthy and actively training. If you are an athlete training or competing at a high altitude (5,000 feet or more above sea level), raise your vitamin-E intake during training or competition to the upper end of the PDI range for men and women competing at high altitudes. If you are an athlete recovering from an injury or surgery, you, too, should keep your intake temporarily higher than normal.

Vitamin K

The body's need for vitamin K was suspected for years, but it was only in 1989 that the vitamin was given an RDA value. Researchers had observed in 1929 that newly hatched chickens on diets containing only the known essential nutrients developed hemorrhagic disorders (disorders marked by excessive bleeding). A decade later, in 1939, scientists isolated vitamin K and established its role in blood clotting.

There are several compounds that display vitamin-K activity. Phylloquinone, also known as vitamin K_1, is the principal one. It occurs naturally in green plants. Other compounds are menaquinone, also known as vitamin K_2, which is produced in the human intestines by bacteria; and menadione, called vitamin K_3, which is synthetically produced. Menadione is manufactured both in a fat-soluble form, which is about twice as potent as phylloquinone, and in water-soluble forms.

Vitamin K's major function is the formation of prothrombin, a substance that is vital for blood clotting. Without vitamin K, the blood-clotting process cannot be initiated. Since athletes undergoing strenuous training are constantly damaging tissue, they would not be remiss in taking supplemental vitamin K to ensure an adequate daily intake.

Deficiency

Vitamin-K deficiency can lead to a decrease in the amount of prothrombin made by the body and an increase in the tendency to hemorrhage (bleed profusely). Luckily, deficiency of vitamin K is rarely encountered in healthy individuals eating a balanced diet, although it can develop in persons who do not eat enough green vegetables or who are taking medications that interfere with the growth of intestinal bacteria. Most instances of vitamin-K deficiency are found in infants. Supplemental vitamin K is sometimes given to patients before surgery to aid in blood clotting. Aspirin can interfere with the metabolic pathways in which vitamin K is involved and can thus prevent normal blood clotting.

Excessive Intake

Excessive intake of vitamin K, even for extended time periods, has not readily produced toxic side effects in adults. However, excessive dosages given to laboratory animals and infants have caused hemolytic anemia (separation of the hemoglobin from red blood cells). The water-soluble forms of menadione (vitamin K_3) obviously have wider margins of safety than do the fat-soluble synthetic form and the natural forms.

Food and Supplement Sources

The forms of vitamin K that are commonly used in supplements are phylloquinone (vitamin K_1) and menadione (vitamin K_3). Look for supplements that contain both.

The chief food sources of vitamin K are green leafy vegetables. Small amounts are also found in milk and dairy products, eggs, cereal, fruits, and vegetables.

Also an important source of vitamin K is the intestinal tract, where the nutrient is made by bacteria. However, this supply is difficult to evaluate and may or may not be a major source.

Estimated Safe Range of Intake

The estimated safe range of intake for vitamin K for adults is 80 to 600 micrograms per day.

Performance Daily Intake

The PDI of vitamin K for men and women who are healthy and actively training is 80 to 180 micrograms.

Athletic Performance Goals

Studies support the adequate intake of vitamin K for the maintenance of overall health. However, few studies have been conducted on vitamin K's direct effects on athletic performance, and current research does not support the practice of taking megadoses of vitamin K for the improvement of performance. Keep your daily vitamin-K intake from food and supplement sources to within the PDI guidelines.

THE WATER-SOLUBLE VITAMINS

The water-soluble vitamins include vitamins B_1 (thiamine), B_2 (riboflavin), B_3 (niacin), B_5 (pantothenic acid), B_6 (pyridoxine), B_{12} (cobalamin), and C, as well as folate and biotin. Vitamin C has been in the spotlight for many years and is best known for its ability to combat colds and its function as an antioxidant. The B vitamins basically act as coenzymes and are involved in the metabolism of fat, protein, and carbohydrates.

The water-soluble vitamins are not normally stored in the body in any significant amounts. Therefore, they must be consumed in constant daily amounts to avoid depletion and interference with normal metabolic functioning.

Vitamin B_1 (Thiamine)

Vitamin B_1, as thiamine pyrophosphate (TPP), is also called thiamine. In the body, thiamine joins with phosphate to form TPP. Vitamin B_1 is water soluble and not readily absorbed by the body.

Thiamine, the same as the other B vitamins, is converted in the body into coenzymes that aid in carbohydrate metabolism. Since athletes tend to eat more carbohydrates than nonathletes do, their need for thiamine is greater. Thiamine also functions in the production of ribose, which is needed for the synthesis of RNA and DNA and for appetite stimulation. It also helps maintain the integrity of nervous-system functioning, which is extremely beneficial for athletes. Endurance athletes have reported improvements in performance from ingesting increased amounts of thiamine.

Deficiency

The symptoms of thiamine deficiency include abnormalities in carbohydrate metabolism, fatigue, loss of appetite, constipation, depression, confusion, poor coordination, and beriberi. Beriberi is the traditional disease associated with prolonged thiamine deficiency. Its primary symptoms involve the cardiovascular and nervous systems. They include muscle weakness, atrophy, heart failure, and depression. Thiamine deficiency is also observed in persons who drink alcohol excessively.

Excessive Intake

Thiamine toxicity is rarely reported in healthy adults, since intake of over 300 milligrams per day is considered safe and excess thiamine is cleared out by the kidneys. In fact, in one study, oral doses of 500 milligrams of thiamine taken daily for one month were found to be nontoxic. This does not mean, however, that consuming megadoses of thiamine all year round will bring increased benefits. What it does mean is that higher doses in season may be beneficial.

Food and Supplement Sources

The forms of thiamine that are the most commonly used in supplements are thiamine hydrochloride and thiamine mononitrate. The two forms seem to perform equally well.

The food sources of thiamine include brewer's yeast, peas, pork, wheat germ, whole-grain pasta, peanuts, beans, organ meats, and fortified grain and cereal products.

Estimated Safe Range of Intake

The estimated safe range of intake for thiamine for adults is up to 300 milligrams per day.

Performance Daily Intake

The PDI of thiamine for men and women who are healthy and actively training is 30 to 300 milligrams.

Athletic Performance Goals

Studies support the adequate intake of thiamine for the maintenance of overall health and athletic performance. Keep your daily thiamine intake from food and supplement sources to within the PDI guidelines. Increase your thiamine intake as you increase your activity level. Some research has supported the practice of taking megadoses of thiamine by endurance athletes for three to five days before competition for acute improvement of performance. The amounts of thiamine reportedly used were 300 to 900 milligrams per day. However, additional research is needed to verify the results and to determine the exact range of intake. Other research has indicated that supplemental thiamine may significantly improve firing accuracy in marksmen.

Vitamin B$_2$ (Riboflavin)

Vitamin B$_2$, also known as riboflavin, is involved in energy production and cellular respiration. In the body, riboflavin functions primarily as part of two coenzymes—flavin mononucleotide (FMN) and flavin adenine dinucleotide (FAD). These two coenzymes are involved in many oxidation-reduction reactions, which are processes that produce energy from carbohydrates, fatty acids, and some amino acids. Because of riboflavin's role in these energy-producing reactions, it is a vital nutrient for the health of all tissues, particularly the skin, eyes, and nerves.

Apart from its essential functions, riboflavin taken in amounts of 10 milligrams per day has been reported to lower neuromuscular irritability after electrical stimulation of the muscles. This indicates that riboflavin taken in higher amounts may improve muscular excitability and bring about better overall performance.

Deficiency

The symptoms of riboflavin deficiency include inflamed lips, cracked skin, reduced growth, hair loss, cataracts, generalized seborrheic dermatitis (a skin condition), and behavioral changes such as depression, moodiness, nervousness, and irritability. Since riboflavin is essential to the functioning of vitamins B$_3$ and B$_6$, a deficiency often causes some symptoms that are actually a result of these other nutrients not operating effectively.

Excessive Intake

Excessive intake of riboflavin does not appear to produce toxic side effects. Riboflavin is considered nontoxic even in doses far greater than the RDA value.

Food and Supplement Sources

The form of riboflavin that is used in supplements is the pure form.

The food sources of riboflavin include brewer's yeast, meat, poultry, fish, dairy products, nuts, fortified grain products, wheat germ, kidney, liver, and green vegetables, especially broccoli, asparagus, spinach, and turnip greens.

Estimated Safe Range of Intake

An estimated safe range of intake has not been established for riboflavin, since no toxicity has been observed. However, 1,000 milligrams per day is the recommended maximum for adults.

Performance Daily Intake

The PDI of riboflavin for men and women who are healthy and actively training is 30 to 300 milligrams.

Athletic Performance Goals

Studies support the adequate intake of riboflavin for the maintenance of overall health and athletic performance. However, current research does not support the practice of taking megadoses of riboflavin for the improvement of athletic performance. Keep your daily riboflavin intake from food and supplement sources to within the PDI guidelines.

Vitamin B$_3$ (Niacin)

Vitamin B$_3$, called niacin, is a water-soluble vitamin of the B-complex family that can be used for both nicotinic acid and niacinamide (nicotinamide), two forms of the vitamin. Niacin is functionally active in the body as two very important coenzymes—nicotinamide adenine dinucleotide (NAD) and nicotinamide adenine dinucleotide phosphate (NADP). NAD and NADP are present in every body cell and play a part in many vital metabolic processes including energy production, glycolysis, carbohydrate and protein metabolism, fatty-acid synthesis, and reduction of cholesterol and fatty acids in the blood. Niacin can be synthesized by the body from the amino acid tryptophan. However, as discussed in Chapter 3, tryptophan is often a limiting amino acid, and its function as a niacin producer should be minimized by supplying the body with supplemental niacin on a daily basis.

Niacin's ability to control cholesterol brought it major acclaim as a miracle nutrient in the 1980s and resulted in its widespread use in megadose quantities. The nicotinic-acid form of niacin seems to lower the cholesterol and fatty-acid blood levels better than the niacinamide form does, but nicotinic acid used in amounts greater than 50 milligrams per day causes the capillaries to dilate, resulting in what has become known as niacin flush. This flushing involves itching, burning, and reddening of the skin. Niacin flush has not been observed with niacinamide.

Note that although niacin is essential for cellular respiration, it clearly reduced performance on several occasions in research on energy production conducted with athletes. The higher amounts of niacin that the researchers administered to the athletes before exercise caused glycogen to be depleted at a faster rate and resulted in earlier onset of fatigue. Niacin apparently blocks the release of fatty acids from adipose tissue, the tissue that stores fat, making fatty acids less available as a source of energy during exercise. Taking megadoses of niacin therefore should be avoided by endurance athletes. However, another study indicated that consuming high dosages of niacinamide before anaerobic (without oxygen) exercise may improve performance. This is probably because anaerobic athletes get more of their energy from glycogen, and the faster release of glycogen from muscle stores may result in greater power output. More research is warranted in this area. The amounts of niacin that were used in these studies ranged from 50 milligrams taken over three days to 200 milligrams taken two hours before exercise.

Deficiency

The symptoms of niacin deficiency include depression, confusion, headaches, an elevated fatty-acid blood level, fatigue, and pellagra. Pellagra is a disease characterized by dermatitis, inflamed mucous membranes, and dementia.

Excessive Intake

Intake of nicotinic acid in amounts greater than 50 milligrams per day may cause niacin flush. Taking megadoses of either nicotinic acid or niacinamide may cause early onset of fatigue. In general, however, intake of niacin in amounts of up to 1,000 milligrams is considered safe. Higher dosages should be administered only by health-care practitioners.

Food and Supplement Sources

Nicotinic acid and niacinamide are both available as individual supplements. Both are also commonly included in multivitamin supplements. Both forms of niacin should be taken on a daily basis.

The food sources of niacin include liver, brewer's yeast, lean meats, whole grains, nuts, legumes, and potatoes.

Estimated Safe Range of Intake

An estimated safe range of intake has not been established for niacin, since no toxicity has been observed. However, 1,000 milligrams per day is the recommended maximum for adults.

Performance Daily Intake

The PDI of niacin for men and women who are healthy and actively training is 20 to 100 milligrams.

Athletic Performance Goals

Studies support the adequate intake of niacin for the maintenance of overall health and athletic performance. However, current research does not support the practice of taking megadoses of niacin for the improvement of athletic performance. Keep your daily niacin intake from food and supplement sources to within the PDI guidelines. In fact, if you are an endurance athlete, keep your niacin intake to below 30 milligrams per day, especially before events.

Vitamin B$_5$ (Pantothenic Acid)

Vitamin B$_5$, more commonly known as pantothenic acid, is another water-soluble member of the B-complex family. It has many important metabolic functions, primarily as a component of coenzyme A. Coenzyme A is important in the Krebs cycle and in the metabolism of fatty acids. Pantothenic acid's metabolic functions are vital in the release of energy from carbohydrates and fatty acids. The vitamin is also involved in steroid and cholesterol synthesis. In addition, according to studies, it may enhance performance for endurance athletes when taken in amounts ranging from 30 to 2,000 milligrams per day for short periods of time.

Deficiency

The symptoms of pantothenic-acid deficiency include weakness, irritability, burning feet, vomiting, and insomnia.

Excessive Intake

Excessive intake of pantothenic acid does not appear to produce toxic side effects. In fact, research subjects were given doses as high as 10,000 milligrams per day for six weeks without showing symptoms. However, ingestion of 10,000 to 20,000 milligrams per day may result in diarrhea or water retention. Intake at these excessive levels is not recommended.

Food and Supplement Sources

The form of pantothenic acid that is used in supplements is D-calcium pantothenate. Pantothenic acid is a common ingredient in multivitamin supplements, but it is not frequently found as a supplement by itself.

The food sources of pantothenic acid include potatoes, eggs, pork, beef, fish, milk, whole wheat, whole-grain cereal, and most fruits and vegetables.

Estimated Safe Range of Intake

The estimated safe range of intake for pantothenic acid for adults is up to 1,000 milligrams per day.

Performance Daily Intake

The PDI of pantothenic acid for men and women who are healthy and actively training is 25 to 200 milligrams.

Athletic Performance Goals

Studies support the adequate intake of pantothenic acid for the maintenance of overall health and athletic performance. Keep your daily pantothenic-acid intake from food and supplement sources to within the PDI guidelines. Some research has supported the practice of taking megadoses of pantothenic acid by endurance athletes for short periods of time (seven to fourteen days) before competition for the improvement of performance. The amounts that reportedly enhanced performance were up to 2,000 milligrams per day. However, additional research is needed to determine the optimum intake for this short-term use.

Vitamin B$_6$ (Pyridoxine)

Vitamin B$_6$, also called pyridoxine, is an essential vitamin that is known in athletic circles for its role in amino-acid metabolism. It occurs in nature in three forms—pyridoxine, pyridoxal, and pyridoxamine. In the body, it is converted to its active forms—pyridoxal phosphate (PLP) and pyridoxamine phosphate (PMP).

Pyridoxine functions primarily in transamination reactions, processes in which an amino group is transferred from an amino acid to a molecule, usually to produce another amino acid. Due to pyridoxine's role in the metabolism of protein and amino acids, its requirement by the body increases as protein intake is increased. Pyridoxine is also involved in the conversion of linoleic acid to arachidonic acid, glycogenolysis (glycogen breakdown), energy production, and synthesis of red blood cells.

Studies using pyridoxine with athletes have had results similar to those using niacin with athletes due to pyridoxine's tendency to increase the body's utilization of its glycogen stores and to decrease its use of fatty acids. Taking megadoses of pyridoxine should therefore be avoided by endurance athletes. However, as with niacin, there is some evidence that consuming high doses of pyridoxine before short-term anaerobic exercise may enhance performance. Again, this is probably because anaerobic athletes, such as weight lifters, sprinters, and shot-putters, get more of their energy from stored glycogen, and faster glycogen release may result in greater power output. Athletes going through the glycogen-depletion phase of a carbohydrate-loading program can increase depletion of their glycogen stores with as little as 8 milligrams of pyridoxine per day. Pyridoxine has also reportedly increased the exercise-induced rise in GH, which is another potential benefit for power athletes.

Deficiency

The symptoms of pyridoxine deficiency include depression, skin disorders, poor wound healing, anemia, fatigue, and convulsive seizures.

Excessive Intake

While pyridoxine is relatively nontoxic and amounts of up to 2,000 milligrams per day are considered safe, massive dosages (2,000 to 6,000 milligrams per day) taken over several months have been reported to cause nervous-system disorders. The symptoms include tingling and numbness in the arms and legs.

Food and Supplement Sources

The form of pyridoxine that is most commonly used in supplements is pyridoxine hydrochloride.

The food sources of pyridoxine include chicken, fish, kidney, liver, eggs, rice, soybeans, bananas, lima beans, peanuts, and walnuts.

Estimated Safe Range of Intake

An estimated safe range of intake has not been established for pyridoxine, since no side effects have been observed in adults with doses of up to 2,000 milligrams per day. However, large amounts taken daily over several months may cause problems with the nervous system.

Performance Daily Intake

The PDI of pyridoxine for men and women who are healthy and actively training is 20 to 100 milligrams.

Athletic Performance Goals

Studies support the adequate intake of pyridoxine for the maintenance of overall health and athletic performance. However, current research does not support the practice of taking megadoses of pyridoxine for the improvement of athletic performance. Keep your daily pyridoxine intake from food and supplement sources to within the PDI guidelines. In fact, if you are an endurance athlete, keep your pyridoxine intake to below 30 milligrams per day, especially before events.

Vitamin B_{12} (Cobalamin)

Vitamin B_{12} is only one part of the nutrition picture, but it is a very important part, playing an essential role in maintaining athletic performance. It is regarded as the primary energy vitamin. In fact, a common practice among athletes is to get vitamin-B_{12} shots during the season. Vitamin B_{12}, also known as cobalamin, is really a group of cobalt-containing compounds that display vitamin-B_{12} activity. The predominant forms of B_{12} in the body are hydroxocobalamin, enosylcobalamin, and methylcobalamin.

Vitamin B_{12} functions in the body in new cell growth, nerve-tissue development, folate metabolism, DNA synthesis, and energy production. It is necessary for the synthesis of red blood cells and, therefore, for the prevention of anemia. Studies conducted in the 1980s on nonathletes experiencing tiredness are credited with initiating the current practices of taking megadoses of B_{12} and injecting B_{12} that are so widespread among athletes. These studies used only vitamin-B_{12} injections, though; the benefits of consuming megadoses of B_{12} have not yet been substantiated by research. Furthermore, various studies examining the strength and endurance effects of B_{12} have not shown the vitamin to provide any immediate bene-

fits. To date, vitamin B_{12}'s primary functions are metabolic.

Researchers are currently focusing their attention on a coenzyme form of B_{12} called cobamamide. Cobamamide is being touted as an anabolic form of B_{12} that is comparable to anabolic steroids. A study conducted on children with growth disorders showed that cobamamide can improve growth. Anabolic growth effects in healthy adults have not been proven. According to athletes, however, cobamamide raises the perceived energy level and increases appetite. Therefore, the use of coenzyme B_{12} along with vitamin B_{12} is recommended for athletes.

Deficiency

The symptoms of vitamin-B_{12} deficiency include fatigue, irritability, loss of appetite, constipation, headaches, tongue soreness, and pernicious anemia. Pernicious anemia is a disease characterized by the defective production of red blood cells. Vitamin B_{12} deficiency is rarely caused by a lack of the nutrient in the diet; rather, most B_{12} deficiencies are attributed to poor absorption. Before vitamin B_{12} can be absorbed, it must be activated, which is done by a substance secreted by the stomach called intrinsic factor. Malabsorption is usually the cause of pernicious anemia due to the body's inability to manufacture intrinsic factor. Vitamin-B_{12} injections are the treatment of choice, since injected B_{12} does not need intrinsic factor for activation and absorption.

Excessive Intake

Excessive intake of vitamin B_{12} does not appear to produce toxic side effects. However, taking megadoses is not recommended, since there may be performance-inhibiting effects yet to be discovered.

Food and Supplement Sources

The form of vitamin B_{12} that is used in supplements is cyanocobalamin. The other forms of vitamin B_{12} are not recommended for supplemental use.

Vitamin B_{12} becomes unstable when it is exposed to light, so make sure that you buy B_{12} in a light-protected bottle. Also look for cobamamide (Dibencozide) in light-protected containers.

The food sources of vitamin B_{12} include lamb, beef, herring, mackerel, pork liver, oysters, poultry, clams, eggs, and tofu.

Estimated Safe Range of Intake

An estimated safe range of intake has not been established for vitamin B_{12}, since no side effects have been observed in adults with doses of up to 500 micrograms per day.

Performance Daily Intake

The PDI of vitamin B_{12} for men and women who are healthy and actively training is 12 to 200 micrograms.

Athletic Performance Goals

Studies support the adequate intake of vitamin B_{12} for the maintenance of overall health and athletic performance. However, taking megadoses of vitamin B_{12} is not recommended. Keep your daily vitamin-B_{12} intake from food and supplement sources to within the PDI guidelines.

Biotin

Biotin is another water-soluble member of the B-vitamin family. It is a sulfur-bearing vitamin that is manufactured by intestinal bacteria. Because biotin is produced in the body, deficiency is rare.

Biotin is involved in new cell growth, fatty-acid synthesis, glucose formation, protein synthesis, energy production, and urea formation. It aids in the utilization of the B vitamins and promotes healthy hair, skin, sweat glands, nerve tissue, and bone marrow. However, biotin is not reported to have any effects on athletic performance.

Deficiency

Biotin deficiency can be caused by a low dietary intake of the nutrient or by consumption of large amounts of a biotin-binding glycoprotein found in raw egg whites. The symptoms of biotin deficiency include nausea, vomiting, depression, pallor, anemia, hair loss, high blood sugar, insomnia, loss of appetite, muscular pain, soreness of the tongue, increased serum cholesterol, loss of muscle tone, and a dry, scaly dermatitis.

Excessive Intake

Excessive intake of biotin in doses as high as 10,000 micrograms per day does not appear to produce toxic side effects.

Food and Supplement Sources

The form of biotin that is used in supplements is the pure form. Biotin is a common ingredient in multivitamin supplements, but it is not frequently found as a supplement by itself.

The food sources of biotin include liver, egg yolks, soy flour, cereal, brewer's yeast, nuts, cauliflower, milk, and legumes.

Estimated Safe Range of Intake

An estimated safe range of intake has not been established for biotin, since no side effects have been observed in adults with doses of up to 10,000 micrograms per day.

Performance Daily Intake

The PDI of biotin for men and women who are healthy and actively training is 125 to 300 micrograms.

Athletic Performance Goals

Studies support the adequate intake of biotin for the overall maintenance of health. However, current research does not show any athletic-performance benefits from the intake of biotin. Keep your daily biotin intake from food and supplement sources to within the PDI guidelines.

Folate

Folate, also called folacin, is another water-soluble B vitamin. It is a group of compounds that have nutritional properties similar to those of folic acid. These compounds function metabolically as coenzymes that transport carbon molecules from one compound to another in amino-acid metabolism and nucleic-acid synthesis. In this way, folate is very important as a cofactor in DNA and RNA formation, protein synthesis, and cellular replication. Folate also stimulates the formation of red blood cells and vitamin B_{12}. In particular, folate affects tissues that grow rapidly, such as the skin, the lining of the gastrointestinal tract, the bone marrow, and regenerating muscle tissue. Studies have also indicated that increasing folate intake during pregnancy reduces the incidence of premature birth and birth defects.

Studies with athletes using high dosages of folate have not revealed immediate performance-enhancing effects. Taking megadoses of folate is not recommended, nor is it easily possible, as supplements containing over 800 micrograms of folate per dose can be obtained only by prescription. Athletes in general will benefit from higher-than-average folate intake, and bodybuilders may find faster recovery and growth rates with even higher doses.

Deficiency

The symptoms of folate deficiency include anemia, birth defects, tongue soreness, gastrointestinal disorders, growth disorders, fatigue, poor memory, and megaloblastic anemia. Megaloblastic anemia is a disease characterized by abnormal forms of the precursor cells of red blood cells.

Excessive Intake

Excessive intake of folate may result in side effects such as kidney damage, a lowered zinc level, and convulsive seizures in persons with epilepsy.

Food and Supplement Sources

The form of folate that is used in supplements is folic acid.

The food sources of folate include beef, lamb, pork, chicken liver, eggs, asparagus, whole wheat, deep-green leafy vegetables, salmon, and brewer's yeast.

Estimated Safe Range of Intake

An estimated safe range of intake has not been established for folate, since levels of over 1,200 micrograms per day have been found to be safe for adults. However, supplements supplying more than 800 micrograms per dose can be obtained only by prescription.

Performance Daily Intake

The PDI of folate for men and women who are healthy and actively training is 400 to 1,200 micrograms.

Athletic Performance Goals

Studies support the adequate intake of folate for the maintenance of overall health and athletic perfmance.

Keep your daily folate intake from food and supplement sources to within the PDI guidelines.

Vitamin C

Scurvy is the dreaded disease that sailors, explorers, and other travelers used to develop when deprived of fresh fruits and vegetables for prolonged periods of time. It has been written about time and again in the scientific literature and in novels. Doctors eventually discovered that eating limes, lemons, and oranges reverses as well as prevents scurvy. In fact, English sailors were nicknamed limeys because of their frequent consumption of these citrus fruits during long voyages. In the 1930s, scientists isolated vitamin C from citrus fruit and identified it as the substance so helpful to sailors.

Vitamin C, also called ascorbic acid, is primarily a water-soluble antioxidant that cannot be synthesized by the human body. Neither is it stored in the body in any significant amount. Therefore, it is an essential vitamin. In addition, a slightly altered form of ascorbic acid, called dehydroascorbic acid, is present in the diet. This oxidized form also displays some vitamin-C activity.

Vitamin C first came into the spotlight when Dr. Linus Pauling, the esteemed Nobel Prize–winning biochemist, advocated its use to help prevent the onset of the common cold. Today, it is touted as a general cure-all by many people. It has multiple functions as a cofactor and coenzyme. It is involved in the formation and maintenance of collagen, a protein that is an important component of skin, ligaments, and bones. It helps heal wounds, may help fight infections, and promotes healthy capillaries, gums, and teeth. It prevents the oxidation of folate, aids in the intestinal absorption of iron, and assists in the metabolism of tyrosine and phenylalanine. It protects cells from free-radical damage and blocks the production of nitrosamines, organic compounds present in various foods and found to produce cancer in laboratory animals. For athletes, studies have indicated that vitamin C plays a part in increasing muscular strength, reducing the blood-lactate level, and sparing glycogen.

Deficiency

A deficiency of vitamin C can lead to scurvy, a serious disease characterized by weakening of the collagenous tissues and structures such as the skin, tendons, and cartilage, resulting in widespread hemorrhaging from capillaries. Scurvy is rarely seen in adults in the United States, but it is sometimes observed in infants and the elderly.

Excessive Intake

Excessive intake of vitamin C (usually more than 3,000 milligrams per day) has been associated with such side effects as headaches, frequent urination, diarrhea, and nausea. Taking megadoses of the vitamin has become common practice among persons looking for both the proven and the speculative health benefits. As is true for all vitamins, consuming vitamin C in excessive dosages for long periods of time is not recommended.

Food and Supplement Sources

The primary form of vitamin C that is used in supplements is synthetic ascorbic acid. Other forms that are used are buffered vitamin C and mineral ascorbates such as calcium and magnesium ascorbate. A natural form of vitamin C is supplied by rose hips, but it is very expensive in comparison to the synthetic form. Look for supplements that contain both ascorbic acid and vitamin C from rose hips. In addition, look for vitamin-C supplements that contain the bioflavonoids, which may increase the absorption of vitamin C. (For a discussion of the bioflavonoids, see page 102.)

There is also a patented form of vitamin C available called ester C polyascorbate. According to independent studies financed by the manufacturer, it may have a higher bioavailability than the other forms of vitamin C. This makes it an especially good choice for individuals suffering from chronic illnesses such as cancer or AIDS.

The food sources of vitamin C include fruits and vegetables, especially citrus fruits, green and red peppers, collard greens, broccoli, spinach, tomatoes, potatoes, and strawberries.

Estimated Safe Range of Intake

The estimated safe range of intake for vitamin C for adults is 60 to 5,000 milligrams per day.

Performance Daily Intake

The PDI of vitamin C for men and women who are healthy and actively training is 800 to 3,000 milligrams.

Athletic Performance Goals

Studies support the adequate intake of vitamin C for the maintenance of overall health and athletic performance. However, current research does not support the practice of taking megadoses of vitamin C for the improvement of athletic performance. Keep your daily vitamin-C intake from food and supplement sources to within the PDI guidelines. Increase your vitamin-C intake as you increase your activity level to make sure you get adequate antioxidant benefits, especially if you are an endurance athlete. Some individuals also increase their intake levels to several thousand milligrams a day when they feel a cold or the flu coming on.

7. MINERALS

MORE MICRO PERFORMANCE FACTORS

Minerals have long been regarded as nutrients essential for proper health and vigor. As scientific equipment grows in sophistication, scientists continue to discover additional minerals that are vital to health. An example of the types of minerals that are still being isolated is trace minerals, which are needed in only very small amounts.

Minerals are inorganic elements that are required by the body. They are supplied either as a part of a mineral-organic compound, such as copper lysinate, or in an inorganic form, such as potassium chloride. While minerals are found throughout the body, they make up only about 4 to 6 percent of the body. They are, however, important because of their many structural and metabolic functions. They are components of tissues, as calcium is of bone. They are parts of organic molecules, as iodine is of thyroxine and iron is of hemoglobin. In ionic form, they occur in bodily fluids such as blood and cellular fluid, as does the group referred to as the electrolytes.

For enhanced athletic performance, minerals are just as important as vitamins. However, current research indicates that while athletes generally have higher mineral requirements than nonathletes do, they derive no clear benefits from taking megadose amounts. Most minerals are not immediately lethal if consumed in overdose amounts, but special care must still be exercised when taking them in supplemental form. Athletes need increased amounts because of the greater metabolic demands caused by their physical activity and to replenish the minerals they lose through sweat and excretion. However, for maximum performance, healthy, active adults should stay within the PDI guidelines. With few exceptions, current research does not support the practice of taking megadoses of minerals for the improvement of athletic performance.

Inadequate intake of minerals is associated with decreased athletic performance, so you must make sure that you consume the amounts that you in particular need. Additionally, if you do not get adequate amounts of the important structural minerals, such as calcium, your skeleton and connective tissues may become weakened, resulting in increased susceptibility to injury. For the best results, obtain your minerals from a combination of food and supplement sources. While food offers a variety of minerals, supplements supply them in precise amounts and in highly bioavailable forms.

In this chapter, we will discuss the minerals. Minerals are commonly referred to as minerals, trace minerals, or electrolytes. The minerals include calcium, magnesium, and phosphorus. The trace minerals include boron, chromium, copper, fluoride, germanium, iodine, iron, manganese, molybdenum, selenium, vanadium, and zinc. Chloride, potassium, and sodium are the major electrolytes, but calcium and magnesium also act as such. We will review the functions of all these minerals, how they improve athletic performance, their food and supplement sources, and the problems induced by their deficiency and excess intake. For each mineral, we will also provide the published safe range of intake and the PDI. For the RDIs, see Appendix E.

THE MINERALS

The minerals—calcium, magnesium, and phosphorus—are the major elements found in the body. They are taken in supplemental form generally in the range of milligrams to grams, usually at dosages of over 100 milligrams. Minerals are inorganic nutrients and play a role in the body in several ways. For example, they are found as soluble salts in bodily fluids and cells, serve as members of organic molecules, and function as structural components of bone and teeth. For the most part, excessive intake of a mineral will quickly result in some type of side effect. You should therefore make an extra effort to keep your mineral intake to within the recommended guidelines and avoid experimenting with megadoses.

Calcium

The average adult body contains approximately 1,200 grams of calcium, 99 percent of which is located in the skeleton. Calcium is found in the skeleton primarily as calcium phosphate. This is why the intake of both calcium and phosphorus are important to the integrity of bone tissue. Calcium also occurs in the body in ionic form and as calcium carbonate.

In addition to its role as the primary nutrient needed for bone formation and maintenance, calcium also plays essential roles in nerve conduction, nerve-impulse transmission, heart rate, muscle contraction, cell-membrane permeability, and blood clotting. It also functions as a coenzyme. Recently, calcium was connected to the control of blood pressure in some individuals.

In bone formation and maintenance, a positive calcium balance—that is, more calcium absorbed than excreted—is required for the proper mineralization of bone. This positive balance must be maintained during the growth years and throughout adulthood. Until recently, most medical authorities believed that after the age of thirty, building more bone tissue became impossible. However, research has now proven what many sports-fitness scientists already knew—exercise and the proper dietary intake of calcium result in increased bone density in adults of all ages. For athletes, these findings mean that an adequate calcium level must be maintained year-round, from childhood through the senior years. This translates into eating a diet high in calcium and taking a multi-vitamin-and-mineral supplement that includes calcium from good sources as well as all the calcium cofactors—vitamin D, boron, copper, manganese, and zinc.

Deficiency

Researchers have determined that calcium deficiency is more common than previously thought. Dietary surveys indicate that both athletes and nonathletes consume inadequate amounts of calcium. This can result in poor bone formation or the onset of a bone disease such as osteoporosis. Poor calcium intake can also cause muscle cramping and a reduced energy level. Rickets and stunted growth are also potential disorders related to a calcium-deficient diet.

Besides the total intake of calcium being low, the calcium in many diets is poorly absorbed. The same as other minerals, calcium occurs in different forms, some of which are absorbed by the body better than others. In fact, researchers have estimated that young adults absorb only 20 to 40 percent of the calcium they take in from food sources. This is another reason daily calcium supplements are vital.

Excessive Intake

Excessive intake of calcium does not appear to produce any major toxic side effects in adults aside from constipation and an increased risk of urinary-stone formation. A high calcium intake may interfere with the absorption of iron, zinc, magnesium, and other minerals. A very high calcium intake for a long period of time may lead to problems with renal functioning.

Food and Supplement Sources

The preferred forms of calcium that are used in supplements are calcium carbonate, calcium citrate, calcium malate, and calcium glycinate.

The food sources of calcium include dairy products such as milk, cheese, ice cream, sour cream, cottage cheese, and yogurt, as well as broccoli, kale, collard greens, oysters, shrimp, salmon, clams, calcium-precipitated tortillas, calcium-fortified foods, and antacid preparations.

Estimated Safe Range of Intake

The estimated safe range of intake for calcium for adults is 1,200 to 4,000 milligrams per day.

Performance Daily Intake

The PDI of calcium for men and women who are healthy and actively training is 1,200 to 2,600 milligrams.

Athletic Performance Goals

Studies support the adequate intake of calcium for the maintenance of overall health and athletic performance. However, current research does not support the practice of taking megadoses of calcium for the improvement of athletic performance. Keep your daily calcium intake from food and supplement sources to within the PDI guidelines.

Magnesium

Most of the magnesium that is present in the body is located in the bones, muscles, and soft tissues. Altogether, the average adult body contains about 24 grams of magnesium. Magnesium plays many metabolic and structural roles. It helps form bone and teeth, functions in muscle tissue and the nervous system, and activates enzymes. It assists calcium and potassium uptake, glycolysis, and many other metabolic processes. Athletes should note that several studies have shown that supplementing the diet with moderate amounts of magnesium (200 to 400 milligrams) improves several performance factors including endurance and strength. Researchers have also observed that athletes who increase their physical activity tend to deplete their magnesium stores. This seems to be especially true of endurance athletes.

Deficiency

Magnesium deficiency is rarely reported, but the symptoms include muscle weakness, irritability, nausea, and depression. Of interest to women, studies show that suboptimum intake of magnesium can cause or increase premenstrual discomfort. This can be corrected with magnesium supplementation.

Excessive Intake

Excessive intake of magnesium rarely produces toxic side effects. Healthy individuals seem to be able to tolerate magnesium well. Large amounts of magnesium (3,000 to 5,000 milligrams) have a laxative effect, and several laxative products contain magnesium compounds for this purpose. In addition, persons with abnormal renal functioning may suffer hypermagnesemia, which is marked by symptoms including depression, nausea, vomiting, and hypotension (abnormally low blood pressure).

Food and Supplement Sources

The forms of magnesium that are used in supplements are magnesium oxide, magnesium glycinate, and magnesium carbonate. Magnesium supplements should also contain calcium in a magnesium-to-calcium ratio of 1 to 2—for example, 300 milligrams of magnesium to 600 milligrams of calcium.

The food sources of magnesium include green vegetables, whole grains, nuts, legumes, oatmeal, and fruit.

Estimated Safe Range of Intake

The estimated safe range of intake for magnesium for healthy adults is up to 3,000 milligrams per day.

Performance Daily Intake

The PDI of magnesium for men and women who are healthy and actively training is 400 to 800 milligrams.

Athletic Performance Goals

Studies support the adequate intake of magnesium for the maintenance of overall health and athletic performance. However, current research does not support the practice of taking megadoses of magnesium for the improvement of athletic performance. Keep your daily magnesium intake from food and supplement sources to within the PDI guidelines.

Phosphorus

The same as calcium, phosphorus is an important part of bone, plus it plays several other significant roles in the body. Phosphorus is present in bone at a phosphorus-to-calcium ratio of 1 to 2—for example, 300 milligrams of phosphorus to 600 milligrams of calcium. In addition, it is found in lipids, proteins, nucleic acids, and other mediums in the body and is present in ionic form in cellular fluid. Among its functions, phosphorus is involved in cell-membrane permeability, metabolism of fats and carbohydrates, modulation of enzyme activity, phospholipid transportation of fatty acids, and synthesis of collagen. It also plays a vital role in the formation of ATP and creatine phosphate (CP), the phosphate compounds that store the chemical energy of the body.

Most diets normally supply adequate amounts of phosphorus, about 1,500 milligrams per day. Even so, some supplementation is recommended for athletes. Phosphate loading may also prove beneficial to certain athletes. Due to phosphate's role in cellular energy storage, phosphate loading has been studied as far back as the early 1900s. During World War I, German troops were fed diets and supplements high in phosphorus to improve their physical performance and to reduce fatigue. More recent research has verified the benefits of short-term phosphate loading, mostly for endurance athletes. The effects on power athletes are less clear, but research indicates that short-term phosphate loading may also improve endurance in anaerobic activities.

Deficiency

Because phosphorus is present in most foods, deficiency is rarely reported in adults. However, it has been observed in cases of malnutrition and in clinical settings among the ill. The symptoms of long-term phosphorus deficiency include poor bone formation, growth disorders, weakness, anorexia, and malaise.

Excessive Intake

Excessive intake of phosphorus has been reported to adversely affect calcium metabolism and to stimulate bone loss.

Food and Supplement Sources

The form of phosphorus that is used in supplements is the pure form. Because phosphorus is plentiful in the diet, its supplemental intake should be restricted to only 100 to 300 milligrams per day. If you are on a low-calorie diet, you may wish to consume a little more from supplement sources. Look for a supplement that has both phosphorus and calcium. The best choice is a supplement that contains phosphorus and calcium as parts of a complete multi-vitamin-and-mineral formulation.

While phosphorus is found in most foods, the best food sources are protein-rich foods and cereal grains. Good sources include milk, fish, eggs, asparagus, bran, brewer's yeast, corn, legumes, nuts, meats, poultry, salmon, and sesame, sunflower, and pumpkin seeds.

Estimated Safe Range of Intake

The estimated safe range of intake for phosphorus for adults is up to 4,000 milligrams per day for short periods of time.

Performance Daily Intake

The PDI of phosphorus for men and women who are healthy and actively training is 800 to 1,600 milligrams.

Athletic Performance Goals

Studies support the adequate intake of phosphorus for the maintenance of overall health and athletic performance. Keep your daily phosphorus intake from food and supplement sources to within the PDI guidelines. Research has supported the practice of taking megadoses of phosphorus, particularly by endurance athletes, for three days before competition for the improvement of performance. The dosage reportedly used was 1,000 milligrams of sodium phosphate four times per day. However, do not practice phosphate loading for more than three days, since the side effects have not been clearly established and the blood-phosphorus level remains high for several days after loading.

THE TRACE MINERALS

The trace minerals compose a subcategory of minerals that is open to interpretation. The minerals that we categorize as trace minerals include boron, chromium, copper, fluoride, germanium, iodine, iron, manganese, molybdenum, selenium, vanadium, and zinc. We call these substances trace minerals because their recommended dosages are in the microgram to milligram range. Some authorities base their classification of trace minerals on the nutrients' levels in the body, not on intake levels. Therefore, in other books and reference sources, you may see what we call a trace mineral listed as a mineral or an ultratrace mineral (a mineral taken in extremely small dosages).

What is more important than a mineral's classification is its function in the body. The trace minerals have a diversity of functions. Some act as cofactors and are required to activate other molecules; others are important parts of organic molecules; and still others have multiple functions. Whatever the function a trace mineral may display, however, maintenance of consistent intake is important. The same as the minerals, trace minerals taken in excessive amounts can cause toxic side effects. Therefore, make sure you stay within the recommended ranges of intake and do not experiment with taking megadoses.

Boron

Boron is a trace mineral that occurs in the body in small amounts. Despite this, it has been established as an essential mineral in humans. Boron appears to have several functions. In addition to influencing calcium, phosphorus, and magnesium metabolism, it affects parathyroid-hormone action, membrane functionality, and bone formation. Some researchers also believe that it increases testosterone production, a function that has won it the attention of athletes in recent years. According to a study published in 1987, supplemental boron increased the testosterone levels in postmenopausal women. However, translating this effect for younger adult males and females is speculative at best. A study in 1992 conducted with bodybuilders taking 2.5 milligrams of boron per day for seven weeks did not show any increases in testosterone levels, nor any significant increases in lean body mass or strength over the placebo group. Further research is needed to determine boron's exact benefits for athletes.

Deficiency

Boron deficiency has never been reported in a human. Because boron is required in such small quantities, it is obtained in adequate amounts from most diets.

Excessive Intake

Excessive intake (5,000 to 10,000 milligrams) of boron may result in side effects such as nausea, vomiting, diarrhea, dermatitis, lethargy, nervous-system irritability, renal failure, and shock.

Food and Supplement Sources

The preferred forms of boron that are used in supplements are boron tri chelate, boron glycinate, and boron citrate. Note that many supplements containing high amounts (some even more than 1,000 milligrams) of boron are currently being marketed and should be avoided until further research determines if these levels are indeed safe and effective.

The food sources of boron include leafy vegetables, fruit, nuts, and grains.

Estimated Safe Range of Intake

The estimated safe range of intake for boron for adults is up to 40 milligrams per day.

Performance Daily Intake

The PDI of boron for men and women who are healthy and actively training is 6 to 12 milligrams.

Athletic Performance Goals

Studies support the adequate intake of boron for the maintenance of overall health and athletic performance. However, current research does not support the practice of taking megadoses of boron for the improvement of athletic performance. Keep your daily boron intake from food and supplement sources to within the PDI guidelines.

Chromium

Chromium is another nutrient that has lately been receiving a lot of attention from the media. This is because it is being touted as everything from a muscle-building anabolic-steroid alternative to the mira-cle fat-loss aid of the 1990s. The fact is, however, that Madison Avenue has once again blown things out of proportion. In addition, manufacturers of the different forms of chromium have declared war on each other. But all that this three-ring circus has produced is massive confusion over what chromium is and what it does.

Chromium is merely another essential nutrient that the body requires for proper health and functioning. Its major role is as a potentiator of insulin—that is, it helps insulin do its job. Chromium also assists in the formation, structural maintenance, and metabolism of the nucleic acids. It helps fatty-acid and cholesterol formation in the liver and, according to some studies, may help lower cholesterol. Furthermore, chromium-deficient diets have been linked to higher incidences of diabetes and heart disease.

It is chromium's role as an insulin potentiator that has brought it the recent media attention, however. Early researchers found that chromium helps lower the blood-sugar level. Because of this, chromium has become known as a glucose tolerance factor. Chromium performs this function by helping glucose and amino acids circulating in the bloodstream to be taken up by the cells at a higher rate. This does not necessarily mean that the level of insulin is increased, nor does it mean that chromium has a direct effect on muscle building, the way testosterone does, or on fat loss, the way GH does. It just means that increasing the dietary chromium level should help improve insulin functioning. The cells use glucose and amino acids for energy and growth. If insulin functioning is not 100-percent efficient, the glucose and amino acids in the bloodstream circulate back to the liver and are possibly converted to fat. Insulin malfunctioning can also lead to the development of diabetes, heart disease, or another metabolic disorder.

Chromium's role in insulin functioning does not make it an anabolic agent either. Rather, chromium is an important cofactor for energy production and tissue growth and repair. For the athlete, adequate chromium intake is essential. Several studies have shown that taking supplemental chromium in association with a training program and good diet has helped increase the rate of muscle gain as well as the rate of fat loss. At the same time, however, other studies have reported no significant improvements in muscle building or fat loss.

Deficiency

Researchers in the 1950s first discovered chromium's essential role in nutrition when they fed chromium-deficient diets to laboratory animals and noticed the development of glucose intolerance. Further experiments resulted in the linking of low amounts of chromium in the diet with impaired glucose tolerance, certain forms of diabetes, poor appetite control, and heart disease.

Excessive Intake

Chromium toxicity is rarely reported, since chromium levels are low in food sources.

Food and Supplement Sources

The preferred forms of chromium that are used in supplements are chromium dinicotinate glycinate, chromium picolinate, and chromium polynicotinate.

The food sources of chromium include meat, mushrooms, liver, bread, brewer's yeast, black pepper, cheese, beer, brown rice, and potatoes.

Estimated Safe Range of Intake

The estimated safe range of intake for chromium for adults is up to 1,000 micrograms per day.

Performance Daily Intake

The PDI of chromium for men and women who are healthy and actively training is 200 to 600 micrograms.

Athletic Performance Goals

Studies support the adequate intake of chromium for the maintenance of overall health and athletic performance. However, current research does not support the practice of taking megadoses of chromium for the improvement of athletic performance. Keep your daily chromium intake from food and supplement sources to within the PDI guidelines.

Copper

Copper is a trace mineral with several important functions. Copper is present in many enzymes. It is important in the formation of collagen and is involved in melanin synthesis, myelin (nerve-fiber sheath) formation, immune functioning, glucose metabolism, and cholesterol metabolism. It also funtions in energy production, a role that attracted the attention of athletic researchers in the 1980s. It is part of cytochrome oxidase, an enzyme that is important in the production of energy. Copper is also part of superoxide dismutase (SOD), an antioxidant. In this last role, it is vital in the protection of the body at the cellular level, for performance, and for recovery.

Deficiency

The symptoms of copper deficiency include anemia, bone abnormalities, reproductive-system failure, abnormal skin pigmentation, decreased arterial elasticity, low SOD activity, and malformation of connective tissues.

Excessive Intake

Excessive intake of copper may result in side effects such as nausea, vomiting, hepatic necrosis (death of liver cells), and abdominal pain. It may also lead to death, especially in individuals with a hereditary disorder called Wilson's disease. Wilson's disease is characterized by the accumulation of copper in the body, leading to problems involving the liver, kidneys, eyes, and nervous system.

Food and Supplement Sources

The preferred forms of copper that are used in supplements are copper lysinate and copper gluconate. The recommended source is a multi-vitamin-and-mineral supplement that includes copper.

The food sources of copper include nuts, seafood, cocoa, chocolate, meat, mushrooms, and organ meats, especially liver.

Estimated Safe Range of Intake

The estimated safe range of intake for copper for adults is up to 10 milligrams per day.

Performance Daily Intake

The PDI of copper for men and women who are healthy and actively training is 3 to 6 milligrams.

Athletic Performance Goals

Studies support the adequate intake of copper for the

maintenance of overall health and athletic performance. However, current research does not support
the practice of taking megadoses of copper for the
improvement of athletic performance. Keep your
daily copper intake from food and supplement
sources to within the PDI guidelines.

Fluoride

The role of fluoride in the prevention of tooth decay
is well known. Less well known is the fact that fluoride has also been associated with increased bone
integrity. Fluoride is found not only in the teeth but
also, in very small amounts, in the bones and soft tissues. According to some research, in fact, maintaining
a good fluoride intake may help reduce osteoporosis.
For the athlete, however, fluoride has not been related to any increase in athletic performance. Its importance lies in the maintenance of good teeth for proper eating and the upkeep of a healthy skeleton. The
primary sources of fluoride are the public water supply and the diet. The link between low levels of fluoride in the water supply and increased tooth decay led
to the practice of adding fluoride to the water in areas
without naturally occurring fluoride. Fluoride supplements are also available but only by prescription.

Deficiency

Fluoride deficiency has been linked to increased
tooth decay and may be a factor in osteoporosis.

Excessive Intake

Excessive intake of fluoride may result in side effects
such as mottled teeth. It may also affect bone health,
kidney functioning, and possibly muscle and nerve
functioning. High intake (5,000 to 10,000 milligrams)
of sodium fluoride has been reported to result in death.

Food and Supplement Sources

The form of fluoride that is used in supplements is
sodium fluoride. Fluoride supplements are available
only by prescription. Fluoride is also included in
some prescription multi-vitamin-and-mineral supplements.

Fluoride is found in most foods in very low
amounts. It is present in tea in moderate amounts. In
fact, a dietary survey conducted in the United
Kingdom found that tea was the main source of fluoride for adults there, accounting for 1.3 milligrams
of the average total daily intake of 1.8 milligrams.

Estimated Safe Range of Intake

An estimated safe range of intake has not been established for fluoride.

Performance Daily Intake

No PDI value has been established for fluoride.

Athletic Performance Goals

No athletic performance goals have been established
for fluoride.

Germanium

Germanium is a relatively obscure trace mineral that
has been studied only in very recent times and primarily in Japan. Kazuhiko Asai, a Japanese researcher,
found that an intake of 100 to 300 milligrams of germanium a day helps increase the energy level, stimulates an adaptogenic response, improves circulation,
has an antitumor effect, reduces the cholesterol level,
combats certain viral infections, acts as a painkiller,
and helps improve arthritis and rheumatism. It
appears that one of the ways germanium works in the
body is by increasing the body's oxygen supply. An
increased oxygen supply has many beneficial effects.

However, despite all its apparent health benefits,
germanium is no longer available as a supplement in
the United States. Perhaps because the supplement,
known as germanium-32, worked so well, it was classified as a "new drug" by the FDA and ordered to be
put through the proper approval process in the 1980s.
The testing has not yet been finished, and a completion date has not been set. Luckily, several herbs that
are commonly used to treat health problems are good
sources of germanium. (For a list of the herbs, see
"Food and Supplement Sources" of germanium on
page 94.) It is interesting to note that these herbs have
been used for hundreds of years to promote energy,
assist healing, and prevent disease. Therefore, to take
advantage of germanium's health benefits, include
one or more of these herbs in your daily diet.

Deficiency

Germanium deficiency has never been reported in a
human.

Excessive Intake

Excessive intake of germanium does not appear to produce toxic side effects.

Food and Supplement Sources

Germanium currently is not available as a supplement in the United States.

The best food sources of germanium are ginseng, garlic, and aloe. Other sources include shiitake mushrooms, onions, comfrey, and boxthorn seed.

Estimated Safe Range of Intake

No estimated safe range of intake has been established for germanium.

Performance Daily Intake

No PDI value has been established for germanium.

Athletic Performance Goals

No athletic performance goals have been established for germanium.

Iodine

Iodine, form-wise, is the simplest mineral that occurs in the body. Its function is also simple. Iodine is found in two thyroid hormones—thyroxine and triiodothyronine—and is therefore required for the proper functioning of the thyroid gland. The thyroid helps regulate metabolism, energy production, growth, and overall physical performance.

Deficiency

Since iodine is essential only for thyroid-gland functioning, a deficiency of iodine is associated with thyroid-gland disorders. The classic symptom of iodine deficiency is goiter, which is a condition manifested by enlargement of the thyroid gland. Cretism, a disorder marked by mental retardation and dwarfism, results from an iodine deficiency present at birth and left untreated.

Excessive Intake

Excessive intake of iodine may result in side effects such as rash, headache, a metallic taste in the mouth, and thyroid-gland dysfunction.

Food and Supplement Sources

Iodine is supplied in supplements through kelp concentrate. The recommended source is a multi-vitamin-and-mineral supplement that includes iodine. Iodized salt can also be considered a supplemental source of iodine. However, most people try to avoid increasing their salt intake.

The food sources of iodine include iodized salt, seafood, cod, cod-liver oil, halibut, oysters, kelp, spinach, meat, and dairy products.

Estimated Safe Range of Intake

The estimated safe range of intake for iodine for adults is up to 1,000 micrograms per day.

Performance Daily Intake

The PDI of iodine for men and women who are healthy and actively training is 200 to 400 micrograms.

Athletic Performance Goals

Studies support the adequate intake of iodine for the maintenance of overall health and athletic performance. However, current research does not support the practice of taking megadoses of iodine for the improvement of athletic performance. Keep your daily iodine intake from food and supplement sources to within the PDI guidelines.

Iron

Iron is best known for its role as a part of hemoglobin, a carrier of oxygen in the body. It also is a constituent of myoglobin, a form of hemoglobin found in muscle tissue, and of a number of enzymes. Iron is primarily stored in the body in the bone marrow, spleen, and liver. When iron intake is low, the body depletes these stores, which results in the development of anemia, but only after a grace period. However, when anemia does occur due to severe iron depletion, it takes a long time to cure. For the athlete, this can be extremely detrimental. Dietary surveys report that many athletes consume diets low in iron. Female athletes, endurance athletes, and athletes on low-calorie diets are especially prone to iron deficiency.

Deficiency

The most common symptom of iron deficiency is anemia. Anemia causes a reduction in the oxygen-carrying capacity of the blood, which results in decreased athletic performance. Additionally, iron deficiency has been linked to impaired immune-system functioning, which increases susceptibility to disease.

Excessive Intake

Excessive intake of iron may lead to toxicity, which is potentially harmful, especially in young children. If the amount is large enough, it may even lead to death. Each year, a few thousand cases of iron poisoning are reported in the United States. Several of these cases result in death. The deaths are usually of very young children who ate large quantities of iron-containing supplements. The lethal dose for a one- to two-year-old child is about 3,000 milligrams. For adults, the lethal dose ranges from 200 to 250 milligrams per 1 kilogram (2.2 pounds) of body weight. Oral dosages of about 200 milligrams can cause abdominal cramping, constipation or diarrhea, and nausea.

Excessive intake of iron may also cause certain liver disorders. In addition, individuals with idiopathic hemochromatosis, a rare hereditary disorder, absorb iron at a higher rate than normal and slowly accumulate high iron stores. This may lead to problems with the liver and other organs.

Food and Supplement Sources

Supplements have become a primary source of iron for most people concerned with iron intake. However, the correct form of supplemental iron is required for safety, absorption, and efficacy. The preferred forms of iron that are used in supplements are ferrous fumarate and iron glycinate. The recommended source is a multi-vitamin-and-mineral supplement that includes iron.

The food sources of iron include red meat, poultry, fish, iron-fortified foods, liver, molasses, nuts, clams, chocolate, legumes, and bread.

Estimated Safe Range of Intake

The estimated safe range of intake for iron for adults is up to 80 milligrams. However, higher amounts are sometimes given under medical supervision.

Performance Daily Intake

The PDI of iron for men and women who are healthy and actively training is 25 to 60 milligrams.

Athletic Performance Goals

Studies support the adequate intake of iron for the maintenance of overall health and athletic performance. However, current research does not support the practice of taking megadoses of iron for the improvement of athletic performance. In fact, high dosages of iron (200 to 300 milligrams or more per day) may have detrimental effects. Keep your daily iron intake from food and supplement sources to within the PDI guidelines.

Manganese

Manganese is another trace mineral with several important functions. Manganese is required for energy production. In addition, it is a component of enzymes and the antioxidant SOD, aids in bone and connective-tissue formation, helps collagen synthesis, and facilitates carbohydrate metabolism. Manganese's role in the formation of bone and connective tissue is of particular importance to athletes. The strength and maintenance of bone and connective tissue are essential for performance. Manganese can benefit injury prevention and recovery. Maintaining the body's SOD supply is also an important function linked to manganese. SOD is a powerful antioxidant that helps protect the body against free-radical damage.

Deficiency

Manganese deficiency is rarely reported, but the symptoms include growth disorders, poor formation and maintenance of bone and connective tissue, low SOD production, and disturbed energy production. Because manganese is essential in bone and cartilage formation and is a component of SOD, deficiency can also lead to certain degenerative diseases such as osteoporosis and arthritis.

Excessive Intake

Manganese toxicity is rarely reported in healthy adults.

Food and Supplement Sources

The preferred forms of manganese that are used in supplements are manganese arginate, manganese glycinate, and manganese gluconate. The recommended source is a multi-vitamin-and-mineral supplement that includes manganese.

The food sources of manganese include Brussels sprouts, spinach, peas, turnip greens, wheat germ, meat, beets, bananas, corn, lettuce, barley seeds, and whole-grain foods such as oatmeal and buckwheat.

Estimated Safe Range of Intake

The estimated safe range of intake for manganese for adults is up to 50 milligrams per day.

Performance Daily Intake

The PDI of manganese for men and women who are healthy and actively training is 15 to 45 milligrams.

Athletic Performance Goals

Studies support the adequate intake of manganese for the maintenance of overall health and athletic performance. However, current research does not support the practice of taking megadoses of manganese for the improvement of athletic performance. Keep your daily manganese intake from food and supplement sources to within the PDI guidelines.

Molybdenum

Molybdenum is a trace mineral that is found in the body in extremely small amounts. Despite this, it is recognized as an essential nutrient and is required by the body for the maintenance of good health. Molybdenum is present in enzymes such as xanthine oxidase, sulfite oxidase, and aldehyde oxidase. These compounds are involved in energy production, nitrogen metabolism, and uric-acid formation.

Deficiency

Molybdenum deficiency has never been reported in a human. Because molybdenum is required in such small quantities, it is obtained in adequate amounts from most diets.

Excessive Intake

Excessive intake (15,000 or more micrograms daily for several months) of molybdenum may result in side effects such as gout, growth disorders, and a lowered copper level.

Food and Supplement Sources

Among the forms of molybdenum that are used in supplements are molybdenum chelate and sodium molybdate. The recommended source is a multi-vitamin-and-mineral supplement that includes molybdenum.

The food sources of molybdenum include milk, beans, bread, cereal, and organ meats. The amount of molybdenum found in a food can vary considerably with the region.

Estimated Safe Range of Intake

The estimated safe range of intake for molybdenum for adults is up to 600 micrograms per day.

Performance Daily Intake

The PDI of molybdenum for men and women who are healthy and actively training is 100 to 300 micrograms.

Athletic Performance Goals

Studies support the adequate intake of molybdenum for the maintenance of overall health and athletic performance. However, current research does not support the practice of taking megadoses of molybdenum for the improvement of athletic performance. Keep your daily molybdenum intake from food and supplement sources to within the PDI guidelines.

Selenium

Selenium's antioxidant activity in the body is well known. Selenium is a vital component of an antioxidant enzyme called glutathione peroxidase. Glutathione peroxidase protects the body against free radicals, in particular hydroperoxides. In this role as an antioxidant, selenium helps prevent damage to the body's tissues, cells, and molecules, which can lead to reduced risk of degenerative diseases such as heart disease, arthritis, and certain cancers. For athletes, this antioxidant activity is important for the protection of tissues, shortening of recovery time, and protection against the extra free-radical load created by exercise. The few studies done on the use of supplemental selenium by athletes reported encouraging findings of a reduction in lipid peroxidation. This translates into reduced tissue damage.

Deficiency

Low intake of selenium can have widespread adverse effects due to the reduction of the body's defenses against hydroperoxide free radicals. The symptoms of selenium deficiency include hair loss, growth disorders, pancreatic problems, muscular discomfort, and weakness.

Excessive Intake

Excessive intake of selenium may result in side effects such as fingernail and toenail changes, hair loss, fatigue, abdominal pain, nausea, increased dental caries, diarrhea, and irritability. Some studies have reported side effects starting with dosages of 5,000 micrograms per day, and dosages of as little as 1,000 micrograms per day may cause fingernail fragility.

Food and Supplement Sources

The preferred form of selenium that is used in supplements is selenomethionine. The recommended source is a multi-vitamin-and-mineral supplement that includes selenium.

The food sources of selenium include Brazil nuts, meat, seafood, kidney, liver, and whole grains such as whole wheat, oats, and millet. The selenium content of a food is dependent upon the selenium content of the soil where the food is from. This includes both foods grown in the soil and products from animals that were fed locally grown foods.

Estimated Safe Range of Intake

The estimated safe range of intake for selenium for adults is up to 1,000 micrograms per day.

Performance Daily Intake

The PDI of selenium for men and women who are healthy and actively training is 100 to 300 micrograms.

Athletic Performance Goals

Studies support the adequate intake of selenium for the maintenance of overall health and athletic performance. However, current research does not support the practice of taking megadoses of selenium for the improvement of athletic performance. Keep your daily selenium intake from food and supplement sources to within the PDI guidelines.

Vanadium

Vanadium is another trace mineral that has become popular among athletes, especially bodybuilders and power athletes, who are reported to be heavy users of vanadium supplements. The interest is due to vanadium's function in glucose metabolism, its role as an insulin cofactor, and even its potential ability to mimic the action of insulin. Marketing executives are using these functions as the basis for claims that the mineral is an anabolic-steroid alternative that increases protein synthesis and reduces fat. Vanadium is known to inhibit cholesterol synthesis. In addition, research has shown that it is needed for cellular metabolism, for the formation of bones and teeth, and for growth and reproduction.

Deficiency

Vanadium deficiency may be linked to cardiovascular disease, kidney disease, reproductive disorders, and infant mortality. Vanadium is not easily absorbed in the body. In addition, smoking decreases the body's uptake of vanadium.

Excessive Intake

Excessive intake of vanadium may lead to toxicity. The symptoms include black discoloration of the tongue, slowed growth, diarrhea, hypoglycemia, and anorexia. If the intake is excessive enough, it may even lead to death. Currently, less than 1,000 micrograms are found in most supplements, although many bodybuilding products contain as much as 30,000 micrograms. Harmful levels have not been clearly established, but consuming more than 1,000 micrograms of vanadium per day for long periods of time is not recommended and should be done only under careful medical supervision.

Food and Supplement Sources

The average adult diet supplies about 10 to 20 micrograms of vanadium per day. If you choose to take supplemental vanadium, do not exceed this range. Furthermore, since vanadium is one of the more toxic minerals, restrict its supplemental use to a few weeks at a time. The preferred forms of vanadium that are used in supplements are vanadium, vanadyl sulfate, and vanadate.

The food sources of vanadium include dill, fish, olives, meat, radishes, snap beans, vegetable oil, and whole grains.

Estimated Safe Range of Intake

No estimated safe range of intake has been established for vanadium.

Performance Daily Intake

No PDI value has been established for vanadium.

Athletic Performance Goals

No athletic performance goals have been established for vanadium.

Zinc

In athletic circles, zinc has acquired the reputation of being one of the primary healing nutrients and a major contributor to male fertility. Zinc plays many important metabolic roles in the body. It is part of various metalloenzymes (mineral-containing enzymes) that function in growth, testosterone production, DNA synthesis, cell replication, fertility, reproduction, and prostate-gland functioning. It occurs in ionic form in cells, assists in the synthesis of molecules, and serves as a component of enzymes. For athletes, maintaining proper zinc intake is vital, especially for the growth and repair of muscle tissue to meet the recovery demands of training. Dietary surveys conducted among athletes show that low zinc intake is common, especially by endurance athletes, athletes on low-calorie diets, power athletes, bodybuilders, and female athletes. At the same time, very few studies have been conducted to examine the effects of zinc supplementation on performance, although one study did show that an effect is increased muscle endurance. Further research will reveal additional benefits for performance. Note that taking too much zinc may impair performance. Zinc's role in healing and testosterone production should not lead you to think that taking more of the mineral is better. It is not. Stick to the PDI guidelines for zinc intake; do not take megadoses.

Deficiency

The symptoms of zinc deficiency include growth disorders, loss of appetite, skin changes, immune-system disorders, delayed sexual maturation, night blindness, and impaired healing.

Excessive Intake

Excessive intake of zinc may result in side effects such as a lowered HDL level, inhibition of copper absorption, nausea, gastrointestinal disorders, headaches, dizziness, and other metabolic disturbances.

Food and Supplement Sources

The preferred forms of zinc that are used in supplements are zinc citrate and zinc arginate. Zinc supplementation is especially recommended for athletes, who tend to consume diets that are high in protein, fiber, or both. Diets high in these macronutrients can impair zinc absorption, and zinc supplementation can ensure adequate zinc intake.

The food sources of zinc include meat, wholegrain products, liver, eggs, seafood, herring, oysters, oatmeal, and maple syrup.

Estimated Safe Range of Intake

The estimated safe range of intake for zinc for adults is up to 80 milligrams per day.

Performance Daily Intake

The PDI of zinc for men and women who are healthy and actively training is 15 to 60 milligrams.

Athletic Performance Goals

Studies support the adequate intake of zinc for the maintenance of overall health and athletic performance. However, current research does not support the practice of taking megadoses of zinc for the improvement of athletic performance. Keep your daily zinc intake from food and supplement sources to within the PDI guidelines.

THE ELECTROLYTES

Sodium, potassium, and chloride are collectively referred to as the electrolytes. An electrolyte is an ion that is required by the body to regulate the electric charge and flow of water between the cells and the bloodstream. Sodium, potassium, and chloride are considered the primary electrolytes in the body, although a number of other minerals also display electrolyte activity. Some authorities count magnesium as a primary electrolyte, but we are treating it separately here due to its unique nonelectrolyte functions and supplement requirements. (For a discussion of magnesium, see page 88.)

Chloride

Chloride is the body's most important extracellular-fluid anion. An anion is a negatively charged molecule. Extracellular fluid is any fluid that is found in areas of the body outside the cells, such as interstitial fluid, lymph, and blood. Chloride plays an essential role in controlling fluid balance and blood acid-base (pH) balance. It is also a component of the stomach's digestive-juice secretions, which are required for the formation of hydrochloric acid.

Deficiency

Chloride deficiency is rarely observed, but the symptoms include dizziness, fainting, and reduced performance. It generally occurs only under conditions of severe dehydration, during prolonged periods of exercise without proper hydration or electrolyte replenishment, or with renal disease.

Excessive Intake

Excessive intake of chloride may result in side effects such as hypertension and problems with fluid balance.

Food and Supplement Sources

Many tablet and capsule supplements contain chloride as part of the hydrochloric molecule that is a common part of some of the ingredients. Powder and liquid supplements usually contain just minor amounts of chloride.

In foods, chloride is supplied mostly as sodium chloride. Table salt and processed foods are by far the primary sources.

Estimated Safe Range of Intake

An estimated safe range of intake has not been established for chloride.

Performance Daily Intake

The PDI of chloride for men and women who are healthy and actively training is 1,500 to 4,500 milligrams.

Athletic Performance Goals

Studies support the adequate intake of chloride for the maintenance of overall health and athletic performance. However, current research does not support the practice of taking megadoses of chloride for the improvement of athletic performance. Keep your daily chloride intake from food and supplement sources to within the PDI guidelines.

Potassium

Potassium functions in the body primarily as an intracellular-fluid cation. A cation is a positively charged ion. Intracellular fluid is any fluid that is found within a cell. As an intracellular cation, potassium is essential to all living cells. It helps maintain fluid balance and functions in nerve transmission, muscle contraction, and glycogen formation.

Deficiency

Because potassium is present in most foods, deficiency is rarely reported. However, deficiency has been observed in cases of inadequate dietary intake due to malnutrition and depletion due to dehydration. A common cause of potassium depletion is prolonged use of diuretics, which promote potassium excretion via the kidneys. The symptoms of potassium deficiency include anorexia, nausea, drowsiness, weakness, and cardiac dysrhythmia.

Excessive Intake

Excessive intake (18,000 milligrams or more) of potassium can cause acute hyperkalemia, which may lead to cardiac arrest and possibly even death. Hyperkalemia is a condition in which the blood-potassium level is abnormally high, usually due to a failure by the kidneys to excrete the potassium.

Food and Supplement Sources

The average adult diet supplies about 2,500 to 3,400 milligrams of potassium per day. Individuals who consume high amounts of fruits and vegetables may even take in as much as 11,000 milligrams of potassium per day. However, if you are concerned that your potassium intake may be low, look for a multi-vitamin-and-mineral supplement that contains potassium. The forms of potassium that are used in supplements are potassium chloride, potassium ascorbate, and potassium–amino acid complexes.

The best food sources of potassium are fruits and vegetables.

Estimated Safe Range of Intake

An estimated safe range of intake has not been established for potassium.

Performance Daily Intake

The PDI of potassium for men and women who are healthy and actively training is 2,500 to 4,000 milligrams.

Athletic Performance Goals

Studies support the adequate intake of potassium for the maintenance of overall health and athletic performance. Keep your daily potassium intake from food and supplement sources to within the PDI guidelines. If you are an athlete who does not eat fruits and vegetables, take a multi-vitamin-and-mineral supplement that contains potassium. If you are an athlete who trains for long hours in a hot climate or experiences profuse water loss through sweating, you, too, should take a multi-vitamin-and-mineral supplement that contains potassium. However, taking megadoses of potassium is not recommended.

Sodium

While potassium is the body's main intracellular cation, sodium is the body's main extracellular cation. Sodium helps regulate the body's volume of extracellular fluids, particularly the blood. It also helps regulate the pressure of these fluids, aids the active transport of nutrients across cell membranes, and assists the uptake of some nutrients in the intestines. In addition, it functions in muscle contraction and nerve-impulse transmission.

Deficiency

Because sodium is present in most foods, deficiency is rarely reported. It generally occurs only under conditions of severe dehydration, during prolonged periods of exercise without proper hydration or electrolyte replenishment, or with renal disease. The side effects include dizziness, fainting, and reduced performance.

Excessive Intake

Excessive intake of sodium may result in side effects such as hypertension, problems with fluid balance, and edema.

Food and Supplement Sources

Most tablet and capsule supplements are sodium-free. Powder and liquid supplements usually contain some sodium.

In foods, sodium is supplied mostly as sodium chloride, although sodium bicarbonate and monosodium glutamate also contribute a good share. Table salt and processed foods are by far the primary sources.

Estimated Safe Range of Intake

An estimated safe range of intake has not been established for sodium.

Performance Daily Intake

The PDI of sodium for men and women who are healthy and actively training is 1,500 to 4,500 milligrams.

Athletic Performance Goals

Studies support the adequate intake of sodium for the maintenance of overall health and athletic performance. However, current research does not support the practice of taking megadoses of sodium for the improvement of athletic performance. Keep your daily sodium intake from food and supplement sources to within the PDI guidelines. Although athletes have higher requirements for sodium due to excessive sweating and increased physical activity, their higher food intake usually supplies enough additional sodium.

8. METABOLITES AND HERBS
THE NEW PERFORMANCE FACTORS

In addition to the macronutrients and traditional micronutrients (vitamins and minerals), several other substances have been shown to benefit performance and health. These items fall into the remaining categories of metabolites and herbs. Metabolites are substances that take part in metabolism. Some are produced in the body as part of the metabolic process, while others are derived from food sources. Some are now also available in supplemental form. Even though the body is able to make many of these substances, loading up on them allows athletes to prevent shortages during exercise and to have an immediately available supply on hand. Much of the pioneering research to determine which metabolites are important to athletes was conducted in clinical settings using both individuals with metabolic disorders and patients recovering from injuries or surgery. The researchers discovered that the subjects not only overcame their disorders but often went on to attain a state of health better than what they had started with. Studies conducted with athletes demonstrated that certain metabolites improve such athletic-performance factors as strength, agility, speed, and aerobic capacity.

Also discussed in this chapter are the popular athletic herbs. The use of herbs in sports is on the rise because when athletes use the correct herbs, they can influence their performance and health. While hundreds of herbs are available in health-food stores and herbal shops, we have singled out the ones that are favored by athletes. An extensive table provides an overview of these herbs, giving brief descriptions of their athletic uses and purposes, the plant parts used, and a selection of other names. Comments and cautions are also included.

Metabolite and herbal supplements are sold in health-food stores, pharmacies, and gyms and through mail-order catalogs and professional trainers. As their popularity continues to grow, some are even making their way onto supermarket shelves. Metabolites and herbs are available as single-ingredient formulations and as part of multi-vitamin-and-mineral formulations. They come in tablet, powder, and liquid forms.

To have an ergogenic effect, most must be ingested in large amounts for short periods of time or taken daily in smaller amounts for longer periods of time to build up stores in the body. Many of the supplements are expensive, and care should be taken to select products manufactured by reputable companies. If one product is much cheaper than similar products, it is probably of a lesser quality.

Use caution when taking any dietary supplement. To be extra safe, keep a record of your daily intake. For the dosage you should take, see your sport-specific plan in Part Four. Competitive athletes should also check with the organization that governs their sport to make sure that the supplement ingredients are acceptable. This is especially important when using herbal supplements, which may include a banned substance, such as ephedra. Ephedra is unacceptable for athletic use because it contains ephedrine and pseudoephedrin.

METABOLITES

The metabolites include a diversity of substances. By definition, a metabolite is a product of metabolism. This means that anything made in the body is a metabolite. Thousands of metabolites are produced by the human body. At present, however, science has determined that only the following metabolites benefit athletic performance in any measurable way.

Beta-Hydroxy Beta-Methylbutyrate

Beta-hydroxy beta-methylbutyrate (BHBM) is one of the newer metabolite supplements to gain popularity. It is being touted as an aid to muscle gain when used in association with a weightlifting program.

Beta-hydroxy beta-methylbutyrate seems to be a breakdown product of the amino acid leucine and may play an important role in protein metabolism. Studies have indicated that when it is taken in supplemental amounts, it boosts nitrogen retention, thereby helping the body to hang onto more amino acids, which are necessary for muscle growth and repair. BHBM therefore may be useful for individuals training to increase muscle mass. According to studies, supplemental amounts ranging from 1,500 to 4,000 milligrams yield positive results. However, if you choose to try BHBM, use it as part of a rounded supplement program, not alone.

Bicarbonate

Bicarbonate is a member of a group of metabolites that has been creating excitement in the sports world in recent years. Known as blood buffers, these metabolites are substances that help maintain the pH balance in the blood. When the blood becomes too acidic due to lactic-acid buildup, fatigue sets in and performance is impaired. Bicarbonate, in particular sodium bicarbonate, is the blood buffer that has gotten most of the attention.

Many studies have reported that sodium bicarbonate produces ergogenic effects in individuals repeatedly exercising to capacity, for several seconds to several minutes. These ergogenic effects have all been confirmed in studies performed with sprinters and world-class rowers. Large amounts of sodium bicarbonate are needed, however—about 100 milligrams for every 1 pound of lean body mass. This means that if you had, for example, 150 pounds of lean body mass, you would need about 15,000 milligrams of sodium bicarbonate. The exact dosage would depend on whether you experienced any side effects, which include diarrhea, nausea, cramps, and flatulence. If you suffered no side effects, you could take your dosage on an empty stomach one hour before your activity. If you experienced gastrointestinal side effects, you would do better starting two hours before your activity and taking one-fourth of your dosage with water every fifteen minutes. Sodium-bicarbonate loading also packs the body with a few thousand milligrams of sodium, so be careful if you have blood-pressure problems or hypertension.

The Bioflavonoids

The bioflavonoids are a group of naturally occurring plant compounds that are associated with vitamin C. They actually improve vitamin-C absorption. The bioflavonoids have been proven to strengthen capillary walls and thereby prevent capillary damage. They may also have an anti-inflammatory effect and anti-cataract activity. They exhibit antioxidant activity and help reduce destruction of vitamin C. The ergogenic effects of the bioflavonoids have not yet been tested, but this group of plant compounds has been noted to improve recovery and to provide nutritional support for athletes healing from injury.

The major bioflavonoids that are available in supplemental form are rutin, hesperidin, citrus, quercetin, flavone, and the flavonols. All are water soluble and found in fruits, such as citrus fruits, grapes, plums, apricots, cherries, blackberries, and rose hips. The recommended daily dosage for each is 200 to 2,000 milligrams.

Carnitine

Carnitine is an organic compound that is often considered an amino acid but that is actually classified as an amine. An amine is a nitrogen-containing compound in which at least one hydrogen atom has been replaced with a hydrocarbon radical. Carnitine can be made by the body when sufficient amounts of lysine, methionine, iron, and vitamins B_1, B_6, and C are available. A deficiency of any of these nutrients can lead to a carnitine deficiency. Carnitine is also available from dietary sources, mainly meat and other foods of animal origin. As a supplement, carnitine is available as D-carnitine, L-carnitine, DL-carnitine, and acetyl-L-carnitine. The preferred form is L-carnitine.

Carnitine's primary role in the body is helping to transport fatty acids into the mitochondria. Studies have shown that supplemental L-carnitine raises the level of carnitine in the resting muscles. Other research has demonstrated that it promotes certain improvements in athletic performance including increased endurance, a reduced blood-lactate level during exercise, and improved anaerobic-strength output. Supplementation with L-carnitine may also help increase the rate of fat loss, but more studies need to be conducted to clearly establish this.

Studies support L-carnitine supplementation by competitive athletes who are intensively training. Benefits, however, have not been reported for athletes who participate in low-intensity activities. Despite this, both endurance and power athletes can benefit from L-carnitine. Dosages of 1,000 to 3,000 milligrams per day for several weeks before competition have reportedly yielded performance benefits. Carnitine loading, using dosages of 2,000 to 5,000 milligrams of L-carnitine per day for one week before competition, has also enhanced performance.

Choline

Choline, often classified as a member of the B-complex family, is an essential vitamin that can be synthesized in the body. It is a lipotropic agent, involved in fatty-acid metabolism and the prevention of fat deposition in the liver. Choline is a component of lecithin and a part of all cell membranes and lipoproteins. It is also used by the body to make acetylcholine, a neurotransmitter that is critical for optimum nervous-system functioning. More research is necessary to determine the exact effects of choline on athletic performance.

Exercise, however, is known to affect choline, depleting the body's supply, which theoretically can decrease the production of acetylcholine and hurt the nervous system. Choline deficiency may also impact the liver, memory, and growth. Luckily, choline deficiency is rarely seen in humans, since the average adult diet supplies about 400 to 900 milligrams of choline per day. While no RDA has been set for choline, the PDI of choline for men and women who are healthy and actively training is 600 to 1,200 milligrams. Intake of 2,000 or more milligrams per day may result in side effects such as diarrhea, depression, and dizziness.

Choline is found in a number of foods including lecithin, egg yolks, liver, soybeans, most fatty foods, meat, whole grains, asparagus, green beans, spinach, and wheat germ. It is also available in supplement form as choline bitartrate, choline dihydrogen citrate, and phosphatidylcholine. In addition, it is a common ingredient in multi-vitamin-and-mineral supplements, lipotropic supplements, and lecithin supplements.

Coenzyme Q_{10}

Coenzyme Q_{10} is also known as ubiquinone. It has a history of clinical use with people suffering from cardiovascular disorders. In addition, studies conducted with athletes report ergogenic effects such as improved physical performance in endurance events. Coenzyme Q_{10}'s safety and effectiveness are well established.

Coenzyme Q_{10} is found in all mitochondria. It participates in the manufacture of ATP and may even act as a limiting factor in the energy-producing process. In addition, Q_{10} has recently been identified as a powerful antioxidant and cell-membrane stabilizer.

As an endurance enhancer, coenzyme Q_{10} espe-cially benefits long-distance athletes. The recommended daily dosage of Q_{10} for its ergogenic effects is 60 to 300 milligrams. For all athletes, the recommended dosage of Q_{10} for its antioxidant effects is 10 to 60 milligrams per day.

Colostrum

Colostrum is the special milk that is secreted by mammals after they give birth. It contains important growth factors, immune-system compounds, and other nutrients that help the new offspring get a jump-start on life. Colostrum production slows down forty-eight to seventy-two hours after birth.

Commercial colostrum, which is primarily bovine (cow) colostrum, has been on the market for a long time and, like cow's milk, is consumed by humans. While the benefits of colostrum for newborns are clearly understood, the benefits for human adults are of growing interest. Dr. Bernard Jensen, a pioneer in the field of nutrition, is one of the great proponents of colostrum, which he calls "white gold." Colostrum's clearly proven benefits are to the digestive system. Its immunoglobulins (Ig's) and growth factors—in particular, its insulin-like growth factors (IGFs)—help keep the lining of the digestive system healthy. They also assist with the maintenance of the intestine's "good bacteria," which help keep the "bad bacteria" in check. Studies with adults and children have shown that colostrum combats severe diarrhea. In athletes, colostrum helps normalize the gastrointestinal system and reduces diarrhea. This leads to better digestion and better absorption of other nutrients, which means better nitrogen balance and recovery. (For a discussion of nitrogen balance, see page 34.) Additionally, the Ig's in colostrum can benefit the immune system. Athletes' immune systems are constantly being stressed by exercise.

The second-level benefits that colostrum has to offer are less certain but are supported by indirect evidence and case studies. The IGFs found in colostrum are known to be critical in the promotion of growth and have been clinically shown to improve nitrogen balance and to increase muscle growth. This is why colostrum exists in mother's milk during the critical first few days of lactation (milk production). The voluminous research data on these powerful growth factors is compelling. Without exception, studies document how two of the most important growth factors found in colostrum, insulin-like growth factor I (IGF-I) and insulin-like growth factor II (IGF-II), enhance DNA and protein synthesis. IGF-I and IGF-II are the healing properties of colostrum. Their muscle-building and connective-tissue-repair characteristics are biochemically unsurpassed. They are essential ingredients in muscle growth, primarily through their roles in the repair and conversion of broken-down muscle fibers.

All told, colostrum has potential as a component in the athlete's diet. Please note, however, that if you choose to take a colostrum supplement, you should look for a standardized product, since the Ig content does tend to vary. We have found colostrum with an Ig content of 26 to 33 percent to be ideal. Colostrum is available as a supplement both alone and as part of a formulation.

Creatine

Creatine is manufactured in the body during protein metabolism. It is also present in food and available in supplemental form as creatine monohydrate. Creatine monohydrate is consumed to increase the body's stores of creatine and creatine phosphate (CP). CP is produced in the body by the combination of creatine and phosphate. In the body, CP is stored in muscle tissue along with ATP. Together, CP and ATP store the chemical energy of the body. The more energy they store, the better the muscles can perform in short-term maximum-strength events.

The body uses CP to quickly replenish ATP, a process that takes just seconds. Creatine loading can therefore bring about improved training intensity and recovery in anaerobic sports involving all-out effort for short periods of time (a few seconds). Dosages of creatine monohydrate that have reportedly been used for this purpose range from 1,000 to 24,000 milligrams per day. For long-term building-up of the creatine level, the recommended daily dosage is 8 milligrams for every 1 pound of lean body mass, or about 1,000 to 2,000 milligrams total. For short-term creatine loading, take 80 to 160 milligrams for every 1 pound of lean body mass, or about 10,000 to 24,000 milligrams total, every day for several days.

Dehydroepiandrosterone

Dehydroepiandrosterone (DHEA) entered the dietary-supplement market during the last few years as, among other things, a longevity substance. However, take note that DHEA is not for everyone; most health authorities do not recommend it for individuals under the age of forty. The DHEA level declines with age, and younger people do not seem to benefit from supplemental DHEA because their bodies are already making enough. Note, too, that DHEA is banned by many sports governing bodies.

DHEA is a hormone produced mainly by the adrenal glands. In men, it is also produced in the testes as an intermediate in testosterone production; and in women, it is also produced in the ovaries as an intermediate in estrogen production. DHEA seems to be a weak androgen (a steroid hormone that promotes masculine characteristics), and it has also been reported to induce growth of body hair in men and women. However, in a study using men between the ages of twenty and twenty-five, supplemental DHEA did not increase testosterone levels but did appear to help decrease body fat and increase lean body mass. Conversely, in another study, an increase in androgen levels was reported in postmenopausal women given supplemental DHEA, as was an increase in body-hair growth during the study period. Another study, this one using both men and women, did not report any significant changes in lean body mass or body fat but did report an overall improvement in the feeling of well-being. This last study also reported a possible anabolic effect—an increase in the IGF-I level. IGF-I is an important growth promoter in muscles, especially in individuals undergoing intensive training. (For a discussion of IGF-I, see "Colostrum" on page 103.)

Studies with athletes have not yet been reported. Going by the results of the studies just mentioned, medically unsupervised DHEA use by young male athletes is not warranted, and use by female athletes and by male athletes over age forty may have some beneficial physical and physiological effects. Other reported benefits of DHEA include immune-system enhancement, anticancer activity, antidepressant action, enhancement of mental functioning, and longevity in laboratory animals. The amounts used in studies have varied, but benefits have been reported in the 25-to-100-milligram range. *A word of caution:* Do not take supplemental DHEA if you are a man who may have prostate cancer or a women who may have breast cancer, a reproductive cancer, or a reproductive disorder.

Gamma Oryzanol and Ferulic Acid

Gamma oryzanol is a substance extracted from rice-bran oil that reportedly promotes a variety of metabolic effects. These metabolic effects include increased endorphin release, antioxidant activity, lipotropic action, stress reduction, GH stimulation, increased growth, and improved recovery. Ferulic acid (FRAC) is part of the gamma-oryzanol molecule and is also available as a supplement. The metabolic effects of FRAC include increased strength, improved recovery, reduced muscle soreness, reduced sensation of fatigue, and decreased catabolic effects by cortisol.

While research is sparse, athletes report beneficial results from the supplemental use of gamma oryzanol and ferulic acid. Daily dosages of 10 to 60 milligrams of ferulic acid and/or 300 to 900 milligrams of gamma oryzanol have been reported to have no toxic side effects. Ferulic acid appears to be about thirty times more bioavailable then gamma oryzanol, but some scientists believe that the sterol molecule to which the ferulic acid is bound is integral to the efficient transport of the ferulic-acid molecule.

For best results, take supplemental gamma oryzanol and/or ferulic acid before workouts on training days and in the morning on nontraining days.

Glucosamine

Glucosamine as a supplement is widely heralded as an effective treatment for arthritis. It is also beneficial to connective tissue. The body contains several types of connective tissue. These different types of connective tissue make up the tendons, ligaments, intervertebral discs, pads between the joints, cell membranes, and cartilage. Connective tissue has two components. The chief component is collagen, which is the most common protein in the body, making up one-third of the body's total protein volume. The other component is proteoglycan (PG), which forms the "framework" for collagenous tissue. PGs are huge structural macromolecules comprised mainly of glycosaminoglycans (GAGs), which are long chains of modified sugars. The principal GAG in PG is hyaluronic acid, of which 50 percent is glucosamine.

Over thirty years of research has gone into understanding how glucosamine acts as a precursor in GAG synthesis. Scientists have long known that ingesting purified glucosamine from connective tissue allows the body to bypass the step of converting glucose to glucosamine. Following are some of the findings from the research studies:

☐ Glucosamine is absorbed 95-percent intact through the gut wall.

☐ About 30 percent of orally administered glu-

cosamine is stored by the body for later synthesis of more connective tissue.

☐ In human clinical trials, glucosamine given orally in doses of 750 to 1,500 milligrams daily initiated a reversal of degenerative osteoarthritis of the knee after two months. The normalization of the cartilage was documented through biopsies of the tissue.

☐ Of greater concern to athletes, glucosamine taken orally gives injured connective tissue the precursor that is the most critical in the rebuilding of its collagenous matrix.

☐ Glucosamine is the preferred substance in synthesizing PG, which forms the framework of connective tissue.

☐ According to in vitro research, glucosamine increases the production of GAG, the most important molecule in PG, by 170 percent.

Supplemental glucosamine clearly aids in the synthesis of connective tissue. All athletes need a supplement that can do this, as the repair and growth of connective tissue is never-ending. For this purpose, take 500 to 2,000 milligrams of glucosamine per day.

Glycerol

Glycerol is a three-carbon-atom molecule that is the backbone of triglycerides and phospholipids. Triglycerides consist of three fatty acids attached to a glycerol molecule, and phospholipids consist of two fatty acids attached to a glycerol molecule, with a phosphate-containing compound attached to the third carbon atom. (For discussions of triglycerides and phospholipids, see Chapter 4.) When glycerol is removed from these fats by hydrolysis, it is a clear, syrupy liquid. The liquid has been utilized in a variety of ways over the years, but it is especially popular as an emollient in skin-care products and cosmetics and as a sweetening agent in pharmaceuticals.

As a supplement, glycerol has been found by researchers to possibly help the body remain better hydrated. Studies have shown that athletes training for prolonged periods (more than one hour) are able to run cooler and longer when they ingest a water-glycerol mixture. Preliminary studies have suggested that glycerol acts like a sponge, absorbing water into the bloodstream and holding it there. However, researchers are still trying to determine appropriate dosages; the current estimates range from 10 to 60 grams, taken with the amount of water recommended for the activity, over a period of a few hours. (For general hydration guidelines for athletes, see page 59.)

A word of caution: Some side effects, including bloating, nausea, and lightheadedness, have been reported with glycerol use. If you choose to try a glycerol-containing beverage, test it out at least several times before competition to see how your body reacts to it.

Inosine

Inosine is a naturally occurring substance found in all human tissues, particularly in the skeletal and cardiac muscles. It is involved in the regeneration of ATP, promoting its synthesis and replenishment. It also stimulates the production of 2,3 diphosphoglycerate (2,3 DPG), which is one of the substances essential in the transportation of oxygen molecules from red blood cells to muscle cells for cellular energy production. In addition, inosine is believed to enhance muscle growth, improve immune response and resistance to infection, and act as a vasodilator, increasing blood flow. It reportedly improves strength, resulting in the ability to lift more weight, finish more repetitions, and engage in better workouts. Endurance athletes have also reported benefits. However, because inosine contains nitrogen and can add to the production of uric acid, individuals with kidney problems or gout should not use inosine.

The recommended dosage of inosine is 5 to 10 milligrams for every 1 pound of lean body mass. For an individual with a lean body mass of 140 pounds, this works out to a total of 700 to 1,400 milligrams. When loading inosine before competition, take it in combination with creatine monohydrate and its cofactors for the best results. Furthermore, take it forty-five to sixty minutes before exercising. The form of inosine is also important. The best is inosine hypoxanthine riboside (inosine HXR), followed by betaglycosidic nucleoside of D-ribose and hypoxanthine, as well as hypoxanthine riboside. Do not use any other form, such as inosinic acid. Store inosine in a moisture-proof bottle in a dry location.

Inositol

Inositol, the same as choline, is often classified as a member of the B-complex family. It is correctly called myo-inositol and is generally considered to be a nonessential vitamin because it is synthesized by most animals, including humans. Also like choline, inositol is a lipotropic agent. It assists fatty-acid metabolism, carbohydrate metabolism, and calcium functioning. A deficiency of inositol can lead to a buildup of fat in the liver and may affect the nervous system. Inositol is not reported to have any effects on athletic performance.

Although no RDA value has been set for inositol, a PDI for men and women who are healthy and actively training has been established at 800 to 1,200 milligrams per day. Intake above 1,200 milligrams has not produced any toxic side effects in healthy individuals. The average adult diet supplies about 1,000 milligrams of inositol per day.

Inositol is found in foods such as heart, whole grains, fruit, milk, nuts, meat, and vegetables. It is available in supplement form as myo-inositol (pure inositol) and is also commonly included in multi-vitamin-and-mineral supplements and lipotropic supplements.

Melatonin

Melatonin is another substance produced by the body that has recently appeared in supplement form in health-food stores. Supplemental melatonin has not been shown in any tests to directly improve athletic performance, but it has been shown to indirectly improve performance by stimulating certain bodily processes. Melatonin's main function is improving sleep. According to studies, it helps people to fall asleep quicker, stay asleep, and enjoy a more restful sleep. Furthermore, it does this without causing sleep hangover, which is an aftereffect of most sleep medications.

Melatonin is the body's natural sleep substance. Researchers have determined that when the sun sets, the body's melatonin level begins to rise. At dawn, the body's melatonin level begins to drop again. There are times, however, when the body's natural melatonin production may be upset. Traveling across time zones disrupts melatonin production, causing what is commonly known as jet lag. Nervousness before a big athletic event affects melatonin production, as does the stress of training. Staying up late to study for a test can also be disruptive because, according to researchers, lamplight may be enough to supress proper melatonin production.

Millions of people have been using supplemental melatonin during the past few years with no apparent side effects. The amounts used successfully in studies have ranged from .5 to 3.0 milligrams. However, until researchers determine the effects of long-term supplemental use of melatonin on the body's natural melatonin-production capabilities, the best advice is to be judicious in your selection of dosage and frequency. Do not use melatonin every night.

Octacosanol

Octacosanol is a component of wheat-germ oil and is used by athletes for its performance benefits. Some athletes take octacosanol as an individual nutrient, while others consume it as a part of wheat-germ oil, which also contains vitamin E, the essential fatty acids, and plant sterols. Among octacosanol's benefits are improved neuromuscular functioning, improved reaction time, improved endurance, improved muscle glycogen storage, and reduced effects of stress.

Supplementation with both octacosanol and wheat-germ oil on a daily basis is recommended during the season and preseason. Dosages of octacosanol of 1,000 to 2,000 micrograms and more per day have been used in studies with humans with no toxic side effects.

HERBS

Herbs have been utilized by humans for centuries. Some herbs are used as seasonings in cooking, while others are used for very specific medicinal purposes. Some herbs, such as ginseng, act as adaptogens. (For a discussion of these special substances, see "Adaptogens," below.) The study of herbs and the practice of prescribing them for health and performance have become a real science. Many herbs have powerful components that can be of great benefit. In fact, the pharmaceutical industry got its start when druggists began isolating these components and making them available in their purer forms. Herbalists believe, however, that the other components in an herb are pre-

sent to enhance the primary components' beneficial effects and to offset their undesirable actions. They feel that an herb should be used in its complete form to allow the body to benefit from the balanced package provided by nature. Many people believe that herbs are just as effective as medications and do not have the side effects.

Herbs do offer many health and performance benefits, but they must be used with care. Some herbs should be used for only short periods of time, to help heal the body of an illness or to treat a symptom. Some herbs should not be combined with certain medications or other herbs, since their primary components may interact negatively. Some herbs should be avoided by competitive athletes, since they contain a substance, such as caffeine, that may be banned by sports governing organizations. (For a discussion of caffeine, see page 108.) Furthermore, not all plants are beneficial to humans. Some herbs are toxic, even deadly, especially if used for prolonged periods of time. Before you use any herb for more than two to three months, seek the advice of a knowledgeable health-care practitioner or a competent herbalist. Including herbal preparations in your performance-nutrition program can prove advantageous if you use them correctly—or disastrous if you do not.

In general, the bitter-tasting herbs are medicinal and the pleasant-tasting herbs are less toxic. Plant roots and bark are naturally fungicidal and bactericidal, since if they were not, they would be destroyed in the ground. In addition, the active components in herbs tend to be most potent when the herbs are freshly picked. At the same time, roots, bark, and other herb parts can remain potent for years if they are properly dried and stored.

Herbalism tends to be geographic in practice, as herbalists have direct access only to the herbs growing in their local areas. Luckily, however, these different areas all seem to have herbs that serve the same pur-

Adaptogens

Adaptogen is a term coined by Russian researchers to describe a substance that helps increase the body's resistance to adverse influences, both physical and environmental. An adaptogen is a cure-all. To be a true adaptogen, a substance must be safe for daily use, increase the body's resistance to a wide variety of

factors, and have a normalizing action in the system. Adaptogens are useful to healthy individuals as an aid for coping with daily stresses and as a tonic support that helps the body normalize itself when it is ill. The herb Siberian ginseng is an example of an adaptogen.

Caffeine

Caffeine is a naturally occurring compound that belongs to a group of substances called methylxanthines. It is found in coffee, tea, chocolate, cola, and several herbs including guarana and yerba maté. Although caffeine occurs naturally in food, it is classified as an over-the-counter drug. Many people use it, in both food form and pill form, as a stimulant or to increase alertness. It performs these functions by exciting the nervous system. It also acts as a diuretic, rouses the cardiac muscle tissue, encourages thermogenesis, and increases lipolysis. Lipolysis is the process in which lipids are broken down into their constituent fatty acids.

A good part of the world's population relies on a caffeinated beverage every morning. However, for athletes, caffeine offers much more than a good morning drink. Studies clearly show that caffeine can benefit performance. Caffeine preferentially increases the body's use of fatty acids for energy, which in turn helps spare glycogen. As a nervous-system stimulant, it provides a mental boost that helps athletes through rigorous training sessions. Research even shows that caffeine can increase the rate of fat loss.

The down side of caffeine is that it can cause dependency and alter physiology. For these reasons, it is banned by some sports governing bodies and by the International Olympic Committee at certain blood levels. Caffeine works by stimulating the nervous system to increase production of the excitatory neurotransmitters. If an individual takes too much caffeine, or takes it for prolonged periods of time, the precursor nutrients that produce these excitatory neurotransmitters become depleted, which causes a feeling of mental burnout. Caffeine's diuretic effects are also detrimental, especially for endurance athletes.

Ahtletes should use caffeine sparingly and only periodically, to get a mental boost to enhance workouts. Athletes who wish to take caffeine as an ergogenic aid before competition must first check on the legality of caffeine in their sport. Researchers recommend 200 to 400 milligrams (about 3 to 5 cups of coffee) one hour before competition. However, before consuming any caffeine, make certain that you are well enough hydrated to offset the diuretic effects.

poses. There are two main herbal approaches that are popular today. In one approach, herbs are used for their specific active ingredients, such as the caffeine in guarana. In the other approach, which is Asian, herbs are used to balance the body's flow of energy. Both approaches have advantages, and a practitioner of either can help you improve your health and performance.

How to Use Herbs

Herbs can be used picked fresh from the ground, their leaves, bark, and roots utilized in their natural forms or made into tablets, capsules, liquids, powders, extracts, tinctures, ointments, or oils. The whole leaves, berries, seeds, roots, flowers, and bark can be dried and used. Whole herbs or herbal parts can also be purchased fresh or dried, and most herbs are available in health-food stores in their most popular forms.

For long-term use, the most convenient form of herbal remedy made at home is tea. The water dilutes the powerful components of the herb; and the tea, especially if it is mild, can be used every day as a tonic and for general well-being. To prepare an herbal tea, place the herbs in a ceramic or glass mug or teapot; do not use metal. Use about 1 to 3 teaspoons of herbs per cup of boiling water. Heat the water in a nonaluminum kettle and, when it boils, pour it over the herbs. Let the herbs steep for at least five minutes but for no longer than ten minutes. If you prefer a stronger tea, increase the amount of herbs rather than the steeping time, since steeping herbs for more than ten minutes produces a bitter-tasting tea. Strain the tea before drinking it.

The other forms in which herbs can be used include the following:

☐ *Compress.* A compress is a cloth soaked in a warm or cool herbal solution. To use the compress, apply it directly to the injured area.

☐ *Decoction.* A decoction is a tea made from the bark, roots, seeds, or berries of a plant. However, instead of steeping the herb, simmer it for about twenty to thirty minutes, unless instructed otherwise for the particular herb you are using. Do not boil the herb.

☐ *Essential oil.* An essential oil is the oil derived from an herb through steam distillation or cold pressing. The essential oil is usually mixed with vegetable oil or water and used as an inhalant, douche, tea, mouthwash, ear wash, or eyewash. It can also be used externally on burns and abrasions and for massage purposes. Essential oils combine readily with the skin's natural lipids. They should never be used internally except under the direction of a health-care practitioner or herbalist trained in their use.

☐ *Extract.* An extract is made by hydraulically pressing an herb and then soaking it in alcohol or water. The excess liquid is allowed to evaporate, yielding a concentrated extract. Extracts are the most effective way in which herbs can be used, especially for people with severe illnesses or malabsorption problems. Both alcohol- and water-based, extracts generally should be diluted in small amounts of water before being used internally. (For a discussion of alcohol, see below.)

☐ *Herbal vinegar.* An herbal vinegar is a vinegar mixed with an herb. Place the herb in raw apple-cider vinegar, rice vinegar, or malt vinegar and let the mixture stand for least two weeks.

☐ *Infusion.* An infusion is similar to a tea but is made from the leaves, flowers, or other delicate parts of the plant. Boil water and steep the plant parts for five to ten minutes; do not boil the herbs.

☐ *Ointment.* An ointment is a salve made by adding one part herbal extract, tea, pressed juice, or powder to four parts heated petroleum jelly, lard, or a similar substance. Apply the ointment directly to the affected area.

☐ *Poultice.* A poultice is a hot, soft, moist mass of herbs tied in a piece of muslin or other loosely woven cloth. Ground or granulated herbs are the best. Place the poultice directly on the affected area and let it remain in place until it cools. Do not reheat a cooled poultice. Instead, replace it with a fresh poultice.

☐ *Powder.* A powder is the useful part of the herb ground up. Once ground, the herb can be made into capsules or tablets.

☐ *Syrup.* A medicinal syrup is a basic syrup to which herbs have been added. A simple recipe is to boil the herbs in honey or supermarket syrup. Strain the mixture through a piece of cheesecloth before using it.

☐ *Tincture.* A tincture is an alcohol solution mixed with an herb. Add powdered herb to alcohol, then add enough water to make a 50-percent alcohol solution. Let the mixture stand for two weeks, shaking the bottle once or twice a day, then strain the mixture before using it.

To store herbs or any of the mixtures or solutions described above, use colored-glass or ceramic jars or bottles. Never store herbs or herbal preparations in clear-glass containers. Sunlight can destroy an herb's potency.

For a brief description of the most popular athletic herbs and their primary actions and uses in sports, see Table 8.1 on page 110. If several different herbs are recommended for a certain disorder, you can alternate among them. This way, you can obtain the other benefits of each herb, plus you can determine which herb works the best with your bodily chemistry and for your particular needs.

Alcohol

While alcohol is an important component of herbal tinctures and some extracts, its use as a beverage on a regular basis should be avoided by athletes and other persons interested in fitness. A glass of wine may benefit the heart, but a six pack of beer or a bottle of Scotch whiskey will slow the reflexes, dull the senses, and possibly even cause physical problems such as addiction or liver damage. Alcohol is a drug. According to statistics, alcohol is the number-one drug used by college athletes. This is really not surprising, since it relaxes the body, reduces tension, and turns an athlete into a "party animal." Some men boast that alcohol acts as an aphrodisiac and prolongs the ability to engage in sexual intercourse. Others notice that it inhibits sexual performance. For the athlete, the effects of alcohol are clear: *Alcohol dulls the senses and impairs performance.*

The best advice is to completely avoid the use of alcohol during the season. If you choose to drink alcoholic beverages, do so in moderation. Consume no more than one drink per day. This does not mean abstaining from alcohol for six days and drinking a six pack of beer on Saturday night. Recovering from the adverse effects of alcohol takes more time and energy than does recovering from a strenuous training session. Do not drink alcohol during the two weeks prior to any major competition. Alcohol has damaging effects on the liver that adversely affect metabolism and slow down the reaction time of the nervous system. As you can see, drinking alcohol is completely counterproductive to the goals of an athlete.

Table 8.1. The Most Popular Athletic Herbs

Herb	Other Names	Parts Used	Athletic Actions and Uses	Comments
Alfalfa	Buffalo herb, lucerne, purple medic.	Flowers, leaves, petals, sprouts.	Benefits cardiovascular system, alleviates pain.	To benefit from vitamin content, use fresh, raw form. Sprouts are especially good.
Aloe	*Aloe vera,* Barbados aloe, Curacao aloe.	Pulp from insides of succulent leaves.	Supports immune system, counteracts effects of aging, assists digestion, alleviates pain, promotes recovery and tissue repair.	Before using, dab small amount behind ear or on underarm. If stinging or rash result, do not use.
Astragalus	Huang qi.	Roots.	Supports immune system, benefits cardiovascular system, increases energy level, promotes recovery and tissue repair.	*Caution:* Do not use if you have a fever.
Barberry	Berberis, European barberry, jaundice berry, pepperidge, pepperidge bush, sowberry.	Bark, berries, roots.	Supports immune system, assists digestion, alleviates pain, promotes recovery and tissue repair.	*Caution:* Do not use if you are pregnant.
Black cohosh	Black snakeroot, bugbane, bugwort, cimicifuga, rattleroot, rattleweed, richweed, squawroot.	Rhizomes, roots.	Eases stress reactions, benefits cardiovascular system, alleviates pain, helps menstrual pain and problems.	*Caution:* Do not use if you are pregnant or have a chronic disease.
Blue cohosh	Beechdrops, blueberry, blue ginseng, papoose root, squaw root, yellow ginseng.	Roots.	Helps menstrual pain and problems.	*Caution:* Do not use during first two trimesters of pregnancy.
Burdock	Bardana, burr seed, clotbur, cocklebur, grass burdock, hardock, hareburr, hurrburr, turkey burrseed.	Roots, seeds.	Supports immune system, alleviates pain, promotes recovery and tissue repair.	*Caution:* Interferes with iron absorption when used internally.
Cayenne	Capsicum, hot pepper, red pepper, Africa pepper, American pepper, bird pepper, chili pepper, Spanish pepper, Zanzibar pepper.	Berries.	Eases stress reactions, supports immune system, benefits cardiovascular system, assists digestion, alleviates pain.	Can be used both internally and topically for pain relief. *Caution:* Do not use for prolonged periods. Keep away from eyes. Used as a pretraining stimulant.

Herb	Other Names	Parts Used	Athletic Actions and Uses	Comments
Celery	Garden celery, wild celery.	Juice, roots, seeds.	Alleviates pain, benefits muscle tissue.	*Caution:* Do not use in large amounts if you are pregnant.
Chamomile	Camomile, Roman camomile, garden camomile, ground apple, low camomile, whig plant.	Flowers.	Eases stress reactions, supports immune system, assists digestion, improves sleep, promotes recovery and tissue repair.	*Caution:* Do not use if you are allergic to ragweed.
Dandelion	Blowball, cankerwort, lion's tooth, priest's crown, puffball, swine snout, white endive, wild endive.	Leaves, roots, tops.	Counteracts effects of aging, assists digestion, increases energy level, promotes recovery and tissue repair.	The root can be roasted and used as coffee substitute.
Echinacea	Coneflower, narrow-leaved purple coneflower, Sampson root.	Leaves, roots.	Supports immune system, promotes recovery and tissue repair.	For internal use, freeze-dried form or alcohol-free extract is best. *Caution:* Do not use if you are allergic to plants in the sunflower family.
Ephedra	Ma huang, Chinese ephedra.	Stems.	Aids fat loss, increases energy level.	Active ingredient is ephedrine. Banned by most sports governing bodies worldwide, so avoid if you are a competitive athlete. *Caution:* Do not use if you are pregnant, take a monoamine oxidase inhibitor, or have an anxiety disorder, glaucoma, heart disease, high blood pressure, or history of stroke.
Evening primrose	Common evening primrose, fever plant, field primrose, king's cureall, night willow-herb, scabish, scurvish, tree primrose, primrose.	Oil from seeds, whole plant.	Supports immune system, benefits cardiovascular system, assists digestion, alleviates pain, helps menstrual pain and problems.	A natural estrogen promoter.

Herb	Other Names	Parts Used	Athletic Actions and Uses	Comments
Garlic	Clove garlic.	Bulbs.	Eases stress reactions, benefits cardiovascular system.	Aged extract is the best form. Odorless supplements are available.
Ginger	African ginger, black ginger, race ginger.	Rhizomes, roots.	Benefits cardiovascular system, relieves nausea.	Internal use of large amounts may upset stomach.
Ginkgo	*Ginkgo biloba.*	Leaves.	Benefits cardiovascular system, counteracts effects of aging, improves memory.	Initial use may result in mild headache. For best results, use for at least two weeks.
Ginseng (Chinese, American, Siberian)	Korean ginseng, Asiatic ginseng, wonder-of-the-world.	Roots.	Eases stress reactions, supports immune system, counteracts effects of aging, improves sleep, promotes recovery and tissue repair.	Siberian belongs to different botanical family than Chinese and American, but properties and uses are similar. Ginseng–royal jelly is a traditional combination for energy. Use 200–1,000 milligrams per day of standardized ginseng or ginseng–royal jelly during season and preseason. Inclusion in multi-vitamin-and-mineral supplement indicates superior product. *Caution:* Do not use if you have hypoglycemia, high blood pressure, or heart disease.
Goldenseal	Eye balm, eye root, ground raspberry, Indian plant, jaundice root, orangeroot, tumeric root, yellow puccoon, yellowroot.	Rhizomes, roots.	Eases stress reactions, supports immune system, benefits cardiovascular system, assists digestion, promotes recovery and tissue repair, helps menstrual pain and problems.	For best results, alternate goldenseal with echinacea or other herbs recommended for your disorder. *Caution:* Do not use if you are pregnant. Do not use for prolonged periods. Use with caution if you have a history of cardiovascular disease, diabetes, or glaucoma.
Gotu kola	Indian pennywort.	Nuts, roots, seeds.	Supports immune system, increases energy level, promotes recovery and tissue repair.	Topical use may cause dermatitis.

Herb	Other Names	Parts Used	Athletic Actions and Uses	Comments
Guarana		Bark, leaves.	Increases energy level.	Active ingredient is caffeine. Works best when combined with other herbs and nutrients in custom-blended energy supplements. Also used in weight-loss supplements. *Caution:* Do not use if you are pregnant or have an anxiety disorder, glaucoma, heart disease, high blood pressure, or history of stroke. Keep use to a minimum.
Hawthorn	English hawthorn, May bush, May tree, quickset, thorn-apple tree, whitethorn.	Berries, flowers, leaves.	Eases stress reactions, benefits cardiovascular system, assists digestion, benefits muscle tissue, lowers blood pressure.	
Hops	European hops, common hops.	Berries, flowers, leaves.	Eases stress reactions, improves sleep.	Used in herbal sleeping preparations.
Kava kava	Kava.	Roots.	Eases stress reactions, improves sleep, alleviates pain; reduces anxiety.	Use for only a few days per week. Do not use during few days before competition, unless sport requires mental focus and steady hand. Best used in evening. *Caution:* May cause drowsiness. If drowsiness becomes a problem, discontinue use or reduce dosage.
Kola nut	Kola tree, caffeine nut, guru nut.	Seeds.	Increases energy level.	Contains more caffeine than coffee beans.
Licorice	Licorice root, sweet licorice, sweet wood.	Roots.	Benefits muscle tissue.	*Caution:* Do not use if you are pregnant or have diabetes, glaucoma, heart disease, high blood pressure, severe menstrual problems, or history of stroke. Do not use for more than seven consecutive days, as this can cause high blood pressure.
Milkweed	Common milkweed, common silkweed, cottonweed, silkweed, silky swallow-wort, swallow-wort, Virginia silk.	Roots.	Counteracts effects of aging, promotes recovery and tissue repair.	*Caution:* Toxic in large amounts, especially for children.

Herb	Other Names	Parts Used	Athletic Actions and Uses	Comments
Passion flower	Maypops, passion vine, purple passion flower.	Flowers, whole plant.	Eases stress reactions, benefits cardiovascular system, improves sleep.	*Caution:* Do not use in large amounts if you are pregnant.
Plantain	Common plantain, broad-leaved plantain, dooryard plantain, greater plantain, round-leaved plantain, way bread, white man's foot.	Leaves, whole plant.	Aids fat loss, promotes recovery and tissue repair.	Young leaves are delicious in salads.
St. Johnswort	Amber, goatweed, Johnswort, Klamath weed, Tipton weed.	Flowers, leaves, stems.	Eases stress reactions, helps menstrual pain and problems.	*Caution:* Internal use in large amounts may heighten sun sensitivity, especially in fair-skinned people. Interferes with absorption of iron and other minerals.
Skullcap	Blue skullcap, blue pimpernel, helmet flower, hoodwort, mad-dog-weed, side-flowering skullcap.	Whole plant.	Eases stress reactions, benefits cardiovascular system, improves sleep, alleviates pain.	
Valerian	Fragrant valerian, allheal, English valerian, German valerian, great wild valerian, heliotrope, setwall, vandal root, Vermont valerian, wild valerian.	Rhizomes, roots.	Eases stress reactions, benefits cardiovascular system, improves sleep, helps menstrual pain and problems.	Water-based extract is the best form.
Willow	White willow, salicin willow, withe, withy.	Bark.	Alleviates pain.	*Caution:* May interfere with absorption of iron and other minerals when used internally.
Yarrow	Milfoil, noble yarrow, nosebleed, sanguinary, soldier's woundwort, thousandleaf, soldier's herb.	Berries, leaves.	Supports immune system, assists digestion, alleviates pain, helps menstrual pain and problems.	*Caution:* Interferes with absorption of iron and other minerals when used internally.
Yellow dock	Curled dock, garden patience, narrow dock, sour dock, rumex, sad dock.	Leaves, roots.	Supports immune system, assists digestion, promotes recovery and tissue repair.	
Yerba maté	Holly, maté, Paraguay tea, yerba, South American holly.	Leaves, twigs.	Increases energy level.	

114

9. FOOD AND DIETARY SUPPLEMENTS
GETTING THE NUTRIENTS YOU NEED

The food and dietary supplements that we consume as part of our daily diets contain the many nutrients described in the foregoing chapters in different combinations and amounts. Food and supplements also come in a variety of forms. Food can be found whole, frozen, canned, or aged. Supplements come in forms such as pills, tablets, capsules, liquids, and powders.

The growing variety of food and supplement choices often leaves us feeling bewildered and forced to do a lot of trial-and-error shopping. In this chapter, we will examine the different types of nutrient sources available, so that you can become familiar with all your options and can target the "right stuff" for you.

ALL FOOD IS NOT CREATED EQUAL

Food in general, as just mentioned, varies considerably in nutritional content. For example, meat is high in protein but has almost no carbohydrates. Carrots are high in beta-carotene but have just trace amounts of protein. To take this even further, the nutritional content of one specific food item can also vary considerably—that is, the nutrients in a specific item can vary from location to location and even within the same location from year to year. This means that a potato grown in Idaho does not necessarily have the same nutritional content as a potato grown in Maine. This variation in nutritional content has formed the basis of one of the major flaws in all the popular dietary approaches, which have always tended to assume that a potato is a potato, no matter what. In the past, compensating for the fluctuation in nutrients was difficult. Today, however, with the help of modern food technology, meeting an athlete's special nutritional needs can be more effectively accomplished. The special food preparations and sports supplements now available are more standard and reliable and make reaching performance-nutrition goals easier and more economical.

Planning a nutritious diet is still far from effortless, however. Some foods are healthier than others. The term *wholesome* is supposed to be reserved for foods that are fresh, healthy, and packed with nutrients. Instead, it is used by many marketing executives to describe all kinds of foods, even high-fat baked goods. In response to the growing demand by consumers for truly wholesome foods, health foods and health-food stores have popped up everywhere during the last few decades. It is estimated that there are about 10,000 health-food stores in the United States alone. But even good foods need to be eaten in moderation. A common misconception is that any food found in a health-food store is good and can be eaten in unlimited quantities. Well, eating too much of even a good thing can be unhealthy. If you check labels, you will see that many health foods are high in fat, albeit unsaturated fat. Whether saturated or unsaturated, fat is one nutrient to keep to a minimum. The primary good foods to buy—in health-food stores and downtown supermarkets—are fresh fruits and vegetables, whole grains and cereals, and lean meats, fish, and poultry.

In addition to fresh, whole foods, there are also processed foods. In some respects, processed foods are similar to supplements—they are both made from specific combinations of ingredients. However, this is where the similarities end. Processed foods, such as canned foods, frozen foods, bread, and snack foods, are generally extremely poor nutrient sources. Most are high in fat or sodium, and most have had their nutrients cooked or otherwise processed out. For example, the ever-growing snack-food category contains foods with too much fat, sugar, and sodium. Cookies and other sweets are full of fat and sugar; and salty snacks, such as potato chips and corn chips, are high in fat and sodium. Most canned foods are also high on the rotten-food list because their vitamins and other heat-sensitive nutrients have been cooked out. And processed foods in general are loaded with a host of additives, preservatives, and other unhealthy chemicals. As a group, processed foods offer the worst nutrition.

Is there anything good at all about processed foods? Just one thing—they generally taste good, which is what keeps us coming back for more. Scientists speculate that the reason we crave snack foods is their fat, sugar, and sodium contents. Early humans did not crave these nutrients. These nutrients were not as plentiful at the dawn of civilization, when humans had to hunt and gather their food. Over the years, however, as our food-gathering methods and diets evolved, our taste buds and cravings did, too. Now we crave fat, sugar, and sodium, which causes us to seek out foods that contain these ingredients and to consume them in large amounts. This is why most of us can eat a pound of potato chips in one sitting but cannot stand to eat even one piece of raw broccoli. If you are striving for maximum performance, you must exercise willpower over what you eat. Stay away from junk foods and processed foods. Concentrate on eating the *good* stuff.

UNDERSTANDING FOOD LABELS

How do you know what you are getting from the foods you eat? This is a good question, but it can be difficult to answer. Take a look at the foods in your kitchen. While most of the products in your pantry and refrigerator have lists of ingredients, and some also say how many calories and nutrients they supply per serving, many foods do not offer any nutritional information. Whole foods—the good foods that should constitute the major portion of your diet, such as eggs, fresh fruits, fresh vegetables, and lean meats—do not have labels. Figuring out exactly what your diet supplies can therefore develop into a full-time undertaking.

You can cut your efforts in half, however, by learning which foods are good sources of the particular nutrients you need and by keeping the list handy for when you plan your menus and go to the supermarket. To begin, keep track of what you eat. Read the labels of the foods that have one, and look up the foods without labels in a nutrition guide such as *The Nutribase Complete Book of Food Counts.* By doing this, you can decide if you need to add a particular food to your diet—or if you need to drop one. You can also see how many calories and fat grams your favorite foods contain, as well as how low in calories and fat most fruits and vegetables are.

Under the FDA's nutrition-labeling regulations, manufacturers must provide certain ingredient and nutritional information on the labels of all their packaged foods. By convention, the ingredients of a product are listed in descending order of predominance. If water is the most prevalent ingredient in a food, then it is the first ingredient listed on the label. The specific amount of each ingredient is not provided, however. Therefore, the label must include such additional facts as the number of calories per serving, the macronutrient content, and the selected micronutrient content of the product.

The Nutrition Facts label that the FDA began requiring manufacturers to display on foods and supplements in 1993 has its good points and its bad points. The label is very different from the labels that food products used to carry and is designed to help consumers make better food choices. For one thing, the label focuses more on fat, detailing the specific number of calories from fat that a product has per serving and what percentage this number is of an average daily diet of 2,000 calories. In addition, all the information on the label is presented in a standardized form, making it easier to compare different products and to see how a certain product fits into your overall diet. Serving sizes also have been standardized, as have the terms describing calorie, fat, and cholesterol contents, such as *fat free, low fat, lean, light* or *lite,* and *cholesterol free.* The labels additionally present the amount of dietary fiber per serving.

On the negative side, the nutrition information that is presented is generalized for the population at large and does not address the needs of any specific group, such as athletes. Furthermore, the Daily Value (DV) system that is being used does not supply values for all the nutrients, with the ones that are supplied based on the government's Recommended Dietary Allowances (RDAs), which feature vitamin and mineral amounts that are even lower than previous recommendations. (For a discussion of the DVs, see "The Nutritional Alphabet Soup" on page 4.) The nutrition information is therefore incomplete for many products.

Most consumers find some parts of the Nutrition Facts label to be helpful and other parts to be useless. Athletes generally feel that the most useful bits of information are the total calories and the macronutrient information. Because not all the micronutrients are listed, it is impossible to use the labels alone to determine whether you are meeting your micronutrient needs.

FOOD-GROUP APPROACH TO NUTRITION— IS IT VALID FOR ATHLETES?

Nutritionists recognize that most people will not spend the necessary time each day calculating the exact nutritional content of each of their meals. To provide an easy-to-follow system for the general population, they developed the food-group approach to nutrition. (For a discussion of the food-group approach, see "What Is Nutrition?" on page 2.) The food-group approach, which has been reworked several times through the decades to take into account the latest nutritional findings, is useful in many respects. However, while it can be used to help design specialized diets for people with certain illnesses, such as diabetes and gastrointestinal disorders, it does not address the needs of athletes.

To help athletes meet their special diet requirements, we present modified basic daily guidelines in each sport-specific plan in Part Four. Instructions for modifying your diet for fat loss or muscle gain are given in chapters 13 and 14, respectively, and sample daily diets are presented in Appendix C. We recommend that you also purchase appropriate fitness software or consult a personal trainer to help you diversify your meals and to assist you in keeping track of your food intake, your training, and the changes in your body composition.

SUPERFOODS—DIETARY SUPPLEMENTS ARE BORN

When people think of dietary supplements, they tend to relate them more to drugs than to food. This is due partly to the way supplements look, since many come in forms such as tablets and capsules, and partly to where they originated, since they were first used in clinical settings. Rather, dietary supplements are superfoods and supernutrients, not drugs. According to the Dietary Supplement Health and Education Act, passed by the U.S. Congress in 1994, they constitute a category of their own—dietary supplements. In addition to creating this separate category, the new act also allowed more informational and educational materials about supplements to be distributed to consumers. However, it prevented manufacturers from making therapeutic claims for their products, even though the claims may be accurate. In general, the 1994 act has been welcomed by nutritionists, since the new dietary-supplement category has helped reduce the gray area between the food and drug categories.

The birth of dietary supplements as an independent category was a long time coming. For many decades, dietary supplements were used only in med-

ical applications. Doctors and clinical nutritionists fed special nutrient solutions to patients as part of their overall efforts to restore health. These intravenous solutions delivered mixtures of nutrients directly into the patients' bloodstreams. Today, health-care practitioners prescribe supplements for a plethora of health reasons. Prime recipients are postsurgical patients, children, senior citizens, and pregnant women. In addition, many hospitals have adopted the use of dietary supplements to accelerate healing due to recent research that demonstrated the rapid recovery of surgical patients who were given supplements.

The success of these clinical applications did not automatically catapult supplements into the mass market, however. In fact, serious research was not undertaken until the 1950s, and even then, the researchers were initially allowed to use just laboratory animals, not humans. This early research produced a good deal of knowledge about the nutrition, growth, and health of laboratory animals, however, and once the hypotheses were tested, formulations for humans were made. Among the first formulations were what came to be known as chemically defined diets. These diets, which were really nothing more than liquid meals containing full profiles of the amino acids, vitamins, minerals, fatty acids, and other nutrients that are necessary for life, eventually led to the development of the first nutrition-related products to make the foray from a clinical setting into the supermarket—liquid weight-loss products.

In the 1960s, the field of human nutrition got a boost from the nutritional research conducted as part of the space program. When scientists from the National Aeronautics and Space Administration (NASA) were preparing to send astronauts into space for the first time, they had no idea how the human digestive system would react to a zero-gravity environment. They also wanted to ensure that the astronauts had nutritionally complete diets, but they needed to reduce the amount of bodily wastes produced during missions. For the first time, scientists were given the funding to use healthy, athletic individuals in their studies and to concentrate on how to maximize performance. Because the astronauts were subjected to numerous experiments that necessitated the periodic measuring of their body weights, blood chemistries, and caloric outputs, a lot of vital information on nutrition and human physiology ended up being gathered.

Ever since the 1960s, the use of dietary supplements has become increasingly widespread. New categories of products are constantly being developed as researchers continue to discover how supplemental nutrients can benefit health and performance. One of the first categories of sports supplements was powder weight-gain drinks. These products are used by bodybuilders, athletes in general, and teenagers who wish to put on body weight. There is also an emerging subculture of nonathletes who use these supplements for health reasons. (For a list of reasons to take supplements, see "Why Take Dietary Supplements?" below.) Supplements are used by just about every person in the United States at some point in life, and their use is constantly increasing. Sports nutrition represents one of the largest and fastest-growing supplement categories, since athletes know that they can improve their performance when they use superfoods as part of their total sports-nutrition program.

DIETARY SUPPLEMENTS VERSUS FOOD

Dietary supplement is a general term that refers to a concentrated source of nutrients that is usually prescribed to be taken in addition to the daily diet to increase nutrient intake. Dietary supplements come in many forms, such as tablets, capsules, and powders.

They can be simple single-ingredient tablets, more complicated multi-ingredient formulations, or concentrated foods. They are thought of as *superfoods* and *designer foods* because they are high in nutrients and designed to meet certain nutritional goals. Dietary supplements are also referred to as *supplements*, *food supplements,* and *nutritional supplements.*

Some supplements are seen by consumers as regular foods. An example of these are sports-nutrition drinks, which come in liquid and powder forms, similar to bottled and powdered iced teas. However, sports-nutrition drinks are formulated to fulfill special athletic needs by providing specific nutrients; iced tea is not. Alternatively, although a certain kind of pasta may be made of a mixture of nutrient-enriched semolina and water, it would not be considered a supplement despite the added nutrients. At the same time, some sports-nutrition companies have designed special pastas that are higher than normal in protein, lower than normal in fat, and enriched with vitamins and minerals not ordinarily found in pasta. So, while a supplement's form ususally distinguishes it from food, there is some overlap. (For a full discussion of the major supplement forms, see page 119.)

There are also many differences between the way food supplies nutrients and the way supplements do.

Why Take Dietary Supplements?

If you are still unsure whether you should take dietary supplements, perhaps one of the following reasons will persuade you:

☐ Supplements supply measurable amounts of nutrients.

☐ Supplements make up for the poor nutritional contents of many of the foods we eat.

☐ Supplements ensure that we get adequate amounts of the essential nutrients.

☐ Supplements replace nutrients destroyed by poor diet, smoking, alcohol consumption, drug use, and pollution.

☐ Most supplements are either calorie- and fat-free or very nearly so.

☐ Special supplements are available for individuals with food allergies.

☐ Stress can increase the body's need for certain nutrients, which can be easily obtained from supplements.

☐ Pregnant women require a reliable supply of all the essential nutrients and extra supplies of nutrients such as iron, folic acid, calcium, zinc, and vitamin D.

☐ Lack of sunlight is common in many parts of the northern hemisphere and necessitates a higher dietary intake of vitamin D.

☐ The elderly need dietary supplementation due to low food intake and poor digestion.

☐ Supplemental amounts of protective nutrients such as the antioxidants can slow the effects of aging, prevent cellular damage, and deter the development of a number of other disorders.

☐ Supplements can help prevent or cure the nutritional deficiencies that are commonly found in athletes.

☐ Supplements can ensure optimum supplies of nutrients for maximum athletic performance.

If you are still not convinced, ask around. Every person you talk to will probably give you another good reason to add dietary supplements to your daily nutrition program.

Food supplies random amounts of nutrients, while supplements supply controlled amounts. Food supplies nutrients indiscriminately, while supplements target specific needs. Table 9.1, right, summarizes some of the major differences between food and supplements as sources of nutrients.

To make matters even more confusing, some foods, such as certain herbs, have drug uses as well as supplement uses; some supplements are foods that also have drug uses; and some drugs contain food derivatives and supplemental nutrients. What to call the use of these substances therefore often causes debate. For example, many professionals would consider the use of a single amino acid to be drug use, while nutrition experts would consider it to be a form of nutritional therapy. Because of this, the definitions of *food, dietary supplement,* and *drug* are not as clearcut as you may think. (For the definitions, see "Some Useful Definitions" on page 120.)

The idea that anything used to prevent or treat a disease should be called a drug is crazy. Both foods and supplements can have very powerful effects in disease treatment and prevention, but they should not be considered drugs. Furthermore, there are many drugs that actually interfere with the absorption of nutrients and produce harmful side effects. Often, a special diet and supplement regimen should be an integral part of a therapy based on drugs. The food, supplements, and medications can boost each other's effectiveness for the ultimate goal of maximum health and performance.

MAJOR SUPPLEMENT FORMS

Dietary supplements come in a variety of forms. Using terminology from the pharmaceutical industry, these supplement forms can also be referred to as delivery systems. They are called delivery systems because they deliver the nutrients into the body.

The major forms that dietary supplements come in include the following:

☐ *Pills, tablets, and caplets.* Pills, tablets, and caplets are all powdered nutrients that have been pressed by machine into their characteristic shapes. By manufacturing definitions, pills, tablets, and caplets are all different. Pills are generally smaller than tablets and are made by pharmacists who use procedures of their own devising. Caplets are tablets that are shaped like capsules. Originally, caplets were tamperproof, one-

Table 9.1. Food Sources Versus Supplement Sources of Nutrients

Food Sources	Supplement Sources
Provide random amounts of nutrients.	Provide controlled amounts of nutrients.
Supply nutrients indiscriminately.	Supply nutrients for targeted purposes.
Supply small, inconsistent amounts of nutrients.	Supply concentrated, specific amounts of nutrients.
Supply nutrients of varied bioavailability.	Are designed to supply highly bioavailable nutrients.
Contain calories.	Usually have no calories or a controlled number of calories.
May have a disagreeable taste.	May have no taste (especially tablets).
Can be time consuming to prepare.	Are convenient to use.
Often are more expensive.	Often are less expensive.
Must usually be purchased without retailer assistance in supermarkets.	Can be purchased with retailer assistance in health-food stores.
Usually come with no instructions regarding use for their nutritional content.	Usually have instructions on the label.
May need to be overeaten to supply even the minimum amounts of nutrients.	Do not need to be overeaten to supply the correct amounts of nutrients.

piece capsules with a hard outer layer and loosely bound contents.

The main form used for supplements today is the tablet. Tablets can be made in many sizes, although there is an upper limit based on the maximum size that a person can safely swallow. Tablets also have longer shelf lives, typically three to five years. In addition, tablets can deliver their contents in several different ways. Some tablets are designed to release their contents quickly, others allow sustained release of

Some Useful Definitions

The following are some useful definitions to keep in mind as you read about food, drugs, and dietary supplements:

☐ *Food.* An edible substance that, when taken into the body, provides nourishment for growth and health by supplying the body with calories and nutrients.

☐ *Dietary supplement.* A product (other than tobacco) that is intended to supplement the diet and that contains one or more of the following dietary ingredients—a vitamin, a mineral, an herb or other plant substance, an amino acid, a substance that increases total dietary intake, or a concentrate, metabolite, constituent, or extract.

☐ *Drug.* A chemical compound that is administered to humans or animals as an aid in the diagnosis, treatment, or prevention of a disease. It can also be used to relieve pain or to control or improve a physiological or pathological condition.

☐ *Nutraceutical.* A food or dietary supplement that is designed for uses other than essential nutrition, such as clinical applications or to treat or prevent a disease. It could be considered a sort of over-the-counter supplement for which specific therapeutic or health claims can be made.

☐ *Phytochemical.* A compound of plant origin that has beneficial health functions, such as disease prevention. Also called *phytonutrient*.

For more definitions of terms useful in the study of sports nutrition, see the "Glossary" on page 383.

their contents, and even others feature timed release. Sustained-release tablets release their nutrients slowly and continuously over an extended period of time. Timed-release tablets release their nutrients in spurts over several hours. Some tablets have an enteric coating, which delays digestion of the tablet until it passes from the stomach into the intestines. Chewable tablets are also available, primarily for children. All these features give tablets an edge over pills and caplets. However, these features also necessitate that tablets be made by experienced manufacturers. Do not assume that all tablets will be digested as expected. If you ever find that a tablet has just "passed through" your system, switch brands.

☐ *Capsules and gelatin capsules.* Capsules are small, digestible containers filled with powdered nutrients. In general, dietary-supplement capsules can be quickly digested. They do not offer sustained release of their contents, and very few feature timed release. Today, capsules do not have the advantages they did decades ago, when tablets were less dynamic. In fact, they now hold no real advantage over tablets.

Gelatin capsules, which are also called soft gels and gel caps, were developed to hold liquid supplements, such as lecithin, cod-liver oil, or vitamin E. The container is made of gelatin and can be soft or hard. Gelatin capsules generally are quickly digested and absorbed. Many people prefer them over regular capsules, pills, tablets, and caplets because they are easier to swallow.

An interesting fact to note is that the material used to make capsules and gelatin capsules is animal in origin. Only recently have some companies developed vegetarian capsules and soft gels. While this first fact is of importance mainly to strict vegetarians, a second interesting fact has implications for everyone. After gelatin capsules are made, they are sent through a wash tunnel to have any residues cleaned away. However, some of these wet-wash processes use a hazardous solvent, and even though the solvent theoretically evaporates from the soft gel, a small amount of residue is believed by some health authorities to remain. This is ironic, since dietary supplements are used primarily to promote health. Recently, several companies developed a dry-cleaning process that employs a rotating drum and absorbent cloths. As the gelatin capsules move through the drum, they are patted dry by the cloths. This new method is preferred over the old, but it may leave the soft gels sticky.

☐ *Powder supplements.* Powder supplements are powdered nutrients designed to be added to a liquid such as water, juice, or milk. They are formulated for a variety of purposes and contain a wide diversity of nutrients. The most common powder supplements are protein powders, diet powders, energy powders, and weight-gain powders. Powder supplements are a convenient way to get high-quality nutrients in exact amounts and exactly when needed. Many athletes have very busy schedules and have trouble fitting in five to six complete meals each day. They find powder supplements to be convenient high-density sources of nutrition that meet their individual needs.

☐ *Liquid supplements.* Liquid supplements include protein drinks, sports rehydration drinks, meal-replacement drinks, herbal extracts, herbal tinctures, and liquid vitamins and minerals. The most common types in athletic circles are carbohydrate drinks and weight-gain drinks.

☐ *Bars.* The bar form of supplement offers convenience and portability. It slips easily into pockets and pocketbooks, and makes the trip to work, school, or practice without fuss or muss. Most bars are also downright delicious. Manufacturers use the bar form for a variety of purposes. Primarily, bars can be a high-density source of nutrition. They are a good source of the macronutrients—fat, protein, and carbohydrates—and usually are also packed with a good sampling of micronutrients.

These are the primary forms that dietary supplements come in. You may occasionally encounter a product that seems to be different. However, when you think about the categories just discussed, you will most likely find that the product slips easily into one. For example, spray vitamins are a liquid supplement. According to the 1994 act, dietary supplements must be intended for ingestion—that is, swallowed and received by the stomach. For now, therefore, the use of other delivery systems—such as nasal sprays, injectables, and suppositories—with dietary supplements is severely limited.

MAJOR CATEGORIES OF SPORTS SUPPLEMENTS

If you had walked into a health-food store or sporting-goods store twenty years ago, you probably would have found a few cans of dust-covered weight-gain powder sitting on a shelf hidden in the back of the store. But if you walk into any major health-food store today, you will find half the store dedicated to the hundreds of different sports supplements that are now available. At first glance, you may think that many of these products are targeted at the bodybuilding crowd. Closer inspection reveals, though, that there are sports supplements for every kind of athlete. In fact, it is interesting to note that the products marketed as bodybuilding supplements are most often used by any athletes who want to build muscle or improve the nutritional quality of their diets. Very few bodybuilding supplements are actually used by competitive bodybuilders.

The bodybuilder is generally considered the pioneer of maximum nutrition and the perfect representation of maximum health. Bodybuilders exercise daily, eat right, and look great. Because of this, athletes traditionally turn toward bodybuilders for advice on nutrition and training. During the 1970s, all kinds of athletes began to use sports and bodybuilding supplements. As the demand for these products grew, so did the number of manufacturers. For this reason, hundreds of brands are now available. With a little guidance, you will be able to use any sports supplement to your benefit and make it a vital part of your nutrition plan.

In this section, we will review the major sports-supplement categories. Our intention is not to provide a critical analysis or description of every sports supplement available, but instead to help you understand in general what the products are, what they have to offer, and how they relate to each other. (For a list of the most popular sports supplements taken by athletes, see "And the Survey Says . . ." on page 122.) In Part Four, we will offer specific guidelines on nutrient intake and will recommend the amounts you should take as part of your total nutrition plan.

The following are the major categories of sports supplements currently available in health-food stores:

☐ *Multi-vitamin-and-mineral supplements.* Multi-vitamin-and-mineral supplements make up a very large sports-supplement category because most supplement manufacturers have at least a few products that fall into it. Multi-vitamin-and-mineral supplements are designed to provide athletes with mixtures of the essential and nonessential nutrients, mostly vitamins and minerals. Typically, the nutrients are supplied in amounts larger than the RDAs to meet the special metabolic demands of athletes. Most of the preparations include a full profile of vitamins and minerals, as well as some metabolites and amino acids. These nutrients may be divided between several tablets and capsules, which are packaged together either in kits of several bottles or in convenient multipacks. (For a discussion of kits, see page 124.) We highly recommend that you use one of these products every day as directed. Select a product that offers either a supply of tablets to be taken with each meal or sustained-release tablets to be taken in the morning. The best products contain a full profile of vitamins and minerals, plus adaptogenic herbs such as ginseng. Superior products

---

And the Survey Says . . .

"What supplements should I take?" is a simple question with a complex answer. The best advice we can give you is to follow the guidelines outlined in your sport-specific plan in Part Four. You might also find some guidance from the results of a survey we conducted among certified fitness trainers. The results were originally published as part of the article "Performance Nutrition: A Review of Performance Nutrition," featured in the June 1995 issue of *BodyCraft Magazine.* Among the certified fitness trainers we surveyed:

☐ 84 percent said they used multi-vitamin-and-mineral supplements.

☐ 53 percent said they used liquid or powder protein supplements.

☐ 49 percent said they used amino-acid supplements.

☐ 37 percent said they used liquid or powder energy supplements.

☐ 33 percent said they used BCAA supplements.

☐ 30 percent said they used liquid or powder weight-gain supplements.

☐ 27 percent said they used energy supplements.

☐ 24 percent said they used L-carnitine supplements.

☐ 24 percent said they used lipotropic or fat-burning supplements.

☐ 20 percent said they used creatine supplements.

☐ 13 percent said they used inosine supplements.

The survey also revealed that most of the respondents spent $30 to $60 per month on sports supplements. The range of money spent was $10 to $250 per month.

---

give dosage recommendations based on body weight and activity level.

☐ *Multi-amino-acid supplements.* Multi-amino-acid supplements are another popular category of sports supplement. For many years, multi-amino-acid products were very valuable to athletes. This was because they contained full profiles of the amino acids in their free forms, which elevated the biological value of the protein obtained from dietary sources. (For a discussion of biological value, see page 33.) Another benefit was that the products could be consumed in between meals to ensure a constant high pool of amino acids in the blood for recovery, repair, and tissue-growth purposes. The formulations typically consisted of tablets or capsules that included all of the essential and nonessential amino acids in their pure, crystalline forms.

Today, however, free-form amino-acid formulations are not allowed to include L-tryptophan. (For a discussion of the FDA's banning of L-tryptophan, see "The Ban on Tryptophan" on page 45.) And since L-tryptophan is missing, the products are not full profile and are basically useless. Nowadays, therefore, your best bet is to look for products that are made from whole proteins, such as casein or egg, which include L-tryptophan and are therefore full profile. The product should contain mostly di- and tri-peptide amino acids and be high in the BCAAs.

☐ *Special-use amino-acid supplements.* Several amino acids and amino-acid combinations have histories of use in clinical applications. For example, for several decades, health-care practitioners have been giving the BCAAs to traumatized patients to help improve recovery. Since the early 1980s, athletes have been using them to compensate for the BCAAs broken down for energy during intense training and to support growth and repair following training. Other popular special-use amino-acid supplements include L-arginine and L-ornithine, L-arginine-pyroglutamate and L-lysine hydrochloride, L-aspartic acid, L-glutamic acid, glycine, L-lysine, L-phenylalanine, and L-tyrosine. (For complete discussions of all of these amino acids, see Chapter 3.)

Take special-use amino-acid supplements with a glass of water or fruit juice to get them into your system quickly. Take them on an empty stomach, so that they will not have to compete with other amino acids for absorption. Since quick and full absorption are important, choose powder supplements, capsules, or quick-release tablets. Generally, the recommended dosage is 1,000 to 4,000 milligrams. Higher dosages may produce side effects such as diarrhea. Use care if you have a stomach disorder, since some of these amino acids may irritate the stomach wall. And do not take any special-use amino-acid supplement for an extended period of time, since harmful side effects may result.

□ *Antioxidant supplements.* Since the discovery that antioxidants protect the body from free-radical damage at the cellular level, a variety of antioxidant supplements for athletes have appeared on the market. These supplements contain ingredients such as vitamin A, beta-carotene, vitamin C, vitamin E, and selenium. Because antioxidants intercept free radicals, athletes like to take extra dosages during and after exercise for additional protection against tissue damage. Antioxidants also protect against the damage caused by oxygen itself, which is taken up by the body in increased amounts during exercise. In addition, antioxidants can reduce the damage caused by the many metabolic waste products generated during physical activity. Antioxidant supplements are generally found in tablet or capsule form.

□ *Lipotropic and fat-burning supplements.* The lipotropic and fat-burning supplements are formulations for athletic and weight-loss purposes. They function by controlling appetite or by increasing fat metabolism. The lipotropics are a group of nutrient cofactors that are taken to prevent fatty buildup in the liver and to ensure that the body metabolizes fat efficiently. The fat burners are nutrient cofactors that help facilitate the metabolism of fat. Ingredients that are commonly found in lipotropic and fat-burning supplements are choline, inositol, L-carnitine, L-taurine, DL-methionine, DL-phenylalanine, and chromium. Other common ingredients are betaine, an alkaloid used to treat muscular degeneration, and herbs such as ephedra, guarana, and brindall berry. Lipotropic and fat-burning supplements are generally available in tablet or capsule form.

□ *Energy supplements.* Energy supplements are pills, tablets, or capsules composed of various combinations of vitamins, minerals, and herbs. They utilize herbs rather than the drug forms of the herbal substances because FDA regulations prohibit mixing drugs that are involved in energy production or alertness promotion with one another or with vitamins, minerals, or other potential energy factors. For example, a common ingredient in energy supplements is the herb guarana, which is high in caffeine. If you decide to use an energy supplement, you must keep in mind that most of them are designed to stimulate mental energy and to provide energy-metabolizing cofactors. Chronic use of these formulations can cause the nervous system to become nutrient depleted from over-stimulation. In addition, supplements that supply caffeine or ephedrine from herbs also have a drying effect on the body and lungs, so you must make sure to keep your fluid intake high. If you wish to enhance your mental or physical energy levels, concentrate on improving your total nutrition program and positive thinking. Use energy supplements sparingly. Remember that the most important energy factors are loaded glycogen stores and a high-carbohydrate diet.

□ *Herbal supplements.* Herbal supplements come in many forms, including tablets, capsules, gelatin capsules, liquids, and tinctures. They offer a wide variety of herbs in single-ingredient and combination forms. Many authorities maintain that the best herbal supplements are alcohol-based extracts; water-based extracts lack the alcohol-soluble components of the herbs. Capsules and tablets are also good delivery systems for herbs. For a complete discussion of herbs and herbal supplements, see Chapter 8.

□ *Liquid and powder weight-gain supplements.* Weight-gain products are one type of sports supplement that many people feel they can live without but that are, in fact, among the biggest moneymakers in the health-food industry. Millions of teenagers and athletes each year train to build muscle, and the sports-nutrition companies have developed a wide range of weight-gain products to help them along. What all of these liquid and powder weight-gain supplements have in common are high amounts of simple and complex carbohydrates, moderate amounts of protein, and a host of vitamins, minerals, and metabolites. Many are also low or very low in fat, and most range from 220 calories to over 1,200 calories per 8-ounce serving.

Several sports-nutrition companies have of late been engaged in a "calorie race," which has resulted in the development of megacalorie weight-gain products. These superhigh-calorie products boast 2,000, 3,000, and even more than 4,000 calories. On the surface, this may be appealing; from a practical standpoint, however, the body can handle only perhaps 800 to 1,600 calories per meal. Furthermore, according to the directions that accompany these products, the calories are spread over several servings. Therefore, unless you are a "hard gainer" (someone who has trouble gaining weight or building muscle mass), a lean teenager going through a growth spurt, a bodybuilder who has reached a plateau, or a long-distance athlete, you should evaluate these products on a per-weight basis, looking at what nutrients they offer ounce for ounce. What you will most likely discover is that the more calories a product has, the fewer nutrients it has per serving. Instead of using the product with the most calories, you might find that a better choice is using more servings of a product that has fewer calories but more nutrients. In addition, before making a final selection, take a close look at the protein content to make sure that a high-quality protein source, such as whey or egg, is included.

☐ *Liquid and powder weight-loss supplements.* Liquid and powder weight-loss supplements are simply nutrient drinks that are low in calories, usually about 120 calories per serving, and used to replace meals. However, even though they are intended for athletes, they are not really appropriate, since they are just spinoffs of the very low calorie diet drinks used by health-care practitioners to help extremely obese patients lose weight. They do not take into account the kind of weight to be lost, the quality of the weight loss, or the maintenance of maximum performance. Nor do they take into consideration muscle mass, strength, endurance, or stamina. While athletes who need to lose excess body fat can make limited use of these products, they really need to take a more specialized approach. For a full discussion of effective fat-loss techniques for athletes, see Chapter 13.

☐ *Liquid and powder protein supplements.* Liquid and powder protein supplements became popular in the 1970s when they were used by millions of people for weight-loss purposes. However, many people used these protein drinks as their sole source of nourishment, and several people eventually died. The bad press almost put an end to these products. Today, athletes are the main consumers of protein supplements. For athletes, liquid and powder protein supplements are excellent sources of pure protein for special purposes. They also offer easy ways to increase the protein content of a meal or snack. These products are useful as a quick supply of 20 to 30 grams or more of protein per serving.

☐ *Liquid and powder energy supplements.* Liquid and powder energy supplements were developed as convenient sources of carbohydrates. They also include protein and energy-related micronutrients. They offer a wide variety of nutrients to meet different metabolic demands. Liquid and powder energy supplements usually contain from 90 to 400 calories per serving. Endurance athletes should stick to the lower-calorie drinks during competitions, since the more concentrated a drink is, the longer it takes to get into the system. The higher-calorie drinks should be reserved for consumption a few hours before and directly after physical activity.

☐ *Nutrition bars.* The sports-nutrition bar is perhaps one of the best nutrition inventions yet. Counter to its high-fat, sugar-laden, empty-calorie cousin, the candy bar, the sports-nutrition bar is a scientifically formulated food that provides precise nutrition. There are a variety of nutrition bars designed for a number of purposes. Among the more popular are diet bars, energy bars, weight-gain bars, and protein bars. Calorie-wise, sports-nutrition bars contain from 90 to over 1,200 calories. They generally are made of high-quality ingredients, supply high levels of carbohydrates and protein, and are very low in fat. Each type of bar also includes important micronutrient cofactors that complement the intended metabolic purpose. We highly recommend daily use of this important supplement product.

In addition to the major categories of sports supplements, a number of minor categories compete for shelf space in health-food stores. Among them are liquid supplements and herbal preparations designed for purposes too numerous to list. Some powder supplements include everything but the kitchen sink, and a number of truly mysterious liquids combine herbs and minerals for a "daily tonic." Other products are formulations delivered in spray, sublingual (under the tongue), dropper, or lozenge form.

Appearing on shelves in the early 1980s were kits, primarily complete kits of supplements for bodybuilders. The most sophisticated kits today include three or more different kinds of dietary supplements. Most also include a manual covering diet and training. Some offer video cassettes, audio cassettes, skinfold calipers, and charts for tracking progress. The diversity of kits has grown in recent years. Now the shelves feature kits for advanced bodybuilders, beginning to intermediate bodybuilders, strength builders, athletes who wish to lose fat, fitness exercisers who wish to lose fat, and anyone who wishes to lose fat.

There are even some kits to help athletes improve their performance. The majority of kits supply supplements for two to eight weeks. They offer a convenient and often economical approach that integrates training, nutrition, and dietary supplementation.

When testing out the different sports supplements and kits to find the ones that work the best for you, do not sacrifice your budget dollars to experimenting with unproven products if it means that you will not be able to afford the more reliable products. You should also be careful for health reasons when trying exotic preparations. Keep track in a journal of how the different supplements make you feel and of any side effects you may experience, such as dizziness, nosebleeding, or blurred vision. Ideally, you should consult a trained herbalist before using an herbal extract. When used properly, herbal supplements can be very helpful.

ECONOMICS OF SPORTS NUTRITION

A good diet is usually cheaper than a diet that is hit-or-miss and includes a high amount of restaurant and fast foods. However, because athletes generally consume about twice as much food as nonathletes do, use more supplements, drink more beverages, and eat more protein, their grocery bills can get out of hand. The best approach is to plan your menus ahead of time and to look for coupons and sales. You could also form a food cooperative with some friends and pool your buying power with the local health-food stores.

When planning your nutrition program, keep in mind that you will need a lot of carbohydrate and protein foods. Look for sales and purchase these foods in bulk. Instead of buying a few pieces of chicken or meat every few days, buy a whole chicken and larger cuts of meat. Do the same with potatoes and pasta. Also, switch to drinking water instead of expensive beverages that are made mainly of water anyway. Buy fresh vegetables and fruits on sale and freeze them for the future.

When you dine out, select a restaurant with a salad bar or buffet of good-quality foods. This way, you will get more food for your money and will have a wide selection from which to choose. When buying supplements, take advantage of sales. Save up some money and purchase several bottles of each supplement you normally use. You can save hundreds of dollars per year if you plan and shop for your foods and supplements the correct way.

Good nutrition does not have to be complicated or expensive. If you arm yourself with knowledge before you hit the supermarket or health-food store, the aisles of foods and dietary supplements staring back at you will seem far less intimidating. Take it one step further and prepare yourself with a concrete nutrition plan and shopping list, and you will emerge from the store confident in your purchases and with change still jingling in your wallet.

PART TWO

ANATOMY, DIGESTION, AND METABOLISM

10. CELLS, TISSUES, AND SYSTEMS

The pages of this book, magazine articles on sports nutrition, and other health media, as well as locker-room companions, doctors, trainers, and coaches, all share something in common—a terminology relating to the human body and its parts. In this chapter, we will discuss the fundamental units of the body, anatomical terms, and concepts commonly encountered in sports science. This introduction to the basics of human anatomy will be followed by a discussion of the digestive system in Chapter 11 and a primer on body composition and metabolism in Chapter 12. These three chapters together will hopefully give you a fundamental knowledge that will help you to better utilize the material presented in Parts Three and Four.

CELLS

The human body is an incredible biological phenomenon comprised of several interdependent systems that are responsible for maintaining life. For example, the skeletal muscle system depends on the nervous system to fire off muscle contractions. It also needs the cardiovascular system to provide it with nourishment and to carry away the metabolic waste products. These complex systems are made of fundamentally simpler units, or building blocks. The digestive system is composed of a number of different organs, which in turn are composed of a variety of tissues, which in turn are composed of cells of different forms and functions.

Cells are the fundamental units of life. About 100 trillion cells somehow organize themselves to compose a human body. They include such cells as striated muscle cells, which can be several inches long and have the unique ability to shorten in length, thereby causing muscle contraction, and fat cells, which are small and round and store fatty acids for energy.

Another magnificent characteristic of cells is that they can reproduce themselves. In fact, cells can arise only from pre-existing cells. The complex human body originates from the union of just two cells—the female egg cell and the male sperm cell. These sex cells merge to form one larger cell, called a zygote. The zygote divides and forms two cells. The two zygote cells divide to form four cells, which then divide. Even when a relatively fixed amount of cells is reached, the division continues, with the new cells replacing old or dead cells.

Cell division happens automatically. All we have to do is eat food to give our bodies nourishment to stay alive. But by eating the *proper* foods, we can help our bodies work better. For example, scientists have suspected for years that a byproduct of metabolism, the free radical, can damage cellular structures and molecules. Free radicals also become more prevalent during periods of strenuous activity or fat loss. Antioxidant nutrients tend to scavenge free radicals. They combine with and help stabilize free radicals, thus preventing damage. Vitamin A, beta-carotene, vitamin C, vitamin E, copper, manganese, selenium, and zinc have all been shown to have antioxidant activity. (For a discussion of free radicals and antioxidants, see Chapter 5.)

Every cell in the human body also has its own anatomy and physiology. These subcellular structures are called organelles. The organelles that each cell typically contains are the cell membrane, nucleus, ribosome, endoplasmic reticulum, Golgi apparatus, lysosome, and mitochondrion.

Cell Membrane

The cell membrane is the outer boundary of the cell. Also called the plasma membrane, it is a complex structure composed mainly of protein and a phospholipid bilayer. The phospholipid bilayer is made of glycerol, two fatty acids, and a phosphate group. The cell membrane therefore is a double-walled structure with proteins embedded in its bilayer sheets.

The fatty acids give the cell membrane its nutritional significance. They make fats an important part of the diet. We should not eat too much fat, but at the same time, we need to consume at least a minimum amount. Fats are especially important for athletes who are training to build muscle mass and for long-distance athletes, whose metabolisms burn up tremendous amounts of fatty acids.

The cell membrane is semipermeable. It allows certain molecules to be transported through it, and it also actively transports certain compounds through itself by itself. These abilities allow the cell to have control over what substances and how much of each substance comes inside. Additionally, the cell membrane allows the cell to rid itself of undesirable compounds while retaining desirable ones.

Nucleus

The nucleus is the control center of the cell. It is located in the approximate middle of the cell and is slightly darker than the surrounding material. The nucleus is essentially a cell within a cell, contained in its own membrane and housing the cell's DNA. Strands of DNA form chromosomes, which contain all of an individual's genetic information in the form of genes. Human cells contain two sets of twenty-three chromosomes, one set from each parent, for a total of forty-six individual chromosomes or twenty-three pairs. The chromosomes are suspended in a liquid called the nucleoplasm. The membrane surrounding the nucleus is called the nuclear membrane. The liquid between the cell membrane and the nuclear membrane is called the cytoplasm, or cytosol, and is the site of many metabolic processes, including gluconeogenesis (synthesis of glucose from noncarbohydrate sources), fatty-acid synthesis, and glycolysis. (For a discussion of two genetic terms that often cause confusion, see ("Is My Foot Size a Phenotype or Genotype?" below.)

The main function of the nucleus is to initiate the production of substances needed by the cell. It does this by signaling the necessary genes to make copies of themselves. These copies are then carried by messenger RNA from the nucleus to the cytoplasm, where they are used as a template to produce the desired substance. Another important function of the nucleus is to initiate cell division. During cell division, every chromosome must be duplicated so that the new cell contains all twenty-three pairs of chromosomes.

Ribosome

A ribosome is an extremely small, spherical organelle composed of protein and RNA. It is by far the most numerous organelle. Some ribosomes are scattered throughout the cytoplasm, while others are attached to the surface of another organelle, the endoplasmic reticulum. The ribosomes in the cytoplasm are the site of the protein synthesis in the cell. The blueprint for the protein is delivered to the ribosome by messenger RNA, and the amino acids are helped into place by transfer RNA. The ribosomes on the endoplasmic reticulum synthesize compounds that are used outside the cell, such as hormones and digestive enzymes.

Endoplasmic Reticulum

The endoplasmic reticulum (ER) is a network of canals within the cytoplasm. There are two types of ERs—one is rough and one is smooth. Rough ER has ribosomes attached. Protein and other molecules are made in rough ER and are transported through the ER canal network either to other parts of the cell or out of the cell. Smooth ER does not have ribosomes attached and its function is less clear, although it may be the site of steroid synthesis in the testes and adrenal glands. Evidence also indicates that lipid and cholesterol metabolism occur in the smooth ER of liver cells.

Is My Foot Size a Phenotype or Genotype?

As genetics has grown in popularity during the last thirty years as a subject of discussion, it has brought into popular use a host of scientific terms. Two of these terms, *genotype* and *phenotype,* are also commonly misused. *Genotype* refers to the genetic information stored in the chromosomes. *Phenotype* refers to the actual physical characteristics, such as eye color and foot size, that a person possesses.

It is believed that phenotype is the result of genotype plus environment. Some phenotypic characteristics, such as eye color, cannot be influenced by the environment. However, other characteristics, such as body weight and athletic performance, can be controlled. Examples of environmental factors are physical surroundings, climate, food, activity, and stress. In conclusion, your genotype is fixed, but the expression of your genes (your phenotype) is dynamic.

Golgi Apparatus

The Golgi apparatus consists of stacks of tiny, oblong sacs embedded in the cytoplasm near the nucleus. Recent research has presented convincing evidence that the Golgi sacs are responsible for the synthesis of carbohydrate molecules. These carbohydrate molecules then combine with the protein molecules made in the ER to form glycoproteins. Enzymes, hormones, antibodies, and structural proteins are all examples of glycoproteins.

As the amount of glycoprotein produced within a Golgi sac increases, the sac becomes inflated. When the sac is fully inflated, small spheres form along its surface, become filled with the glycoproteins, and break away. The spheres then transport their glycoprotein cargoes out of the cell and into the bloodstream, for use by other cells.

Lysosome

A lysosome is another saclike structure. Unlike a Golgi sac, however, it changes in size and shape according to its degree of activity. It starts out small and grows as its activity increases.

Lysosomes house a variety of enzymes that catalyze (initiate) and direct all the major biochemical reactions in the cell. These enzymes are capable of breaking down all of a cell's main components, including its protein, fat, and nucleic acid. In this way, lysosomes prevent the digestion of whole cells by containing and isolating these important cellular digestive enzymes. The breakdown products formed inside a lysosome are used as the raw materials for the synthesis of new molecules or for energy. Lysosomes also help to engulf and destroy bacteria that enter the cell.

Mitochondrion

Next to the nucleus, the mitochondrion is probably the best known and most discussed organelle. In the athletic arena, this is due to its role in the generation of energy. Called the cell's powerhouse, a mitochondrion is a small, complex organelle that is shaped like a sausage. It consists of a smooth outer membrane surrounding an inner membrane, forming a sac within a sac. The inner membrane is folded like an accordion, and the inward folds of the inner membrane are called the cristae.

Mitochondria are the storehouses for one of the body's most important molecules, adenosine triphos-

phate, as well as for the enzymes involved in cellular metabolic activities, including ATP production. ATP stores the energy that is used to power biological functions. Specifically, nutrients such as glucose and fatty acids are made of carbon atoms linked together by chemical bonds. When the catabolic enzymes from the inner mitochondrion membrane help break these chemical bonds, energy is released. This energy is trapped and stored in ATP molecules within the mitochondrion, thereby becoming available to the body in a form that it can utilize.

TISSUES

While cells are the fundamental units of life, tissues are the fundamental units of function and structure of the human body. Tissues are defined as an aggregation of cells that work together to perform a common function. For example, cells in the adrenal glands form a tissue that produces several adrenal hormones, including aldosterone and hydrocortisone. Muscle tissue, which has the ability to shorten in length, is made up of special long muscle cells called muscle fibers.

Despite the complexity of the human body, the tissues that form it can be separated into five basic groups. These basic tissues that make up the entire body are epithelial tissue, connective tissue, muscle tissue, nervous tissue, and reproductive tissue.

Epithelial Tissue

Epithelial tissue is found throughout the body. It forms the continuous external layer over the whole body known as the skin, composes the topmost layer of the majority of the body's inner cavities, and makes up the body's several glands. On the surface of the body, the epithelial tissue's main function is to protect the underlying cells from bacteria, adverse chemicals, and dehydration. On the inside, its main functions are absorption and secretion.

The primary types of epithelial tissue are:

☐ *Squamous epithelium.* This tissue is composed of one layer of flat cells. It helps form the linings of the mouth, esophagus, blood vessels, and lymphatic vessels. Substances can pass through this type of tissue very easily.

☐ *Cuboidal epithelium.* This tissue is composed of cube-shaped cells and is found in the lining of the renal tubule (a section of the kidney).

131

☐ *Columnar epithelium*. This tissue is composed of cells that resemble columns, or pillars. It is found throughout the body, forming the linings in the digestive tract and respiratory tract. Its main functions are secretion and absorption. Some columnar tissue also has small hairs, called cilia, which move rhythmically to sweep materials by, such as in the respiratory tract, where the cilia keep foreign matter out of the lungs.

☐ *Glandular epithelium*. This tissue secretes mucus and hormones. It comes in a variety of shapes, such as spheroids, columns, and cubes, and forms glands such as the salivary and thymus glands.

Epithelial tissue is categorized according to the shape of the cells that compose it.

Connective Tissue

The same as epithelial tissue, connective tissue is found throughout the body. As its name implies, connective tissue's main function is to connect. Some kinds of connective tissue join other tissues to each other, some kinds join muscle to bone, and some connect bone to bone. Another function of connective tissue is to support.

Connective tissue is composed of cells embedded in a nonliving matrix. Some connective tissues are like a soft gel that is firm but flexible, while others are hard, tough, and rigid. This is due to the matrix. Bone is cells within a hard, calcified matrix, while blood consists of cells suspended within a fluid matrix. The matrix is made of water, protein, carbohydrates, and a mixture of salts. Among the fibers and cells embedded in the matrix are elastic fibers for elasticity, collagen fibers for strength, reticular fibers for support, microphages and white blood cells for fighting infections, fat cells for storage, and plasma cells for antibody production.

There are certain kinds of connective tissue that are more important than other kinds to athletes. They include the following:

☐ *Cartilage*. This tissue forms the foundation of bone tissue. It contains more matrix than cells and is like a firm gel in consistency. The three types of cartilage are elastic cartilage, which is found in the ear and eustachian tube; fibrous cartilage, which is the tough cartilage found in the disks between the bones of the spine; and hyaline cartilage, which is the hard cartilage found at the ends of bones and in the nose, larynx, and trachea. Mature cartilage does not contain blood vessels or nerves. It is fed through small holes that allow nutrients to seep in.

☐ *Bone*. This tissue forms the skeleton, which supports and protects the body. It both resembles and differs from cartilage. Like cartilage, bone has more matrix than cells. But in bone, the matrix is calcified and hardened rather than gel-like. This is because the matrix contains calcium salts and a large number of collagen fibers. Bone tissue and bone marrow also have numerous blood vessels, which continually deliver food and oxygen to the cells within the matrix and carry waste products away.

☐ *Tendons and ligaments*. These tissues are the strongest connective tissues. They are flexible but sturdy. This is because their matrices are made of both collagen fibers and reticular fibers. Collagen fibers are tough, while reticular fibers are fine, occurring in networks to support delicate structures such as capillaries and nerve fibers. Tendons connect muscles to bones and other structures. They can be thick, like the Achilles tendon, or thin, like the poneurosis (the thin layer of tissue that covers the skull). Ligaments join bone to bone, usually as joints.

Some other types of connective tissue are the reticular tissue of the spleen, lymph nodes, and bone marrow, which acts as a filter for blood and lymph; areolar tissue, a loose connective tissue that links organs and binds the skin to underlying muscle tissue; and adipose tissue, which contains fat and is found under the skin throughout the body as protection, insulation, support, and a food reserve. Also classified as connective tissues are blood, bone marrow, and lymph.

Because connective tissue consists of only a few cells and mostly nonliving matrix, it has a very limited capacity for regeneration. This is one reason why tendon and ligament injuries often require surgery. However, proper nutrition and strength training can help make connective tissue stronger and more resistant to injury. One nutritional therapy that is well documented in the research literature is the supplemental use of glucosamine. (For a discussion of glucosamine, see page 105.)

Muscle Tissue

Muscle tissue makes up approximately 43 percent of a man's body weight and 34 percent of a woman's body weight. Some 620 muscles work together, with the support of the skeletal system, to create motion. An additional 30 or so help food to pass through the digestive system, help blood to circulate, and help a number of internal organs to operate. In exercise physiology, muscles are the main operative tissue, expending energy, generating waste products, and requiring substantial nutrition.

The main function of muscle tissue is contraction. Muscle contraction is caused by either involuntary stimuli or voluntary stimuli. Voluntary muscle tissue is controlled by the somatic nervous system. Its contraction can be voluntarily controlled. The major voluntary muscle tissues are the skeletal muscles. Involuntary muscle tissue is controlled by stimuli from the autonomic nervous system. Its contraction cannot be voluntarily controlled, except in rare instances. The body's eternal pump, the heart, is an example of involuntary muscle tissue.

Muscles also vary in appearance when observed under a microscope. This is due to differences in their underlying cellular structures. Some muscle tissue appears striated, while other muscle tissue appears smooth. Based on these functional and structural differences, muscle tissue is divided into the following types:

☐ *Skeletal muscle tissue.* This tissue is striated-voluntary muscle tissue. It is attached to the bones and the eyeballs and is found in the upper third of the esophagus. Skeletal muscle tissue functions to move the bones and the eyes. It also moves food down the esophagus during the first part of swallowing. It is made of long muscle cells (muscle fibers) that are unique in that they contain many nuclei. Characteristically, skeletal muscle tissue cannot sustain prolonged contraction, as it fatigues easily.

☐ *Cardiac muscle tissue.* This tissue is striated-involuntary muscle tissue. It is found in just one spot in the body—the wall of the heart. It functions to contract the heart and pump blood through the body. Cardiac muscle cells are often branched and their nuclei are more centered than those of skeletal muscle cells. Cardiac muscle cells have a tendency to branch into and fuse with each other. Fortunately, cardiac muscle tissue does not fatigue easily; it makes do with the period of rest in between contractions. Even during periods of intensive exercise, the skeletal muscles fatigue before the heart does.

☐ *Smooth muscle tissue.* This tissue is smooth-involuntary muscle tissue. It is found in the walls of the tube-shaped organs of the digestive, respiratory, reproductive, and urinary systems. It is also found in the walls of the blood vessels and large lymphatic vessels, in the ducts of glands, within the eyeballs, and in the erector muscles that are attached to some hair follicles. Smooth muscle tissue helps substances move along their respective tracts, changes the diameter of blood vessels, moves substances along the glandular ducts, changes the diameter of the pupil and the shape of the lens, and holds hair erect. Like skeletal muscle cells, smooth muscle cells are elongated. However, they differ from skeletal muscle cells because they have pointed ends and only one nucleus. Smooth muscle tissue also contracts more slowly than striated muscle tissue does and therefore does not fatigue as easily.

For a further discussion of muscle tissue, especially skeletal muscle tissue, see Chapter 14.

Nervous Tissue

Nervous tissue is responsible for the control of the bodily functions. It is found in the brain, spinal cord, and nerves. Nervous tissue is composed of the following types of cells:

☐ *Neurons.* These cells conduct nerve impulses, register sensory impulses, and conduct motor impulses. They consist of a nucleus surrounded by cytoplasm. They also have two kinds of projections—dendrites, through which the impulses enter, and an axon, which carries the impulses away from the cell. The point where two neurons make contact is called the synapse.

☐ *Neuroglia.* These cells, also called glial cells, make up the special connective tissue of the central nervous system. They include four kinds of cells—oligodendrocytes, astrocytes, ependymal cells, and microglia. They help supply the neurons with nutrients and function in the neurons' embryological growth and orientation.

☐ *Neurosecretory cells.* These cells manufacture and secrete substances that produce effects elsewhere in the body.

Neurons are the primary cells composing the nervous tissue. However, for every neuron, there are about five to ten neuroglia. In fact, neuroglia make up about 40 percent of the cells in the brain and spinal cord.

Reproductive Tissue

The final kind of tissue is the one responsible for the propagation of the species. Reproductive tissue, as its name implies, is composed of cells that specialize in producing the next generation. These cells are the ovum (egg cell) in females and the spermatozoon (sperm cell) in males. Ova are spherical in shape and contain yolk to feed the developing offspring from the instant of fertilization until the baby is able to obtain food in an alternative way.

SYSTEMS

All of the tissues just discussed interact in one way or another to form functional body units referred to as systems. Technically, the body is one living system made up of subsystems. However, for academic purposes, anatomists and physiologists refer to the subsystems as systems.

As already mentioned, the various systems that make up the body are interdependent—that is, although each system can be separated from the rest, without the other systems, it cannot carry out its functions to completion. For example, if the skeletal muscle system were disconnected from the nervous system, nerve impulses might travel through neurons but would not be able to stimulate muscle contraction.

The human body is generally recognized as being composed of nine major systems. These systems are the skeletal system, skeletal muscle system, nervous system, respiratory system, cardiovascular system, digestive system, urinary system, reproductive system, and endocrine system.

Skeletal System

The skeletal system consists of all the bones in the body, plus the joints formed where the bones are attached to each other. The predominant tissues are bone, cartilage, ligaments, and hemopoietic tissue (the bone-marrow and lymphatic tissue in which blood cells and platelets are formed). The basic functions of the skeletal system are support, protection, movement, and hemopoiesis (production of blood cells and platelets).

Skeletal Muscle System

The skeletal muscle system includes all of the body's skeletal muscles and tendons, which are nourished by the cardiovascular system and controlled by the somatic nervous system. The main function of the skeletal muscle system is the voluntary movement of the body. The skeletal muscles also serve, to a limited extent, as storage tissue for protein (amino acids). However, breakdown of this tissue for its protein stores is detrimental for athletes and beneficial in general only during periods of starvation. (For a three-part diagram of the muscles of the human body, see Appendix F on page 379.)

Nervous System

The nervous system is the network of cells that carries nerve impulses throughout the body to help the body operate. It is divided into the central nervous system, which consists of the brain and spinal cord, and the peripheral nervous system, which is composed of all the remaining nervous tissue. The peripheral nervous system includes the autonomic nervous system, which is further divided into the sympathetic and parasympathetic nervous systems. The nervous system's two main functions include providing memory and integrating bodily functions, communication, and control.

Respiratory System

The respiratory system consists of the nose, pharynx, larynx, trachea, bronchi, and lungs. Its purpose is to connect the trillions of cells that make up the human body with the gaseous environment outside the body. The respiratory system provides a conduit for the intake of oxygen and the expulsion of carbon dioxide and water. It needs the cardiovascular system to complete its functions—transferring oxygen from the lungs to the bloodstream and then to the cells, and transferring carbon dioxide and water from the cells to the bloodstream and then out of the body.

Cardiovascular System

The cardiovascular system, also called the circulatory system, consists of the heart, veins, arteries, and lymphatic system. The lymphatic system is considered part of the cardiovascular system because it is composed of a group of vessels, called the lymphatics, that move a fluid, called lymph, through the body. The cardiovascular system performs a vital pickup and delivery service for the body. By means of the blood it circulates through the body, it picks up food and oxygen from the digestive and respiratory systems and delivers them to the cells. From the cells, it picks up waste products and delivers them to the excretory organs, such as the kidneys. It also picks up the hormones secreted by the glands of the endocrine system and delivers them to their target tissues. Directly or indirectly, the cardiovascular system helps every cell of the body to function.

Digestive System

The digestive system is also called the alimentary canal or gastrointestinal system. It consists of the mouth, esophagus, stomach, small intestine, large intestine, and rectum. Several accessory organs are connected to or exist in the digestive system. They include the pancreas, liver, and gallbladder. The main function of the digestive system is to break down food into a form in which it can be digested and absorbed. Another function is the transportation and excretion of waste products. (For a complete discussion of the digestive system, see Chapter 11.).

Urinary System

The urinary system consists of a pair of kidneys, a pair of ureters, a bladder, and a urethra. The kidneys filter waste products from the blood, maintain the body's electrolyte and pH balances, influence blood pressure, and play a role in homeostasis. They also reabsorb 97 to 99 percent of the substances needed by the body that they initially filtered out. The waste products that the kidneys selectively remove from the blood and do not reabsorb are transported to the bladder by the ureters. The bladder collects and stores these waste products in the form of urine. When the bladder is filled, the urine is expelled from the body through the urethra.

Reproductive System

The reproductive system consists of those organs whose primary purpose is to produce offspring. In males, these organs function to produce viable sperm. They include a pair of testes, which produce sperm and testosterone; a pair of seminal vesicles, which store the sperm until ejaculation; a prostate gland, which helps produce semen, a nutritional fluid that helps the sperm to survive in the vagina; and a pair of

bulbourethral glands, which secrete an alkaline fluid that mixes with the semen. Various ducts tie these organs together.

In females, the reproductive system consists of those organs that work to produce fertile eggs and that provide an internal environment suitable for a fertilized egg to develop into a baby. It includes a pair of ovaries, which contain unfertilized eggs; a pair of fallopian tubes, which carry one egg a month down to the uterus; a uterus, which is where the fertilized egg becomes implanted; the cervix, which is the neck of the uterus and protects the developing fetus from bacteria and other invaders; and the vagina, which functions as the vestibule for the erect penis. The female reproductive system is much more complex than the male's.

Endocrine System

The endocrine system consists of a number of glands that produce a variety of hormones. The glands do not have ducts and secrete their hormones directly into the bloodstream. The hormones are carried by the bloodstream to where they are needed, producing their effects away from the glands in which they were produced. The glands of the endocrine system include the adrenal glands, pancreas, parathyroid glands, pituitary gland, thymus gland, thyroid gland, ovaries (in females), and testes (in males). The hormones they secrete include the following:

☐ *Adrenocorticotropic hormone (ACTH)*. Secreted by the pituitary gland. Stimulates the secretion of hormones by the adrenal glands.

☐ *Aldosterone*. Secreted by the adrenal glands. Regulates the blood-mineral levels and increases the bodily fluid levels.

☐ *Antidiuretic hormone (ADH)*. Secreted by the pituitary gland. Regulates water absorption by the kidneys and causes arteriole constriction.

☐ *Estrogen*. Secreted by the ovaries. Functions in the development of feminine characteristics.

☐ *Follicle stimulating hormone (FSH)*. Secreted by the pituitary gland. Stimulates testosterone secretion and sperm development in males and egg production and estrogen secretion in females.

☐ *Glucagon*. Secreted by the pancreas. Increases the blood-sugar level, converts fat and protein to glucose, and increases the blood-potassium and -phosphate levels.

☐ *Growth hormone (GH)*. Secreted by the pituitary gland. Helps regulate metabolism and stimulates both hard- and soft-tissue growth.

☐ *Hydrocortisone*. Secreted by the adrenal glands. Regulates the metabolism of protein, carbohydrates, and fat.

☐ *Insulin*. Secreted by the pancreas. Decreases the blood-sugar level, promotes glycogen storage, and decreases the blood-potassium and -phosphate levels.

☐ *Luteinizing hormone (LH)*. Secreted by the pituitary gland. Stimulates progesterone secretion by the ovaries, prepares the uterus for the fertilized egg, and aids in the development of the mammary glands.

☐ *Oxytocin*. Secreted by the pituitary gland. Stimulates uterine contractions during childbirth and milk ejection after birth.

☐ *Parathyroid hormone (PTH)*. Secreted by the parathyroid glands. Increases the blood-calcium level and decreases the blood-phosphate level.

☐ *Prolactin*. Secreted by the pituitary gland. Stimulates milk secretion by the mammary glands.

☐ *Testosterone*. Secreted by the testes. Functions in the development of masculine characteristics and aids in the development of the male sex organs.

☐ *Thymus hormone*. Secreted by the thymus gland. Stimulates antibody production in the lymphoid tissue and liver.

☐ *Thyroid stimulating hormone (TSH)*. Secreted by the pituitary gland. Stimulates the secretion of hormones by the thyroid gland.

☐ *Thyroxine*. Secreted by the thyroid gland. Increases the metabolic rate.

The same as the nervous system, the endocrine system's main functions are control, communication, and integration of bodily functions. However, the endocrine system uses secretions (hormones) to accomplish these purposes, rather than impulses, the way the nervous system does. In addition, its responses are much slower than those of the nervous system.

The complexity of the human body can be staggering. However, once you start thinking about the body as an organized system, with subsystems that carry out different functions and that are composed of cells performing specialized jobs, it becomes much easier to understand. Just think of a corporation with departments manned by skilled workers performing specific duties. The body is complicated but logical, and the logic makes it comprehensible. The terminology of anatomy and physiology add another degree to that comprehension, as well as providing the color that "brings the body to life."

11. DIGESTION AND ABSORPTION

Most people enjoy eating. In fact, the average person eats several hundred pounds of food every year. When you think about it, it is amazing that all we have to do to survive is shovel some food into our mouths and drink some liquid; our bodies do the rest. If you eat just for survival, this approach is fine. But if your goals are to extend your life and improve your athletic performance, you need to do a little more. Learning about digestion is a start.

In this chapter, we will discuss the basics of digestion. For discussions of the digestion of carbohydrates, protein, and lipids in particular, see Chapters 2, 3, and 4, respectively.

THE DIGESTIVE SYSTEM

The digestive system is the body's life-support connection with the external environment. When food is eaten, the digestive system breaks it down into useful molecules to supply the body with the energy it needs for life and the building blocks it needs for growth. Digestion, therefore, is the process in which food is broken down through chemical and physical means.

The digestive system starts with the mouth, runs some twenty-five feet through the trunk of the body, and ends with the anus. It is basically a strong muscular tube lined with epithelial tissue and specialized cells. Its functions include:

☐ Receipt, mastication (chewing), and transport of ingested foodstuffs.

☐ Secretion of the acids, mucus, digestive enzymes, bile, and other materials needed to break down foodstuffs.

☐ Digestion of foodstuffs.

☐ Absorption of nutrients.

☐ Transport, storage, and excretion of waste products.

Other names for the digestive system are the alimentary canal, the gastrointestinal system, and the gut.

Physically, the digestive system is quite complex and remarkable. It is composed of several anatomically different structures—the mouth, esophagus, stomach, small intestine, large intestine, and rectum. In addition, it includes accessory organs—such as the pancreas, liver, and gallbladder—that perform essential functions during the digestive process.

Mouth

The mouth is the gateway to the digestive tract. When you take a bite of food, that food enters your digestive system. To begin the digestive process, the mouth performs four functions with the food.

First, in the mouth, the food is physically broken apart and reduced in size through chewing. Thorough chewing is vital to the digestive process. By thoroughly chewing your food, you get the full benefit of the digestive enzyme ptyalin, which begins the chemical breakdown of starch (carbohydrates). Chewing also physically reduces the food and prepares the other macronutrients for digestion, so that the stomach can perform its functions easier.

Second, the mouth mixes the food with saliva to form a moist mass called a bolus. The saliva lubricates the food for its journey down the esophagus to the stomach. It also supplies the enzyme ptyalin, as well as mucus, which makes the food particles stick together.

Third, the mouth cools or warms the food to the appropriate temperature for digestion. The temperature of the bolus is important, since enzymes function at their best within a narrow temperature range. For humans, this range is around body temperature. Also, cold food can cause the stomach to empty its contents too quickly, thus reducing digestive efficiency. One exception is before and during exercise, when drinking cold fluids and causing the stomach to empty faster will help the body rehydrate more quickly.

Fourth, the major function of the mouth is to initiate swallowing when the bolus is ready. Swallowing passes the masticated food mass through the pharynx and into the esophagus.

Esophagus

The esophagus is the transport conduit for food and water that extends from the pharynx to the stomach. When the bolus enters the esophagus, an involuntary wave of muscle contractions is triggered and propels the food mass down into the stomach. These muscle contractions are known as peristalsis. The peristaltic waves travel down the esophagus at a rate of about 3 inches per second.

At the base of the esophagus is a ringlike muscle called the esophageal sphincter. Once the bolus has traveled through the esophagus, the esophageal sphincter relaxes to let the food pass into the stomach. At the same time, the esophageal sphincter also prevents other food from spurting out of the stomach and back up into the esophagus. If it is weakened or malfunctions, however, it may not succeed. The acidic contents of the stomach may thus shoot up into the esophagus and cause the unpleasant, bitter sensation in the throat that is known as heartburn. Despite its name, heartburn has nothing to do with the heart except for the discomfort that may develop in the chest area. To reduce stress on the esophageal sphincter and prevent heartburn, eat your meals in a sitting position and do not overfill your stomach with food or liquid.

Stomach

The stomach is a muscular sac about 2 quarts in size. Its primary functions are to digest food through chemical secretions and physical churning, to store the food, and then to gradually release the food into the small intestine.

The stomach secretes several substances that help break down food. Intrinsic factor binds with vitamin B_{12} and aids the later absorption of that vitamin in the small intestine. The hormone gastrin helps regulate other stomach secretions during digestion. And the digestive enzymes rennin, pepsin, and lipase either break down or begin the breakdown process of several nutrients. Rennin prepares casein (milk protein) for breakdown by pepsin; pepsin breaks down protein in the presence of hydrochloric acid; and lipase breaks down fat molecules.

Hydrochloric acid is another secretion of the stomach. It catalyzes pepsin activity, which sets protein metabolism into motion. In addition, it helps keep the stomach relatively free of bacteria and assists in the maintainance of a low pH balance there. A mucous coating protects the stomach wall against the hydrochloric acid and also acts as a lubricant.

When carbohydrates, protein, and fat are consumed individually, they leave the stomach at different rates. Carbohydrates empty from the stomach the quickest. Protein is the next quickest to leave, and fat is the slowest. However, when carbohydrates, protein, and fat are consumed together, they take the longest to empty from the stomach. It normally takes the stomach one to four hours to empty, depending upon the amount and kinds of foods that were eaten.

While nutrients are absorbed primarily from the intestines, some can be absorbed from the stomach. In general, alcohol, glucose, water, aspirin and some other medications, and several vitamins, including vitamin B_3, can be absorbed from the stomach. Of particular interest are water and glucose, whose ability to be at least partially absorbed from the stomach enables their quick replenishment during exercise. Because of this, glucose is included as an ingredient in some popular sports drinks, along with fructose, which is more slowly absorbed, and complex carbohydrates, which release glucose slowly and steadily. Glucose ingestion can help spare the body's glycogen supply during exercise, but the glucose must be ingested within a half hour of beginning the exercise or it can cause an influx of insulin that can upset energy production during the exercise.

The stomach only begins the process of breaking down complex molecules into their smaller components, such as protein into amino acids. The breakdown process, called hydrolysis, is continued in the intestines. The partially digested material from the stomach is called chyme and enters the small intestine in squirts through the pyloric sphincter muscle.

Small Intestine

If the small intestine were stretched out to its full length, it would measure about 12 feet. The small intestine is divided into three main sections—the duodenum, the jejunum, and the ileum. The duodenum is connected to the stomach and makes up the first section. Some absorption takes place there, but the duodenum's main functions are the continued breakdown of food and its storage. The majority of nutrient absorption takes place in the second and third sections of the small intestine—the jejunum and the ileum, respectively.

To accomplish complete absorption, the small intestine has a very unique anatomy. Instead of being smooth, like skin, the inside of the small intestine is lined with special cells called villi. Villi are very small, fingerlike projections that cover the entire inner surface of the intestine. Each villus has a blood vessel running into it. When food passes through the small intestine, the nutrients pass through the cells of the villi and are absorbed into the villi blood vessels. They then travel through the bloodstream to the liver.

Another transport system is also present in the villi. This second system is the lymphatic system. In addition to a blood vessel, a small projection called a lacteal extends into each villus. The lacteals absorb fat. About 60 to 70 percent of all ingested fat is absorbed by the lacteals and transported to the liver through the lymphatic system. Unlike the circulatory system, however, the lymph system has no pump to move things along. Materials are transported by muscle contractions and passive flow. The remaining ingested fat, consisting primarily of shorter-chain fatty acids, is taken up by the blood vessels and transported through the bloodstream to the liver, where it is processed for use as energy. This is why short- and medium-chain triglycerides do not convert easily to body fat, which in turn is why they have become so popular among athletes. (For discussions of the triglycerides and fatty acids, see page 50.)

Large Intestine and Rectum

If the large intestine, also called the colon, were stretched out, it would measure about 3 feet long. Even though it is shorter than the small intestine, it is divided into more sections. The first section is called the cecum and begins where the ileum ends. The 3-inch-long, wormlike appendage known as the appendix is also located here. After the cecum comes the section known as the ascending colon, so named because it ascends toward the liver. After a left turn comes the transverse colon, which travels transversely, or horizontally, across the upper abdomen. Just below the spleen, the colon turns downward and becomes known as the descending colon. At the groin, it makes another turn and is called the sigmoid colon. Following a final turn is the rectum, which terminates with the anus.

The large intestine is the site of the final absorption of water, minerals, and vitamins. It is the home to bacteria whose metabolism helps produce nutrients such as vitamin K. It is also the storage facility for the waste products of digestion. These waste products, known as fecal matter, further decompose when they meet up with the large intestine's bacteria. The result often includes the production of gas.

When peristalsis occurs, the colon empties its contents into the rectum, which triggers defecation. Normally, the rectum is empty. The more fiber there is in the diet, the softer the feces are and the easier the defecation process is.

Pancreas

The pancreas, an endocrine gland situated beside the small intestine near the stomach, is an accessory organ of the gut. It produces several substances that are important for the digestion and absorption of the nutrients that are secreted into the small intestine. It also produces two substances that help control carbohydrate metabolism—insulin and glucagon.

Insulin is secreted into the bloodstream during a meal. It helps mediate the transport of glucose and amino acids through cell membranes. It also fosters lipogenesis (the formation of fat). Therefore, insulin has an anabolic function.

Glucagon is the functional opposite of insulin. It initiates a series of reactions that lead to the breakdown of glycogen for the purpose of releasing glucose into the bloodstream for energy. During exercise, the blood-sugar level is increased to help raise the energy level. Insulin and glucagon work together in a seesaw fashion to maintain the appropriate blood-sugar level.

Liver

Digestion is not complete until the nutrients extracted from the food moving through the stomach and intestines are delivered to the liver and then released into the bloodstream. The liver is one of the larger organs of the body, weighing in at about 4 pounds. It is connected directly to the intestines by the portal vein. Through the portal vein, the nutrients that are taken up from the intestines are delivered directly to the liver. Fats that travel through the lymphatic system first go into the bloodstream and then circulate to the liver for processing. In general, the nutrients are then control-released from the liver into the general circulation.

The liver has many important functions. Among

them, it processes the digested nutrients, extracting them and then either releasing them for immediate use or storing them for later use. It also changes nutrients into other substances that the body needs and stores these substances until they are needed. In addition, it converts glucose that is not required for immediate energy into glycogen for storage, and converts the stored glycogen back into glucose when energy is needed. The glycogen stored in the liver is used mainly to supply the brain with energy.

Gallbladder

The gallbladder is located directly under the liver and acts as the storage depot for the major substance secreted by the liver—bile. Bile is a solution composed of cholesterol, bile salts, lecithin, and the pigments bilirubin and biliverdin. It is concentrated by the gallbladder and released into the small intestine as needed for digestion. Bile is essential for the functioning of the digestive enzyme lipase, for the digestion and absorption of fats, and for the assimilation (conversion into living tissue) of calcium. It is necessary for the absorption of the fat-soluble vitamins and for the conversion of beta-carotene to vitamin A. It also plays a role in peristalsis.

FACTORS AFFECTING DIGESTION

Eating should not be taken for granted. The proper digestion of food requires good eating habits. To get the most mileage out of your meals, observe the following points:

☐ Eat slowly and chew your food thoroughly.

☐ Remain in an upright position when eating; do not eat while lying down.

☐ Eat five or more moderately sized meals instead of three large meals.

☐ Remain calm while you eat. For example, do not fight at the table and do not watch television. Nervousness can affect the movements of the digestive system and cause gastrointestinal disturbances.

☐ Give your digestive system a chance to function. Do not engage in strenuous physical activity directly after eating.

☐ Avoid foods that may irritate your stomach, such as hot spices and alcohol.

If you have any digestive-system complaints, try improving your eating habits. You could also try one of the digestive aids that are available, or you might find that a simple change in your food intake does the trick. However, if the digestive complaint does not seem to improve, consult your health-care practitioner. *A word of caution:* If you are experiencing abdominal pain, excessive gas, blood in the stool, or any gastrointestinal irregularity, seek medical attention immediately.

DIGESTIVE AIDS

Supplements for the digestive system have been around for centuries. Digestive tonics and teas have been in use for thousands of years. Of particular interest to the athlete are digestive-enzyme formulations, digestive herbs, and intestinal-bacteria supplements.

Digestive-Enzyme Formulations

Digestive-enzyme formulations in special forms for athletes are just hitting the market. For example, enzyme preparations for protein digestion are now available. Digestive-enzyme formulations are made with enzymes that act as catalysts for the breakdown of food components. (There are also enzymes that catalyze building-up processes or speed up biochemical reactions.) Under normal circumstances, the digestive system is quite efficient. However, since athletes tend to eat more than the normal amount of food, and since extra activity speeds up the movement of food through the digestive tract, an athlete's digestive efficiency may be severely compromised. Moreover, after the age of thirty, digestive irregularities become more common.

The enzymes used in digestive-enzyme formulations can be of plant or animal origin. Some plant enzymes that are commonly used are bromelin (from pineapple), papain (from papaya), protease, lipase, amylase, cellulase, and lactase. Bromelin has also become popular as a nutritional aid for healing and for the reduction of inflammation. A common enzyme of animal origin is pancreatin. Hydrochloric acid is also often used as a digestive aid by individuals whose stomach secretions of the acid have slowed down.

Digestive enzymes are available as capsules, tablets, and enteric-coated tablets. The capsules and regular tablets are reportedly more effective than the enteric-coated tablets because they release their ingredients into the system more quickly. The enteric-coated tablets may not dissolve early enough in the intestines to promote digestive action. In addition, animal-pancreatic enzymes function better as digestive aids than plant enzymes do, according to comparisons done using people with digestive problems. The blood levels of the nutrients were monitored and the animal-pancreatic enzymes were found to improve nutrient absorption.

When shopping for digestive-enzyme formulations, check the listed potency. Also note the ingredients; lipase, trypsin, chymotrypsin, and protease are common. Always take digestive enzymes with meals or as directed on the label.

A word of caution: If you have a gastrointestinal disorder, do not use a digestive-enzyme formulation except under the supervision of a health-care practitioner.

Digestive Herbs

Along with digestive enzymes, a variety of herbs have a history of use as appetite stimulants, appetite depressants, or overall digestive aids. Many athletes find that their appetites lag behind what they should be. If you cannot seem to eat everything you should, try taking some herbal supplements designed to stimulate the appetite or improve digestion. Digestive stimulants also often increase pancreatic secretion and gastric function.

Some herbs that are commonly used as appetite stimulants or overall digestive aids are blessed thistle, feverfew, gentian, ginseng, quassia, sabal palmetto, sweet flag, and Virginia snakeroot. Herbs that act as appetite depressants are brindall berry, chamomile, fennel, and red clover.

Intestinal-Bacteria Supplements

Within everyone's intestinal tract live billions of microscopic bacteria called lactobacilli. Lactobacilli are any of the rodlike bacteria of the genus *Lactobacillus* that ferment lactic acid from carbohydrates. *L. acidophilus* are present in the human intestines at birth. About two weeks later, they are joined by *L. bifidus*. Both these bacteria are called friendly bacteria because they help maintain proper intestinal functioning and overall health. They benefit the health of the entire body by suppressing the growth of harmful bacteria in the intestines, by playing a role in the pro-

duction of a variety of nutrients, and by maintaining the intestinal environment for proper nutrient absorption.

Acidophilus and bifidus (also known as bifidobacteria) are both available in supplement form, and at least one should be taken daily, especially if you suffer from frequent gastrointestinal disorders or are taking a course of antibiotics. Antibiotics wipe out good bacteria along with the bad, upsetting the balance of these microorganisms in the intestines. A high level of unhealthy flora can result in a high level of ammonia, which can irritate the intestinal membranes and seep into the bloodstream. The result can be all kinds of toxic reactions, such as nausea, decreased appetite, vomiting, constipation, excessive gas, allergies, and yeast infections. Acidophilus or bifidus supplements will bring balance back to the intestines by replenishing the good flora, plus they will help detoxify the system, thus relieving some of the strain on the liver.

Acidophilus and bifidus supplements are available in tablet, capsule, and powder forms. The enteric-coated tablets are a good delivery system because stomach enzymes can digest the bacteria. The powder form is also good. However, avoid the capsules, since they may contain moisture, which could activate the bacteria in the bottle and cause them to starve to death. The bacteria can also die from high temperatures, so store the supplements in a cool, dry place, such as the refrigerator. Do not freeze them.

When shopping for acidophilus or bifidus supplements, check the label for the number of active bacteria per daily dose. The range should be in the millions to billions. The best product has one strain of organisms, with at least one billion organisms per gram. If you are lactose intolerant, look for a nondairy formula. No matter what type of supplement you purchase, take it with water on an empty stomach in the morning and one hour before each meal, or as directed on the label. If you are taking antibiotics, do not take the acidophilus or bifidus together with the medication.

FIBER AND DIGESTION

The importance of fiber has been common knowledge for several years now. A high fiber intake improves bowel function, reduces the chances for bowel cancer, lowers the blood-cholesterol level, and helps stabilize the blood-sugar level. It also helps dieters, providing a feeling of satiety that reduces

Feed Me!

The body has developed an intricate communication system for sending "I am full" and "I am hungry" signals to the brain. Hunger pangs are the body's signal that it wants to be fed. But what exactly are hunger pangs and what causes them?

Research using human subjects and a device that measures stomach contractions has provided some answers. When the subjects felt hunger pangs, they signaled the researcher, who then made a mark on the printout from the measuring device. The marks showed that the hunger pangs were caused by increased contractions of the empty stomach.

The scientific evidence on what triggers hunger pangs is less clear. The stomach contractions that cause hunger pangs are not controlled by the nervous system, since hunger pangs still occur when the gastric nerves are cut. However, the sugar content of the blood may play a role in hunger pangs. When the blood-sugar level drops, hunger pangs kick in. But in conditions of outright starvation, hunger pangs gradually come less frequently. This may be due to ketones, which are produced during the incomplete metabolism of fatty acids.

While some of the puzzle is still unsolved, the question of how to control hunger pangs is partially answered. Maintaining an adequate blood-sugar level is one proven way. This is why including complex carbohydrates in the diet is a good nutritional practice. Foods such as rice, potatoes, and pasta provide the body with a slow, steady stream of glucose.

Another part of the puzzle that has still to be solved is why contractions of the empty stomach cause pangs and contractions of the full stomach do not.

---

overeating. (For a discussion of hunger pangs, see "Feed Me!" above.) Despite all this, however, nutrition surveys indicate that daily fiber intake has dropped in the United States during the past sixty years.

While exact recommendations have not been determined, many health officials and nutritionists recommend consuming 40 to 60 grams of dietary fiber per day. There are several ways to reach this intake goal. One is to eat more high-fiber foods. Make sure that your diet includes whole-grain cereals and flours, brown rice, all kinds of bran, fresh fruits, dried prunes, nuts, seeds (especially flaxseeds), beans, lentils, peas, and raw fresh vegetables. A good trick is to buy organic produce and eat it unpeeled. Another trick is to add extra bran to cereal and baked goods. For a list of foods that contain approximately 10 grams of dietary fiber, see "Fiber 10 Foods for Athletes" on page 28.

There are also several fiber supplements available in supermarkets, pharmacies, and health-food stores. Popular are the psyllium-seed products, such as Metamucil. Psyllium seed is a grain grown in India that is a good intestinal cleanser and stool softener. The ground psyllium is mixed with liquid and consumed as a beverage. Fiber supplements that are more natural and less processed are also available and can be purchased in health-food stores.

Maintaining a healthy digestive system is an important part of any performance-nutrition program. A healthy digestive system properly and completely breaks down food, fully and appropriately releasing the nutrients that the body needs to function effectively. Understanding digestion and the digestive system will help as you plan your diet and supplement programs, as well as when you try to correct any ills that may befall you.

12. BODY COMPOSITION AND METABOLISM

As an athlete, you need to know more about your body than your bathroom scale or a height-weight chart can tell you. To meet your sport-specific goals, you need to mold and sculpt your body. You must know how much body fat and lean body mass you have. You must know how your body responds to nutrition and training. What is your metabolic set point? How many calories does your body need? Are you getting enough protein?

In this chapter, we will discuss body composition and how to estimate body-fat percentage and lean body mass. We will also review metabolism and how to estimate daily caloric requirement. Once you have read through the chapter, you can estimate your own body composition and caloric needs with the help of the step-by-step instructions within the chapter. Transfer your results to the Personal Inventory form provided in Appendix A.

BODY COMPOSITION

Body composition refers to the fat and lean-tissue makeup of the body. Determining your body composition is an important part of your personal assessment. An excessive level of body fat is associated with reduced athletic performance and an array of health problems including heart disease, cancer, and diabetes. Knowing your body composition also helps you determine your primary training goal—fat loss, muscle gain, or body-composition maintenance.

Several methods of measuring body composition are currently in popular use. While none of the methods is 100-percent accurate, each helps you estimate how much of your body is fat and how much is lean tissue. Four measurements are important—total pounds of body fat, total pounds of lean body mass, and body fat and lean body mass as percentages of total body weight. Lean body mass is all of a body's bones, muscles, organs, blood, and water—all of the bodily tissues apart from body fat. Occasionally, the term *fat-free mass* is used interchangeably with *lean body mass*.

Keeping a record of your body composition is a mandatory part of your performance-nutrition program. Knowing your body composition and weight is necessary for determining your daily caloric requirement. Fluctuations in body weight result from changes in muscle mass, body fat, and/or water weight. To keep track of which ones are causing your weight changes, you should measure your body composition at least three times a week during the season and once a week during the off-season. You may be surprised to discover that while your total body weight remains the same, your lean body mass is increasing and your body fat is decreasing. If this happens during the season, especially at the beginning of the season, it is most likely due to the rigors of training. After the season ends and your activity level declines, you may find your lean body mass decreasing and your body fat increasing while your total body weight remains the same. In general, short-term (day-to-day) fluctuations in weight come primarily from water-weight changes. Longer-term (week-to-week) fluctuations generally come from either muscle-mass or body-fat changes. Alterations in bone density are difficult to determine, but in general, if you are healthy and well nourished, your bone density will remain relatively constant.

It is important to note, however, that none of the methods for determining body composition is precise. In fact, every one of the measurement methods currently in use has a margin of error of several percentage points. This is because the reference values are based on data collected several decades ago using cadavers that represented neither athletes nor a good cross-section of racial groups. The human body varies considerably. The best that any method can do is provide *relative* measurements of body fat and lean body mass.

The primary methods for determining body composition that are currently being used are:

☐ *Anthropometry.* Anthropometric methods of body-composition analysis are the easiest to use and require the smallest monetary investment. These methods include the height-weight charts compiled by insurance companies and tables such as body-mass indexes and waist-hip ratios. All of these methods were developed before scientists realized that body-fat percentage is a better method for determining state of health. In addition, most athletes cannot use these charts because the ratios were developed for the population at large and based on data compiled using average people. For example, athletes cannot use height-weight charts because their extra muscle mass always makes them too heavy for their height.

☐ *Hydrostatic weighing.* The method that has become the all-time favorite procedure for analyzing body composition is hydrostatic weighing (underwater weighing). The principle on which it is based is very simple—lean body mass is *more* dense than water and fat is *less* dense than water. Therefore, the more fat you have, the less you will weigh under water; the more muscle you have, the more you will weigh under water. Once you have been weighed under water, your body composition is calculated accordingly.

☐ *Skin-fold measurement.* Measuring skin folds is also a very popular way to analyze body composition. It is inexpensive, easy to learn, quick, and reliable. It measures the thickness of the adipose tissue (the anatomical fat found in between the skin and muscle) on the theory that the more fat there is, the thicker the skin fold will be. Since skin-fold measurements can be easily taken with special skin-fold calipers, researchers have compiled a vast database using a diversity of individuals. Through this, they realized that different methods of analysis are needed for different kinds of people. For example, younger people tend to have harder adipose tissue than older people do and therefore need different mathematical formulations for calculating percent as well as amount of body fat. In addition, different measurement procedures and calculations are needed for the two sexes because men carry their body fat differently than women do. If you have a skin-fold analysis performed, make sure that the technician is trained and uses methods appropriate for your age and sex.

Also note that a variety of skin-fold calipers are used. Some calipers are designed to measure only one site, while others are designed to measure twelve or more sites. The more sites that are measured, the more accurate the analysis is. However, you can get a reliable estimate of your body composition based on the measurement of just three or four sites. Skin-fold calipers of good quality cost about $150 to $350, but plastic skin-fold calipers can be purchased for less than $40. Plastic calipers tend to be less accurate, but they are useful for keeping track of changes in skin-fold measurements. Look for calipers with a parallel-jaw design and constant spring tension. Constant spring tension helps you apply the same force on your body each time you use the calipers.

☐ *Bioelectrical impedance or conductivity.* The bioelectrical methods of measuring body composition are based on the principle that water conducts electricity better than fat does. Because muscle has a high water content and fat has a very low water content, the rate at which the body conducts or impedes electricity can be used to estimate body composition. A variety of bioelectrical devices are available, but many are extremely expensive, costing thousands of dollars. Hand-held versions that give instant readings have also been developed but are intended for the population at large and use calculations for average people.

Recent scientific reviews of the bioelectrical methods indicate that they are extremely unreliable. Use one of these methods only in addition to a more reliable method. Methods based on ultrasound or infrared light are similar to the bioelectrical methods and also should not be used as a sole method of analyzing body composition.

Visual methods and the time-honored "pinch an inch" are also useful. If you look lean, have good muscle definition, and cannot grab a handful of fat around your stomach, you most likely have an average or below-average body-fat percentage.

Some athletes may wish to go one step further and determine precisely how much muscle is included in their lean muscle mass. These athletes may find one of the laboratory methods well worth the time and expense. A popular one measures the amount of creatinine excreted from the body. Creatinine is a waste product of creatine metabolism and is normally passed in the urine. Scientists have determined that there is a direct relationship between the amount of muscle mass an individual has and the amount of creatinine he or she excretes. Since lean body mass consists of all the tissues except body fat, measuring the amount of creatinine in the urine provides a precise measurement of how much muscle mass the lean body tissue includes. However, the creatinine-excretion method requires the services of a physician, since urine samples must be collected over a period of time and analyzed by a trained technician.

Hydrostatic weighing, skin-fold measurement, and laboratory analysis are all good ways to determine and keep track of body composition. The best way, however, is to use at least three different measurement methods to get a comparative analysis. You can then pick one method and use it on a regular basis to keep track of changes. We recommend having yourself hydrostatically weighed three times during the season and using the Quick Method for Determining Body Composition (see below) a few times per week. We also recommend measuring your skin folds three times a week. In addition, especially during the season, you should weigh yourself every day in the morning on an empty stomach, before *and* after exercise, *and* in the evening before bedtime.

QUICK METHOD FOR DETERMINING BODY COMPOSITION

The following method for determining body composition is known as the Quick Method because it takes just a few minutes to do. The equipment needed is a bathroom scale, tape measure, and calculator. If possible, use a tape measure with a spring-tension device to help keep human error to a minimum.

The Quick Method was developed specifically for athletes. It is really two methods—one for male athletes and one for female athletes. Both the male and female methods utilize mathematical constants that researchers have determined account for the fixed parameters of the body such as the bones, body cavities, organs, lung volume, and connective tissues. The same as the other methods, however, the Quick Method is still not 100-percent accurate. While the constants allow us to get a more reliable estimate of a body's fat content versus lean body mass, the results may still be off by 4 percent or more. However, the Quick Method will enable you to immediately determine your approximate body composition, which will allow you to calculate your daily caloric requirement.

The Quick Method for Determining Body Composition for men is as follows:

1. Weigh yourself (in pounds) in the nude. Multiply your total body weight by 1.082, which is men's weight constant one. Then add 94.420, which is men's weight constant two. The result is your weight factor.

(Total body weight x 1.082) + 94.420 = Weight factor

2. Measure your waist (in inches) at your navel. Multiply your waist measurement by 4.150, which is the men's waist constant. The product is your waist factor.

Waist measurement x 4.150 = Waist factor

3. Subtract your waist factor from your weight factor. The difference is your pounds of lean body mass.

Weight factor – Waist factor = Lean body mass

4. Subtract your lean body mass from your total body weight. The difference is your pounds of body fat.

Total body weight – Lean body mass = Body fat

5. Multiply your body fat by 100, then divide the result by your total body weight. This is the standard equation for obtaining a percentage. The result is your body-fat percentage.

(Body fat x 100) ÷ Total body weight = Body-fat percentage

6. Subtract your body-fat percentage from 100 percent. The difference is your lean-body-mass percentage.

100 percent – Body-fat percentage = Lean-body-mass percentage

For an example of how one man used this formula to determine his body composition, see "How Muscular Am I?" on page 146.

The Quick Method for Determining Body Composition for women is similar to the formula for men. The steps are as follows:

1. Weigh yourself (in pounds) in the nude. Multiply your total body weight by 0.732, which is women's weight constant one. Then add 8.987, which is women's weight constant two. The result is your weight factor.

(Total body weight x 0.732) + 8.987 = Weight factor

2. Measure your wrist (in inches) at its fullest point. Divide your wrist measurement by 3.140, which is the women's wrist constant. The result is your wrist factor.

Wrist measurement ÷ 3.140 = Wrist factor

3. Measure your abdomen (in inches) at your navel. Multiply your abdominal measurement by 0.157,

How Muscular Am I?

If you are a man who would like to figure out how much lean body mass and body fat you have, use the Quick Method for Determining Body Composition that is described on page 145. John used the method and found it to be not only quick but easy. His calculations, detailed below, show exactly how to follow the formula.

John is a weekend golfer who has been entering amateur tournaments since high school. He is an excellent golfer, but he wants to improve. His goal is to leave his office job and turn professional. Perhaps he can even become the next Tiger Woods. But to reach his goal, John needs to become more serious about his nutrition and training programs. His first step is to determine his body composition, so that he can plan an appropriate diet and workout. John weighs 205 pounds and has a waist measurement of 35 inches. Following are his calculations:

1. First, John takes his total body weight (205 pounds) and multiplies it by 1.082 (men's weight constant one). Then, he adds the product (221.810) to 94.420 (men's weight constant two). The result (316.230) is his weight factor.

205	Total body weight
× 1.082	Men's weight constant one
221.810	
+ 94.420	Men's weight constant two
316.230	Weight factor

2. Next, John takes his waist measurement (35 inches) and multiplies it by 4.150 (the men's waist constant). The result (145.250) is his waist factor.

35	Waist measurement
× 4.150	Men's waist constant
145.250	Waist factor

3. John takes his weight factor (316.230) and subtracts his waist factor (145.250). The difference (170.980 pounds) is his lean body mass.

316.230	Weight factor
− 145.250	Waist factor
170.980	Lean body mass

4. John takes his total body weight (205 pounds) and subtracts his lean body mass (170.980 pounds). The difference (34.020 pounds) is his body fat.

205.000	Total body weight
− 170.980	Lean body mass
34.020	Body fat

5. Using the standard equation for obtaining a percentage, John takes his body fat (34.020 pounds) and multiplies it by 100, then he divides the product (3,402.000) by his total body weight (205 pounds). The result (16.595 percent) is his body-fat percentage.

34.020	Body fat
× 100	Percent
3,402.000	
÷ 205	Total body weight
16.595	Body-fat percentage

6. Finally, John takes his body-fat percentage (16.595 percent) and subtracts it from 100 percent. The difference (83.405 percent) is his lean-body-mass percentage.

100.000	Percent
− 16.595	Body-fat percentage
83.405	Lean-body-mass percentage

John has 170.980 pounds of lean body mass, according to step 3, and 34.020 pounds of body fat, according to step 4. His body fat is 16.595 percent of his total body weight, according to step 5, and his lean body mass is 83.405 percent, according to step 6.

How Lean Am I?

There are many benefits to knowing precisely what your body composition is. If you are a woman and you need or want to know how much lean body mass you have or what your body-fat percentage is, use the Quick Method for Determining Body Composition that is described on page 145. Jane used the formula, and the information it yielded was invaluable in her efforts to improve as a horsewoman. Use her calculations, as a model for your own.

Jane had been riding horses since she could first sit up-right in a saddle. She owned her own horse, and she took care of him like a favorite child. She had been competing in shows since she was in grade school. However, as her thirtieth birthday was approaching, she found that posting and jumping were taking a little more effort. Her trainer suggested that she improve her nutrition and training program.

The first thing Jane needed to do was figure out her body composition. Knowing her exact body-fat percentage, Jane could then determine her caloric and macronutrient requirements. Jane weighed 130 pounds and had a 6.25-inch wrist, 27-inch abdomen, 38-inch hips, and 10-inch forearms. Following are her calculations:

1. First, Jane took her total body weight (130 pounds) and multiplied it by 0.732 (women's weight constant one). Then, she added the product (95.160) to 8.987 (women's weight constant two). The result (104.147) was her weight factor.

130		Total body weight
× 0.732		Women's weight constant one
95.160		
+ 8.987		Women's weight constant two
104.147		Weight factor

2. Next, Jane took her wrist measurement (6.25 inches) and divided it by 3.140 (the women's wrist constant). The result (1.990) was her wrist factor.

6.25		Wrist measurement
÷ 3.140		Women's wrist constant
1.990		Wrist factor

3. Jane took her abdominal measurement (27 inches) and multiplied it by 0.157 (the women's abdominal constant). The product (4.239) was her abdominal factor.

27		Abdominal measurement
× 0.157		Women's abdominal constant
4.239		Abdominal factor

4. Jane took her hip measurement (38 inches) and multiplied it by 0.249 (the women's hip constant). The product (9.462) was her hip factor.

38		Hip measurement
× 0.249		Women's hip constant
9.462		Hip factor

5. Jane took her forearm measurement (10 inches) and multiplied it by 0.434 (the women's forearm constant). The product (4.340) was her forearm factor.

10		Forearm measurement
× 0.434		Women's forearm constant
4.340		Forearm factor

6. Jane took her weight factor (104.147) and added her wrist factor (1.990), subtracted her abdominal factor (4.239), subtracted her hip factor (9.462), and added her forearm factor (4.340). The result (96.776 pounds) was her lean body mass.

104.147	Weight factor
+ 1.990	Wrist factor
106.137	
− 4.239	Abdominal factor
101.898	
− 9.462	Hip factor
92.436	
+ 4.340	Forearm factor
96.776	Lean body mass

7. Jane took her total body weight (130 pounds) and subtracted her lean body mass (96.776 pounds). The difference (33.224 pounds) was her body fat.

130.000	Total body weight
− 96.776	Lean body mass
33.224	Body fat

8. Using the standard equation for obtaining a percentage, Jane took her body fat (33.224 pounds) and multiplied it by 100, then she divided the product (3,322.400) by her total body weight (130 pounds). The result (25.557 percent) was her body-fat percentage.

33.224	Body fat
x 100	Percent
3,322.400	
÷ 130	Total body weight
25.557	Body-fat percentage

9. Finally, Jane took her body-fat percentage (25.557 percent) and subtracted it from 100 percent. The difference (74.443 percent) was her lean-body-mass percentage.

100.000	Percent
− 25.557	Body-fat percentage
74.443	Lean-body-mass percentage

Jane had 96.776 pounds of lean body mass, according to step 6, and 33.224 pounds of body fat, according to step 7. Her body fat was 25.557 percent of her total body weight, according to step 8, and her lean body mass was 74.443 percent, according to step 9.

which is the women's abdominal constant. The product is your abdominal factor.

Abdominal measurement x 0.157 = Abdominal factor

4. Measure your hips (in inches) at their fullest point. Multiply your hip measurement by 0.249, which is the women's hip constant. The product is your hip factor.

Hip measurement x 0.249 = Hip factor

5. Measure your forearm (in inches) at its fullest point. Multiply your forearm measurement by 0.434, which is the women's forearm constant. The product is your forearm factor.

Forearm measurement x 0.434 = Forearm factor

6. Add your weight factor to your wrist factor, subtract your abdominal factor, subtract your hip factor, and add your forearm factor. The result is your pounds of lean body mass.

Weight factor + Wrist factor – Abdominal factor
– Hip factor + Forearm factor = Lean body mass

7. Subtract your lean body mass from your total body weight. The difference is your pounds of body fat.

Total body weight – Lean body mass = Body fat

8. Multiply your body fat by 100, then divide the result by your total body weight. This is the standard equation for obtaining a percentage. The result is your body-fat percentage.

(Body fat x 100) ÷ Total body weight
= Body-fat percentage

9. Subtract your body-fat percentage from 100 percent. The difference is your lean-body-mass percentage.

100 percent – Body-fat percentage
= Lean-body-mass percentage

For an example of how one woman used this formula, see "How Lean Am I?" on page 146.

NORMAL RANGES OF BODY-FAT PERCENTAGE

Once you have figured out what percentage of your body is composed of fat, check Table 12.1, right, to see if you fall into the normal range. Table 12.1 presents the overall normal ranges and desirable ranges of body-fat percentage for male and female athletes and nonathletes. Do not get frustrated if you do not fit into the normal range, however. Every person is an individual, and the guidelines are not meant for everyone. In fact, different authorities designate different ranges as "normal." Plus, different kinds of athletes have different ranges. (For a sampling of the average body-fat percentages of different athletes, see Table 13.1 on page 165.)

Sports scientists tend to agree, however, that too high a body-fat percentage impairs performance and jeopardizes health. At the same time, too little body fat also threatens performance and health. In fact, studies have shown that the essential body fats, such as the lipids of the bone marrow and central nervous system, may be compromised if the body-fat percentage is kept too low. For males, 5 to 7 percent is usually considered the minimum, while for females, 11 to 14 percent is the minimum. If you find yourself at either extreme of your appropriate overall range, contact your health-care practitioner to rule out a medical cause and any negative consequences.

BODY TYPES

Body type is the result of genetic and environmental factors. The genetic factors exert the dominant influence, since they are inherited and on the whole cannot be changed. The environmental factors include influences such as training and nutrition.

Scientist W. H. Sheldon noticed that human bodies tend to fall into three general types. These body types—or somatotypes, as he called them—are the mesomorphic type, which is muscular; the ectomorphic type, which is slim and linear; and the endomor-

Table 12.1. Overall Normal and Desirable Ranges of Body-Fat Percentage

	Overall Normal Range	Desirable Range
Males		
Athletes	5%–16%	6%–12%
Nonathletes	10%–22%	12%–16%
Females		
Athletes	11%–28%	12%–18%
Nonathletes	16%–32%	18%–28%

Note: This chart is based on estimates for adults.

phic type, which is fat and round. Sheldon devised a system of classifying individual bodies using a three-digit number in which the first digit rates the degree of endomorphy, the second digit rates the degree of mesomorphy, and the third digit rates the degree of ecotmorphy. All three digits are between 1 and 7, with 1 indicating a low degree and 7 a high degree. Using the system, an extreme endomorph is rated 711, an extreme mesomorph is rated 171, and an extreme ectomorph is rated 117. The classic bodybuilder's body is 171.

Most individuals are dominant in one somatotype but also display characteristics of the other two. An average person is rated around 333 to 444. Elite, world-class athletes usually have a mesomorphic rating of 5 to 7, an endomorphic rating of 1 to 3, and an ectomorphic rating of 1 to 4. This indicates that elite athletes tend to be predominantly mesomorphic, which makes sense, since mesomorphs have a higher percentage of muscle mass, the primary tissue involved in athletic performance. This does not mean that ectomorphs and endomorphs cannot become superior athletes, however. Endomorphs and ectomorphs just need to put a little more effort into their training and diet, to build more muscle mass and to keep their percentage of body fat within the desirable range for their sex and sport.

If you are a competitive athlete, you should consider having your somatotype determined by a trained professional. Knowing your somatotypic classification will help you to better understand your genetic predisposition and better plan your sports-nutrition program. To find someone trained in the somatotypic system, contact your health-care practitioner.

ESTIMATING BASAL METABOLIC RATE

How many times have you wondered, "How many calories should I eat?" Or, "How can I lose weight?" Or, "What should I eat?" The key to answering any of these questions is figuring out how many calories your body needs.

The body's rate of energy expenditure is referred to as its metabolic rate. A body's metabolic rate is its total daily caloric expenditure. There are several traditional scientific methods for determining metabolic rate. One measures oxygen consumption, since the amount of oxygen inhaled and the amount of carbon dioxide exhaled are direct results of energy expenditure and indirect reflections of metabolism. These lab-

oratory methods require sophisticated equipment, however, and are out of the average person's reach. Therefore, sports scientists have devised a number of easy formulas and handy charts to serve as everyday reference tools for anyone interested in estimating his or her daily caloric requirement. These formulas and charts are presented and explained in the following pages. However, as you read through them, keep in mind that they each contain a margin of error. Even the most sophisticated laboratory methods may yield daily caloric requirements that are too high or too low. This is why it is important to keep track of your body composition—to enable you to fine-tune your caloric intake based on your specific individual metabolic rate. In addition, bear in mind that ectomorphs usually require more energy than the charts estimate and endomorphs usually require less, so these individuals may need to adjust their estimates by a few hundred calories to maintain their desired body-composition or performance goals. (Mesomorphs usually require just about what the charts estimate.)

Everybody expends a different amount of energy each day. The amount of energy that is spent depends on factors such as physical activities and diet. However, a person's basic metabolic rate, called the basal metabolic rate (BMR), or basal metabolism, remains relatively constant from day to day. The BMR is the rate at which the body expends energy for maintenance activities such as keeping the body alive and the organs functioning. It is the lowest during sleep. However, most methods measure BMR during waking hours, but under controlled conditions—that is, with the person resting in a room kept at a specific temperature. *Basal metabolic rate* therefore is an estimate of the number of calories a person would burn over twenty-four hours while lying down but not sleeping in a room that is neither too hot nor too cold. That same person's *actual metabolic rate* would be estimated by adding to the BMR the caloric costs of all the activities he or she engages in throughout the day. The actual metabolic rate takes a person's real life into account, at least as best as possible.

The formula to get a rough estimate of BMR is different for men than for women. For men, the formula is:

BMR (in calories) = 1.0 x body weight (in kilograms) x 24 hours

To convert your weight to kilograms, multiply your weight in pounds by .45. For example, if you weigh

200 pounds, multiply 200 by .45 to get 90 kilograms. To get your BMR, multiply 90 (your body weight in kilograms) by 1.0 to get 90, then by 24 to get a BMR of 2,160 calories.

The formula to get a rough estimate of BMR for women is:

BMR (in calories) = .9 x body weight (in kilograms) x 24 hours

A woman who weighs 130 pounds would first convert her weight to kilograms by multiplying it by .45. She would find her weight to be 58.5 kilograms. Next, to get her BMR, the woman would multiply 58.5 kilograms by .9 to get 52.65, then by 24 to get a BMR of 1,264 calories (rounded up from 1,263.6 calories). Women multiply by .9 rather than by 1.0 the way men do because they have more body fat and less muscle mass than men do, which means that, pound for pound, they burn fewer calories than men do.

Both these formulas are reasonably accurate for individuals with average body-fat percentages (approximately 20 percent for men and 28 percent for women). Individuals with higher body-fat percentages have lower BMRs because, the same as women in general, they have less muscle tissue to burn calories. Individuals with lower body-fat percentages have higher BMRs because their bigger muscles burn more calories. Energy requirements above the BMR depend on daily activity level and can be as low as 130 percent of BMR and as high as over 200 percent.

ESTIMATING AVERAGE DAILY CALORIC REQUIREMENT

There are several ways to estimate average daily caloric requirement, but as always, some are more accurate than others. Most people have seen the tables that supply the hourly caloric costs of various activities. These tables tell you, for example, that bowling uses 215 calories per hour, cooking uses 240 calories per hour, and gardening uses 295 calories per hour. What these charts generally fail to mention, is that the estimates are for an average adult male. If you are not an average adult male, the counts are meaningless.

Better ways for athletes to estimate average daily caloric requirement are the Hour-by-Hour Method and the Daily Caloric Requirement Guide. The Hour-by-Hour Method is the better of these two, but both result in estimates that come as close to exact as possible with this kind of approach.

The Hour-by-Hour Method

Of the various methods for determining average daily caloric requirement, the Hour-by-Hour Method is one of the more intricate, but, as just mentioned, it is also one of the more accurate. Basically, the Hour-by-Hour Method involves determining your hourly BMR, estimating your caloric expenditure for every hour in an average day, and adjusting the results for your body-fat percentage. (For an example of an hourly caloric breakdown, see ("How Active Am I?" on page 151.) More specifically:

1. Have your body-fat percentage determined by a trained professional using hydrostatic weighing or skin-fold measurement, or determine your own body-fat percentage using skin-fold measurement or the Quick Method described on page 145.

2. Take your body-fat percentage from step 1, above, and determine your lean-factor multiplier using Table 12.2 on page 152. For example, if you were a 130-pound woman with 28-percent body fat, you would find the "Females" column in Table 12.2 and run your finger down the column until you came to the "28%–38%" row. Moving your finger straight across the row to the right, you would find that you have a lean factor of 3 and a lean-factor multiplier of 90 percent, or .9.0.

3. Determine your hourly BMR by calculating your daily BMR using the appropriate formula (see "Estimating Basal Metabolic Rate" on page 149) and dividing your daily BMR by 24. (Or, you could just omit the final step in that calculation in which you multiply by 24.) Adjust your hourly BMR for your body-fat percentage by multiplying it by your lean-factor multiplier from step 2. If desired, round off your adjusted hourly BMR to the nearest whole number. For example, by following the formula, our 130-pound woman with 28-percent body fat would find that her BMR was 1,264 calories. Dividing that BMR by 24, she would find that her hourly BMR was 52.667 calories. To adjust this hourly BMR for her 28-percent body fat, our woman would multiply the 52.667 calories by .90, her lean-factor multiplier from step 2. This would show that her adjusted hourly BMR is 47.400 calories, which can be rounded out to 47 calories.

4. Make a photocopy of Appendix B on page 343, or draw a table just like Jane's table on page 151. In the first column, under "Hour," the twenty-four hours of the day should be listed in one-hour increments.

How Active Am I?

Estimating your daily caloric requirement using the Hour-by-Hour Method on page 150 looks like a complex process, but with the step-by-step instructions and Tables 12.2 and 12.3, the process is a breeze. Jane, our equestrian from page 146, found that the calculations were easy, quick, and well worth the effort. Knowing how many calories she expends on an average day allowed her to plan a diet that helped her attain the results she wanted—improved body composition, improved energy, and improved equestrian performance.

The table below shows Jane's work. On an average day, Jane sleeps until 7 A.M. Between 7 and 9 A.M., she dresses, eats breakfast, and travels to work. From 9 P.M. to 5 P.M., Jane earns a living as a sales clerk, doing a fair amount of walking and lifting along with waiting on customers. At noon she has a chance to rest, though, taking lunch until 1 P.M. When she leaves work at 5 P.M., she heads for the stable or gym. At about 6 P.M., Jane goes home, where she prepares dinner and then cleans up afterwards. She relaxes in front of the television for a while, then goes to bed at around 11 P.M. Note that Jane weighs 130 pounds and has 26-percent body fat, a lean factor of 3, and a basal metabolic rate of 47 calories per hour.

Jane's Sample Hourly Caloric Breakdown

Hour	Activity	Percent of BMR	Calories Used
Midnight–1 A.M.	Sleeping	−22%	47 x .78 = 37
1–2 A.M.	Sleeping	−22%	47 x .78 = 37
2–3 A.M.	Sleeping	−22%	47 x .78 = 37
3–4 A.M.	Sleeping	−22%	47 x .78 = 37
4–5 A.M.	Sleeping	−22%	47 x .78 = 37
5–6 A.M.	Sleeping	−22%	47 x .78 = 37
6–7 A.M.	Sleeping	−22%	47 x .78 = 37
7–8 A.M.	Light activity	270%	47 x 2.70 = 127
8–9 A.M.	Light activity	270%	47 x 2.70 = 127
9–10 A.M.	Moderate activity	360%	47 x 3.60 = 169
10–11 A.M.	Moderate activity	360%	47 x 3.60 = 169
11 A.M.–Noon	Light activity	270%	47 x 2.70 = 127
Noon–1 P.M.	Moderate activity	360%	47 x 3.60 = 169
1–2 P.M.	Moderate activity	360%	47 x 3.60 = 169
2–3 P.M.	Moderate activity	360%	47 x 3.60 = 169
3–4 P.M.	Moderate activity	360%	47 x 3.60 = 169
4–5 P.M.	Moderate activity	360%	47 x 3.60 = 169
5–6 P.M.	All-out training	720%	47 x 7.20 = 388
6–7 P.M.	Moderate activity	360%	47 x 3.60 = 169
7–8 P.M.	Light activity	270%	47 x 2.70 = 127
8–9 P.M.	Moderate activity	360%	47 x 3.60 = 169
9–10 P.M.	Very light activity	120%	47 x 1.20 = 56
10–11 P.M.	Very light activity	120%	47 x 1.20 = 56
11 P.M.–Midnight	Sleeping	−22%	47 x .78 = 37
		Daily total	2,825 calories

5. In the second column, under "Activity," note the general type of activity that you engage in during each hour on a normal day. Use Table 12.3, right, as your guide. For example, if you normally sleep between midnight and 1 A.M., mark down "Sleeping" for that hour. If you generally meet your friends for a game of football or tennis between 6 and 7 P.M., mark down "Sports" for that hour.

6. In the third column, under "Percent of BMR," transfer the appropriate percentage from Table 12.3 for each activity noted in the second column. For example, if you are a man who has "Sleeping" marked in the second column for the hour of midnight to 1 A.M., mark down "−20%" in the third column. If you are a woman who has "Very heavy activity" marked in the second column for the hour of 7 to 8 P.M., mark down "540%" in the third column.

7. In the last column, under "Calories Used," calculate your caloric expenditure for each hour. (Or, do your calculations on scratch paper and transfer the results to your table.) To do this, multiply your adjusted hourly BMR from step 3 by the appropriate BMR-percentage multiplier from Table 12.3. For example, if you are like our sample woman from step 3 whose adjusted hourly BMR is 47 calories and you engage in light activity between 7 and 8 A.M., you would multiply the 47 calories by 2.70 for an hourly caloric expenditure of 126.90 calories, which can be rounded up to 127 calories.

8. To get your average daily activity level, add up the calories in the fourth column. The sum is the total number of calories you use on an average day.

While the Hour-by-Hour Method may seem complex, it really is not. You will need to set aside about an hour to do the work, but you will need this time more for writing than calculating. In fact, you may even find the method to be so simple, you will

Table 12.3. Energy Expenditure Guide

Percent of BMR		BMR-Percentage Multiplier		Activity
Males	Females	Males	Females	
−20%	−22%	.80	.78	Sleeping.
0%	0.1%	1.00	.99	Resting—lying down totally relaxed but not sleeping.
200%	120%	2.00	1.20	Very light activity—sitting, studying, talking, just a little walking.
300%	270%	3.00	2.70	Light activity—typing, teaching, lab or shop work, some walking.
400%	360%	4.00	3.60	Moderate activity—walking, jogging, gardening.
500%	450%	5.00	4.50	Heavy activity—heavy manual labor such as digging or tree felling, climbing.
600%	540%	6.00	5.40	Very heavy activity—fitness-oriented weight training, aerobic dance, cycling.
700%	630%	7.00	6.30	Sports—vigorous extended athletic competition such as football or racquetball.
800%	720%	8.00	7.20	All-out training—extremely high intensity weight training with little rest in between sets or exercises.
900%	810%	9.00	8.10	Extended maximum effort—extremely high intensity and high endurance athletic competition such as a triathlon or cross-country skiing.

Table 12.2. Lean Factors and Lean-Factor Multipliers

Body-Fat Percentage		Lean Factor	Lean-Factor Multiplier
Males	Females		
10%−<14%	14%−<18%	1	100% (1.00)
14%−<20%	18%−<28%	2	95% (.95)
20%−<28%	28%−<38%	3	90% (.90)
28% and over	38% and over	4	85% (.85)

The symbol < means "less than."

decide to make separate breakdowns of your work-days and off days, or of your workout days and rest days. But whether you make one hour-by-hour breakdown for all seven days of the week or a different one for each day, you will find that the time you spend on the task is well worth the effort.

Daily Caloric Requirement Guide

Another good way to estimate average daily caloric requirement utilizes the Daily Caloric Requirement Guide presented in Table 12.4, below. This method is not as reliable as the hour-by-hour approach, but it is quick and relatively accurate. To use the Daily Caloric Requirement Guide, find the total weight that is closest to yours. For example, if you weighed 217 pounds, you would find the 220-pound weight class. If you weighed 133 pounds, you would find the 130-pound weight class. Note that each weight class on the table also has the average BMRs of a male and female of that weight listed directly below, in the first column on the left.

After finding your weight class, find your lean factor in the second column. If necessary, first figure out your lean factor using Table 12.2. Each weight class has all four lean factors listed.

Next, run your finger across the row with your lean factor until you find your activity level. If you engage in:

☐ Very light activity such as sitting, studying, talking, or just a little walking, your activity level is 130 percent.

☐ Light activity such as typing, teaching, lab or shop work, or some walking, your activity level is 155 percent.

☐ Moderate activity such as walking, jogging, gardening, an active job, or training for one to two hours, your activity level is 165 percent.

☐ Heavy activity such as heavy manual labor (for example, digging, tree felling, or construction work) or participating in sports activities for two to three hours, your activity level is 200 percent.

☐ Very heavy activity such as a combination of moderate and heavy activities for eight or more hours plus sports activities for two to four hours, your activity level is 230 percent.

When you reach the column with your activity level, make sure that you stop on the calorie count appropriate for your sex. This estimated daily caloric requirement is not as precise as what you

Table 12.4. Daily Caloric Requirement Guide

Basal Metabolic Rate (BMR)	Lean Factor	Average Daily Activity Level (in calories)									
		130%		155%		165%		200%		230%	
		Males	Females	Males	Females	Males	Females	Males	Females	Males	Females
For a total weight of 100 pounds:											
Males burn	1	1,418	1,277	1,691	1,522	1,800	1,620	2,182	1,964	2,509	2,259
1,091 calories	2	1,347	1,213	1,606	1,446	1,710	1,539	2,073	1,866	2,384	2,146
Females burn	3	1,276	1,149	1,521	1,370	1,620	1,458	1,964	1,768	2,258	2,033
982 calories	4	1,205	1,085	1,437	1,294	1,530	1,377	1,858	1,669	2,133	1,920
For a total weight of 110 pounds:											
Males burn	1	1,560	1,404	1,860	1,674	1,980	1,782	2,400	2,160	2,760	2,484
1,200 calories	2	1,482	1,334	1,767	1,590	1,881	1,693	2,280	2,052	2,622	2,360
Females burn	3	1,404	1,264	1,674	1,501	1,782	1,604	2,160	1,944	2,484	2,236
1,080 calories	4	1,326	1,193	1,581	1,423	1,683	1,515	2,040	1,836	2,346	2,111
For a total weight of 120 pounds:											
Males burn	1	1,701	1,531	2,029	1,826	2,160	1,944	2,618	2,356	3,010	2,709
1,309 calories	2	1,616	1,454	1,928	1,735	2,052	1,847	2,487	2,238	2,860	2,574
Females burn	3	1,531	1,378	1,826	1,643	1,944	1,750	2,356	2,120	2,709	2,438
1,178 calories	4	1,446	1,301	1,725	1,552	1,836	1,652	2,225	2,003	2,559	2,303

Basal Metabolic Rate (BMR)	Lean Factor	Average Daily Activity Level (in calories)									
		130%		155%		165%		200%		230%	
		Males	Females	Males	Females	Males	Females	Males	Females	Males	Females
For a total weight of 130 pounds:											
Males burn	1	1,843	1,659	2,198	1,978	2,340	2,105	2,836	2,552	3,261	2,935
1,418 calories	2	1,751	1,576	2,088	1,879	2,223	2,000	2,694	2,424	3,098	2,788
Females burn	3	1,659	1,493	1,978	1,780	2,106	1,895	2,552	2,297	2,935	2,641
1,276 calories	4	1,567	1,410	1,868	1,681	1,989	1,789	2,411	2,169	2,772	2,495
For a total weight of 140 pounds:											
Males burn	1	1,985	1,788	2,367	2,131	2,520	2,269	3,054	2,750	3,512	3,163
1,527 calories	2	1,886	1,699	2,249	2,024	2,394	2,156	2,901	2,613	3,336	3,005
Females burn	3	1,787	1,608	2,130	1,917	2,268	2,041	2,749	2,474	3,161	2,847
1,375 calories	4	1,687	1,520	2,012	1,811	2,142	1,929	2,596	2,338	2,985	2,689
For a total weight of 150 pounds:											
Males burn	1	2,127	1,915	2,536	2,283	2,699	2,430	3,272	2,946	3,763	3,388
1,636 calories	2	2,021	1,819	2,409	2,169	2,564	2,309	3,108	2,799	3,575	3,219
Females burn	3	1,914	1,724	2,282	2,055	2,429	2,187	2,945	2,651	3,387	3,049
1,473 calories	4	1,808	1,628	2,156	1,941	2,294	2,066	2,781	2,504	3,199	2,880
For a total weight of 160 pounds:											
Males burn	1	2,269	2,042	2,705	2,435	2,879	2,592	3,490	3,142	4,014	3,613
1,745 calories	2	2,156	1,940	2,570	2,313	2,735	2,462	3,316	2,985	3,813	3,432
Females burn	3	2,042	1,838	2,435	2,191	2,591	2,332	3,141	2,827	3,613	3,251
1,571 calories	4	1,929	1,736	2,299	2,070	2,447	2,203	2,967	2,671	3,412	3,071
For a total weight of 170 pounds:											
Males burn	1	2,412	2,170	2,875	2,587	3,061	2,754	3,710	3,338	4,267	3,839
1,855 calories	2	2,291	2,062	2,731	2,458	2,908	2,616	3,525	3,171	4,054	3,647
Females burn	3	2,171	1,953	2,588	2,329	2,655	2,479	3,339	3,005	3,840	3,456
1,669 calories	4	2,050	1,845	2,444	2,199	2,602	2,341	3,154	2,837	3,627	3,263
For a total weight of 180 pounds:											
Males burn	1	2,553	2,297	3,044	2,739	3,241	2,916	3,928	3,534	4,517	4,064
1,964 calories	2	2,425	2,182	2,892	2,602	3,079	2,770	3,732	3,357	4,291	3,861
Females burn	3	2,298	2,068	2,740	2,466	2,917	2,625	3,535	3,182	4,065	3,659
1,767 calories	4	2,170	1,952	2,587	2,328	2,755	2,479	3,339	3,004	3,839	3,454
For a total weight of 190 pounds:											
Males burn	1	2,694	2,425	3,213	2,891	3,420	3,077	4,146	3,730	4,768	4,290
2,073 calories	2	2,559	2,304	3,052	2,746	3,249	2,923	3,939	3,544	4,530	4,076
Females burn	3	2,424	2,183	2,892	2,603	3,078	2,770	3,731	3,358	4,291	3,862
1,865 calories	4	2,290	2,061	2,731	2,457	2,907	2,615	3,524	3,171	4,053	3,647
For a total weight of 200 pounds:											
Males burn	1	2,837	2,553	3,382	3,044	3,600	3,241	4,364	3,928	5,019	4,517
2,182 calories	2	2,695	2,425	3,213	2,892	3,420	3,079	4,146	3,732	4,768	4,291
Females burn	3	2,553	2,298	3,044	2,739	3,240	2,916	3,928	3,535	4,517	4,065
1,964 calories	4	2,411	2,170	2,875	2,587	3,060	2,755	3,709	3,339	4,266	3,839

Basal Metabolic Rate (BMR)	Lean Factor	Average Daily Activity Level (in calories)									
		130%		155%		165%		200%		230%	
		Males	Females	Males	Females	Males	Females	Males	Females	Males	Females
For a total weight of 210 pounds:											
Males burn	1	2,978	2,681	3,551	3,196	3,780	3,402	4,582	4,124	5,269	4,743
2,291 calories	2	2,829	2,547	3,373	3,036	3,591	3,232	4,353	3,918	5,006	4,506
Females burn	3	2,680	2,412	3,196	2,876	3,402	3,062	4,124	3,711	4,742	4,269
2,062 calories	4	2,531	2,279	3,018	2,717	3,213	2,892	3,895	3,505	4,479	4,032
For a total weight of 220 pounds:											
Males burn	1	3,120	2,808	3,720	3,348	3,960	3,564	4,800	4,320	5,520	4,968
2,400 calories	2	2,964	2,668	3,534	2,668	3,762	2,668	4,560	4,104	5,244	4,720
Females burn	3	2,808	2,527	3,348	3,023	3,564	3,207	4,320	3,888	4,968	4,471
2,160 calories	4	2,652	2,387	3,162	2,846	3,366	3,029	4,080	3,672	4,692	4,223
For a total weight of 230 pounds:											
Males burn	1	3,262	2,935	3,889	3,500	4,140	3,726	5,018	4,516	5,771	5,193
2,509 calories	2	3,099	2,788	3,695	3,325	3,933	3,540	4,767	4,290	5,482	4,933
Females burn	3	2,936	2,642	3,500	3,150	3,726	3,353	4,516	4,065	5,193	4,674
2,258 calories	4	2,603	2,495	3,306	2,975	3,519	3,167	4,265	3,839	4,905	4,414
For a total weight of 240 pounds:											
Males burn	1	3,403	3,063	4,058	3,652	4,320	3,887	5,236	4,712	6,021	5,419
2,618 calories	2	3,232	2,910	3,855	3,469	4,104	3,693	4,974	4,476	5,720	5,148
Females burn	3	3,063	2,756	3,652	3,287	3,888	3,499	4,712	4,241	5,419	4,877
2,356 calories	4	2,893	2,604	3,449	3,104	3,672	3,304	4,451	4,005	5,118	4,606
For a total weight of 250 pounds:											
Males burn	1	3,545	3,192	4,227	3,805	4,500	4,051	5,454	4,910	6,272	5,647
2,727 calories	2	3,368	3,032	4,016	3,615	4,275	4,285	5,181	4,665	5,958	5,365
Females burn	3	3,191	2,971	3,804	3,424	4,050	3,645	4,090	4,418	5,645	5,080
2,455 calories	4	3,013	2,713	3,593	3,234	3,825	3,443	4,636	4,174	5,331	4,800
For a total weight of 260 pounds:											
Males burn	1	3,687	3,319	4,396	3,957	4,679	4,212	5,672	5,106	6,523	5,872
2,836 calories	2	3,503	3,153	4,176	3,759	4,445	4,001	5,388	4,851	6,197	5,578
Females burn	3	3,318	2,986	3,956	3,561	4,211	3,790	5,105	4,594	5,871	5,284
2,553 calories	4	3,134	2,821	3,737	3,363	3,977	3,580	4,821	4,340	5,545	4,991
For a total weight of 270 pounds:											
Males burn	1	3,829	3,446	4,565	4,109	4,859	4,374	5,890	5,302	6,774	6,097
2,945 calories	2	3,638	3,274	4,337	3,904	4,616	4,155	5,596	5,037	6,435	5,792
Females burn	3	3,446	3,101	4,109	3,698	4,373	3,936	5,301	4,771	6,097	5,487
2,651 calories	4	3,255	2,929	3,880	3,493	4,130	3,718	5,007	4,507	5,758	5,182

would get with the Hour-by-Hour Method, but it is adjusted for your weight, lean factor, activity level, and sex.

HOMEOSTASIS

In Chapter 11, we discussed how the body procures nutrients for growth, maintenance, energy, repair, and life sustenance. Digesting foodstuffs and absorbing nutrients are not the body's only tasks, however. It also must initiate and monitor an astounding number of chemical reactions to accomplish these tasks, controlling each reaction to prevent over- or underproduction of the end product. To do this, it needs its many components—all the cells, tissues, and systems discussed in Chapter 10—to work together in a highly organized manner. It must maintain balance by continually adjusting its many physiological control mechanisms. This tendency of the body to keep an internal equilibrium is called homeostasis.

The term *homeostasis* was coined in the early twentieth century by American physiologist Walter Bradford Cannon. A good example of homeostasis is the body's constant maintenance of an internal temperature of 98.6°F. If physical exertion or external heat cause the body's temperature to rise, the brain sends a signal to the body to increase its rate of sweating. When the sweat evaporates, it carries away the extra heat. If external cold causes the body's temperature to drop, the brain sends a signal to the body to shiver to generate more heat. Other metabolic functions under homeostatic control are the production of hormones and the maintenance of their proper levels of concentration, maintenance of proper serum-oxygen and carbon-dioxide levels, maintenance of pH balance in the blood and cells, control of the water content of the blood and cells, maintenance of the blood-sugar and other blood-nutrient levels, and maintenance of the metabolic rate.

The concept of homeostasis is of special interest to athletes. Indeed, it is vital that athletes be in equilibrium with the environmental stimuli imposed upon them. For example, consider how muscles change in response to different training programs. If you spend most of your time lifting heavy weights, your muscles will grow larger. A shift will take place in your homeostasis. The simple action of lifting a weight will cause more protein to be synthesized in the muscles being exercised. In addition, your hormone levels will change to accommodate the growth, and the muscle

fibers will increase in size to accommodate the storage of more ATP and CP. On the other hand, if you choose to jog every day, your muscles will take a different form. They will develop a higher aerobic-endurance capacity, form more fat-burning muscle fibers, and develop a higher capacity to use oxygen in energy production.

Homeostasis is also affected by nutrition. Eating too much of the wrong foods or too little of the right foods can cause a shift in balance. Eating too much fat or too many calories can cause the body to become fat. Not eating enough protein can cause the muscles to be cannibalized. Not eating enough carbohydrates can cause early onset of fatigue. For optimum homeostasis and metabolism, eating the right nutrients in the right amounts at the right times is critical.

ANABOLISM AND CATABOLISM

The many biochemical processes that make up the body's metabolism can be grouped into two general categories—anabolism and catabolism. Anabolism is the building up of complex molecules, while catabolism is their breakdown. To build molecules and sustain life, the body needs energy. It gets this energy from the breakdown of nutrients such as glucose and fatty acids. So, for molecular construction to occur, molecular destruction must go on at the same time to release the energy required to drive the biochemical reactions. When anabolism exceeds catabolism, net growth occurs. When catabolism exceeds anabolism, net loss occurs.

Anabolism includes the chemical reactions that cause different molecules to combine to form larger, more complex ones. The net result of anabolism is the creation of new cellular material, such as enzymes, proteins, cells, cell membranes, and tissues. Anabolism is necessary for growth, maintenance, and tissue repair.

Catabolism includes the chemical reactions that break down complex molecules into simpler ones for energy production, for recycling of their molecular components, or for their excretion. If energy is produced, it is stored as glycogen or fat. Recently, the trend in sports nutrition has been to focus on anti-catabolic training methods and nutrients. For example, when the muscles are strenuously trained and the muscle fibers are damaged, cortisol is released at a higher level, speeding up the breakdown of tissues. Nutrients such as L-glutamine have been shown to reduce the effects of cortisol, resulting in reduced tissue breakdown. Antioxidants and a number of phyto-chemicals also have anticatabolic effects, as does good nutrition in general. By reducing the rate of catabolism, anabolism is increased, resulting in faster recovery, a higher level of performance, and an increased growth rate.

Metabolism includes only the chemical changes that occur within the tissue cells of the body. It does not include changes to any other substances, such as foodstuffs going through the digestive tract. The body needs many nutrients to function optimally. A slight deficiency of even one vitamin can slow down metabolism and cause chaos throughout the body. The body builds thousands of enzymes to drive the metabolism in the direction dictated by activity and nutrition. So, if you generally train several hours a day, you had better make sure that your diet contains the nutrients it needs to fuel its many metabolic pathways.

THE METABOLIC SET POINT

The metabolic set point is the average rate at which an individual's metabolism runs. During an intensive study of weight loss, researchers discovered that the body seeks to maintain a certain base rate of metabolism. This set point is controlled by genetics and environmental factors, but research has demonstrated that it can be changed through dietary means and physical activity.

The existence of a metabolic set point causes the body to also have a body-composition set point. People with a slow metabolism seem to store fat easily, while people with a fast metabolism seem to be able to eat whatever they want and never get fat. However, studies have demonstrated that going on a low-calorie diet causes the body to lower its metabolic set point in an effort to conserve energy. The body actually resets itself to burn fewer calories. Exercising tends to keep the metabolic rate up, and exercising aerobically tends to cause the body to burn more fat for energy.

FOOD AND METABOLISM

Food also influences metabolism. Diets that are low in fat and high in protein and carbohydrates can increase the BMR. The processing of the excess protein seems to require additional energy. Certain substances found in food also increase the metabolic rate. Prime examples are caffeine and ephedrine. Because of this, the herbs ephedra, which contains ephedrine, and guarana, which contains caffeine, are popular ingredients in supplements called metabolic boosters. Metabolic boosters, also known as thermogenic aids, are substances whose digestion causes the body to produce more than the normal amount of heat (energy).

A common question among athletes is which of the macronutrients—carbohydrates, protein, or lipids—is the primary producer of energy. The answer is not easy to determine because it varies from person to person. However, researchers have devised a method for calculating the specific "fuel mix" that is used by a particular person. Called the respiratory quotient (RQ), the method measures the ratio of fat, carbohydrates, and protein that is burned for energy.

The RQ compares the volume of carbon dioxide exhaled to the volume of oxygen inhaled. Because different amounts of oxygen are used to burn fat, carbohydrates, and protein, this ratio can indicate which macronutrient is the predominant energy source. According to research, persons consuming a normal diet derive about 40 to 45 percent of their energy from fatty acids, 40 to 45 percent from carbohydrates, and 10 to 15 percent from protein. When the diet is high in carbohydrates, more energy comes from carbohydrates. When the diet is low in carbohydrates and high in fat, more energy comes from fat.

Training intensity also affects which energy source is primary. During exercise, a training intensity below 60 percent of VO_2 max (the maximum rate at which oxygen can be consumed) causes fatty acids and carbohydrates to be equal sources of energy. The more the training intensity is increased above 60 percent of VO_2 max, the more carbohydrates are used for energy. When the training intensity reaches 100 percent of VO_2 max, a rate that can be sustained for only a few minutes, carbohydrates become the sole source of energy. Keep in mind that amino acids, particularly the BCAAs, are also used for energy during both exercise and rest. During exercise, they may even supply as much as 10 percent of energy.

In general, physical conditioning causes the body to obtain more energy from fatty acids. However, more energy is also obtained from protein in trained individuals. Carbohydrates are always used for energy. In research comparing trained individuals with untrained individuals, both groups used mostly carbohydrates for fuel during exercise, but the trained individuals used more fatty acids than the untrained individuals did. High-intensity exercise causes the use of more carbohydrates for energy, while low- to moderate-intensity exercise causes the use of more fatty acids in addition to the carbohydrates. Fatty acids are the predominant energy source during rest.

THE ENVIRONMENT AND METABOLISM

The environment also exerts an influence on metabolic rate. When you are exposed to cold, your body increases its metabolic rate to keep your body temperature constant and to prevent shivering. You begin to shiver when your core temperature drops. Shivering is actually a series of involuntary muscle contractions intended to create heat in the body.

When you are exposed to colder-than-normal temperatures for several days, your body compensates by increasing its BMR to run hotter than average. When the weather begins to warm up, you may find that even a 60°F day is hot because your metabolism has been running so much faster. After several days of becoming accustomed to the warmer climate, however, your body decreases its BMR once again and you eventually find 80°F weather to feel the same as the 60°F weather formerly did.

EXERCISE AND METABOLISM

Exercise influences metabolism by affecting the body's anatomy, physiology, and biochemical makeup. Different kinds of exercise promote different kinds of changes. Exercise type, duration, and intensity are all important factors that shape the body.

Low-intensity exercise, which is usually long in duration, promotes the development of slow-twitch muscle fibers and stimulates the use of the oxidative energy systems. Slow-twitch muscle fibers are called into action when endurance is needed, since they produce a steady, low-intensity, repetitive contraction. (For a complete discussion of slow- and fast-twitch muscle fibers, see page 174.) In general, aerobic exercise causes increases in the mitochondria density of muscle cells, especially of slow-twitch muscle fibers, and in the percentage of slow-twitch muscle fibers. It also causes increases in the number of capillaries and in cardiac output. At the same time, aerobic exercise causes decreases in the percentage of fast-twitch muscle fibers, in the resting heart rate, in body fat, and in muscle size.

High-intensity exercise, which is usually short in duration, promotes the development of fast-twitch muscle fibers and stimulates the use of the nonoxida-

tive energy systems. Fast-twitch muscle fibers are called into action when strength and power are needed, since they contract quickly, providing short bursts of energy. Some of the major changes resulting from anaerobic exercise, such as heavy-weight lifting, are increases in the size and percentage of fast-twitch muscle fibers, in the ability to tolerate higher blood-lactate levels, and in the enzymes involved in the nonoxidative phase of glycolysis. Other changes are increases in the levels of ATP, CP, creatine, and glycogen in resting muscles and of GH and testosterone after short bouts (forty-five to seventy-five minutes) of intensive weight training.

ENERGY METABOLISM

Energy metabolism consists of a series of chemical reactions that break down foodstuffs and thereby produce energy. The body traps about 20 percent of the energy that is produced and releases the remaining 80 percent as heat. This is why the body heats up during exercise.

Energy production in the human body revolves around the rebuilding of ATP molecules after they have been broken down for energy. ATP is the molecule that stores energy in a form that the body can use. This rebuilding of ATP molecules is accomplished in a number of ways, all of which correlate to the four main purposes for which energy is utilized during athletic performance—power, speed, strength, and endurance—and to the four basic types of physical activity—strength-power, sustained power, anaerobic power-endurance, and aerobic endurance.

When resting, the body derives most of its energy from the oxidative energy systems. But when physical activity begins, the nonoxidative energy systems kick in. When the exercise level becomes very intense, the nonoxidative immediate energy systems predominate. First, the ATP reserves in the muscle cells are drafted. However, these ATP reserves are depleted instantly—within a second. Therefore, if the exercise level remains very intense, resting CP stores are called upon, regenerating the ATP molecules, which can then continue to serve as the primary fuel. If the exercise level still remains very intense, the next nonoxidative energy system, glycolysis, jumps in. Nonoxidative glycolysis functions during near-maximum efforts lasting up to about one and a half minutes. It helps maintain the intensity of the muscle contractions, even though the muscles' force output becomes diminished. When an ATP molecule releases its energy to power a muscle contraction, it is reduced to 1 adenosine-diphosphate (ADP) molecule and 1 phosphate atom. In nonoxidative glycolysis, a glucose molecule is split in half to regenerate ADP back to ATP. Every glucose molecule releases enough energy to regenerate 2 ATP molecules. Nonoxidative glycolysis also results in the formation of lactic acid. Glycolysis takes place in the cytoplasm of a cell. Since the amount of free glucose in a cell is generally low, the glucose that is used is usually derived from the breakdown of glycogen. During intensive exercise, the oxidative energy systems also supply energy, but they contribute a much smaller share.

As the intensity of the exercise is reduced and the duration is increased—generally to more than three or four minutes—the oxidative energy systems begin to prevail once more. The oxidative systems include oxidative glycolysis and beta oxidation. In oxidative glycolysis, when the glucose molecule is split in half, it forms 2 molecules of pyruvate. These pyruvate molecules enter the Krebs cycle, a process in which short chains of carbon atoms from glucose, fatty-acid, or protein molecules are broken down and the energy that is released is used to regenerate ATP molecules. The breakdown products of the Krebs cycle are then shuffled into the electron transport system, a process in which electrons are passed between certain protein molecules, releasing energy that is used to regenerate additional ATP molecules. The complete catabolism of 1 molecule of glucose yields about 36 ATP molecules. In beta oxidation, fatty acids are metabolized. Each fatty-acid molecule is broken down into 2 carbon acetyl fragments. The acetyl molecules then combine with coenzyme A to form acetyl-coenzyme A (acetyl-CoA). The acetyl-CoA molecule is shuffled to the Krebs cycle and broken down, yielding energy to regenerate ATP. Oxidative energy metabolism is a slower process than nonoxidative energy metabolism, but it more completely breaks down the energy molecules—for example, glucose and fatty acids—and generates a lot more energy. The complete breakdown of 3 molecules of fatty acids containing 18 carbon atoms each yields about 441 ATP molecules.

GLYCOGEN DEPLETION AND THE METABOLISM OF FATIGUE

Glycogen is essential for good performance in both anaerobic and aerobic activities. Muscles that are being strenuously exercised rely on glycogen to power their

strength-generating muscle contractions. In aerobic-endurance activities, the primary fuel is fatty acids, but glycogen is also utilized. In fact, fat catabolism works better when carbohydrates are metabolized at the same time. Research on aerobic-endurance exercise and work performance has shown that when glycogen is depleted in the body, fatigue sets in. Therefore, adequate carbohydrate intake and glycogen replenishment are vital factors for peak energy output.

Glycogen depletion is just one factor that contributes to the onset of fatigue, however. Some other factors are ATP and CP depletion, accumulation of lactic acid, buildup of calcium ions in the muscles, oxygen depletion, dehydration, and decreased blood pH. The proper conditioning of the body to enable it to appropriately utilize the preferred energy systems is also important. If the body is poorly conditioned, it cannot properly use the energy systems appropriate for the activity, which can lead to early onset of fatigue. To avoid this, focus your physical-conditioning efforts on developing the primary energy systems needed for your sport or fitness activity. In addition, make sure that your diet supplies the ideal fuel mix to enhance your physical conditioning. (For nutrition guidelines appropriate for your activity, see your sport-specific plan in Part Four.)

MONITORING METABOLISM

Through the 1980s, there were no affordable or easy-to-use home testing tools for measuring key metabolic parameters. The 1990s, however, have witnessed the introduction of two such tools, with others soon to come. The first home testing tool introduced to the athletic market was a product called NitroStix. Developed by a group of inventors and scientists led by innovator Robert Fritz, NitroStix consists of diagnostic sticks that measure nitrogen balance. (For a discussion of nitrogen balance, see page 34) Persons interested in athletics or fitness can now monitor their nitrogen balance on a daily basis in the privacy of their homes to determine if their protein intake is sufficient. They can also see if their nutrient intake from food and supplement sources is adequate. A newly developed product that combines testing for nitrogen balance with testing for fat metabolism takes this home-diagnostic ability one step further. Both these home testing kits measure the amount of metabolites excreted from the body via the urine.

Testosterone and cortisol levels are the focus of

another useful test developed by Robert Fritz, in conjunction with eminent sports physiologist Dr. Thomas D. Fahey. This test uses the saliva to determine testosterone and cortisol levels in the body. The concept reportedly was originally developed by Russian scientists and may have been one of the best-kept training secrets of Russian athletes. The test works by determining the ratio of testosterone to cortisol. Cortisol is a hormone that stimulates the breakdown of bodily tissues. A high level of cortisol in the body is an indicator of stress and overwork. Testosterone, on the other hand, is a powerful hormone that stimulates the building of tissues, especially muscle tissue. In a well-conditioned individual, the testosterone level is almost constant. Therefore, by looking at your testosterone-to-cortisol ratio, you can determine if you have been overtraining. For example, if your testosterone-to-cortisol ratio is high, your cortisol level is low and you can handle a rigorous training day. If, however, your ratio is low, your cortisol level is high and your body needs rest or low-intensity training.

There is a lot to be learned from the intimate connection between body composition and metabolism. As this chapter has demonstrated, physical activity and nutrition directly effect body composition and athletic performance. In Part Three, we will discuss how to structure your nutrition program to improve your body composition and fine-tune your performance.

PART THREE

FINE-TUNING
YOUR PERFORMANCE

13. GUIDE TO EFFECTIVE FAT LOSS

For many athletes, there comes a time when a modification in body composition—weight gain or weight loss—is desired. This is also true for fitness exercisers and "just plain folks." No matter which category you fall into, for maximum performance and results, you need to specifically target any modifications you attempt to make in your body composition. This means that if you wish to lose weight, your actual goal is to lose fat. If you wish to gain weight, your actual goal is to gain muscle. As it turns out, the best way to attain these goals is the same for athletes, fitness exercisers, and the average Joe.

There are thousands of products and services available designed to aid fat loss or muscle gain. They include books, video cassettes, audio cassettes, magazines, nutritional products, exercise equipment, packaged meals, support groups, and seminars. Billions of dollars are spent on these items each year by people who want to lose or gain weight. Most of these people not only do not reach their goals, they also lose out in terms of wasted time and money, impaired athletic performance, and diminished health and energy.

In this chapter, we will discuss what we have found to be the best way to lose fat whether you are a competitive athlete, fitness exerciser, or armchair quarterback. Fat loss is not something everyone needs, but if your body-fat percentage is too high, reducing that percentage is a first step in fine-tuning your performance. Other steps—which, again, may or may not be appropriate for you—are muscle building, covered in Chapter 14, and carbohydrate loading, examined in Chapter 15. In Chapter 16, we will discuss several final topics pertinent to winning athletic performance, such as medical support and psychological techniques, and we will "put together" the information from Parts One, Two, and Three for a performance-improvement formula appropriate for anyone interested in sports, fitness, or health.

THE BEST WAY TO LOSE WEIGHT

Losing weight has become an American pastime, and

Americans have learned a lot about it along the way. When we were trying to determine the optimum fat-loss approach for athletes and fitness exercisers, we reviewed the traditional methods to get an overview of the field. It soon became evident that the traditional fat-loss approaches are extremely varied and are not intended for athletes. The traditional methods were developed primarily for people who need to lose weight quickly for health reasons or who would just like to trim down for appearance's sake.

There are three main ways to lose weight—dehydration, lean-body-mass loss, and fat loss. Dehydration as a method of weight loss is not recommended. Despite this, wrestlers and other athletes who need to "make weight" often use this method as a last-minute resort. Losing a few pounds just before a competition to make it into a specific weight class may not be harmful as long as the body's initial state of hydration was good. In most cases, the body can be rehydrated directly after the weigh-in. However, do not rely on dehydration to lose more than a few pounds (usually less than 3 percent of your total body weight), and do not stay dehydrated for more than several hours or cause dehydration through heat stress. Ideally, steer clear of dehydration as a method for making weight.

Lean-body-mass loss is a result of cutting back on food intake by too many calories, losing weight too fast, not eating the macronutrients in the proper ratio, or not exercising properly. It is due primarily to the breakdown of muscle tissue, but it can also be caused by a reduction in bone or connective tissue. Lean-body-mass loss, therefore, is a very detrimental type of weight loss. It also causes a lowering in the BMR and jeopardizes body structure and function.

The best way to lose weight is targeted fat loss. A proper fat-loss program also increases lean-body-mass percentage. An increase in lean-body-mass percentage can come from losing fat and keeping the amount of lean body mass the same, which results in a lower percentage of body fat and higher percentage of lean body mass. Or, it can come from actually increasing lean body mass, which results in an even greater increase in lean-body-mass percentage and decrease in body-fat percentage.

In its crudest form, weight loss can be accomplished by cutting back on the amount of food that is consumed, perhaps even cutting it out almost completely (outright starvation). When caloric intake is less than caloric output, the body must liberate energy from its tissues and stores. While reducing total calories does result in weight loss, it also causes a significant amount of lean body mass to be lost in the process. A decrease in lean body mass means an increase in body-fat percentage, which also means a drop in BMR. You should *never* try to lose fat using a crash diet, starvation diet, or any of the faddish approaches that have been common in the sports-nutrition industry. Weight-loss clinics, meal-replacement drinks, diet pills, and other common means are often in themselves incapable of meeting the athlete's sophisticated fat-loss requirements.

An interesting note: Meal-replacement drinks usually cause an initial drop in weight that is attributed mostly to a loss of water weight and gastrointestinal bulk. Additionally, they often cause diarrhea, which causes dehydration and adversely affects performance.

When following our Targeted Fat Loss Program, dieters are often surprised at how easy losing fat can be. In fact, if you follow the guidelines properly, you may not even realize that you are on a fat-loss program, because you will be eating just about the same amount of food as you would on a weight-maintenance plan.

THE TARGETED FAT LOSS PROGRAM

Our Targeted Fat Loss Program is not a plan of specific daily menus utilizing magic weight-loss foods that add up to a "one size fits all" total daily caloric count. On the contrary, it is a *set of guidelines* that individual dieters can adapt to their particular situations and needs. The goal is not to lose a certain number of pounds in a certain number of weeks or months. It is not to attain some arbitrary weight goal set by a coach or weight class. Rather, the goal of your personal Targeted Fat Loss Program is to reach a reduced body-fat percentage that is both realistic and can be achieved within your time constraints.

Our Targeted Fat Loss Program is also dynamic in that it can be adapted to the time of year. Ideally, you should make any body-composition changes during your off-season. This way, the focus of your preseason and in-season nutrition and training programs can be maximization of performance. Most elite athletes follow this approach, since roller-coaster fluctuations in body composition during the season can affect performance adversely.

To individualize our Targeted Fat Loss Program for your specific needs, first determine your body-composition goal. The best way to do this is to consult a competent professional such as your health-care practitioner or a trained nutritionist. You can also refer to Table 12.1 on page 148, which gives the overall normal and desirable ranges of body-fat percentage for male and female athletes and nonathletes, and Table 13.1 on page 165, which provides the body-fat percentages for a variety of elite athletes. Next, estimate how long it will take you to reach your goal and plan when to begin and end your program. The best time to end your program (reach your goal) is two months before your season begins. This will give you ample opportunity to adjust to your new body composition before starting competition. Depending on the amount of fat you want to lose, the program can take from several weeks to several months.

To lose fat during the off-season or preseason, simply follow the dietary guidelines outlined in your sport-specific plan in Part Four but reduce your total daily caloric intake by 4 calories per pound of lean body mass. For example, if you are a man who weighs 195 pounds and has 20-percent body fat, your lean body mass is about 156 pounds. Multiply those 156 pounds of lean body mass by 4 calories for a result of 624 calories. This is the number of calories by which you should reduce your total daily caloric intake. Thus, if you are following a weight-maintenance plan of 3,500 calories per day, subtracting 624 calories will give you a total daily caloric intake of 2,876 calories. Since a pound of fat contains 3,500 calories, it will take you about six days to lose 1 pound.

It is possible, of course, to lose fat at a faster rate. However, reducing more quickly will bring with it a loss of lean body mass. A moderate rate will result in a fat loss of about 5 pounds per month. Most experts recommend a slow to moderate rate. Calculate your body composition a few times per week to determine your individual rate of fat loss.

Once you have determined the number of calories to subtract from your daily total, figure out how many calories to subtract from each meal. To continue with our example, if you consume five meals per day, reduce each meal by about 125 calories (one-fifth of 625 calories). Even though you are subtracting calories from your diet, you should not subtract any meals.

The calories that you subtract from your diet should come first from dietary fats, then from simple carbohydrates, and finally from complex carbohydrates. These three calorie sources are the fat-causing culprits. Cut back your intake of fast foods, junk foods, spreads, deserts, pastries, fruit, soda pop, and other sources of fat, sugar, or alcohol. Studies continue to confirm that people who consume high-fat diets tend to put on body fat and have difficulty taking it off, while people who consume low-fat diets generally do not have these problems. Cut back on complex carbohydrates only minimally, since they help maintain the blood-sugar level and provide a steady supply of energy. In addition, when carbohydrates are present in the diet, the body burns fats more efficiently.

The calories that you subtract should not come from protein at all. Amino acids are generally the last source the body turns to for energy, since their primary functions are the building and repair of tissues and compounds. Protein also stimulates thermogenesis, since the body must use more calories to process protein than it derives from protein.

In addition to cutting calories, stick to the core strength-training and endurance-exercise program for your specific sport. If your program does not include daily aerobic activity, add forty minutes of aerobic exercise to your schedule four or five days per week. Aerobic exercise uses mostly fatty acids for fuel, while strength training uses mostly muscle glycogen. Exercising daily will also keep your BMR up, maintain or increase your lean body mass, and keep your fat-burning enzymes at high levels.

To lose fat during the season, follow the same guidelines for the off-season and preseason but aim for a slower rate of loss. Instead of reducing your total daily caloric intake by 4 calories per pound of lean body mass, cut back by 2 calories per pound. You will still lose fat, but you should not suffer adverse effects on your performance.

INTEGRATING TARGETED FAT LOSS WITH PERFORMANCE NUTRITION

Following a sound sports-nutrition program is not always easy, but it is something that every athlete should do. Although eating properly may not be practical, the more you do, the better a competitor you will be.

Table 13.1. Body-Fat Percentages of Different Elite Athletes

Sport	Males	Females
Basketball	7%–12%	14%–20%
Bodybuilding [1]	4%–8%	9%–12%
Football		
Back positions	7%–12%	—
Line positions	10%–15%	—
Gymnastics	4%–8%	10%–12%
Long-distance running	5%–10%	10%–12%
Powerlifting [2]	5%–10%	10%–15%
Soccer	7%–10%	—
Swimming	5%–8%	10%–15%
Tennis	8%–13%	15%–21%
Track and field		
Jumping	7%–10%	10%–13%
Sprinting	4%–8%	10%–13%
Throwing	8%–12%	10%–15%
Weightlifting [2]	5%–10%	10%–15%
Wrestling [2]	4%–8%	—

[1] Elite male bodybuilders are usually closer to the 8-percent level than the 4-percent level. Experts believe that this is due to their putting on extra "mass" via fat deposits within the muscles themselves. However, these same bodybuilders keep their subcutaneous-fat levels extremely low to show their "cuts" (muscular definition).

[2] Athletes in the heavier weight classes typically exceed these guidelines by 3 to 4 percentage points.

Note: The above ranges of body-fat percentage were compiled from profiles of elite athletes.

The following guidelines will help you integrate your Targeted Fat Loss Program with your performance-nutrition program. (For a complete description of the performance-nutrition program recommended for you in particular, see your sport-specific plan in Part Four.) These guidelines will prove beneficial whether you are trying to lose fat, gain muscle, or simply maintain your already-polished physique.

Guideline One: Eat Five Meals a Day

Always eat at least five meals a day. Two or three meals often simply are not enough. If your muscles do not get the calories they need, how will they keep going? They will need to *cannibalize* muscle tissue—the same muscle tissue you sweated so many hours to get! On the flip side, do not think that this guideline gives you license to eat all day long. Overeating, even at just one meal a day, keeps the fat-building enzymes in your body ready to turn any excess food into body fat.

Guideline Two: Maintain Your Proper Macronutrient Ratio

During your preseason and season, make sure that you consume the macronutrients in the ratio recommended for your specific sport in Part Four. During your off-season, you can either continue to consume the same diet or switch to one composed of 20-percent fat, 20-percent protein, and 60-percent carbohydrates. A 20:20:60 diet can also serve as an excellent general diet for people who are more interested in health and fitness than athletic performance.

For a list of food groups and suggested servings that can be used as a general guide when planning your daily food intake on a 20:20:60 diet, see Table 13.2, below. The servings suggested in the table will provide between 2,500 and 3,500 calories per day and are intended for a reference individual who is male, lean, and 175 pounds in weight. If you weigh more or less than this, you can adjust the total calories by adding or subtracting, respectively, about one serving in each food group. Spread your food intake over five to seven meals according to Guideline Three, below.

Guideline Three: Eat According to the Next Three Hours

Whenever you sit down to eat, ask yourself, "What

Table 13.2. Daily Food-Intake Goals for 20:20:60 Diet

Food Group	Suggested Daily Servings*	Sample Serving Sizes
High-protein foods Meat, poultry, and fish	**3–4 servings** Choose lean meats and skinless chicken, turkey, and fish	5–7 ounces of cooked lean meat, poultry, or fish. Count 1 egg, ½ cup cooked beans, or 2 tablespoons peanut butter as 1 ounce.
Complex carbohydrates Bread, cereal, grains, pasta, and starchy vegetables	**11–14 servings** Include several servings of whole-grain products	1 slice bread; ½ hamburger bun or English muffin; 1 small roll, biscuit, or muffin; 4 crackers; ½ cup cooked cereal, rice, or pasta; 1 ounce ready-to-serve cereal.
Vegetables Dark-green leafy vegetables	**5–8 servings** Include a diversity of vegetables	½ cup cooked vegetable; ½ cup chopped raw vegetable; 1 cup raw leafy vegetable such as lettuce or spinach.
Fruits Citrus, melons, berries, and other fruits	**4–6 servings** Choose fresh fruits whenever possible	1 whole fruit such as an apple, banana, orange, or pear; ½ grapefruit; ½ melon wedge; ½ cup berries; ½ cup cooked or canned fruit; ¼ cup dried fruit; ¾ cup juice.
Dairy products Milk, cheese, and yogurt	**2–3 servings** Choose low-fat products whenever possible	8 ounces milk; 1½ ounces cheese; 8 ounces yogurt.
Fats Dietary fats, saturated fats, and cholesterol	Consume as little as possible	
Sweets Sugar and sugar-containing foods	Consume as little as possible	
Fluids Filtered water, diluted fruit juices, and low-calorie beverages.	**8–12 servings**	8 ounces

*For a lean, 175-pound male.

166

am I going to be doing for the next three hours of my life?" Then, eat accordingly. For example, if you will be taking a nap, eat fewer calories than normal. If you will be training, eat more.

When planning your caloric intake for a meal, use the following general guide:

☐ If you will be engaging in a strenuous workout during the next three hours, add 300 calories to your average meal.

☐ If you will be engaging in a moderate workout during the next three hours, add 200 calories to your average meal.

☐ If you will be engaging in vigorous activity during the next three hours, add 100 calories to your average meal.

☐ If you will be engaging in moderate activity during the next three hours, eat an average meal.

☐ If you will be engaging in light activity during the next three hours, subtract 100 calories from your average meal.

☐ If you will be relaxing during the next three hours, subtract 200 calories from your average meal.

☐ If you will be napping during the next three hours, subtract 300 calories from your average meal.

Remember that when you overeat at a meal, the excess calories will be stored as body fat. Therefore, even if you skip a meal, do not make up for it at the next meal. Instead, continue to eat for what you will be doing afterwards.

Guideline Four: Zigzag Your Caloric Intake

Another thing to remember when you are trying to lose fat is to "zigzag" your caloric intake. Zigzagging your total daily calories will help reset your metabolism. If you stay on a reduced-calorie diet for too long, your BMR will drop to conserve energy. Temporarily increasing your caloric intake every several days will help combat this. For a complete discussion of zigzagging, see "Zigzagging Your Caloric Intake," right.

Guideline Five: Take Your Dietary Supplements

The final things to remember are that no matter how hard you try:

☐ You cannot always eat perfectly balanced meals.

☐ You cannot always eat five or more meals a day.

☐ You cannot always get all the nutrients you need from just your diet.

Thanks to today's advanced nutritional and botanical sciences, there are many substances, both man-made and natural, that can help make up for any shortcomings due to your diet or daily life. Supplements are also available that help control appetite or boost metabolism. For a list of recommended supplements, see your sport-specific plan in Part Four. For a list of supplements that double as fat-loss aids, see "Common Supplements Used as Fat-Loss Aids" on page 170.

ZIGZAGGING YOUR CALORIC INTAKE

"I eat like a *bird* and still gain weight!"

"No matter *what* I do, I get fatter and fatter!"

"All I have to do is *smell* food and I put on weight!"

Anyone who has been around the fitness world for any length of time has heard these complaints. Even athletes and bodybuilders preparing for competition often have trouble shedding those last couple of third place–rendering, muscle-masking pounds of adipose.

The intrepid sleuths of academe are also no strangers to these complaints. Researchers have long known that stringent dieting causes a drop in BMR, making it difficult, often impossible, to continue the fat-shedding process. Scientists are finally beginning to garner some hard data in support of what bodybuilders have known for quite some time—that there is a way to lose fat and still maintain a reasonably high BMR to keep the fat-loss process continuing smoothly. The method is called "zigzagging," and it works better than any other fat-loss method known. Why? Because the fat loss is permanent—that is, if you continue to eat five or six smaller meals per day and exercise regularly. Zigzagging also allows you to maintain (or increase) your lean body mass.

Zigzagging, developed and tested by Dr. Hatfield, works by confusing your metabolism. When you reduce your caloric intake and increase your caloric output, you force your body-fat percentage to drop. However, your BMR also drops. To force your BMR back up to a more-normal level, you add calories to your diet again for a brief period of time. Your body-fat percentage climbs, too, but before it can reach its starting level again, you cut your calories once more. Down go your body fat and your BMR. Eat normally again, and up go your BMR and body fat—but, again, the body fat does not go up as high as it was before. You can continue this process until your body-fat percentage is at a healthful level.

By zigzagging your caloric intake, you allow periodic adjustments of your BMR to take place, bringing your metabolism to a level more appropriate for your new (lower) body weight. When your metabolism is running at an appropriate rate, you can begin to lose fat again. If you simply eat a reduced-calorie diet day after day and never give your BMR a chance to adjust, you will find your fat-loss efforts becoming more and more difficult until, in sheer frustration, you binge and add body fat. Zigzagging will also help you get past, or even avoid, the phenomenon called plateauing. A plateau, which usually comes after several pounds have been lost, is the point at which the weight loss stops. When most people hit a plateau, what do they do? They reduce their caloric intake further. This just adds to the problem, causing an additional drop in the BMR. If you instead zigzag your caloric intake up, your metabolism will become readjusted at a higher rate and your body will once again begin to burn more calories.

An important key to zigzagging is weight training. Without weight training, your weight loss may come from both fat and lean body mass. Bigger muscles burn more calories than little muscles do. The more muscle tissue you lose, the less muscle tissue you have to burn calories and the more your ability to lose fat—and to keep it off—is sabotaged. Another key is not to rush. Even with weight training, a starvation diet will cause too much muscle to be lost. Walking is fine for individuals considered chronically obese. For persons who are only slightly overweight, other forms of aerobic exercise are also excellent for maintaining cardiovascular fitness. But weight training stands out as the single best method for ensuring that weight loss comes from fat stores and not from hard-won muscle tissue. Why? Because aerobic training simply does not build muscle to the extent that weight training does. In fact, aerobic training alone tends to reduce lean body mass and cause a drop in BMR. This means that you need to exercise more to burn the same number of calories. In addition, if you gain 5 or 10 pounds of muscle through weight training, you will burn more calories all the time, even when you are asleep.

For the ultimate fat-loss program, combine zigzagging and weight training with moderate aerobic exercise, a healthy diet, and an appropriate supplement program. You will be amazed at how easy it is to lose fat—and how utterly enjoyable it is to keep it off forever!

How to Zigzag Your Caloric Intake

If you decide that you would like to zigzag your caloric intake to aid your fat-loss efforts, you must first figure out your average daily caloric requirement and your reduced daily caloric intake. To figure out how many calories you expend on an average day, see "Estimating Average Daily Caloric Requirement" on page 150. To figure out your reduced daily caloric intake, see "The Targeted Fat Loss Program" on page 164. To zigzag your caloric intake, consume the reduced number of calories for five to six days, then consume your normal number of calories for one to two days. Continue alternating your caloric total until you reach your desired level of body fat.

The length of time it will take you to reach your body-fat goal using the zigzag method will vary with how much fat you wish to lose, your age, and your activity level. Generally, the closer you are to your ideal body-fat percentage, the longer it will take you to lose body fat. The less fat you have left to lose, the more care you need to take to ensure that only fat is lost. Chronically obese individuals will also take longer to lose fat. This is because their BMRs are very low and they are usually unable to engage in strenuous (calorie-burning) exercise until they lose some pounds and build up their heart muscle and strength.

ADDITIONAL TIPS FOR LOSING FAT

The following tips for losing body fat can also be called "keys to sound nutrition." They have become very well known in today's health-conscious society and can almost be considered common knowledge. However, if you find your fat loss slowing down despite your best efforts, you may wish to refresh your memory by glancing through the list. You might find something that you have forgotten or a tip that you have not yet tried.

☐ General tips

• Plan your meals. This will allow you to control your caloric intake and macronutrient ratio.

• Keep a nutrition log to keep track of your food intake. (For a sample log page, see Appendix D on page 373.)

• Eat your meals at approximately the same times

every day. This will keep you from becoming uncontrollably hungry and will increase the efficiency of your digestive system.

• Do not watch television or read the newspaper while eating. People who are distracted during meals tend to overeat and may not chew their food properly.

• Do not skip meals. You need to consume all your recommended meals to sustain your blood-sugar level, to provide the energy you need for your upcoming activities, and to supply the nutrients you need, especially the amino acids necessary for recovery, repair, and growth.

• Do not cut your total daily caloric intake too drastically or you will lose lean body mass as well as body fat.

• Reduce your fat intake to 20 percent or less of your total daily calories. To do this, eat foods that are fat free or have no more than 2 grams of fat per 100 calories. Excess dietary fat is converted to body fat.

• Increase your intake of foods that are high in fiber. High-fiber foods not only satisfy hunger cravings, they also help lower cholesterol and hinder the absorption of fat in the body.

• Increase your intake of complex carbohydrates. Foods such as grains, pasta, and starchy vegetables provide a steady supply of energy, help keep the blood sugar at an appropriate level, and satisfy hunger cravings.

• Eat fresh foods. Fresh foods are high in nutrients and low in additives.

• Eat plenty of vegetables. Vegetables are high in vitamins and low in calories and fat.

• Read nutrition labels.

• Avoid foods that are high in sodium, such as processed foods and snack foods. Sodium causes water retention, which hinders performance and can be hazardous to health.

• Eliminate junk food from your diet. Most junk foods are high in fat, sodium, and sugar. They will do little more than make a roller coaster out of your blood-sugar level, and pump you with artery-clogging saturated fat and water-retaining sodium.

• Use low-fat protein supplements to help meet your daily protein requirement.

• Eat egg whites as a snack in the evening to help reduce hunger pangs.

• Do not use heavy sauces on foods. Sauces tend to be high in calories and fat.

• Break the habit of eating out on a daily basis, especially at fast-food restaurants. Fast foods in particular are usually high in fat, salt, and calories.

• Drink at least eight to ten glasses of water every day to ensure adequate replacement of the fluids lost during exercise. Do not wait until you are thirsty. By then, you will by dehydrated. Do not drink all your water at one time, but spread out your intake throughout the day.

• Use calorie-free beverages such as water, club soda, and flavored seltzer to help maintain your proper level of fluid intake.

• Exercise daily to keep your BMR up and to burn calories.

• Maintain or increase your lean body mass through weight training. Since muscle burns calories, the more muscle you gain, the more calories you will burn and the greater your rate of fat loss will be. Weight training will also increase your bone density and make your tendons and ligaments stronger.

• Maximize the thermogenic effect by keeping your protein intake up, increasing your activity level, and taking the appropriate dietary supplements.

☐ Cooking tips

• Always trim away excess fat and skin from meat and poultry.

• Avoid the use of monosodium glutamate (MSG), which is very high in sodium.

• Do not fry foods or use oil or fat in the cooking process. Instead, bake, broil, or microwave your food. If necessary, use nonstick cooking spray to coat your frying pan or baking dish.

• Use nonstick frying pans, pressure cookers, steamer baskets, and roasting racks to cook. These tools help separate unnecesary fat from food.

• Broiling, baking, and grilling all reduce the fat content of food.

☐ Restaurant tips

• Choose restaurants that offer a variety of foods that are included in your meal plan.

• Study your menu and look for broiled meat or fish. Broiled items tend to be the best choices at restaurants.

• Request that sauces and dressings be served on the side.

• Seafood restaurants offer low-fat meals such as broiled fish.

• At a steak house, order a lean cut of meat such as a filet, ground steak, or skinless chicken breast.

• At a Chinese restaurant, choose steamed vegetables with chicken or beef. Ask that the MSG be omitted.

• Be aware of portions. Restaurant servings tend to vary in size.

• Do not feel that you must always clean your plate. Take your leftovers home for another meal.

☐ Travel tips

• Take along fruit, ready-to-serve cereal, air-popped popcorn, sports drinks, and sports nutrition bars on long car trips.

• Take along a bagged lunch if you know you will be on the road at your normal lunchtime. Do not leave yourself stranded without healthy food.

• Order special meals for airplane trips. Fruit plates and other healthy meals can be ordered through a travel agent.

• Bring bottled water with you to keep up your water intake.

For more tips on how to lose fat or boost your nutrition, reread Part One of this book. Your sport-specific plan in Part Four will also provide guidelines.

FACTORS THAT AFFECT THE RATE OF FAT LOSS

Your rate of fat loss will be affected by a myriad of factors, some of which you will have no control over. For example, men tend to lose fat and gain muscle easier than women do. This is due to hormonal differences. For one thing, men have more testosterone than women, which helps them maintain a higher proportion of muscle mass and a higher BMR than women. At the same time, a woman's hormonal system resists changes in body composition as a protective mechanism that helps conserve energy stores during pregnancy. Women, therefore, lose fat at a slower rate than men do and find it difficult to maintain body-fat levels below 16 percent.

Both men and women experience a slow-down in their rates of fat loss as they age. However, this should not serve to discourage anyone. Rather, it should underscore the importance of establishing realistic, lifelong goals, including to follow a balanced nutrition plan and to exercise and weight train daily.

In addition to gender and age, factors that may affect your rate of fat loss include your body type, genetics, metabolism, nutrition, and exercise program. Ectomorphs (slim, linear types) have the easiest time losing fat, but they have difficulty gaining muscle. Mesomorphs (muscular types) find it easy to both lose fat and gain muscle. Endomorphs (fat, round types) are able to lose fat at a good rate, but they need to watch what they eat and follow a strength-training and aerobic-exercise program. Endomorphs may also find it beneficial to raise their protein intake up to 25 to 30 percent of their total daily calories. (For a discussion of somatotypes, see "Body Types" on page 148.)

JUMP-STARTING YOUR TARGETED FAT LOSS PROGRAM

You may find it helpful to give your Targeted Fat Loss Program a "jump-start" by depleting your glycogen stores. Glycogen depletion encourages greater use of body-fat stores. To deplete your glycogen stores, simply cut out carbohydrates completely for the first day or two of your fat-loss program. Eat plenty of low-calorie vegetables and your full daily quota of protein. This will deplete your muscle glycogen stores and cause a loss in water weight. It will also cause your fat stores to begin burning. Slowly phase carbohydrates back into your diet over the next two to three days.

Jump-start your diet only during your off-season and pre-season. Glycogen depletion can adversely affect performance and therefore should not be done during the season.

COMMON SUPPLEMENTS USED AS FAT-LOSS AIDS

If you want to maximize your fat loss, or if you want to speed up your rate of fat loss because you feel that it is too slow, try adding one or more of the following dietary supplements to your nutrition program:

☐ Anorectics (natural appetite suppressants)— Brindall berry, 1,500 to 3,000 milligrams per day; L-phenylalanine, 250 to 1,000 milligrams per day; L-tyrosine, 250 to 1,000 milligrams per day.

☐ Chromium, 200 to 600 micrograms per day.

☐ Fiber, 30 to 50 grams per day from food and supplement sources.

☐ Herbal bitters—*Gentiana lutea* (liquid drops), used as directed on the bottle.

☐ Herbal lipotropics—Barberry, bearberry, dandelion, milk thistle, wall germander, wild Oregon grape, used as directed on the package.

☐ L-carnitine, 600 to 1,200 milligrams per day.

☐ Lipotropics—Betaine, 200 micrograms; choline, 200 to 500 milligrams; inositol, 200 to 500 milligrams; L-methionine, 500 milligrams.

☐ Natural digestive aids—Bromelin, lipase, papain, protease, 250 to 500 milligrams with each meal.

☐ Thermogenic aids—Caffeine, cayenne, ephedra, fo ti, guarana, mustard seed, used as directed on the package.

Use your chosen fat-loss aids in addition to your regular dietary supplements. Also take a daily multi-vitamin-and-mineral supplement, and drink a protein shake every day as a nutrient-dense snack.

IF NOTHING WORKS

If you cannot seem to lose fat despite your best efforts, you may need to consult your health-care practitioner to determine if you have a medical problem. Overweight and obesity are symptoms of a vast number of physical conditions, such as insulin resistance (resistance of the body against the effects of insulin). Factors such as aging and genetic makeup may also cause overweight or obesity. Pregnancy brings with it added pounds, since the body is caring for an ever-growing fetus. After birth—or, if you breastfeed your baby, after the baby moves on to the bottle or solid food—the pounds will drop off. Stress and emotional disturbances are also well known to wreak havoc with the appetite.

Your appetite control center may be excessively stimulated due to a medical weakness . . . or because of the wonderful cooking aromas drifting down the hallway from your neighbors' apartments every evening. A cold temperature can cause you to crave food because your body needs an insulating layer of fat, or because you are housebound and bored due to the blizzard raging outside. If you do not exercise enough due to health problems or time constraints, or if you lead a sedentary life due to your health or job, you are not burning off the calories that you are consuming. Even poverty can cause weight problems, since the only food you may be able to afford is laden with calories, sugar, and fat but devoid of nutrients.

If you do not know why you are having problems losing weight, consult your health-care practitioner to treat or rule out possible medical causes. Consult a doctor who specializes in medical weight loss, or a nutritionist or personal trainer. Join a self-help group to learn about behavior modification. Most importantly, seek the support of your family and friends in sticking to your prescribed program.

If you still have problems, perhaps you are expecting too much of yourself. Your weight-loss regimen should never be so spartan or strict that you lose interest in it or quit because it is too difficult to maintain. Ease up on yourself and you may find the pounds sliding off.

AN APPROACH FOR LIFE

Athletes and fitness exercisers usually do not have problems losing body fat when they stick to the Targeted Fat Loss Program discussed in this chapter. The primary problems they usually encounter involve the quality of their weight loss. Muscle is lost with gimmick diets. By following the approach presented here, you will easily lose body fat and reach your body-composition goal.

Do not become frustrated if you find it difficult to attain your goal. Give yourself time and use the scientific approaches discussed in the preceding pages. You may find that you have to start your fat-loss program by first gaining muscle—by first adding weight and getting your muscles in shape—and then enlist the aid of those muscles in getting rid of the fat. However, the majority of people who have trouble losing fat need to focus on improving their nutrition.

Most of the general population is on a constant search for a quick-weight-loss gimmick. These people are forever looking for a magic pill or a food that melts away fat. While many gimmick diets do bring about a loss of weight, their success rates are under 10 percent, according to a recent evaluation. This is because they do not use real food and do not advocate sensible exercise. In addition, the weight they take off includes lean body mass. When you lose lean body mass, your BMR drops and your body-fat percentage remains the same or goes up. Avoid weight-loss gimmicks and drugs. Use a well-researched, solid, integrated approach, such as the Targeted Fat Loss Program presented here. The Targeted Fat Loss Program is an approach for life.

14. GUIDE TO EFFECTIVE MUSCLE BUILDING

The bodybuilding market exploded during the 1980s and has continued to grow ever since. Just walk into a health-food store and you will find yourself standing face-to-face with hundreds of muscle-building products. These products range from simple powders to comprehensive kits.

Building muscle is just as scientific an undertaking as losing fat is and requires a specific nutrition and training program. In this chapter, we will discuss how to put together such a program. We will also take a look at the skeletal muscles and how they function. To see where any muscle mentioned in this chapter is located in the body, see Appendix F on page 379.

THE SKELETAL MUSCLES

Muscle tissue, as discussed in Chapter 10, makes up a large part of the human body—43 percent of a man's body by weight and 34 percent of a woman's body by weight. Altogether, the body contains about 650 muscles. The vast majority—about 620 muscles—work in conjunction with the skeletal system to create motion. They are called the skeletal muscles. The remaining 30 muscles, called the cardiac muscles and the smooth muscles, perform such vital functions as pumping the blood through the body and helping a variety of internal organs to operate. In terms of the body's day-to-day functioning, muscle tissue is the most important tissue in the body.

The muscles that are the focus of bodybuilding are the skeletal muscles. The skeletal muscles are classified as striated-voluntary muscles. (For discussions of muscle cells and muscle tissue, as well as of the skeletal muscle system, see Chapter 10.) These types of muscles are called voluntary because their nerve fibers come from the central nervous system, making their contraction voluntarily controlled. They called striated because they appear grainy. The skeletal muscles are the major striated-voluntary muscles.

The main function of muscle tissue is contraction. However, with few exceptions, muscles do not contract individually. Rather, they contract in specific sets or sequences. Even the simplest movements require the contraction of complex sets or sequences of muscles. The production of contractions is controlled by the brain and spinal cord. The orders for contraction are sent through nerve fibers. When the nervous system receives an order for a certain movement, it causes the contraction of the muscles that are required and the neutralization of the muscles that are not required.

Every individual muscle fiber does not have its own "line" to the central nervous system. Instead, impulses from the central nervous system move along a nerve axon, which resembles the trunk of a tree, then branch off to groups of muscle fibers, which contract as units. To coordinate all the movements of a muscle, the central nervous system must be aware of the length of the muscle and the tension of the tendons that attach the muscle to the skeleton. This information is supplied by special sense organs called muscle spindles. Muscles must contract not only rapidly in response to signals from the central nervous system but also with the correct amount of tension to produce an effective mechanical force.

In between a nerve fiber and the surface of a muscle is a gap. When an impulse first reaches a nerve fiber, it triggers the release of a chemical, acetylcholine, from the nerve ending. The acetylcholine passes across the gap and stimulates the membrane of the muscle fiber. The stimulation, in the form of an electric current, moves along the surface of the muscle fiber and causes the muscle to contract. It takes only one one-thousandth of a second for a current to move along the surface of a muscle fiber. Unless another nerve impulse arrives, the muscle fiber stops contracting and relaxes as soon as the current has passed. If the acetylcholine were blocked from passing across the gap, the result would be paralysis.

MECHANICS OF MUSCLE CONTRACTION

To the naked eye, the skeletal muscles appear grainy. This is because they are composed of small fibers (long cells). These fibers are cylinderlike and may be several centimeters long. They are also divided into bands (striations) and thus resemble coins stacked in a pile.

Every individual muscle fiber is surrounded by a thin plasma membrane called a sarcolemma. About 80 percent of each fiber is made of tiny fibrils known as myofibrils, which are the structures that are directly involved in contraction. One fiber can have from several hundred to several thousand myofibrils. The remaining 20 percent of each fiber is made of a jelly-like intracellular fluid called sarcoplasm. The sarcoplasm, which contains many nuclei and other cell constituents, such as mitochondria, is where the biochemical reactions that produce energy take place.

The myofibrils are made of two types of protein—actin and myosin—which take the form of long filaments. The myosin filaments are thick, while the actin filaments are thin. Both kinds of filaments are able to interlock and slide over each other to accommodate stretching of the muscle. During shortening (contraction) of the muscle, they have the ability to slide into one another. In addition, during contraction, cross-links seem to form between the actin and myosin filaments. When the cross-links form, the two filaments move toward one another, which is what causes the muscle to shorten (contract). These cross-links are almost instantaneously broken again, with new cross-links forming further along the two filaments.

Contraction does not always refer to the shortening of a muscle. Technically, it refers to the development of tension within a muscle. There are two major types of contractions. A contraction in which the muscle develops tension but does not shorten is an isometric contraction. A contraction in which the muscle shortens and maintains constant tension is called an isotonic contraction. For example, a man trying to curl a heavy barbell strains against the weight. His arm muscles develop tension but do not shorten because the resistance generated by the barbell is greater than the muscles' tension. This is an isometric contraction. But when the man lightens the barbell by removing some plates, the resistance is decreased and the working muscles shorten as they contract. This is an isotonic contraction. When the muscles shorten by overcoming the resistance, such as when a barbell is being curled up, the isotonic contraction is called a concentric isotonic contraction. When the muscles lengthen and act to maintain constant tension during the lengthening movement, such as when a barbell is slowly being let down, the isotonic contraction is called an eccentric isotonic contraction.

The energy that the muscles use to contract comes from the chemical reaction between the food we eat and the oxygen we breathe. Energy production involves the breakdown of glucose to carbon dioxide and water. As the glucose is broken down, energy is released and used by the muscle protein to cause contraction. The breakdown process requires huge amounts of oxygen, which are often unavailable. Even during intensive exercise, the blood supply often does not have enough hemoglobin to carry sufficient oxygen to the muscles. To compensate, the muscles convert glucose into lactic acid, a process that does not need oxygen but that still supplies ample energy. However, if too much lactic acid is produced before it can be used, it limits the intensity of exercise and ultimately prevents continuation of the exercise at the same concentration. The muscles become fatigued. The excess lactic acid eventually makes its way into the bloodstream and is circulated to the liver, where it can be reassembled into glucose and returned to the bloodstream or stored as glycogen. Some lactic acid may also be converted back into pyruvate, a form in which it can enter the mitochondria and be completely broken down for energy.

The body may also obtain energy from its stores of muscle glycogen. Muscle glycogen is used during high-intensity, low-endurance activities, such as weightlifting. During low-intensity, high-endurance activities, such as long-distance running, the body uses a mixture of glucose from its glycogen stores and fatty acids from its fat stores.

FAST-TWITCH AND SLOW-TWITCH MUSCLE FIBERS

Skeletal muscle tissue is composed of two general types of muscle fibers—fast-twitch and slow-twitch. Fast-twitch muscle fibers are selectively recruited when heavy work is demanded of the muscles, and strength and power are needed. They contract quickly, providing short bursts of energy, and are therefore used for high-intensity, low-endurance activities, such as sprinting, weightlifting, shot-putting, and swinging a golf club. However, fast-twitch muscle fibers become exhausted quickly. Pain and cramps rapidly develop from the buildup of lactic acid, which is a byproduct of the metabolism of this kind of muscle fiber.

Slow-twitch muscle fibers produce a steady, low-intensity, repetitive contraction. They do not tire easily and are recruited when endurance is needed.

Therefore, slow-twitch muscle fibers are used for low-intensity, high-endurance activities, such as long-distance running.

The duration and intensity of your activity will influence the physiology of your muscle tissue and the development of your muscle fibers. Endurance athletes tend to develop a greater percentage of slow-twitch muscle fibers, while power athletes tend to develop a greater percentage of fast-twitch muscle fibers. One reason for this is that in power athletes, the fast-twitch muscle fibers increase in size to store more ATP and CP. ATP and CP are needed for explosive energy. Another reason is that power athletes need more muscle glycogen to fuel their muscles, while endurance athletes need both muscle glycogen and fatty acids.

MUSCLE HYPERTROPHY AND MUSCLE HYPERPLASIA

Muscle hypertrophy is simply enlargement of a muscle due to an increase in the size of the muscle fibers. Muscle fibers increase in size in response to adaptive overload stress—that is, by adjusting to increasingly greater amounts of resistance. This adjustment can take place in several ways. The principal way is by an increase in the number of myofibrils in the individual muscle cells. This probably occurs because a greater total amount of amino acids is transported into the cells, enhancing the cells' incorporation into the muscle proteins that cause contraction. Muscle hypertrophy also results from increases in the sizes and numbers of mitochondria, myoglobin, and capillaries; increases in the amounts of extracellular and intracellular fluid; and fusion between muscle fibers, principally fast-twitch fibers, and their surrounding satellite cells.

Muscle hyperplasia is similar to muscle hypertrophy in that the result is enlargement of a muscle. However, it is different in that it is caused by an increase in the number of muscle fibers. It is also different because its occurrence is a topic of heated scientific controversy. Some researchers have reported the possibility of muscle fibers splitting lengthwise, resulting in the development of new muscle fibers. Other researchers, however, have criticized the methodology used in these studies, and the issue remains unresolved.

THE BEST WAY TO BUILD MUSCLE

The best way to build up the skeletal muscles is to fol-

low the nutrition guidelines given for bodybuilders in Part Four and either a training program designed for your specific sport or one of the weight-training systems described later in this chapter. The same as fat loss, muscle building—except by power athletes—should be undertaken only during the off-season. Even then, athletic performance should not be sacrificed for increases in strength or muscle mass. Set goals for yourself based on your sport and body-composition needs. Once you have added your desired extra muscle mass, you can focus your efforts in the preseason and season on strength training and maximizing your sport performance.

Many "experts" say that building muscle mass is just a matter of increasing your caloric and protein intakes. This is not so. You must first and foremost follow an effective weight-training program, one that is designed specifically for muscle building. Not all weight-training programs result in optimum muscle gain. In fact, most of the weight-training programs that are labeled "strength training" will build some muscle, but focus more on building strength and power. Strength and power are important performance factors, but they can be worked on in the preseason, after the desired muscle mass has been added.

Again, the same as for an effective fat-loss program, set realistic muscle-gain goals and focus on the long-term benefits as they relate to your sport or fitness needs. It makes no sense to gain 30 pounds of muscle by lifting heavy weights for several hours a day only to lose the added muscle mass during the season because your sport demands a different level of muscle mass and performance.

The ability to build muscle mass varies considerably among individuals and depends upon body type, sex, age, and current training status. Mesomorphic men tend to pack on muscle the quickest. Endurance athletes tend to build muscle at a slower rate due to their training regimens and training-induced muscle-fiber contents. So, is it possible to gain 30 pounds of muscle in one year? Yes, but you should not be discouraged if your personal rate of muscle gain is slower.

Following are some important tips to keep in mind when you design your muscle-building program:

☐ During the off-season, follow the nutrition guidelines for bodybuilders in Part Four to most effectively build muscle mass. Then, during the preseason, follow your sport-specific training program to maximize your strength and power for your particular activity.

☐ Measure your body composition weekly. (For a discussion of the different measurement methods, see "Body Composition" on page 143.)

☐ Follow the Targeted Fat Loss Program described in Chapter 13, but instead of subtracting calories from your total daily caloric intake, add 2 calories for every 1 pound of lean body mass. Add the calories to your protein and carbohydrate intakes and leave your fat intake at roughly 20 percent. Divide the added calories equally among all your daily meals. For complete instructions, see Chapter 13.

☐ Eat five to six smaller meals a day to give your body a steady supply of calories and nutrients and to keep your blood sugar at a constant level.

☐ Eat whole foods, which generally are packed with nutrients. Avoid processed foods, which usually have had their nutrients processed out.

☐ Eat high-quality, low-fat proteins, such as egg whites, chicken, turkey, tuna, lean red meat, low-fat dairy products, and low-fat protein supplements.

☐ Since most people have difficulty eating their total required amount of food every day, try consuming a high-protein, low-fat powder weight-gain drink as a snack or as part of a meal.

☐ While you should increase your protein intake, you must be careful not to consume too much protein. The body can effectively digest and assimilate only about 25 to 40 grams of protein per meal.

☐ Eat more complex carbohydrates such as brown rice, whole-grain pasta, potatoes, whole-grain bread, and beans.

☐ For snacks, eat sports-nutrition bars that are low in fat and high in carbohydrates and protein.

☐ Eat dried fruits and nuts for a boost in energy. (However, do not eat these foods directly before working out.)

☐ Consume energy drinks before weight training but just water during weight training.

☐ Wait at least one hour before consuming your post-training meal. Studies show that if you train hard for about an hour, your GH and testosterone levels will reach a peak. However, if you eat during or directly after training, your hormonal responses will be reduced.

☐ Split your weight training into two sessions per day to maximize your hormonal responses.

☐ Do not overtrain. Overtraining, which is defined as cumulative microtrauma, actually stimulates the release of catabolic hormones, such as cortisol, which break down muscle. Weight train at your level of fitness; do not push yourself if you are a beginner. Whether you are a beginner or seasoned athlete, give your body a chance to repair its muscle and connective tissue.

If your goal is to build muscle mass without adding body fat, keep your gain to 2 to 4 pounds of lean body mass per month. The human body usually cannot synthesize muscle tissue any faster than this, even under the most ideal biochemical circumstances. The best way to gain lean body mass but not body fat is to follow the Targeted Fat Loss Program, adding calories instead of subtracting them, as described above. If you combine your efforts with an intensive weight-training program, you should gain about 1 to 4 pounds of muscle mass per month.

Another way to build up your muscle mass but not your body fat is to zigzag your caloric intake. To do this, consume an increased number of calories for four to five days, then consume your normal number of calories for one to two days. When you zigzag up, you will gain a pound of muscle and fat. When you zigzag down again, you will lose the added fat but not the added muscle. If you continue to zigzag for several months, you may be able to increase your muscle mass to elite proportions. Even hard gainers usually discover that increasing muscle mass is easy with zigzagging. Individuals with low body-fat levels, however, may have to increase their total daily calories more than the average person. (For a complete discussion of zigzagging and instructions on how to do it, see "Zigzagging Your Caloric Intake" on page 167.)

WEIGHT TRAINING

The other part of your muscle-building program is weight training. Training methods that employ dumbbells, barbells, hydraulic devices, pressurized-air devices, elastic devices, springs, or any of the machines designed to provide heavy external resistance to musculoskeletal effort all fall into the category of resistance training. According to tradition, however, weight training is limited to those exercises intended to be performed with dumbbells, barbells, or any device designed to simulate traditional dumbbell or barbell movements.

Exercising with dumbbells and barbells, which are

also called free weights, is considered to be the best training method for stimulating muscle gain. However, research indicates that combining free-weight training with machine training is also beneficial. The key is to learn to interpret the results you obtain with each piece of equipment and to determine the appropriate combination of free-weight and machine exercises.

If you have never weight trained or have not done so in a while, or if you have been exercising for just a few months, ease into weight training slowly to maintain safety and to derive maximum benefits. For the first three months, keep your workouts light; do not attempt any high-intensity movements. Never exercise to the point of extreme exhaustion or dizziness. Set realistic goals and pace yourself. Do not overexert yourself, and do not try to lift very heavy weights, even for 1 repetition (rep). Focus on your style, concentrating on achieving good form, and always train with a spotter. If you have muscle soreness that persists for a prolonged period of time or suffer an injury, seek medical attention.

Before beginning a workout, spend a few minutes stretching to limber up your muscles and ligaments. Doing some aerobic exercise is a good way to increase your heart rate and warm up your body at the same time. You should also perform one set of warm-up reps for each individual weight-training exercise, using light weights and slow movements. About 16 to 20 reps are adequate.

In addition to your weight training, you should perform twenty to forty minutes of aerobic exercise three to five times per week. If you are training to decrease your body fat as well as build up your muscles, you should perform forty to sixty minutes of aerobic exercise four to six times per week. Some beneficial types of aerobic exercise are running, interval running, and cycling, as well as using a treadmill, stationary cycle, stair-climbing machine, or cross-country-skiing machine. If you are a beginner, do a low-intensity aerobic exercise, such as walking. As you get into better shape, advance to a higher-intensity aerobic activity, such as running or cycling.

WEIGHT-TRAINING SYSTEMS

Weight training, like most other sports and fitness activities, is not something that can be carried out in a haphazard manner. To be effective, a weight-training program must be planned. Picking just any piece of equipment and doing random exercises for an arbi-

trary number of reps will not bring you the results you want. You need to exercise your muscles in a certain progression, for a certain number of sets and reps, with rest periods of a certain number of minutes in between. As your proficiency and your muscles increase, this may become even more important.

If you are a novice at weight training, seek the advice of a personal trainer. Whether you exercise at home or in a gym, a trainer can custom design a program for you based on your current condition and your goals. One consultation, or a consultation once every several months, may be all that you need. Several good generalized weight-training programs are also available on video cassettes or are described in books.

Today's weight-training programs generally are based on one or a mixture of five popular systems. The systems are the set system, the superset system, the peripheral heart action system, the circuit-training system, and the variable-split system.

The Set System

The set system is perhaps the single most popular weight-training system in use today. This is true among athletes, fitness exercisers, and bodybuilders alike. The set system derives its popularity from its simplicity. Many offshoot programs can be accommodated within the general confines of the set system, and often are.

The simplicity of the set system is hard to match. All you need to do is exercise for the appropriate number of reps and sets, resting for the appropriate amount of time in between the sets, and then move on to the next exercise. For example, to do squats using the set system, do one set of squats and rest for two to three minutes, do a second set of squats and rest for two to three minutes, do a third set of squats and rest for two to three minutes, then move on to the next exercise.

The only negative aspect of the set system is that it cannot be adapted to cardiovascular training, since so many rest periods are required. At the same time, however, the ample rest intervals make the set system the best system for improving strength.

The Superset System

The superset system of weight training is basically the same as the set system except that each superset is composed of two exercises rather than one. The two exercises are anatomically antagonistic (opposite) movements—for example, bench presses, which work the pectorals (pecs), and bent rows, which work the rhomboids. The two exercises are performed back to back, each for the required number of reps, with no rest period in between. A brief rest is taken in between the supersets. A full superset workout is shown in Table 14.1, below.

Antagonistic exercises are alternated in each superset for two reasons. First, doing so ensures that the blood supply is confined to a relatively small anatomical area. This facilitates speedy recovery, since one side can recover while the other side is being worked. Second, by exercising the muscles on both sides of a joint, normal flexibility can be maintained due to a balance being kept in the muscle tone.

The two exercises in each superset are done without resting to keep the heart rate at about 60 to 80 percent of maximum (about 150 beats per minute for younger individuals; lower for older individuals). This helps develop cardiovascular efficiency. The key is to perform the reps rhythmically, with a brief pause of one to two seconds in between each rep. This reduces the pressor response (rise in blood pressure) that is usually inherent in weight training and that tends to negate the cardiovascular benefits.

In between each superset, take a rest that is just long enough to allow the heart rate to fall back to a manageable level (approximately 100 to 120 beats per minute). Repeat each superset the required number of times, then move on to a superset of two new exercises. Make sure that each new pair of exercises is physically far removed from the previous pair. This prevents undue fatigue by ensuring that the same muscles are not used in back-to-back supersets.

The Peripheral Heart Action System

The peripheral heart action (PHA) system could be the single most efficient method for obtaining general fitness that is in popular use today. It was developed by Chuck Coker, inventor of the Universal weight-lifting machine.

In the PHA system, nearly all the components of fitness are served, depending on how the exercises and exercise sequences are arranged. A sample PHA workout is shown in Table 14.2 on page 179. Beginners would probably have difficulty finishing this sample workout because it is extremely rigorous. In fact, if you are new to weight training, you should not try any PHA workout until you have exercised for two to three months using the superset system, circuit-training system, or another system that is not quite as taxing.

To perform a PHA workout, complete the exercises in the first sequence in order and nonstop, doing each exercise for the required number of reps. Repeat the entire sequence two more times, then move on to the second sequence. Perform all of the second sequence three times, then move on to the third sequence. Perform all of the third sequence three times, then do the same with the fourth sequence. Go through the entire workout without resting. However, if your heart rate exceeds the required 140 to 160 beats per minute, slow down or rest briefly.

The principal goals of the PHA system are to increase cardiovascular efficiency, maintain flexibility, increase muscular strength and/or size, and provide a sound foundation for overall fitness. The key, again, is to perform the reps rhythmically, pausing just one to two seconds in between each one. This reduces the pressor response and prevents negation of the cardiovascular benefits.

Note again that each new exercise should work muscles that are far removed from the muscles worked by the previous exercise. At the same time, the exercises in each sequence should traverse the entire

Table 14.1. A Full Workout Utilizing the Superset System*

Superset	Exercises	Muscles Involved
1	Bench presses	Pectorals
	Bent rows	Rhomboids
2	Crunches	Abdominals
	Back raises	Erectors
3	Partial dumbbell presses	Deltoids
	Lat pulldowns	Latissimus dorsi
4	Side bends to the left	Right obliques
	Side bends to the right	Left obliques
5	Triceps extensions	Triceps
	Biceps curls	Biceps
6	Leg extensions	Quadriceps
	Leg curls	Hamstrings

* Repeat each superset twice, with a short rest in between each superset but not between the sets.

Table 14.2. A Full Workout Utilizing the Peripheral Heart Action System*

Sequence 1	Sequence 2	Sequence 3	Sequence 4
Partial dumbbell presses	Lat pulldowns	Bench presses	Bent rows
Crunches	Back raises	Side bends to the left	Side bends to the right
Squats	Leg curls	Leg extensions	Toe raises
Triceps extensions	Biceps curls	Dips	Shrugs

*Repeat each sequence three times without stopping to rest.

body, forcing blood to be shunted up and down the body. This allows the muscles to endure repeated maximal overload (maximum training intensity) by giving them long intervals between being "blitzed" during which they can recover.

The Circuit-Training System

Another excellent system for beginners aspiring to improve their cardiovascular efficiency as well as strength and muscle tone is the circuit-training system. Circuit training consists of a planned course, called a circuit, of different exercises or machines, called stations. The primary objective is to complete the circuit in progressively shorter periods of time. The exercises included in the circuit should help you to either prepare for your sport or eliminate your weaknesses. The more important exercises should be placed early in the circuit, with the less important ones coming later. When you achieve your target time, or as you find new weaknesses cropping up, you can adjust your circuit appropriately.

A circuit may be repeated as many times as desired during one training session. Either repeat each station several times, resting in between sets, or go through the circuit several times nonstop. As always, to reduce the pressor response, perform the reps rhythmically, pausing just one to two seconds in between each one. In addition, to prevent fatigue and to accomplish maximal overload, make sure that each new exercise works out a body area that is far removed from the one worked in the previous exercise.

The Variable-Split System

The variable-split system, also called the ABC system, is perhaps the most advanced weight-training system of all. At the same time, it is extremely versatile and can be used by raw beginners as well as elite bodybuilders and athletes. The variable-split system was developed by Dr. Hatfield, who based the system on the fact that every body part has its own unique recovery ability. One thing that is often overlooked is that you cannot *always* train hard. You have to balance periods of high-intensity training with periods of low-intensity training to give your muscles a chance to rest and recuperate.

Furthermore, not only does each body part require a different amount of rest, but each muscle does, too. In addition:

☐ Larger muscles take longer to recover than smaller ones.

☐ The fast-twitch muscle fibers take longer to recover than the slow-twitch muscle fibers.

☐ Shorter workouts are easier to recover from than longer workouts.

☐ Fast movements take longer to recover from than slow movements.

☐ High-intensity training takes longer to recover from than low-intensity training.

☐ Females take longer to recover than males.

☐ Older individuals take longer to recover than younger individuals.

☐ Lifting movements with negative or eccentric portions take longer to recover from than simple movements.

In the variable-split system, two or three workouts of different intensities are alternated according to a set schedule to give the different muscles and body parts a chance to adequately recover. Beginners can alternate between two workouts—an easy routine and a moderate routine—and more advanced athletes and bodybuilders can alternate between three workouts—an easy, a moderate, and a tough routine. The easy workouts are called A workouts, and the moderate workouts are called B workouts. The all-out, gut-busting, "killer" workouts are called C workouts.

A workouts are characterized by ample rest periods

in between the sets. Resting around two to three minutes is sufficient. Before beginning the workout, do a couple of warm-up sets with light weights (around 30 to 50 percent of your maximum weight). For the workout itself, do three to ten sets of 10 to 12 reps for a maximum effort. If you are an advanced exerciser, you will need to reduce the amount of weight you use so that you can complete the required number of sets. Just make sure that you perform each set with near-maximum effort. When feasible, do each rep with explosive movements. (It is not generally feasible to do calf or forearm exercises with explosive movements, since these muscle groups involve very short ranges of motion.)

A moderate-intensity A workout might consist of the following:

☐ 10 reps for 10 sets using weights around 60 percent of your maximum and explosive movements (10 reps/10 sets/60% max/explosive movements)

A specific routine would be:

☐ Bench presses, 10 reps/10 sets/60% max/explosive movements

B workouts are composed of two or three related exercises or a basic exercise with one or two variations. The primary exercise is done for just a few reps with heavy weights and explosive movements, while the other exercises are done for more reps with lighter weights and more rhythmic movements. As with the A workout, do a couple of warm-up sets of the primary exercise with light weights (around 30 to 50 percent of your maximum weight). For the workout itself, do three to four sets of 5 to 6 reps of the primary exercise using heavy weights (85 percent of your maximum) and explosive movements. For the second exercise, do three to four sets of 12 to 15 reps using moderate weights (70 to 75 percent of your maximum) and rhythmic movements. For the third exercise, do three to four sets of 40 reps using light weights (40 to 50 percent of your maximum) and slow, continuous movements. Take a sufficient rest period (about two to three minutes long) in between each set.

A moderate-intensity B workout might consist of the following:

☐ 5 reps/2–3 sets/85% max/explosive movements

☐ 12 reps/2–3 sets/70% max/rhythmic movements

☐ 40 reps/2–3 sets/40% max/slow, continuous movements

A specific routine would be:

☐ Bench presses, 5 reps/2 sets/85% max/explosive movements

☐ Dumbbell bench presses, 12 reps/2 sets/70% max/rhythmic movements

☐ Dumbbell flyes, 40 reps/2 sets/40% max/slow, continuous movements

C workouts are called *wholistic*. They are performed nonstop, with two or more related exercises combined into one giant set. No rest periods are allowed. Because of this, C workouts are maximum-intensity workouts. After warming up, do the routine wholistically, making smooth transitions between the different exercises, weights, and types of movements. Aim for a total of about 200 reps. If you wish, repeat the wholistic set once, but not more than once.

The high number of reps required in a C workout is achievable because the muscle fibers involved in the explosive movements are not the same ones that are involved in the slower movements. Therefore, while you are doing one exercise, the muscle fibers you used in the previous exercise have a chance to recover. Furthermore, because different muscle fibers are used, different energy systems are also utilized. However, if necessary, beginners can take a minimal rest (about three seconds) in between the sets. They can also reduce their weights by 5 to 10 pounds.

Note that it is not necessary to perform calf exercises wholistically. Instead, wear strength shoes daily to keep your calves sufficiently stressed for long periods of time. In addition, wholistic sets are not used in forearm training, since every time a weight is picked up, the forearm muscles are automatically used in the gripping movement.

A moderate-intensity C workout might consist of the following:

☐ 5 reps/85% max/explosive movements
☐ 12 reps/75% max/rhythmic movements
☐ 5 reps/85% max/explosive movements
☐ 12 reps/75% max/rhythmic movements
☐ 5 reps/85% max/explosive movements

☐ 40 reps/40% max/slow, continuous movements

☐ 5 reps/85% max/explosive movements

☐ 12 reps/75% max/rhythmic movements

☐ 5 reps/85% max/explosive movements

☐ 40 reps/40% max/slow, continuous movements

☐ 5 reps/85% max/explosive movements

A specific routine would be:

☐ Bench presses, 5 reps/85% max/explosive movements

☐ Dumbbell bench presses, 12 reps/75% max/rhythmic movements

☐ Bench presses, 5 reps/85% max/explosive movements

☐ Dumbbell bench presses, 12 reps/75% max/rhythmic movements

☐ Bench presses, 5 reps/85% max/explosive movements

☐ Dumbbell flyes, 40 reps/40% max/slow, continuous movements

☐ Bench presses, 5 reps/85% max/explosive movements

☐ Dumbbell bench presses, 12 reps/75% max/rhythmic movements

☐ Bench presses, 5 reps/85% max/explosive movements

☐ Dumbbell flyes, 40 reps/40% max/slow, continuous movements

☐ Bench presses, 5 reps/85% max/explosive movements

Bench presses, dumbbell bench presses, and dumbbell flyes are, of course, not the only exercises that can be used with Dr. Hatfield's ABC system. The following list offers a good sampling of equally adaptable exercises, grouped by the primary body parts that are worked:

☐ *Chest*—Bench presses (regular or inclined), dumbbell bench presses (regular or inclined), dumbbell flyes (regular or inclined), cable crossovers (for the upper or lower chest), and pec decks.

☐ *Shoulders*—Dumbbell raises (front, lateral, or inverted), seated dumbbell presses (to the middle of the head), upright rows (to the middle of the head), and shrugs (for the trapezius, using dumbbells or a barbell).

☐ *Lower back*—Back extensions (with hips stabilized, moving only the spine).

☐ *Upper back*—Bent rows (with the elbows held close to the sides or pointed outward), long cable pulls (with the elbows held close to the sides or pointed outward), one-arm dumbbell rows, and lat pulldowns.

☐ *Biceps*—Dumbbell curls (using a pronated or supinated grip), barbell curls (using a straight bar or EZ curl bar), scott curls (using dumbbells, a barbell, or an EZ curl bar), seated incline curls (using dumbbells), and cable curls.

☐ *Triceps*—Pushdowns (using a cable), French presses (using an overhead cable, dumbbells, or an EZ curl bar), and nose crushers (using a barbell or EZ curl bar).

☐ *Midsection*—Prestretched crunches, side bends to the left or right (using a dumbbell in one hand), torso twists (machine), and inverted crunches (inclined, bringing the knees to the forehead).

☐ *Upper legs*—Safety squats (for the quadriceps), leg extensions (for the quadriceps), partial stiff-legged deadlifts (prestretch the hamstrings by tilting the pelvis, then lower the bar to the knees), glute-ham raises (for the gluteals and hamstrings), standing leg curls (for the hamstrings), leg presses or hack squats (using any of a variety of machines), squats (any variations, such as erect torso squats, front and side lunges, power squats, Jefferson squats, sissy squats, overhead squats, and Smith machine squats).

☐ *Calves*—Standing calf raises, donkey raises, and seated calf raises.

☐ *Forearms*—Thor's hammer (pronated or supinated grip), spring or ball squeezing (for the grip), wrist curls (seated, with a bar hanging over the knees), and reverse wrist curls (seated, with a bar hanging over the knees).

While the aforementioned exercises are the main resistance exercises, many more are popularly used. Talk to your trainer or check magazine articles or books on weight training.

The beauty of the ABC system, as already explained, is that it works equally well for beginning, intermediate, and advanced weight trainers. If you are a beginning or intermediate exerciser, work out four days a week using A and B workouts only. As

Table 14.3. Sample Workout Schedule for Beginning and Intermediate Exercisers Utilizing the Variable-Split System

Day	Week 1							Week 2						
	1	2	3	4	5	6	7	8	9	10	11	12	13	14
Chest	—	B	—	—	—	A	—	—	B	—	—	—	A	—
Shoulders	—	—	—	A	—	—	B	—	—	—	A	—	—	B
Back	—	B	—	—	—	A	—	—	B	—	—	—	A	—
Biceps	—	—	—	A	—	—	B	—	—	—	A	—	—	B
Triceps	—	B	—	A	—	B	—	—	B	—	A	—	B	—
Midsection	—	—	—	A	—	—	B	—	—	—	A	—	—	B
Upper legs	—	B	—	A	—	B	—	—	B	—	A	—	B	—
Calves	—	—	—	A	—	B	—	—	B	—	A	—	—	B
Forearms	—	B	—	A	—	B	—	—	B	—	A	—	B	—

A = A workout; B = B workout; — = no workout.

you progress, slowly add C workouts to your schedule. Begin with two C workouts per body part per month. For a sample schedule for beginning and intermediate exercisers, see Table 14.3, above.

Effective muscle building is accomplished with proper nutrition and weight training. Only several hours of training per week will bring you visible results within one month's time. Gaining 30 or more pounds of muscle mass in one year is possible for most people. Just make sure that you are consistent in your efforts and follow the guidelines presented in this chapter. If you are interested in advanced bodybuilding, see *Hardcore Bodybuilding: A Scientific Approach,* by Frederick C. Hatfield, Ph.D (Chicago: Contemporary Books, 1993).

15. GUIDE TO EFFECTIVE CARBOHYDRATE LOADING

Several decades ago, it was discovered that when the body's glycogen stores are depleted, fatigue sets in and athletic performance is reduced. However, it was also discovered that when glycogen stores are depleted and then properly replenished, they hold more glycogen than they did originally. These findings have been used to devise several methods of packing more than the normal amounts of glycogen into athletes' muscles. This "glycogen packing" helps endurance athletes compete for longer periods of time without hitting the wall. Today, glycogen packing is called glycogen supercompensation or, more popularly, carbohydrate loading or carbo loading. Other types of athletes now also reap the benefits of carbo loading, and bodybuilders find that the practice gives their visible muscles a fuller, denser, more striated appearance for bodybuilding contests.

In this chapter, we will discuss carbohydrate loading. We will look at carbohydrates and energy and will present three effective carbo-loading methods. We will also look at supplements that help maximize the two phases of carbohydrate loading.

CARBOHYDRATES AND PERFORMANCE

During the 1960s, two Scandinavian researchers, Bergstrom and Hultman, experimented with the different influences that diet can have on glycogen stores and physical endurance. Using a normal mixed-nutrient diet, a carbohydrate-free diet, and a carbohydrate-rich diet, the researchers found that diet can affect exercise capacity in a number of interesting ways. Additionally, they experimented with intensive exercise performed in association with the different diets. What Bergstrom and Hultman discovered was that when their research subjects performed intensive exercise and followed it with a diet low in carbohydrates, exercise capacity was decreased. However, when the research subjects followed this period of glycogen depletion with several days of consuming a diet rich in carbohydrates, their exercise capacity was significantly increased. The researchers also deter-

mined that the latter routine produced a muscle glycogen content that was much higher than that attained when just following a normal mixed-nutrient diet.

The muscles use carbohydrates as their main source of energy during intensive exercise. When carbohydrates are consumed, they are broken down into their component parts, including glucose. The glucose that is not used for energy immediately is converted to glycogen and stored in the muscles and liver for future use. When an energy need arises, the glycogen is converted back to glucose and utilized.

The rate at which the body uses carbohydrates, or glucose, for energy depends upon several factors—level of fitness, whether the activity is aerobic or anaerobic, and diet. It also depends upon the intensity of the activity. At rest, the body burns a combination of carbohydrates and fatty acids. As the body becomes more active, however, carbohydrates become the more important source of fuel for the muscles. At very high training intensities, carbohydrates are the sole source of energy, fueling the powerful contractions of the fast-twitch muscle fibers.

Even though glycogen is the body's more important source of energy, the body's glycogen stores are much more limited than its fatty-acid stores. Because of this, you should always make sure that your glycogen stores are filled to capacity. Once your glycogen supply runs low, or runs out, your body turns to its fatty-acid supply as its sole source of energy and athletic performance is negatively affected. In addition, when its glycogen stores are depleted, the body uses more amino acids from muscle tissue for energy and to manufacture glucose. This increases muscle catabolism. Therefore, the more glycogen your body can store, the better it is for both your health and your performance.

In general, the athletes who benefit the most from carbohydrate loading are endurance athletes. These athletes include long-distance runners, mountaineers, triathletes, cross-country skiers, long-distance cyclists, rock climbers, long-distance swimmers, soccer players, and boxers participating in matches. Athletes competing in day-long tournaments also benefit from carbo loading, as well as from ingesting carbohydrate drinks during the tournament. In general, any athlete participating in an endurance event lasting more than one and a half to two hours benefits highly from carbohydrate loading, as do athletes who train for more than two hours at a stretch. Athletes who derive moderate benefits from carbo loading include football players, sprinters, basketball players, baseball players, downhill skiers, swimmers, rowers, track-and-field athletes, and runners participating in events lasting less than one hour.

In addition to the athletes who practice carbohydrate loading to enhance their performance, bodybuilders use carbo loading to pump up the appearance of their muscles for contests. This is because 3 ounces of water are stored in the muscles along with every 1 ounce of glycogen. Therefore, if bodybuilders can double the amount of glycogen stored in their muscles on the day of a bodybuilding contest, they can make their muscles appear larger and harder while keeping their body fat and subcutaneous water low.

Some athletes should not practice carbohydrate loading at all. Athletes who need to meet weight-class requirements find it difficult to use carbohydrate loading because of the high caloric intake and gain in water weight during the three days before competition. Other athletes find that the extra muscle glycogen and water make their muscles too heavy and stiff, hindering their performance instead of enhancing it. Any athlete considering carbohydrate loading before an important competition should first make a trial run during the off-season or preseason to see how his or her individual body will respond.

METHODS OF CARBOHYDRATE LOADING

The original method of carbohydrate loading was developed by Bergstrom and Hultman, the Scandinavian researchers, as a direct result of their study on the effects of diet on glycogen storage and physical endurance. This Scandinavian method, however, has a major drawback—the glycogen stores are drained to such an extremely low level for two to three days that training may become difficult. Since athletes commonly practice carbohydrate loading before important competitions, they could, ironically, end up hindering their performance.

During the 1980s, a study conducted by researchers Sherman and Costill showed that a modified nutrition-exercise regimen can produce results similar to those of the Scandinavian method but without the severe drawbacks. This newer study indicated that during the six days before competition, athletes should gradually taper down the intensity and duration of their exercise. During the first three of those six days, they should consume a normal mixed-nutrient diet, with about 55 to 60 percent of their total calories coming from carbohydrates. During the final three days, they should switch to a diet in which 70 percent of their total calories come from carbohydrates, with 20 percent coming from fat and 10 percent from protein. This combination of diets, the researchers found, produces a superhigh level of muscle glycogen, similar to the high level that is reached using the traditional carbohydrate-loading method.

We recommend three basic methods of carbohydrate loading that are modified versions of the methods just described. Picking the one that is most suitable for you is up to you and your coach. Combined with the proper training program, each of these modified methods can help you pack 40 to 60 percent more glycogen than normal into your muscle cells. This can provide you with insurance for an improved performance or, if you are a bodybuilder, for a better on-stage appearance.

Carbohydrate loading generally consists of two phases. The two phases are:

1. *Glycogen depletion.* During this phase, the body's glycogen stores are drained by manipulating the diet, moderately restricting caloric intake, and increasing training intensity. The degree to which the stores are drained varies with the method.
2. *Glycogen replenishment.* During this phase, the body's glycogen stores are refilled by reducing training intensity and increasing carbohydrate consumption.

All kinds of carbohydrates can help replenish the glycogen stores. However, before a training session, as well as during the day in general, carbohydrates with low glycemic indexes work the best because they release glucose into the bloodstream slowly, allowing the steady release of insulin that activates glycogen synthetase, the enzyme that is essential for glycogen storage. Carbohydrates with high glycemic indexes raise the blood-sugar level too rapidly, causing wild fluctuations in the insulin level and reducing the effectiveness of carbohydrate loading. During and directly after training, simple carbohydrates work the best. Simple carbohydrates are readily used for energy, thereby sparing muscle glycogen, when they are consumed during the training session; and they replenish glycogen faster, within one to one and a half hours, when they are consumed right after training.

Water consumption is also important during the glycogen-replenishment phase of carbohydrate loading. For each 1 ounce of glycogen that is stored in the muscle cells, about 3 ounces of water are also stored. Therefore, it is vital to keep your water consumption up. For bodybuilders, it is the glycogen-bound water that makes the visible muscles appear denser, fuller, and more striated. No matter what kind of athlete you are, make sure that you drink at least 8 ounces of water with each meal. For more specific hydration guidelines, see "Special Water Needs of the Athlete" on page 59.

Carbohydrate-Loading Method I

The first carbohydrate-loading method is the simplest of the three and does not require following stringent dietary do's and don'ts or completely depleting your glycogen stores. It takes just three days, skipping the glycogen-depletion phase and going directly into glycogen replenishment.

Three days before your competition, consume large amounts of carbohydrates with low glycemic indexes while reducing your intake of refined sugars. (For a list of some common foods and their glycemic indexes, see "The Glycemic Index" on page 29.) Consume simple carbohydrates only during and directly after your training sessions and low-glycemic-index carbohydrates throughout the rest of the day. Keep your macronutrient ratio at each of your five to six daily meals at 15-percent fats, 15-percent protein, and 70-percent carbohydrates. In addition, maintain a reduced training intensity during all three days, with the lowest intensity on the third day. Throughout the three days, take your dietary supplements as directed.

Carbohydrate-Loading Method II

The second carbohydrate-loading method is a little more exacting than the first method but not as rigorous as the third. It takes one week, with the glycogen-depletion phase lasting four days.

One week before your competition, begin depleting your glycogen stores. Do this by training to exhaustion every day and keeping your macronutrient ratio at each of your five to six daily meals at 15-percent fats, 30-percent protein, and 55-percent carbohydrates. Continue this phase for four days.

Three days before your competition, begin replenishing your glycogen stores. Load up on carbohydrates with a glycemic index of up to 49 percent and consume beverages containing simple carbohydrates only during and directly after exercise. In addition, alter your macronutrient ratio to 15-percent fats, 15-percent protein, and 70-percent carbohydrates.

Through all seven days, take your dietary supplements as directed.

Carbohydrate-Loading Method III

The third carbohydrate-loading method is the most rigorous of the three. It takes six days, with the glycogen-depletion phase lasting three days.

Six days before your competition, begin depleting your glycogen stores. Do this by maintaining a very high training intensity and keeping the macronutrient ratio of each of your five to six daily meals at 20-percent fats, 60-percent protein, and 20-percent carbohydrates. With this low carbohydrate intake, you may feel fatigued and weak and might lose potassium and muscle tissue. To avoid these negative effects, make sure that you consume your full quota of calories; do *not* allow yourself to starve! Continue this phase for three days.

Three days before your competition, begin replenishing your glycogen stores. Alter your macronutrient ratio to 15-percent fats, 15-percent protein, and 70-percent carbohydrates and load up on low-glycemic-index carbohydrates. In addition, during the first two days of this second phase, keep your workouts very low in intensity and only thirty minutes in duration. Rest a lot, and do not work out at all on the last day before competition.

Through all six days, take your dietary supplements as directed.

SUPPLEMENTS THAT MAXIMIZE CARBOHYDRATE LOADING

Several dietary supplements have been shown to help maximize glycogen depletion or replenishment when taken in extra amounts. Take these extra supplements or amounts in addition to your regular daily supplements or dosages.

To maximize glycogen depletion, take extra amounts of vitamins B_3 and B_6 two days before beginning the glycogen-depletion phase, then again on the first day of the phase. The recommended extra daily dosage for each supplement is 2 milligrams for every 1 pound of lean body mass. (For directions on how to determine your lean body mass, see "Body Composition" on page 143.) In addition, add a protein supplement to your diet. Protein and vitamins B_3 and B_6 all help increase the rate of glycogen depletion.

To maximize glycogen replenishment, take 2 extra micrograms of chromium for every 1 pound of lean body mass with each of your five to six daily meals. Double your regular vitamin-C and beta-carotene dosages and take a carbohydrate supplement that is fat- and protein-free and consists mainly of glucose polymers and maltodextrin. In addition, take 1,000 to 3,000 milligrams of L-glutamine per day. When you first wake up in the morning and just before you go to bed at night, drink a complex-carbohydrate beverage that has about 400 to 600 calories per serving. In addition, add a fructose beverage to your diet to make sure that your liver glycogen stores are also replenished. Even though fructose has a low glycemic index, however, be careful not to "overdose." Fructose does not help replenish muscle glycogen stores and any excess is converted to fat in the liver.

Carbohydrate loading, the same as other ergogenic aids, has its place in the athlete's repertoire. Practiced appropriately, it can enhance performance or appearance. Overused, it can become ineffective or even detrimental to performance. Scientists recommend that competitive athletes practice carbohydrate-loading methods that stimulate complete glycogen depletion no more than three times a year. Under normal off-season or preseason training conditions, following the nutrition guidelines in your sport-specific plan in Part Four will help your body store sufficient glycogen to get you through even the most grueling training sessions.

16. PUTTING IT ALL TOGETHER

Whether your goal is to win the Olympics or just improve your level of fitness for health reasons, you need to address several factors in your personal performance-improvement program in order to succeed. Primary among those factors are nutritional practices, dietary supplements, warming up and cooling down, strength training, skill training, flexibility training, psychological techniques, medical support, and therapeutic modalities. In this chapter, we will round out our discussions of nutritional practices and dietary supplements, which have been the focus of this book, and we will review those factors that we have not yet examined.

NUTRITIONAL PRACTICES

As this book has stressed from its very first pages, athletes do not eat just to stay alive and healthy; they also eat to excel at their sports. Athletes' diets are designed to assist in the achievement of specific sport and training goals. There are also several special nutritional techniques that help in areas such as endurance and force output, the improvement of which further enhances training and competition efforts.

To put together the nutritional component of your personal performance-improvement program, simply follow the dietary guidelines presented in your sport-specific plan in Part Four. If you wish to lose fat, build muscle, or carbohydrate load to improve performance, see the appropriate chapter in Part Three. Use the Daily Nutrition Log presented in Appendix D to keep track of what you eat. Keeping a record of everything you consume lets you stay on top of your caloric and macronutrient intakes, plus helps when you try to fine-tune your diet. Finally, if possible, consult a nutritionist qualified in sports nutrition for help in adjusting your nutrition program to meet your individual needs. The best kind of nutritionist for an athlete is a certified specialist in performance nutrition. To locate such a nutritionist, or to find out about becoming one yourself, contact the International Sports Sciences Association at (800) 650–4772.

DIETARY SUPPLEMENTS

Many sports scientists and nutritionists believe that "three square meals" a day is ample fare for athletes in heavy training. Other experts dispute this, however, contending instead that the foods athletes consume on a daily basis do not provide them with all the nutrients they need to achieve their performance goals. We agree with the latter viewpoint for four important reasons:

1. Many state-of-the-art dietary supplements have been designed to take the body beyond normal biochemical functioning.

2. No person alive is able to consistently eat "three square meals" a day.

3. A myriad of research reports clearly show that deficiencies *do* exist in athletes' diets for many well-documented reasons.

4. Numerous studies have also shown that many supplements improve health and performance by supplying certain nutrients in amounts that are not attainable from the diet alone.

Athletes use dietary supplements for a number of purposes that go beyond mere survival or gustatory indulgence. Among them are the following:

- ☐ To improve general health and fitness
- ☐ To build muscle mass
- ☐ To lose fat
- ☐ To improve anaerobic energy
- ☐ To improve aerobic energy
- ☐ To reduce pain and inflammation
- ☐ To improve tissue repair
- ☐ To improve recovery
- ☐ To improve mental focus and arousal
- ☐ To improve strength

Each of these purposes is, in fact, included among most athletes' training goals at some point in their careers. It therefore is logical to conclude that athletes train, eat, and use supplements to enhance their planned progression toward their training and competition goals. Indeed, eating a proper diet and taking supplements are seen as part and parcel of a scientifically planned training program. A training program that did not include them would be considered woefully inadequate.

If any of the above purposes are among your training goals, see Table 16.1, below, for a list of recommended supplements. Each of the supplements on the list enjoys at least some support in the research literature. The list is not exhaustive, however, plus some of the supplements that are included on it can be found in more than one category.

In addition to taking supplements for general training goals, you should also take supplements to help meet your sport-specific goals. For a list of these recommended supplements, see your sport-specific plan in Part Four. For detailed information on any of the nutrients listed in Table 16.1 or in Part Four, as well as for dosage recommendations and cautions, see the appropriate chapter in Part One.

Table 16.1. Supplements Recommended for Basic Training Goals

Training Goal:

To improve general health and fitness

Recommended Supplements:

- Multi-vitamin-and-mineral supplement
- Antioxidants (beta-carotene, vitamins C and E, selenium, L-glutathione)
- Immune-system boosters (astragalus, echinacea)
- Individual amino acids (selected according to specific personal health goals)
- Herbal antioxidants (ginkgo, green tea, milk thistle)
- Cardiovascular tonics (black cohosh, cayenne, garlic, ginger, goldenseal, onion, skullcap)
- Adaptogens (Siberian ginseng)
- Essential fatty acids (alpha-linolenic acid, linoleic acid)
- Glucose tolerance factor (chromium)
- Acidophilus, bifidus

Training Goal:

To build muscle mass

Recommended Supplements:

- Low-fat protein drink with egg or whey
- Ornithine alphaketoglutarate
- Branched-chain amino acids
- Glucosamine
- Ferulic acid
- Insulin-like growth factors (from colostrum)
- L-glutamine
- Creatine monohydrate
- Glucose tolerance factor (chromium)
- Inosine
- Growth-hormone stimulators (glycine, L-arginine, L-ornithine)
- Beta-hydroxy beta-methylbutyrate

Training Goal:

To lose fat

Recommended Supplements:

- Meal-replacement drink with balanced content of micro- and macronutrients from high-grade sources
- High-quality, low-fat protein drinks and bars
- Thermogenic aids (ephedra*, guarana*)
- Glucose tolerance factor (chromium)
- Herbal supplements (barberry, brindall berry, wall germander)
- L-carnitine
- Fiber
- Lipotropic supplements (choline, inositol, L-methionine)

Training Goal:

To improve anaerobic energy

Recommended Supplements:

- Energy drink with short- and medium-chain glucose polymers
- Creatine monohydrate
- Blood buffer (sodium bicarbonate)
- Inosine
- Ferulic acid
- Vitamin B_3

Training Goal:

To improve aerobic energy

Recommended Supplements:

- Energy drink with long-chain glucose polymers
- Coenzyme Q_{10}
- Octacosanol
- Ginseng
- L-carnitine

Training Goal:

To reduce pain and inflammation

Recommended Supplements:

- White willow
- Turmeric
- Aloe
- DL-phenylalanine
- Bioflavonoids
- Antioxidants (beta-carotene, vitamins C and E, selenium, L-glutathione)
- Glucosamine
- Gamma linolenic acid

Training Goal:

To improve tissue repair

Recommended Supplements:

- Protein supplements
- Antioxidants (beta-carotene, vitamins C and E, selenium, L-glutathione)
- Ornithine alphaketoglutarate
- Glucosamine
- Turmeric
- Bioflavonoids
- Essential fatty acids (alpha-linolenic acid, linoleic acid)

Training Goal:

To improve recovery

Recommended Supplements:

- Branched-chain amino acids
- Immune-system boosters (astragalus, echinacea)
- L-glutamine
- Glucosamine
- Adaptogens (Siberian ginseng)
- Antioxidants (beta-carotene, vitamins C and E, selenium, L-glutathione)

Training Goal:

To improve mental focus and arousal

Recommended Supplements:

- Caffeine* (coffee*, guarana*, yerba maté*)
- Ephedra*
- Kava kava
- Branched-chain amino acids

Training Goal:

To improve strength

Recommended Supplements:

- Protein drink with egg or whey
- Ornithine alphaketoglutarate
- Branched-chain amino acids
- Insulin-like growth factors (from colostrum)
- L-glutamine
- Creatine monohydrate
- Glucose tolerance factor (chromium)
- Inosine
- Siberian ginseng
- Chinese ginseng

*This supplement is or contains a substance that has been banned by most sports governing bodies, including the International Olympic Committee.

WARMING UP AND COOLING DOWN

If you are like most people, you were first taught about the importance of warming up way back in gym class in grammar school. The older you get and the more you advance in your athletic career, the more important warming up before exercise becomes. Warming up generally consists of doing some calisthenics and stretching, followed by performing your sport event or fitness activity a few times at a slow pace. If you are strength training or taking an aerobics class, start out slowly, picking up your pace after your muscles feel ready. The main purposes of warming up are to raise the body temperature and to limber up the muscles and connective tissues. The recommended warm-up period is fifteen to thirty minutes.

Most trainers also recommend cooling down after exercising. Cooling down consists simply of reducing the intensity of your physical activity gradually, as opposed to just stopping it. The purpose is to ease your breathing and heart rate back to their resting levels. This generally takes only a few minutes and, the same as for warming up, is well worth the time.

STRENGTH TRAINING

Strength, simply defined, is applied force. When you lift a barbell, throw a ball, or even run, you are applying force, or using strength. Different actions use different kinds of strength. For example, some actions use aerobic strength, while others use anaerobic strength.

When most of us think of strength, we think of anaerobic strength—maximum or near-maximum force output that does not require the utilization of oxygen. But, on the energy continuum, this is just one type of strength. The muscles also exert force during aerobic activities. Aerobic-strength training focuses on performing more muscle contractions with less force output. Furthermore, there are linear and nonlinear forms of strength. Linear-strength movements are movements that are performed repetitively without interruption, such as running strides. Nonlinear-strength movements come in bursts, such as the explosive plays of football and the jumping, starting, and dodging movements of basketball and soccer.

Also a component of strength is power. The textbook definition of power is "force times distance divided by time," or "strength plus speed." Sprinters require massive amounts of speed-strength, which demands huge amounts of power output per contraction. Even long-distance runners, whose primary goal is the maintenance of speed, require some strength, which demands at least a modicum of power output per muscle contraction. Any muscle that contracts and relaxes exhibits strength, and every muscle contraction displays some combination of strength, power, speed, and endurance.

To condition the muscles to exert optimum strength and thereby enhance performance, a number of strength-training devices have been developed and are available in gyms or for home use. Best known are free weights. Also popular are the variety of systems that apply resistance to the muscles, such as hydraulic devices, pressurized-air devices, elastic devices, springs, and the host of machines that apply heavy external resistance. All of these devices can be grouped into four major categories of strength-training technologies:

1. *Constant-resistance devices.* These are resistance-training devices in which the amount of weight (resistance) remains the same. Examples are dumbbells, barbells, and some pulley systems.

2. *Variable-resistance devices.* These are resistance-training devices in which the amount of weight (resistance) is increased or decreased during the exercise movement. Examples are the Nautilus and Cybex exercise machines.

3. *Accommodating-resistance devices.* These are variable-resistance devices that have been modified to allow maximum force to be exerted during the range of motion of the exercise movement but keep the speed of motion fixed. Examples are the Com II and Com III exercise machines.

4. *Static-resistance devices.* These are resistance-training devices that are immovable or fixed and designed to be pushed or pulled. They cause the muscles to contract without using motion. They can be used to focus strength development at a particular point in the range of motion. Examples are any of the exercise machines that can be locked into one position.

Another form of strength training includes any exercise in which the body alone is the source of resistance—for example, running, swimming, calisthenics, and aerobic dance. These exercises are called light resistance training. Another category of strength training utilizes machines that apply light external resistance, such as the stationary cycle, rowing machine, and stair-climbing machine.

With all these different training technologies and devices available, it is vital that you follow a program that is appropriate for the strength requirements of your specific sport. Following an incorrect strength-training program can actually hurt your performance. For example, if you are a middle-distance or endurance athlete or fitness exerciser, you should not just go into a gym and start lifting weights like a bodybuilder or power lifter. You will gain strength and, in the beginning, perhaps see some improvement in your performance, but as you continue to develop anaerobic strength, your overall performance will begin to suffer. This does not mean that you should not lift weights at all. Rather, you should train in a way that is appropriate for your sport-specific energetic goals. For example, if you are a basketball player, your goal is to develop a balance of strength and endurance. You would benefit most from lifting moderate weights for a moderate number of repetitions. Lifting heavy weights for a few repetitions would go against your energetic goals and could lead to injury. If you are a mid-distance runner, your primary goal is to develop endurance. Your best results would come from lifting light weights for a high number of repetitions. You should also do some higher-intensity strength training to increase your jumping height but not at the expense of your other running-performance requirements. As a general rule of thumb, sports that require short bursts of power rely mostly on the fast-twitch muscle fibers for energy. Training, therefore, should be high in intensity and short in duration, resulting in a massive physique with big, well-developed muscles that are able to generate tremendous strength, power, and speed. Sports that require endurance rely mostly on the slow-twitch muscle fibers for energy. Training should be longer in duration and lower in intensity, resulting in a slim, light physique with muscles that generate less power per contraction but that can contract effectively for longer periods of time.

As you examine your sport-specific plan in Part Four, these strength and endurance concepts will become more clear to you. The main thing to remember at this point is that every muscle contraction, whether predominately from the slow-twitch or fast-twitch muscle fibers, displays strength, power, speed, and endurance, and your nutrition and training program needs to be structured to maximize the unique energetics of your particular sport. Consult an expert to help you determine which forms of strength training will benefit you the most. Note also that if you wish to participate in more than one sport, you should choose sports that have the same basic energetic profiles.

SKILL TRAINING

To hone your skills, find the best coach that you can. Performing your skills perfectly will almost always help you apply greater force, whether to an object, an opponent, or the ground. Good skills execution involves the efficient activation or inhibition of the appropriate muscles. The muscles must also be activated or inhibited in the proper sequence, which involves accurately judging such factors as position, direction, timing, rate, speed, and effect of force application.

If your goal is to become an elite athlete, you must skill train all year long. A quite sophisticated training concept used by professional and world-class athletes

is periodization. With periodization, the year is divided into phases called macrocycles, with specific training goals set for each period of training. Four macrocycles are usually used, with each one lasting one to four months. Often, the macrocycles are further divided into mesocycles, which are several weeks long, and microcycles, which are several days long. Your specific sport, your skills, and your goals will determine how your year should be divided.

In general, a periodized training program includes the following:

☐ *Macrocycle I.* Developmental phase, four months long. The training focus of this macrocycle should be on developing skills, defining physical-performance parameters, adjusting body composition, and improving weaknesses as well as strengths. The training intensity should be moderate.

☐ *Macrocycle II.* Preparation phase, three months long. This macrocycle immediately preceeds the competitive season. The training focus should be on making final adjustments to body composition (preferably early in the macrocycle) and honing skills. The training intensity should go from moderate to high over the course of the macrocycle.

☐ *Macrocycle III.* Competition phase, four months long. This is the macrocycle during which all the attention to training and good nutrition pays off. The training focus should be on improving skills and physical-performance factors that were found to be lacking after the first few competitions. The training intensity should remain very high throughout the macrocycle.

☐ *Macrocycle IV.* Recovery phase, one month long. The goal of this macrocycle is to maintain fitness and flexibility. The training focus should be on healing injuries using professionally supervised therapeutic and nutrition programs. The training intensity should be low. During this macrocycle, plans for the following year's macrocycle I should be made with input from the coach, trainer, and team physician.

If your season runs longer or shorter than the typical four months used in this example, adjust your schedule by modifying macrocycles I and IV. Do not change macrocycle II, which should always be three months long for the best results.

A year-round training program will help you make steady progress toward your ultimate performance goals. The top athletes in the world train year-round to be their best. If being the best is your goal, find a good coach to help you construct a periodized training program appropriate for your sport, skills, and goals.

FLEXIBILITY TRAINING

The first rule of flexibility is not to overstretch. When joints are stretched beyond their normal range of motion, they may become too loose and may actually become prone to injury. Do not compare your flexibility to anyone else's. Everyone is different, and trying to be as flexibile as someone else can lead to overstretching.

If a particular joint or muscle group is inflexible, it may indicate that injury has occurred or adhesions have formed. Proper medical attention may therefore be necessary. Inflexibility of a particular joint or muscle group may also be the result of a muscle imbalance, which usually takes years to develop. Medical attention plus strength training may be required, and it can take months or even years to correct the problem.

Achieving and maintaining good flexibility is best accomplished by following the entire program outlined in this chapter. Simply stretching as part of your warm-up before exercising may not be enough. A proper diet, strength training, skill training, and therapeutic modalities are all necessary factors.

Some sports and fitness activities require more flexibility training than others. Martial arts and ballet, for example, require a daily program of stretching. Powerlifting, discus throwing, and marathon running require less. Work closely with your coach or trainer to design a flexibility-training program appropriate for your sport.

PSYCHOLOGICAL TECHNIQUES

Self-hypnosis, mental imagery, meditation, visualization, and a number of other "mind strategies" can help you improve your strength and performance in competition and training. They can help you develop a mental edge and a winning mind-set.

Until recently, the powers of the human mind were generally overlooked by our society. Other cultures place limitations on individuals and restrict their mental potential. The human mind has the capacity to store trillions of bits of information, more than the most powerful computers. In fact, according to one progressive educational authority, the human brain has a greater storage capacity than the U.S. National Archives. Sadly, however, most people utilize only a small percentage of their mind's capacity.

When you start to understand what you can do with your mind, you can begin to open your mind to new thoughts and information and expand its utilization. Your mind is more than just a storehouse for knowledge. Your mind also regulates your emotions, your ego, your physical abilities, and your overall vim and vigor. Medical research has determined that the mind even has the ability to heal the body.

For athletes, the mind is a powerful piece of sports equipment. Knowing how to maximize and control your internal forces can offer you a big advantage in sports and life. Most athletes practice some kind of mental technique, even if it is just "psyching themselves up" before a competition. Among the more popular techniques practiced by athletes are meditation, visualization, anchoring, and future pacing.

Meditation

Meditation has been practiced since the beginning of recorded history. However, while the Asian societies and primitive cultures of the world have held onto the practice of meditation as a way of life and health, Western society parted ways with meditation many years ago. Luckily, Westerners are now once again beginning to realize the importance of meditation. In its most fundamental sense, meditation is a technique in which you elevate your state of mind above the conscious to the unconscious. In other words, you clear your mind of all conscious thoughts and enter an altered state of consciousness, a state of relaxation and mental imagery.

Many practitioners look at the anatomical divisions of the brain and ascribe the power to meditate to the right hemisphere. In the contemporary model of the brain, the mind's logical functions (such as speaking, writing, calculating, and worrying) take place in the left hemisphere, while the more creative, visually orientated operations take place in the right hemisphere. Although this simple model of the human brain is constantly being updated and revised, of practical interest to us here is that even modern science recognizes the function and power of the creative right hemisphere. To put it in more practical terms, most people tend to function from the left hemisphere, always preoccupied with jealousy, insecurity, anger, and other negative thoughts that adversely affect their overall state of health and well-being. By meditating, you can open up and develop your powerful creative mind and use techniques such as visualization to help improve your athletic performance and health.

If you are interested in trying meditation, seek the guidance of a trained professional. In addition, read through the following guidelines:

☐ Plan to meditate at a time of day when you can relax and when you are not under the influence of a stimulant such as alcohol, a medication, or a recent meal.

☐ Find a quiet place away from distractions. Turn off the phone and create a comfortable, relaxing environment.

☐ Turn down the lights and sit in a comfortable position. If you wish, meditate in the dark while lying down.

☐ To meditate, first clear your thoughts. If you have trouble, try repeating the same word to yourself or focusing, with your eyes closed, on a bright object that you picture in your mind. Even beginners will find themselves slipping in and out of the meditative state. Your goal is the state between consciousness and unconsciousness, the point where the conscious and unconscious meet.

☐ Work up to meditation sessions lasting thirty to sixty minutes.

Whatever the exact physiological condition is that your body enters into during meditation, one thing is certain—when you are done meditating, you will feel relaxed, refreshed, and renewed. And each time you meditate, the benefits will accrue. You will eventually find your general state of mind to be more controlled and less stressful. Meditation, therefore, is an important stepping stone in the path to total empowerment. When you learn to control your thoughts and emotions, you will be on your way to mastering your sport and defeating your opponents. You will be on your way to success in life.

Visualization

Visualization is the technique of using mental imagery to picture yourself accomplishing a stated purpose. It is almost like daydreaming, but more intense. You can practice it as part of your meditation or you can use it to help reach the meditative state.

Before you begin a visualization session, you must state your purpose. For example, your purpose may be to master a certain move or to prepare yourself mentally for a competition. Once you have stated your purpose, you must set your stage—that is, you must establish your setting and point of view before you bring on the "players." Then, begin the visualization, running a picture of yourself accomplishing your purpose over and over again in your mind. Visualize everything—all the sights, sounds, smells, and feelings. If you are preparing for a contest, visualize the specific moves you will use to defeat your opponent. Visualize everything you anticipate happening.

Visualization can be a powerful tool. Practice it on a weekly basis, for about thirty to sixty minutes per session. Increase your sessions to once a day during the week before a tournament.

Anchoring and Future Pacing

Anchoring and future pacing are mental techniques related to meditation and visualization. Most people have experienced the sensation of having a memory triggered by a sight, sound, smell, or other stimulus. Perhaps a song on the radio makes you remember when you were a child playing with your best friend, or a sunset brings back memories of a romantic moment. Anchoring is a method in which you deliberately associate a stimulus with a particular experience. Your anchor can be a single stimulus, such as an internal verbalization, visualization, feeling, or smell, or it can be a combination of stimuli.

For an athlete, anchoring can be especially useful for tournaments and away games. When you practice in your regular environment, you can make a mental note of what it feels like to perform your moves in your home surroundings. If you win a competition, you can lock into your memory the song that is playing as you accept your trophy. Then, when you are in an unfamiliar environment, you can use your anchor to recreate these feelings, helping yourself to feel at home and reducing the intimidation of being in a strange place. You can recall the sights, smells, and sounds of being where you feel most comfortable and perform at your best.

If you are competing in a foreign environment, get to the location as early as possible. Find a quiet corner, meditate for a while, and visualize defeating your opponent. Then work out for a while, calling up your anchor to help make yourself feel as comfortable as possible. As you become comfortable with using anchoring as a technique, you will develop a routine that works best for you.

Future pacing is the same as anchoring but focuses on future events, such as defeating an upcoming opponent. To future pace, visualize your anticipated performance and relate it to an anchoring stimulus. When the competition finally begins, use the anchor to stimulate yourself to play as well as you visualized. The goal is to do in reality what you picture yourself doing in your mind.

MEDICAL SUPPORT

Medical support is a very important performance factor. Follow-up visits, chiropractic adjustments, and prescription medications are sometimes indicated for athletes in heavy training who have come down with a medical problem. Only qualified sports-medicine specialists are allowed to prescribe such support. Do not hesitate to seek a second opinion if you are not satisfied with a diagnosis or course of treatment prescribed by one doctor. If you have a serious injury, seek the advice of a sports doctor who specializes in your particular injury. Sports medicine is a highly diversified and complex field.

Preventive medicine is also an important factor. More and more research supports the practice of visiting your doctor on a regular basis to keep track of your state of health. In addition, you should also regularly visit a chiropractor and masseuse as part of your preventive program. Keep good records of everything you do.

THERAPEUTIC MODALITIES

Whirlpools, electrical muscle stimulation, massage, ultrasound, intense light, and a host of other therapeutic modalities can have a very positive effect on your training efforts, both directly (the degree of your force output) and indirectly (how quickly you recover from your workout). In other words, pamper yourself. Use these therapeutic modalities to your advantage. When you are hurt, tend to your injury immediately. Utilize all the medical and therapeutic help that you can. There is nothing macho about letting your injuries go unattended. It is much smarter to deal with an injury when it occurs than to suffer with the consequences when it heals incorrectly. Better yet, make your preferred therapeutic modalities a part of your preventive program. Taking time during training for injury prevention may seem bothersome, but it will pay off in the long term.

"If I knew then what I know now."

This is the credo of all athletes. No matter who you are, you can never expect to be the best without 100-percent dedication. Heavy training alone is not always the answer. In fact, training smart is the only way to excel in today's athletic environment. Make every second of your day count. This means seeking the advice of the best coaches and trainers. Go to sport camps whenever you can. In the off-season, join a local sport club to maintain your physical conditioning. Read every book you can on your sport, as well as biographies of champion athletes. If you approach your athletic career with realistic expectations and follow a scientific approach, you will soon be on the road to achieving sports excellence.

PART FOUR

THE
PLANS

AN INTRODUCTION TO THE SPORT-SPECIFIC PLANS

Part Four is the heart and soul of *Dynamic Nutrition for Maximum Performance*. It is the reason for the book's existence. Part Four concisely summarizes all the information in Parts One, Two, and Three, and presents what is pertinent for you in particular. For example, if you are a football player, you can turn to the football plan and learn which of all the nutrients discussed in Part One you should take to help improve your physical fitness in general, your performance on the football field in particular. Furthermore, this sport-specific plan will tell you how much of each recommended nutrient to take and how to structure your diet to meet your particular energy requirements as a football player. If you are a bowler, or a dancer, or a tennis player, you can find this same information in a plan tailored just for you.

Altogether, over a hundred sports and fitness activities, as well as a number of popular recreational activities, are covered in twenty-eight plans in Part Four. We focus on twenty-eight nutrition plans because many sports and fitness activities place similar energy demands on the body and therefore call for basically identical diet and supplement programs. To determine the plan that you should follow, see the "Guide to Locating Your Sport-Specific Plan" on page 198. This guide lists the individual sport and fitness activities covered by the plans and indicates which specific plan provides all the information you need as a player or participant. Note that a number of sports and activities are covered in more than one plan. Use the plan that seems the most appropriate for you. For example, if you look up cycling, you will be directed to the cycling, fitness activities, and triathlon plans. If you are a competitive professional or amateur cyclist, turn to the cycling plan. If you cycle on weekends for fitness or fun, turn to the fitness activities plan. If you cycle as a triathlete, turn to the triathlon plan.

In addition to taking into account the demands of your particular sport or activity, a good performance-nutrition program also factors in your body composition and lifestyle, plus the energy demands of your general-fitness workouts and sport-specific training.

The twenty-eight nutrition plans presented in the following pages do exactly that. Furthermore, the plans are structured for ease of use and for implementation after just several minutes of reading.

Each sport-specific plan presented in Part Four includes the following information:

☐ *Introduction.* Each plan begins with a brief overview of the sport or activity and preliminary information on its dynamics and energy demands.

☐ *Energy sources.* This section begins with a review of the three major systems that the muscles rely on for their energy supply. (For a complete discussion of the immediate, glycolytic, and oxidative energy systems, see "Energy Metabolism" on page 158.) A table, "Where Your Energy Comes From," lists the major skills or events of the sport or activity, or an average workout and/or competition, and shows how much the body relies on each of the energy systems for every item listed. Percentages are often also given for similar sports or activities. Following the energy profile of the sport or activity is a list of factors that you should remember when considering the type of nutritional support to give your training program. The section ends with a statement concerning the aims of the nutrition program.

☐ *Dietary guidelines.* This section is highlighted by an easy-to-read pie chart that details what percentages of your diet should be composed of fat, of protein, and of carbohydrates. The ratio presented in the pie chart flows out of the energy profile presented in the previous section. Some of the sport-specific plans have one pie chart for the entire year, since the macronutrient ratio should remain the same in the season, pre-season, and off-season. Other plans have two or even three pie charts, since the macronutrient ratio should change with the seasons. The section ends with a list of guidelines to help you translate the pie chart into an appropriate daily diet.

☐ *Supplementation guidelines.* This section features two tables designed to guide you in designing an appro-

197

priate supplementation program. The first table, "Recommended Nutrients and Ranges of Intake," lists the nutrients recommended for participants of the particular sport or activity, as well as an intake guideline for each nutrient. The nutrients include vitamins, minerals, amino acids, fatty acids, and metabolites. The second table, "Recommended Sports Supplements and Nutritional Practices," lists the different types of sports supplements available and indicates if they should in the season, preseason, or directly before a competition. The table also addresses the popular nutritional practices of bicarbonate loading, carbohydrate loading, creatine and/or inosine loading, and water loading. *All the recommendations are for individuals who are actively training or exercising.*

The dietary and supplemention guidelines given in each plan in Part Four are intended for healthy adults and teenagers who have completed puberty. However, no matter what condition you are in, if you have any questions about the appropriateness of a suggested supplement or dietary guideline, contact your health-care practitioner. As a cautionary note, you should always consult your physician before starting a new nutrition or training program.

Today, nutrition for maximum performance is truly dynamic. Scientists continue to isolate new, safe, and effective nutrients; researchers continue to discover new functions of and uses for known nutrients; and nutritionists continue to fine-tune dosage recommendations. We have attempted to present the latest information in this book. However, as new findings are released, do not hesitate to incorporate them, if appropriate, into your personal performance-nutrition program. A personal nutrition program should never be static. Your goal is maximum performance. If you continue to climb toward your goal, you will know that you are on the right nutritional track. If you stop short of your goal or begin to backslide, you need to make adjustments based upon your specific needs. Listen to your body. Only you, and the professionals who guide you, can evaluate your growth and progress.

Guide to Locating Your Sport-Specific Plan

Part Four of this book was written with over a hundred sports and fitness activities, plus a number of popular recreational activities, in mind. However, since many sports and fitness activities place similar energy demands on the body and therefore call for basically identical diet and supplement programs, we have chosen to focus on twenty-eight nutrition plans. The following guide will help you find the plan that you should follow. It lists the individual sports and fitness activities covered by the plans and indicates which specific plan provides all the information you need as a player or participant. If more than one plan is listed for your activity, use the one that seems the most appropriate for you. Note that the fitness activities plan is intended primarily for individuals who enjoy the activities discussed in that section for fitness or fun, while the other plans are geared more towards competitive professionals and amateurs.

Sport or Activity	Sport-Specific Plan to Follow	Sport or Activity	Sport-Specific Plan to Follow
Acrobatics	*See* Gymnastics	Ball throwing	*See* Baseball; Track and field
Aerobics	*See* Fitness activities	Ballet	*See* Dancing
Alpine skiing	*See* Skiing	Ballooning	*See* Fitness activities
Amateur boxing	*See* Boxing	Ballroom dancing	*See* Dancing
Archery	*See* Fitness activities	Baseball	*See* Baseball
Arm wrestling	*See* Fitness activities	Basketball	*See* Basketball
Australian football	*See* Football	Baton twirling	*See* Fitness activities
Badminton	*See* Racket sports	Beach volleyball	*See* Volleyball
Balance beam	*See* Gymnastics	Biathlon	*See* Skiing

Sport or Activity	Sport-Specific Plan to Follow	Sport or Activity	Sport-Specific Plan to Follow
Billiards	*See* Fitness activities	Frisbee	*See* Fitness activities
Board sailing	*See* Fitness activities	Golf	*See* Golf
Boating	*See* Fitness activities	Grass skiing	*See* Skiing
Bobsledding	*See* Skiing	Gymnastics	*See* Gymnastics
Bocce	*See* Bowling	Hammer throwing	*See* Track and field
Bodybuilding	*See* Bodybuilding	Handball	*See* Racket sports
Bowling	*See* Bowling	Hang gliding	*See* Fitness activities
Boxing	*See* Boxing	Heptathlon	*See* Track and field
Break dancing	*See* Dancing	High jumping	*See* Track and field
Canadian football	*See* Football	Hiking	*See* Fitness activities
Cheerleading	*See* Fitness activities	Hockey	*See* Hockey
Circus acrobatics	*See* Gymnastics	Horizontal bar	*See* Gymnastics
Climbing	*See* Rock climbing	Horseracing	*See* Equestrian
Court volleyball	*See* Volleyball	Horseshoes	*See* Fitness activities
Cricket	*See* Baseball	Hunting	*See* Fitness activities
Croquet	*See* Fitness activities	Hurdles	*See* Track and field
Cross-country running	*See* Track and field	Hydroplaning	*See* Motor sports
Cross-country skiing	*See* Skiing	Ice dancing	*See* Dancing
Curling	*See* Bowling	Ice skating	*See* Fitness activities
Cycling	*See* Cycling; Fitness activities; Triathlon	Jai alai	*See* Racket sports
Cyclocross	*See* Cycling	Javelin	*See* Track and field
Dancing	*See* Dancing	Jogging	*See* Fitness activities
Decathlon	*See* Track and field	Jousting	*See* Equestrian
Demolition derby	*See* Motor sports	Judo	*See* Martial arts
Disc golf	*See* Golf	Jumping rope	*See* Fitness activities
Discus	*See* Track and field	Karate	*See* Martial arts
Diving	*See* Gymnastics	Kayaking	*See* Fitness activities
Downhill skiing	*See* Skiing	Kickboxing	*See* Martial arts
Drag racing	*See* Motor sports	Lacrosse	*See* Field hockey
Driving	*See* Motor sports	Long jumping	*See* Track and field
Épée	*See* Fitness activities	Luge	*See* Skiing
Equestrian	*See* Equestrian	Mall walking	*See* Fitness activities
Fast dancing	*See* Dancing	Marathon running	*See* Fitness activities; Track and field
Fencing	*See* Fitness activities	Martial arts	*See* Martial arts
Field hockey	*See* Field hockey	Motocross	*See* Motor sports
Figure skating	*See* Fitness activities	Motorboating	*See* Fitness activities
Fishing	*See* Fitness activities	Motorcycling	*See* Motor sports
Floor exercise	*See* Gymnastics	Mountain biking	*See* Cycling
Foil	*See* Fitness activities	Mountaineering	*See* Fitness activities
Football	*See* Football	Netball	*See* Basketball
Formula I racing	*See* Motor sports	Nordic skiing	*See* Skiing
Freestyle skiing	*See* Skiing	Orienteering	*See* Fitness activities

Sport or Activity	Sport-Specific Plan to Follow	Sport or Activity	Sport-Specific Plan to Follow
Paddle tennis	*See* Racket sports	**Soaring**	*See* Fitness activities
Parachuting	*See* Fitness activities	**Soccer**	*See* Soccer
Parallel bars	*See* Gymnastics	**Softball**	*See* Baseball
Pentathlon	*See* Track and field	**Speedskating**	*See* Football
Petanque	*See* Bowling	**Sports-car racing**	*See* Motor sports
Ping pong	*See* Fitness activities	**Squash**	*See* Racket sports
Platform tennis	*See* Racket sports	**Steeplechase**	*See* Track and field
Pole vaulting	*See* Track and field	**Step aerobics**	*See* Fitness activities
Polo	*See* Equestrian	**Stickball**	*See* Baseball
Pool	*See* Fitness activities	**Still rings**	*See* Gymnastics
Power walking	*See* Fitness activities	**Surfing**	*See* Fitness activities
Powerlifting	*See* Powerlifting	**Swimming**	*See* Swimming; Triathlon
Professional boxing	*See* Boxing	**Synchronized swimming**	*See* Swimming
Quarter horse racing	*See* Equestrian		
Racquetball	*See* Racket sports	**Table tennis**	*See* Fitness activities
Rallye	*See* Motor sports	**Tae kwon do**	*See* Martial arts
Relay	*See* Track and field	**Tandem cycling**	*See* Fitness activities
Road racing	*See* Fitness activities; Track and field; Triathlon	**Team handball**	*See* Field hockey
		Tennis	*See* Tennis
Rock climbing	*See* Rock climbing	**Tobogganing**	*See* Skiing
Rodeo	*See* Equestrian	**Track**	*See* Track and field
Rollerblading	*See* Fitness activities	**Trampoline**	*See* Gymnastics
Roller-skating	*See* Fitness activities	**Trekking**	*See* Fitness activities
Rugby	*See* Football	**Triathlon**	*See* Triathlon
Running	*See* Fitness activities; Track and field; Triathlon	**Triple jumping**	*See* Track and field
		Tug of war	*See* Fitness activities
Sailing	*See* Fitness activities	**Uneven parallel bars**	*See* Gymnastics
Scuba diving	*See* Fitness activities	**Unicycling**	*See* Fitness activities
Shooting	*See* Fitness activities	**Vaulting**	*See* Gymnastics
Shot-putting	*See* Track and field	**Volleyball**	*See* Volleyball
Shuffleboard	*See* Bowling	**Walking**	*See* Fitness activities; Track and field
Side horse	*See* Gymnastics		
Skateboarding	*See* Fitness activities	**Water exercising**	*See* Fitness activities
Skeet	*See* Fitness activities	**Water polo**	*See* Swimming
Ski jumping	*See* Skiing	**Water skiing**	*See* Fitness activities
Skiing	*See* Skiing	**Weight throwing**	*See* Track and field
Skin diving	*See* Fitness activities; Swimming	**Weightlifting**	*See* Weightlifting
		Wheelchair basketball	*See* Fitness activities
Snorkeling	*See* Fitness activities; Swimming	**Wheelchair road racing**	*See* Fitness activities
		Wheelchair tennis	*See* Fitness activities
Snowboarding	*See* Skiing	**Wrestling**	*See* Wrestling
Snowmobiling	*See* Motor sports	**Wrist wrestling**	*See* Fitness activities
Snowshoe racing	*See* Skiing	**Yachting**	*See* Fitness activities

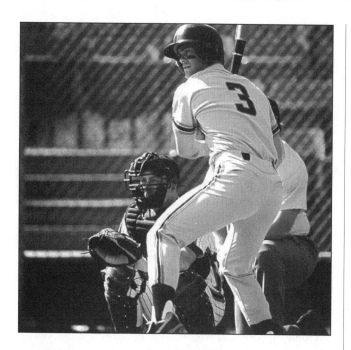

BASEBALL

Also for Ball Throwing, Cricket, Softball, and Stickball

Baseball is a multifaceted game that involves a wide range of skills and movements. It requires not only speed and strength in short, explosive bursts, but also flexibility and agility for throwing, pivoting, and sliding.

It is said that professional scouts look for three elements in a young player—bat speed, throwing ability (the ability to throw forcefully with accuracy), and running speed and quickness. All else, it is said, can be taught by a good coach.

Every bit of your training and diet must reflect these three elements. These elements are what make baseball "ballistic" in nature. In fact, baseball is very "ballistic," so improved recovery and tissue repair plus increased speed and strength are your year-round training and dietary goals. Nutritionally, this means emphasizing short-term energy needs and maximizing the muscles' recovery and tissue-repair processes.

In baseball, the energy output is primarily anaerobic (without oxygen). This does not mean that training for or playing the game is easy, however. Baseball training is extremely intensive and grueling. At the highest levels, baseball speed training forces you to operate at your anaerobic threshold (the point at which you must receive oxygen).

In addition, hitting and throwing require strength and quickness. In baseball, the aim is to make the muscles as strong and as quick as possible. This calls for

specialized training. Furthermore, the incredible force output of baseball, especially coupled with the ballistic aspects of the game, requires the support of a carefully constructed nutrition program.

ENERGY SOURCES OF BASEBALL PLAYERS

The muscles rely on three major systems to supply the energy they need—the immediate, glycolytic, and oxidative energy systems. For short-term energy for explosive-strength output, the muscles depend on the immediate energy systems. The immediate energy systems are nonoxidative—that is, they do not use oxygen. Instead, these systems generate energy through the use of adenosine triphosphate (ATP) and creatine phosphate (CP). CP is produced in the body and stored in the muscle fibers. It is broken down by enzymes to regenerate ATP, which is also stored in the muscle fibers. When the ATP is in turn broken down, the result is a spark of energy that triggers a muscle contraction.

For medium-term energy for repeated near-maximum exertion, the muscles turn to the glycolytic energy systems. In these systems, which are also nonoxidative, glycogen is used to produce energy. Glycogen is the storage form of glucose. It is stored in the liver and muscles, and is readily converted back to glucose when it is needed for energy.

For long-term energy for endurance activities, the muscles use the oxidative energy systems. In these systems, oxygen is used to oxidize long-chain fatty acids, protein, and glucose, which generates energy. For athletes, getting enough oxygen can mean a winning performance rather than a second-place showing.

Every sport involves a variety of skills, and each skill utilizes a unique combination of these three energy sources. The following table lists the major baseball skills and shows how much your body relies on each of the energy sources when you perform them. Percentages are also given for an average game and an average workout, as well as for two similar sports.

WHERE YOUR ENERGY COMES FROM

For Baseball Players		
Energy Systems		
IMMEDIATE	GLYCOLYTIC	OXIDATIVE
Skills		
Batting 100%	0%	0%
Pitching 80%	20%	0%

Energy Systems			
	IMMEDIATE	GLYCOLYTIC	OXIDATIVE
Running	95%	5%	0%
Throwing	100%	0%	0%
Average game	95%	5%	0%
Average workout	80%	20%	0%

For Similar Sports			
Cricket	90%	10%	0%
Softball	90%	10%	0%

When considering the type of nutritional support to give your training program, keep the following factors in mind:

☐ All athletes need to consume high-quality protein several times a day for effective recovery and adequate repair of damaged muscle tissue.

☐ Athletes whose muscles rely substantially on the immediate or glycolytic energy systems should keep their fat intake to a minimum because fat is not an efficient energy source for their intensive training, which is almost exclusively anaerobic in nature. Since the fat calories consumed by these athletes are not generally used for energy, they are stored as body fat.

☐ All athletes should consume a carefully measured amount of high-quality carbohydrates several times a day to ensure an adequate supply of energy.

☐ The carbohydrates in all preworkout meals should consist of foods with low glycemic indexes to ensure that training intensity does not wane and that muscle tissue is not cannibalized for energy. (For the glycemic indexes of some common foods, see page 29.)

The aim of your nutrition program is to make your body healthy enough to accomplish recovery and tissue repair speedily and efficiently—without adding body fat. Your further aim is to do this while maintaining a high strength-to-weight ratio. These aims alone make diet as critical as training for baseball players. You must eat just the right amount of food. Eat the wrong foods or the wrong amounts just a few times too often and you will sabotage your fitness efforts. Even more important, do not be in a hurry. It takes *years* to become a great baseball player. Rush the nutrition and training processes and you will become fat, your recovery rate will decline, and your injury rate will rise.

NUTRITION FOR BASEBALL PLAYERS

Baseball players are power athletes. No matter what position they play, they obtain most of their energy from the immediate energy systems. Therefore, as a baseball player, you need to plan your nutritional intake, from both food and supplement sources, to support the immediate systems. In addition, since your energy expenditure changes in the preseason and off-season, you need to adjust your caloric intake and macronutrient ratio to match. Following are dietary guidelines for baseball players to help you in planning your nutrition program. Supplementation guidelines for baseball players can be found on page 203.

Dietary Guidelines

The following pie charts illustrate how you should divide up your caloric intake to match the energy demands of baseball during the preseason, season, and off-season. They show the target percentages of fat, protein, and carbohydrates that your five to six meals should supply each day.

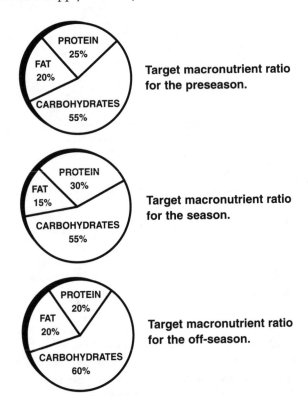

Target macronutrient ratio for the preseason.

Target macronutrient ratio for the season.

Target macronutrient ratio for the off-season.

Note that fat has about 9 calories per gram, while protein and carbohydrates have only 4 calories per gram. Therefore, during the season, if you needed to consume a total of 2,500 calories per day, you would aim for 375 calories (15 percent of your total daily calories) from fat, 750 calories (30 percent of your total daily calories) from protein, and the remaining 1,375 calories (55 percent of your total daily calories) from carbohydrates.

Some other important considerations for baseball players are:

☐ Carbohydrates are the major source of energy for short-term activities. Complex carbohydrates are the best source because they most effectively refill the glycogen stores in the muscles and liver. In addition, they elevate the blood sugar to a level sufficient for long sessions of intensive training.

☐ As a power athlete, you must make sure that you consume adequate amounts of both carbohydrates and protein. If your energy stores become drastically depleted or you experience lactic-acid buildup, you may suffer temporary muscle fatigue. If you do not refill your glycogen stores before your next workout or game, your body may begin breaking down muscle tissue for the protein it needs for energy.

☐ Directly before workouts and games, consume carbohydrate drinks with high glycemic indexes to keep your blood sugar sustained at an appropriate level. This will allow you to train or play intensively without having your explosiveness hindered by fatigue.

☐ As a power athlete, you need to stimulate the storage of glycogen in your muscles while promoting repair and growth of your muscle tissue and inhibiting buildup of body fat. To do this:

• Train anaerobically on a regular basis. Intensive training stimulates increased storage of glycogen in the muscles and liver, which provides additional energy for greater exercise capacity.

• Consume five to six meals a day. Eating several smaller meals rather than three larger ones will keep your blood-sugar level stable throughout the day and will ensure that a supply of protein is always available for your muscles.

• Keep your fat intake to a minimum. Large amounts of fat in your diet will add to your body fat and will cause you to lose minerals through frequent urination.

• Consume low-glycemic-index foods about two to three hours before workouts and games. These foods help sustain the blood-sugar level.

• Drink plenty of water. Not only will this practice

reduce your chances of becoming dehydrated, but every ounce of glycogen that is stored within the muscles needs 3 ounces of water stored along with it. Therefore, remaining properly hydrated will also help prevent weakened muscle contractions.

• Do not eat a new food just before a game. Different people often react differently to the same food. Before a game, eat just those foods that you know your body will handle well.

As a baseball player, you should turn to Appendix C on page 345 for full discussions of the 20:25:55, 15:30:55, and 20:20:60 dietary plans. Also presented are sample daily diets that use common, healthy foods to meet an athlete's energy and caloric needs. Use the directions on page 150 to estimate your average daily caloric requirement. Then use the directions in Chapter 13 or 14 to adjust your diet for off-season fat loss or muscle building, respectively.

Supplementation Guidelines

In addition to eating a proper diet, you should also take dietary supplements to make sure that any nutrients you lose due to sweating or training are replenished. The following tables will help guide you in selecting the supplements appropriate for you. The first table lists the nutrients recommended for baseball players, as well as the range of intake for each nutrient. (For discussions of these nutrients, see Part One.) Note that within the ranges of intake, the lower amounts are for smaller individuals and lower-activity days, while the higher amounts are for larger individuals and higher-activity days.

RECOMMENDED NUTRIENTS AND RANGES OF INTAKE

For Baseball Players	
NUTRIENT	**RANGE OF INTAKE**
VITAMINS	
Vitamin A	8,000–16,000 IU
Beta-carotene	20,000–30,000 IU
Vitamin B₁ (thiamine)	30–120 mg
Vitamin B₂ (riboflavin)	30–120 mg
Vitamin B₃ (niacin)	40–80 mg
Vitamin B₅ (pantothenic acid)	20–100 mg
Vitamin B₆ (pyridoxine)	20–80 mg
Vitamin B₁₂ (cobalamin)	12–120 mcg
Biotin	125–175 mcg

NUTRIENT	RANGE OF INTAKE
Folate	400–800 mcg
Vitamin C	800–2,000 mg
Vitamin D	400–800 IU
Vitamin E	200–600 IU
Vitamin K	60–160 mcg
MINERALS	
Boron	2–8 mg
Calcium	800–1,500 mg
Chromium	200–500 mcg
Copper	1–4 mg
Iodine	100–200 mcg
Iron	15–50 mg
Magnesium	250–650 mg
Manganese	12–35 mg
Molybdenum	100–200 mcg
Phosphorus	150–800 mg
Potassium	50–1,000 mg
Selenium	100–200 mcg
Zinc	15–50 mg
AMINO ACIDS	
L-glutamine	1,000–2,000 mg
FATTY ACIDS	
Alpha-linolenic acid	1,000–2,000 mg
Docosahexaenoic acid (DHA)	250–750 mg
Eiocosapentaenoic acid (EPA)	250–750 mg
Gamma linolenic acid (GLA)	100–400 mg
Linoleic acid	3,000–6,000 mg
METABOLITES	
Bioflavonoids	200–800 mg
Choline	100–600 mg
Creatine monohydrate	4,000–12,000 mg
Ferulic acid	50–100 mg
Inosine	500–1,000 mg
Inositol	100–600 mg
L-carnitine	750–2,000 mg
Octacosanol	1,000–3,000 mcg

IU = international units, mcg = micrograms, mg = milligrams.

The second table lists the different types of sports supplements available and indicates if their use by baseball players is recommended in the preseason, during the season, or directly before a game. The list also includes a number of popular nutritional practices—bicarbonate loading, carbohydrate loading, creatine and/or inosine loading, and water loading.

(For a discussion of any of these supplements or practices, see the appropriate section in Part One or Part Three.)

RECOMMENDED SPORTS SUPPLEMENTS AND NUTRITIONAL PRACTICES

For Baseball Players

	Intake Recommendation		
	PRESEASON	SEASON	PREGAME
SUPPLEMENTS			
Multivitamins	Yes	Yes	No
Multiminerals	Yes	Yes	No
Antioxidants	Yes	Yes	No
Fatty acids	Yes	Yes	No
Metabolites	Optional	Yes	Yes
Branched-chain amino acids	Yes	Yes	Yes
Herbs	Yes	Yes	No
Low-calorie protein drink (200–300 calories)	Yes	Yes	Yes
Carbohydrate drink	Yes	Yes	Yes
Fat-burning supplement	Yes	Optional	No
PRACTICES			
Bicarbonate loading	No	Optional	Optional
Carbohydrate loading	No	No	No
Creatine and/or inosine loading	Optional	Yes	Yes
Water loading	No	No	Optional

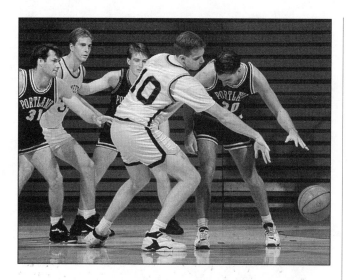

BASKETBALL

Also for Netball

Basketball requires a variety of skills. A basketball player must be a combination sprinter, leaper, and even dancer to execute the fundamental movements of the game. Basketball conditioning, therefore, must take each of these areas into account.

Only the most rigorous nutrition and training program can prepare an athlete for a full-court basketball season. And although you probably will not be training for such a schedule, you can still follow the routines practiced by the professionals to improve your skills and give your conditioning efforts a boost. Increased strength can make you a better basketball player, even if your game is the weekend variety played in the local gymnasium or schoolyard.

Through the careful application of scientific training techniques, you can multiply your on-court effectiveness in all areas of the game. You can improve your jumping ability, sprinting ability, endurance, agility, and ball control, playing better even when you are fatigued. Furthermore, the incredible diversity of skills and energy demands of basketball require the support of a carefully constructed nutrition program.

ENERGY SOURCES OF BASKETBALL PLAYERS

The muscles rely on three major systems to supply the energy they need—the immediate, glycolytic, and oxidative energy systems. For short-term energy for explosive-strength output, the muscles depend on the immediate energy systems. The immediate energy systems are nonoxidative—that is, they do not use oxygen. Instead, these systems generate energy through the use of adenosine triphosphate (ATP) and creatine phosphate (CP). CP is produced in the body and stored in the muscle fibers. It is broken down by enzymes to regenerate ATP, which is also stored in the muscle fibers. When the ATP is in turn broken down, the result is a spark of energy that triggers a muscle contraction.

For medium-term energy for repeated near-maximum exertion, the muscles turn to the glycolytic energy systems. In these systems, which are also nonoxidative, glycogen is used to produce energy. Glycogen is the storage form of glucose. It is stored in the liver and muscles, and is readily converted back to glucose when it is needed for energy.

For long-term energy for endurance activities, the muscles use the oxidative energy systems. In these systems, oxygen is used to oxidize long-chain fatty acids, protein, and glucose, which generates energy. For athletes, getting enough oxygen can mean a winning performance rather than a second-place showing.

Every sport involves a variety of skills, and each skill utilizes a unique combination of these three energy sources. The following table shows how much your body relies on each of the energy sources during an average basketball game.

WHERE YOUR ENERGY COMES FROM

For Basketball Players		
Energy Systems		
IMMEDIATE	GLYCOLITIC	OXIDATIVE
Average game 30%	30%	40%

When considering the type of nutritional support to give your training program, keep the following factors in mind:

☐ All athletes need to consume high-quality protein several times a day for effective recovery and adequate repair of damaged muscle tissue.

☐ Athletes whose muscles rely substantially on the immediate or glycolytic energy systems should keep their fat intake to a minimum because fat is not an efficient energy source for their intensive training, which is almost exclusively anaerobic in nature. Since the fat calories consumed by these athletes are not generally used for energy, they are stored as body fat.

□ Athletes whose muscles rely substantially on the oxidative energy systems can eat more fat because their energy is manufactured through the oxidation of fatty acids. But even these athletes should watch their fat calories if they train aerobically (with oxygen) for less than half an hour at a time.

□ All athletes should consume a carefully measured amount of high-quality carbohydrates several times a day to ensure an adequate supply of energy.

□ The carbohydrates in all preworkout meals should consist of foods with low glycemic indexes to ensure that training intensity does not wane and that muscle tissue is not cannibalized for energy. (For the glycemic indexes of some common foods, see page 29.)

The aim of your nutrition program is to make your body healthy enough to accomplish recovery and tissue repair speedily and efficiently—without adding body fat. Your further aim is to do this while maintaining a high strength-to-weight ratio. These aims alone make diet very important for basketball players. You must eat just the right amount of food. Eat the wrong foods or the wrong amounts just a few times too often and you will sabotage your fitness efforts. Even more important, do not be in a hurry. It takes *years* to become a great basketball player. Rush the nutrition and training processes and your recovery rate will decline and your injury rate will rise.

NUTRITION FOR BASKETBALL PLAYERS

Basketball players are combination power–middle-distance–endurance athletes. No matter what position they play, they obtain almost the same amounts of energy from the immediate, glycolytic, and oxidative energy systems. Therefore, as a basketball player, you need to plan your nutritional intake, from both food and supplement sources, to support all three systems equally. In addition, since your energy expenditure changes in the preseason and off-season, you need to adjust your caloric intake and macronutrient ratio to match. Following are dietary guidelines for basketball players to help you in planning your nutrition program. Supplementation guidelines for basketball players can be found on page 207.

Dietary Guidelines

The following pie charts illustrate how you should divide up your caloric intake to match the energy demands of basketball during the preseason, season, and off-season. They show the target percentages of fat, protein, and carbohydrates that your five to six meals should supply each day.

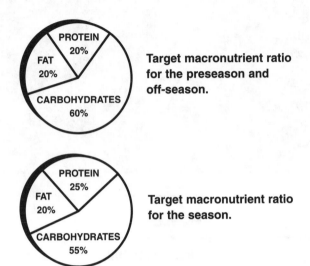

Target macronutrient ratio for the preseason and off-season.

Target macronutrient ratio for the season.

Note that fat has about 9 calories per gram, while protein and carbohydrates have only 4 calories per gram. Therefore, during the season, if you needed to consume a total of 2,500 calories per day, you would aim for 500 calories (20 percent of your total daily calories) from fat, 625 calories (25 percent of your total daily calories) from protein, and the remaining 1,375 calories (55 percent of your total daily calories) from carbohydrates.

Some other important considerations for basketball players are:

□ Carbohydrates are the major source of energy for short-term activities. Complex carbohydrates are the best source because they most effectively refill the glycogen stores in the muscles and liver. In addition, they elevate the blood sugar to a level sufficient for long sessions of intensive training.

□ As a combination power–middle-distance–endurance athlete, you must make sure that you consume adequate amounts of both carbohydrates and protein. If your energy stores become drastically depleted or you experience lactic-acid buildup, you may suffer temporary muscle fatigue. If you do not refill your glycogen stores before your next workout or game, your body may begin breaking down muscle tissue for the protein it needs for energy.

□ Directly before workouts and games, consume carbohydrate drinks with low glycemic indexes to keep your blood sugar sustained at an appropriate level. This will allow you to train or play intensively for longer periods of time.

☐ As a combination power–middle-distance–endurance athlete, you need to stimulate the storage of glycogen in your muscles while promoting repair and growth of your muscle tissue and inhibiting buildup of body fat. To do this:

• Train against your anaerobic threshold (to exhaustion) on a regular basis. Intensive, exhaustive training stimulates increased storage of glycogen in the muscles and liver, which provides additional energy for greater exercise capacity.

• Consume five to six meals a day. Eating several smaller meals rather than three larger ones will keep your blood-sugar level stable throughout the day and will ensure that a supply of protein is always available for your muscles.

• Keep your fat intake to a minimum. Large amounts of fat in your diet will add to your body fat and will cause mineral loss through frequent urination.

• Consume low-glycemic-index foods about two to three hours before workouts and games. These foods help sustain the blood-sugar level.

• Drink plenty of water. Not only will this practice reduce your chances of becoming dehydrated, but every ounce of glycogen that is stored within the muscles needs 3 ounces of water stored along with it. Therefore, remaining properly hydrated will also help prevent weakened muscle contractions and early onset of fatigue.

• Do not eat a new food just before a game. Different people often react differently to the same food. Before a game, eat just those foods that you know your body will handle well.

As a basketball player, you should turn to Appendix C on page 345 for full discussions of the 20:20:60 and 20:25:55 dietary plans. Also presented are sample daily diets that use common, healthy foods to meet an athlete's energy and caloric needs. Use the directions on page 150 to estimate your average daily caloric requirement. Then use the directions in Chapter 13 or 14 to adjust your diet for off-season fat loss or muscle building, respectively.

Supplementation Guidelines

In addition to eating a proper diet, you should also take dietary supplements to make sure that any nutrients you lose due to sweating or training are replenished. The following tables will help guide you in selecting the supplements appropriate for you. The first table lists the nutrients recommended for basketball players, as well as the range of intake for each nutrient. (For discussions of these nutrients, see Part One.) Note that within the ranges of intake, the lower amounts are for smaller individuals and lower-activity days, while the higher amounts are for larger individuals and higher-activity days.

RECOMMENDED NUTRIENTS AND RANGES OF INTAKE

For Basketball Players

NUTRIENT	RANGE OF INTAKE
VITAMINS	
Vitamin A	8,000–16,000 IU
Beta-carotene	25,000–35,000 IU
Vitamin B_1 (thiamine)	40–120 mg
Vitamin B_2 (riboflavin)	40–120 mg
Vitamin B_3 (niacin)	20–40 mg
Vitamin B_5 (pantothenic acid)	20–100 mg
Vitamin B_6 (pyridoxine)	20–80 mg
Vitamin B_{12} (cobalamin)	12–120 mcg
Biotin	125–175 mcg
Folate	400–800 mcg
Vitamin C	800–2,000 mg
Vitamin D	400–800 IU
Vitamin E	200–800 IU
Vitamin K	60–160 mcg
MINERALS	
Boron	2–8 mg
Calcium	800–1,500 mg
Chromium	200–500 mcg
Copper	1–4 mg
Iodine	100–200 mcg
Iron	15–50 mg
Magnesium	250–650 mg
Manganese	12–35 mg
Molybdenum	100–200 mcg
Phosphorus	150–800 mg
Potassium	50–1,000 mg
Selenium	100–200 mcg
Zinc	15–50 mg

NUTRIENT	RANGE OF INTAKE
AMINO ACIDS	
L-glutamic acid	500–1,000 mg
L-glutamine	1,000–2,000 mg
FATTY ACIDS	
Alpha-linolenic acid	500–1,000 mg
Docosahexaenoic acid (DHA)	250–750 mg
Eiocosapentaenoic acid (EPA)	250–750 mg
Gamma linolenic acid (GLA)	100–400 mg
Linoleic acid	2,000–3,000 mg
METABOLITES	
Bioflavonoids	300–800 mg
Choline	200–600 mg
Inositol	200–600 mg
L-carnitine	500–1,500 mg
Octacosanol	1,000–2,000 mcg

IU = international units, mcg = micrograms, mg = milligrams.

The second table lists the different types of sports supplements available and indicates if their use by basketball players is recommended in the preseason, during the season, or directly before a game. The list also includes a number of popular nutritional practices—bicarbonate loading, carbohydrate loading, creatine and/or inosine loading, and water loading. (For a discussion of any of these supplements or practices, see the appropriate section in Part One or Part Three.)

RECOMMENDED SPORTS SUPPLEMENTS AND NUTRITIONAL PRACTICES

For Basketball Players

	Intake Recommendation		
	PRESEASON	SEASON	PREGAME
SUPPLEMENTS			
Multivitamins	Yes	Yes	No
Multiminerals	Yes	Yes	No
Antioxidants	Yes	Yes	No
Fatty acids	Yes	Yes	No
Metabolites	Optional	Yes	Yes
Branched-chain amino acids	Yes	Yes	Yes
Herbs	Yes	Yes	No
Medium-calorie protein drink (300–500 calories)	Yes	Yes	Yes
Carbohydrate drink	Yes	Yes	Yes
Fat-burning supplement	Yes	Optional	No

	Intake Recommendation		
	PRESEASON	SEASON	PREGAME
PRACTICES			
Bicarbonate loading	No	No	No
Carbohydrate loading	No	No	Optional
Creatine and/or inosine loading	No	No	No
Water loading	No	No	Optional

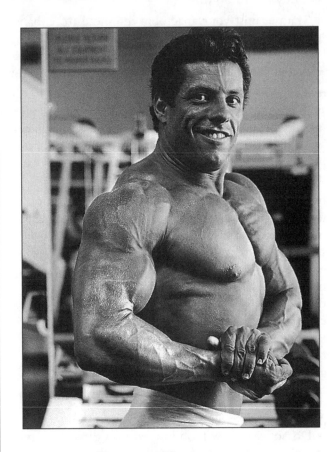

BODYBUILDING

In bodybuilding, the energy output is primarily anaerobic (without oxygen). Lifting weights for 5 to 40 repetitions does not take more than about a minute at the most. This does not mean that training for or competing in bodybuilding contests is easy, however. Training as a bodybuilder is extremely intensive and grueling. At the highest levels, bodybuilding training forces you to operate at your anaerobic threshold (the point at which you must receive oxygen) for up to an hour.

Muscles grow when they are stressed. In bodybuilding, the aim is to make the muscles grow as large as possible. Therefore, adaptive overload stress must be applied to as many muscle cells—and to as many of each cell's elements—as possible. This calls for specialized training. You must use light weights and heavy weights, do fast movements and slow movements, do a high number of reps and a low number of reps, and everything in between. Because of the incredible diversity of energy output that it demands, bodybuilding requires the support of a carefully constructed nutrition program.

ENERGY SOURCES OF BODYBUILDERS

The muscles rely on three major systems to supply the energy they need—the immediate, glycolytic, and oxidative energy systems. For short-term energy for explosive-strength output, the muscles depend on the immediate energy systems. The immediate energy systems are nonoxidative—that is, they do not use oxygen. Instead, these systems generate energy through the use of adenosine triphosphate (ATP) and creatine phosphate (CP). CP is produced in the body and stored in the muscle fibers. It is broken down by enzymes to regenerate ATP, which is also stored in the muscle fibers. When the ATP is in turn broken down, the result is a spark of energy that triggers a muscle contraction.

For medium-term energy for repeated near-maximum exertion, the muscles turn to the glycolytic energy systems. In these systems, which are also nonoxidative, glycogen is used to produce energy. Glycogen is the storage form of glucose. It is stored in the liver and muscles, and is readily converted back to glucose when it is needed for energy.

For long-term energy for endurance activities, the muscles use the oxidative energy systems. In these systems, oxygen is used to oxidize long-chain fatty acids, protein, and glucose, which generates energy. For athletes, getting enough oxygen can mean a winning performance rather than a second-place showing.

Every sport involves a variety of skills, and each skill utilizes a unique combination of these three energy sources. The following table lists five different kinds of average weight-training sets and shows how much your body relies on each of the energy sources when you perform them. Percentages are also given for two kinds of average workouts, as well as for an average contest.

WHERE YOUR ENERGY COMES FROM

For Bodybuilders			
	Energy Systems		
	IMMEDIATE	**GLYCOLYTIC**	**OXIDATIVE**
Average sets			
1–4 reps	90%	10%	0%
5–9 reps	80%	20%	0%
10–19 reps	60%	40%	0%
20–39 reps	50%	50%	0%
40–100 reps	40%	60%	0%
Average contest	50%	50%	0%
Average workouts			
General	60%	40%	0%
Precontest (final week)	80%	10%	10%

When considering the type of nutritional support to give your training program, keep the following factors in mind:

☐ All athletes need to consume high-quality protein several times a day for effective recovery and adequate repair of damaged muscle tissue.

☐ Athletes whose muscles rely substantially on the immediate or glycolytic energy systems should keep their fat intake to a minimum because fat is not an efficient energy source for their intensive training, which is almost exclusively anaerobic in nature. Since the fat calories consumed by these athletes are not generally used for energy, they are stored as body fat.

☐ All athletes should consume a carefully measured amount of high-quality carbohydrates several times a day to ensure an adequate supply of energy.

☐ The carbohydrates in all preworkout meals should consist of foods with low glycemic indexes to ensure that training intensity does not wane and that muscle tissue is not cannibalized for energy. (For the glycemic indexes of some common foods, see page 29.)

The aim of your nutrition program is to make your body healthy enough to accomplish recovery and tissue repair speedily and efficiently—without adding body fat. As a bodybuilder, you must also remain in positive calorie balance—that is, for your muscles to grow, you must eat more than your body needs. These aims alone make diet as critical as training for bodybuilders. You must eat just the right amount of food.

Eat the wrong foods or the wrong amounts just a few times too often and you will sabotage your fitness efforts. Even more important, do not be in a hurry. It takes *years* to become a great bodybuilder. Rush the nutrition and training processes and you will become big—but big and fat instead of big and cut!

NUTRITION FOR BODYBUILDERS

Bodybuilders are power athletes. Their primary energy sources are the immediate energy systems. Therefore, as a bodybuilder, you need to plan your nutritional intake, from both food and supplement sources, to support the immediate systems. In addition, since your energy expenditure changes in the off-season, you need to adjust your caloric intake and macronutrient ratio to match. Following are dietary guidelines for bodybuilders to help you in planning your nutrition program. Supplementation guidelines for bodybuilders can be found on page 211.

Dietary Guidelines

The following pie charts illustrate how you should divide up your caloric intake to match the energy demands of bodybuilding during the preseason, season, and off-season. They show the target percentages of fat, protein, and carbohydrates that your five to six meals should supply each day.

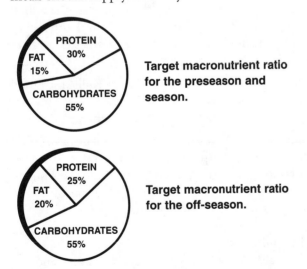

Target macronutrient ratio for the preseason and season.

Target macronutrient ratio for the off-season.

Note that fat has about 9 calories per gram, while protein and carbohydrates have only 4 calories per gram. Therefore, during the season, if you needed to consume a total of 2,500 calories per day, you would aim for 375 calories (15 percent of your total daily

calories) from fat, 750 calories (30 percent of your total daily calories) from protein, and the remaining 1,375 calories (55 percent of your total daily calories) from carbohydrates.

Some other important considerations for bodybuilders are:

☐ Carbohydrates are the major source of energy for short-term activities. Complex carbohydrates are the best source because they most effectively refill the glycogen stores in the muscles and liver. In addition, they elevate the blood sugar to a level sufficient for long sessions of intensive training.

☐ As a power athlete, you must make sure that you consume adequate amounts of both carbohydrates and protein. If your energy stores become drastically depleted or you experience lactic-acid buildup, you may suffer temporary muscle fatigue. If you do not refill your glycogen stores before your next workout or contest, your body may begin breaking down muscle tissue for the protein it needs for energy.

☐ Directly before workouts and contests, consume carbohydrate drinks with high glycemic indexes to keep your blood sugar sustained at an appropriate level. This will allow you to train or compete intensively without having your explosiveness hindered by fatigue.

☐ As a power athlete, you need to stimulate the storage of glycogen in your muscles while promoting repair and growth of your muscle tissue and inhibiting buildup of body fat. To do this:

● Train anaerobically on a regular basis. Intensive training stimulates increased storage of glycogen in the muscles and liver, which provides additional energy for greater exercise capacity.

● Consume five to six meals a day. Eating several smaller meals rather than three larger ones will keep your blood-sugar level stable throughout the day and will ensure that a supply of protein is always available for your muscles.

● Keep your fat intake to a minimum. Large amounts of fat in your diet will add to your body fat and will cause you to lose minerals through frequent urination.

● Consume low-glycemic-index foods about two three hours before workouts and contests. These foods help sustain the blood-sugar level.

● Drink plenty of water. Not only will this practice reduce your chances of becoming dehydrated, but every ounce of glycogen that is stored within the muscles needs 3 ounces of water stored along with it. Therefore, remaining properly hydrated will also help prevent weakened muscle contractions.

• Do not eat a new food just before a contest. Different people often react differently to the same food. Before a contest, eat just those foods that you know your body will handle well.

As a bodybuilder, you should turn to Appendix C on page 345 for full discussions of the 15:30:55 and 20:25:55 dietary plans. Also presented are sample daily diets that use common, healthy foods to meet an athlete's energy and caloric needs. Use the directions on page 150 to estimate your average daily caloric requirement. Then use the directions in Chapter 13 or 14 to adjust your diet for off-season fat loss or muscle building, respectively.

Supplementation Guidelines

In addition to eating a proper diet, you should also take dietary supplements to make sure that any nutrients you lose due to sweating or training are replenished. The following tables will help guide you in selecting the supplements appropriate for you. The first table lists the nutrients recommended for bodybuilders, as well as the range of intake for each nutrient. (For discussions of these nutrients, see Part One.) Note that within the ranges of intake, the lower amounts are for smaller individuals and lower-activity days, while the higher amounts are for larger individuals and higher-activity days.

RECOMMENDED NUTRIENTS AND RANGES OF INTAKE

For Bodybuilders

NUTRIENT	RANGE OF INTAKE
VITAMINS	
Vitamin A	8,000–16,000 IU
Beta-carotene	20,000–30,000 IU
Vitamin B$_1$ (thiamine)	30–120 mg
Vitamin B$_2$ (riboflavin)	30–120 mg
Vitamin B$_3$ (niacin)	40–80 mg
Vitamin B$_5$ (pantothenic acid)	20–100 mg
Vitamin B$_6$ (pyridoxine)	20–80 mg
Vitamin B$_{12}$ (cobalamin)	12–120 mcg
Biotin	125–175 mcg

NUTRIENT	RANGE OF INTAKE
Folate	400–800 mcg
Vitamin C	800–2,000 mg
Vitamin D	400–800 IU
Vitamin E	200–600 IU
Vitamin K	60–160 mcg
MINERALS	
Boron	2–8 mg
Calcium	800–1,500 mg
Chromium	200–500 mcg
Copper	1–4 mg
Iodine	100–200 mcg
Iron	15–50 mg
Magnesium	250–650 mg
Manganese	12–35 mg
Molybdenum	100–200 mcg
Phosphorus	150–800 mg
Potassium	50–1,000 mg
Selenium	100–200 mcg
Zinc	15–50 mg
AMINO ACIDS	
L-arginine	1,000–4,000 mg
L-glutamine	1,000–3,000 mg
L-ornithine	1,000–4,000 mg
FATTY ACIDS	
Alpha-linolenic acid	1,000–2,000 mg
Docosahexaenoic acid (DHA)	250–750 mg
Eiocosapentaenoic acid (EPA)	250–750 mg
Gamma linolenic acid (GLA)	400–800 mg
Linoleic acid	3,000–6,000 mg
METABOLITES	
Beta-hydroxy beta-methylbutyrate	1,500–3,000 mg
Bioflavonoids	200–800 mg
Choline	100–600 mg
Creatine monohydrate	8,000–20,000 mg
Ferulic acid	100–200 mg
Inosine	500–1,000 mg
Inositol	100–600 mg
L-carnitine	750–2,000 mg

IU = international units, mcg = micrograms, mg = milligrams.

The second table lists the different types of sports supplements available and indicates if their use by bodybuilders is recommended in the preseason, during the season, or directly before a contest. The list also includes a number of popular nutritional practices—bicarbonate loading, carbohydrate loading, creatine and/or inosine loading, and water loading. (For a discussion of any of these supplements or practices, see the appropriate section in Part One or Part Three.)

RECOMMENDED SPORTS SUPPLEMENTS AND NUTRITIONAL PRACTICES

For Bodybuilders

	Intake Recommendation		
	PRESEASON	SEASON	PRECONTEST
SUPPLEMENTS			
Multivitamins	Yes	Yes	No
Multiminerals	Yes	Yes	No
Antioxidants	Yes	Yes	No
Fatty acids	Yes	Yes	No
Metabolites	Yes	Yes	No
Branched-chain amino acids	Yes	Yes	Yes
Herbs	Yes	Yes	No
Low-calorie protein drink (200–300 calories)	Yes	Yes	Yes
Carbohydrate drink	Yes	Yes	Yes
Fat-burning supplement	Yes	Yes	Yes
PRACTICES			
Bicarbonate loading	No	Optional	No
Carbohydrate loading	No	No	Optional
Creatine and/or inosine loading	Optional	Yes	Yes
Water loading	No	No	Optional

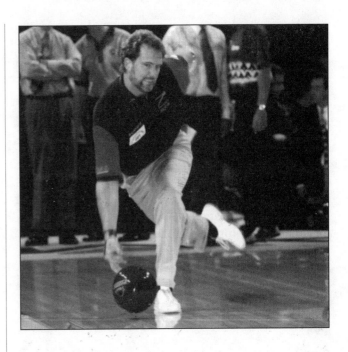

BOWLING

Also for Bocce, Curling, Petanque, and Shuffleboard

In bowling, the energy output is anaerobic (without oxygen). Rolling back-to-back games—sometimes up to twelve or more in a tournament—can be downright draining. The muscles in your bowling hand slowly become fatigued and you begin to lose fine motor control over the ball upon release. Your wrist and forearm muscles tire similarly. Training for bowling tournaments is not easy either. It is grueling and mind-numbing. At the highest levels, bowling forces you to train like an elite athlete, pushing your threshold of both physical and mental fatigue.

While it is not yet the norm for bowlers to follow a specialized training program, it will become so. It is inevitable, since it is part of the quest to become number one in most sports. Furthermore, the energy output of competitive bowling requires the support of a carefully constructed nutrition program.

ENERGY SOURCES OF BOWLERS

The muscles rely on three major systems to supply the energy they need—the immediate, glycolytic, and oxidative energy systems. For short-term energy for explosive-strength output, the muscles depend on the immediate energy systems. The immediate energy systems are nonoxidative—that is, they do not use oxygen.

Instead, these systems generate energy through the use of adenosine triphosphate (ATP) and creatine phosphate (CP). CP is produced in the body and stored in the muscle fibers. It is broken down by enzymes to regenerate ATP, which is also stored in the muscle fibers. When the ATP is in turn broken down, the result is a spark of energy that triggers a muscle contraction.

For medium-term energy for repeated near-maximum exertion, the muscles turn to the glycolytic energy systems. In these systems, which are also nonoxidative, glycogen is used to produce energy. Glycogen is the storage form of glucose. It is stored in the liver and muscles, and is readily converted back to glucose when it is needed for energy.

For long-term energy for endurance activities, the muscles use the oxidative energy systems. In these systems, oxygen is used to oxidize long-chain fatty acids, protein, and glucose, which generates energy. For athletes, getting enough oxygen can mean a winning performance rather than a second-place showing.

Every sport involves a variety of skills, and each skill utilizes a unique combination of these three energy sources. The the following table lists three different kinds of average bowling tournaments and shows how much your body relies on each of the energy sources when you participate in them. Percentages are also given for three similar sports.

WHERE YOUR ENERGY COMES FROM

For Bowlers		
Energy Systems		
IMMEDIATE	GLYCOLYTIC	OXIDATIVE
Average tournaments		
1–10 games 60%	40%	0%
11–20 games 50%	50%	0%
21 or more games 50%	50%	0%
For Similar Sports		
Bocce 80%	20%	0%
Curling 80%	20%	0%
Petanque 80%	20%	0%

When considering the type of nutritional support to give your training program, keep the following factors in mind:

□ All athletes need to consume high-quality protein several times a day for effective recovery and adequate repair of damaged muscle tissue.

□ Athletes whose muscles rely substantially on the immediate or glycolytic energy systems should keep their fat intake to a minimum because fat is not an efficient energy source for their intensive training, which is almost exclusively anaerobic in nature. Since the fat calories consumed by these athletes are not generally used for energy, they are stored as body fat.

□ All athletes should consume a carefully measured amount of high-quality carbohydrates several times a day to ensure an adequate supply of energy.

□ The carbohydrates in all preworkout meals should consist of foods with low glycemic indexes to ensure that training intensity does not wane and that muscle tissue is not cannibalized for energy. (For the glycemic indexes of some common foods, see page 29.)

The aim of your nutrition program is to make your body healthy enough to accomplish recovery and tissue repair speedily and efficiently—without adding body fat. Your further aim is to do this while maintaining a high strength-to-weight ratio. These aims alone make diet as critical as training for bowlers. You must eat just the right amount of food. Eat the wrong foods or the wrong amounts just a few times too often and you will sabotage your fitness efforts. Even more important, do not be in a hurry. It takes *years* to become a great bowler. Rush the nutrition and training processes and you will become fat, you may become overtrained, and your handicap will suffer.

NUTRITION FOR BOWLERS

Bowlers are combination power–middle-distance athletes. They obtain most of their energy from a combination of the immediate and glycolytic energy systems. Therefore, as a bowler, you need to plan your nutritional intake, from both food and supplement sources, to support these nonoxidative systems. In addition, since your energy expenditure changes in the off-season, you need to adjust your caloric intake and macronutrient ratio to match. Following are dietary guidelines for bowlers to help you in planning your nutrition program. Supplementation guidelines for bowlers can be found on page 214.

Dietary Guidelines

The following pie charts illustrate how you should divide up your caloric intake to match the energy demands of bowling during the preseason, season, and off-season. They show the target percentages of fat, protein, and carbohydrates that your five to six meals should supply each day.

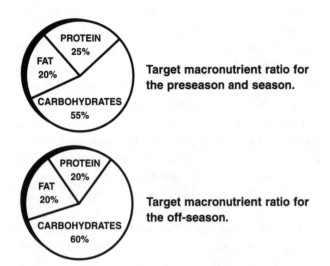

Target macronutrient ratio for the preseason and season.

Target macronutrient ratio for the off-season.

Note that fat has about 9 calories per gram, while protein and carbohydrates have only 4 calories per gram. Therefore, during the season, if you needed to consume a total of 2,500 calories per day, you would aim for 500 calories (20 percent of your total daily calories) from fat, 625 calories (25 percent of your total daily calories) from protein, and the remaining 1,375 calories (55 percent of your total daily calories) from carbohydrates.

Some other important considerations for bowlers are:

☐ Carbohydrates are the major source of energy for short-term activities. Complex carbohydrates are the best source because they most effectively refill the glycogen stores in the muscles and liver. In addition, they elevate the blood sugar to a level sufficient for long sessions of intensive training.

☐ As a combination power–middle-distance athlete, you must make sure that you consume adequate a-mounts of both carbohydrates and protein. If your energy stores become drastically depleted or you experience lactic-acid buildup, you may suffer temporary muscle fatigue. If you do not refill your glycogen stores before your next workout or tournament, your body may begin breaking down muscle tissue for the protein it needs for energy.

☐ Directly before workouts and tournaments, consume carbohydrate drinks with high glycemic index-es to keep your blood sugar sustained at an appropri-

ate level. This will allow you to train or play intensively for longer periods of time.

☐ As a combination power–middle-distance athlete, you need to stimulate the storage of glycogen in your muscles while promoting repair and growth of your muscle tissue and inhibiting buildup of body fat. To do this:

• Train against your anaerobic threshold (to exhaustion) on a regular basis. Intensive, exhaustive training stimulates increased storage of glycogen in the muscles and liver, which provides additional energy for greater exercise capacity.

• Consume five to six meals a day. Eating several smaller meals rather than three larger ones will keep your blood-sugar level stable throughout the day and will ensure that a supply of protein is always available for your muscles.

• Keep your fat intake to a minimum. Large amounts of fat in your diet will add to your body fat and will cause mineral loss through frequent urination.

• Consume low-glycemic-index foods about two to three hours before workouts and tournaments. These foods help sustain the blood-sugar level.

• Drink plenty of water. Not only will this practice reduce your chances of becoming dehydrated, but every ounce of glycogen that is stored within the muscles needs 3 ounces of water stored along with it. Therefore, remaining properly hydrated will also help prevent weakened muscle contractions and early onset of fatigue.

As a bowler, you should turn to Appendix C on page 345 for full discussions of the 20:25:55 and 20:20:60 dietary plans. Also presented are sample daily diets that use common, healthy foods to meet an athlete's energy and caloric needs. Use the directions on page 150 to estimate your average daily caloric requirement. Then use the directions in Chapter 13 or 14 to adjust your diet for off-season fat loss or muscle building, respectively.

Supplementation Guidelines

In addition to eating a proper diet, you should also take dietary supplements to make sure that any nutrients you lose due to sweating or training are replenished. The following tables will help guide you in selecting the supplements appropriate for you. The first table lists the nutrients recommended for bowlers, as well as the range of intake for each nutrient. (For discussions of these nutrients, see Part One.) Note that within the ranges of intake, the lower amounts are for smaller individuals and lower-activity days, while the higher amounts are for larger individuals and higher-activity days.

RECOMMENDED NUTRIENTS AND RANGES OF INTAKE

For Bowlers

NUTRIENT	RANGE OF INTAKE
VITAMINS	
Vitamin A	8,000–16,000 IU
Beta-carotene	20,000–30,000 IU
Vitamin B$_1$ (thiamine)	30–120 mg
Vitamin B$_2$ (riboflavin)	30–120 mg
Vitamin B$_3$ (niacin)	40–80 mg
Vitamin B$_5$ (pantothenic acid)	20–100 mg
Vitamin B$_6$ (pyridoxine)	20–80 mg
Vitamin B$_{12}$ (cobalamin)	12–120 mcg
Biotin	125–175 mcg
Folate	400–800 mcg
Vitamin C	800–2,000 mg
Vitamin D	400–800 IU
Vitamin E	200–600 IU
Vitamin K	60–160 mcg
MINERALS	
Boron	2–8 mg
Calcium	800–1,500 mg
Chromium	200–500 mcg
Copper	1–4 mg
Iodine	100–200 mcg
Iron	15–50 mg
Magnesium	250–650 mg
Manganese	12–35 mg
Molybdenum	100–200 mcg
Phosphorus	150–800 mg
Potassium	50–1,000 mg
Selenium	100–200 mcg
Zinc	15–50 mg
AMINO ACIDS	
L-glutamine	1,000–2,000 mg
FATTY ACIDS	
Alpha-linolenic acid	500–1,000 mg
Docosahexaenoic acid (DHA)	250–750 mg
Eiocosapentaenoic acid (EPA)	250–750 mg
Gamma linolenic acid (GLA)	100–400 mg

NUTRIENT	RANGE OF INTAKE
Linoleic acid	2,000–4,000 mg
METABOLITES	
Bioflavonoids	200–800 mg
Choline	100–600 mg
Creatine monohydrate	4,000–8,000 mg
Ferulic acid	50–100 mg
Inosine	500–1,000 mg
Inositol	100–600 mg
L-carnitine	750–1,500 mg
Octacosanol	3,000–6,000 mcg

IU = international units, mcg = micrograms, mg = milligrams.

The second table lists the different kinds of sports supplements available and indicates if their use by bowlers is recommended in the preseason, during the season, or directly before a tournament. The list also includes a number of popular nutritional practices—bicarbonate loading, carbohydrate loading, creatine and/or inosine loading, and water loading. (For a discussion of any of these supplements or practices, see the appropriate section in Part One or Part Three.)

RECOMMENDED SPORTS SUPPLEMENTS AND NUTRITIONAL PRACTICES

For Bowlers

	Intake Recommendation		
	PRESEASON	SEASON	PRE-TOURNAMENT
SUPPLEMENTS			
Multivitamins	Yes	Yes	No
Multiminerals	Yes	Yes	No
Antioxidants	Yes	Yes	No
Fatty acids	Yes	Yes	No
Metabolites	Optional	Yes	Yes
Branched-chain amino acids	Yes	Yes	Yes
Herbs	Yes	Yes	No
Low-calorie protein drink (200–300 calories)	Yes	Yes	Yes
Carbohydrate drink	Yes	Yes	Yes
Fat-burning supplement	Yes	Optional	No
PRACTICES			
Bicarbonate loading	No	No	No
Carbohydrate loading	No	No	No
Creatine and/or inosine loading	Optional	Yes	Yes
Water loading	No	No	Optional

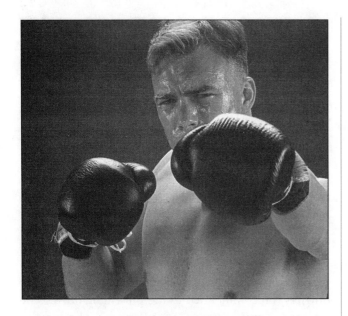

BOXING

Includes Professional and Amateur

Boxing, both professional and amateur, involves a wide range of skills and movements. It requires not only speed and strength in short, explosive bursts, but also a high level of anaerobic-strength endurance, as well as flexibility and agility.

Every bit of your training and diet must reflect these important elements. These elements are what make boxing explosive in nature. In fact, boxing is very explosive, so improved recovery and tissue repair plus increased speed and strength are your year-round training and dietary goals. Nutritionally, this means emphasizing short-term energy needs and maximizing the muscles' recovery and tissue-repair processes.

In boxing, the energy output is primarily anaerobic (without oxygen). This does not mean that training for or competing in boxing is easy, however. You must punch, grapple, dodge, feint, jab, and perform other lightning-quick reflexive movements over and over again, repeatedly testing your tolerance to pain and fatigue, caused by lactic-acid buildup in your muscles. Training for boxing is extremely intensive and grueling. At the highest levels, speed training for boxing forces you to operate at your anaerobic threshold (the point at which you must receive oxygen).

Muscles grow when they are stressed. In boxing, the aim is to make the muscles grow as strong and as quick as possible. This calls for specialized training. Furthermore, the incredible force output of boxing,

expecially coupled with the explosive aspects of the sport, requires the support of a carefully constructed nutrition program.

ENERGY SOURCES OF BOXERS

The muscles rely on three major systems to supply the energy they need—the immediate, glycolytic, and oxidative energy systems. For short-term energy for explosive-strength output, the muscles depend on the immediate energy systems. The immediate energy systems are nonoxidative—that is, they do not use oxygen. Instead, these systems generate energy through the use of adenosine triphosphate (ATP) and creatine phosphate (CP). CP is produced in the body and stored in the muscle fibers. It is broken down by enzymes to regenerate ATP, which is also stored in the muscle fibers. When the ATP is in turn broken down, the result is a spark of energy that triggers a muscle contraction.

For medium-term energy for repeated near-maximum exertion, the muscles turn to the glycolytic energy systems. In these systems, which are also nonoxidative, glycogen is used to produce energy. Glycogen is the storage form of glucose. It is stored in the liver and muscles, and is readily converted back to glucose when it is needed for energy.

For long-term energy for endurance activities, the muscles use the oxidative energy systems. In these systems, oxygen is used to oxidize long-chain fatty acids, protein, and glucose, which generates energy. For athletes, getting enough oxygen can mean a winning performance rather than a second-place showing.

Every sport involves a variety of skills, and each skill utilizes a unique combination of these three energy sources. The following table shows how much your body relies on each of the energy sources during an average professional boxing match and an average amateur boxing match. Percentages are also given for two kinds of average workouts.

WHERE YOUR ENERGY COMES FROM

For Boxers		
Energy Systems		
IMMEDIATE	GLYCOLYTIC	OXIDATIVE
Average matches		
Amateur (up to 3 rounds) 60%	40%	0%

	Energy Systems		
	IMMEDIATE	GLYCOLYTIC	OXIDATIVE
Professional *(up to 15 rounds)*	50%	40%	10%
Average workouts			
Prematch	50%	40%	10%
Off-season	60%	30%	10%

When considering the type of nutritional support to give your training program, keep the following factors in mind:

☐ All athletes need to consume high-quality protein several times a day for effective recovery and adequate repair of damaged muscle tissue.

☐ Athletes whose muscles rely substantially on the immediate or glycolytic energy systems should keep their fat intake to a minimum because fat is not an efficient energy source for their intensive training, which is almost exclusively anaerobic in nature. Since the fat calories consumed by these athletes are not generally used for energy, they are stored as body fat.

☐ All athletes should consume a carefully measured amount of high-quality carbohydrates several times a day to ensure an adequate supply of energy.

☐ The carbohydrates in all preworkout meals should consist of foods with low glycemic indexes to ensure that training intensity does not wane and that muscle tissue is not cannibalized for energy. (For the glycemic indexes of some common foods, see page 29.)

The aim of your nutrition program is to make your body healthy enough to accomplish recovery and tissue repair speedily and efficiently—without adding body fat. Your further aims are to do this while maintaining a high strength-to-weight ratio plus remaining within 3 to 4 percent of your competition body weight. These aims alone make diet as critical as training for boxers. You must eat just the right amount of food. Eat the wrong foods or the wrong amounts just a few times too often and you will sabotage your fitness efforts. Even more important, do not be in a hurry. It takes *years* to become a great boxer. Rush the nutrition and training processes and you will become fat, your recovery rate will decline, and your injury rate will rise.

NUTRITION FOR BOXERS

Boxers are power athletes. They obtain most of their

energy from the immediate energy systems. Therefore, as a boxer, you need to plan your nutritional intake, from both food and supplement sources, to support the immediate systems. In addition, since your energy expenditure changes in the off-season, you need to adjust your caloric intake and macronutrient ratio to match. Following are dietary guidelines for boxers to help you in planning your nutrition program. Supplementation guidelines for boxers can be found on page 218.

Dietary Guidelines

The following pie charts illustrate how you should divide up your caloric intake to match the energy demands of boxing during the preseason, season, and off-season. They show the target percentages of fat, protein, and carbohydrates that your five to six meals should supply each day.

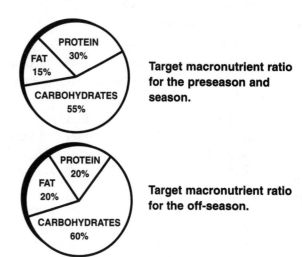

Target macronutrient ratio for the preseason and season.

Target macronutrient ratio for the off-season.

Note that fat has about 9 calories per gram, while protein and carbohydrates have only 4 calories per gram. Therefore, during the season, if you needed to consume a total of 2,500 calories per day, you would aim for 375 calories (15 percent of your total daily calories) from fat, 750 calories (30 percent of your total daily calories) from protein, and the remaining 1,375 calories (55 percent of your total daily calories) from carbohydrates.

Some other important considerations for boxers are:

☐ Carbohydrates are the major source of energy for short-term activities. Complex carbohydrates are the best source because they most effectively refill the glycogen stores in the muscles and liver. In addition, they elevate the blood sugar to a level sufficient for long sessions of intensive training.

☐ As a power athlete, you must make sure that you consume adequate amounts of both carbohydrates and protein. If your energy stores become drastically depleted or you experience lactic-acid buildup, you may suffer temporary muscle fatigue. If you do not refill your glycogen stores before your next workout or match, your body may begin breaking down muscle tissue for the protein it needs for energy.

☐ Directly before workouts and matches, consume carbohydrate drinks with high glycemic indexes to keep your blood sugar sustained at an appropriate level. This will allow you to train or compete intensively without having your explosiveness hindered by fatigue.

☐ As a power athlete, you need to stimulate the storage of glycogen in your muscles while promoting repair and growth of your muscle tissue and inhibiting buildup of body fat. To do this:

• Train anaerobically on a regular basis. Intensive training stimulates increased storage of glycogen in the muscles and liver, which provides additional energy for greater exercise capacity.

• Consume five to six meals a day. Eating several smaller meals rather than three larger ones will keep your blood-sugar level stable throughout the day and will ensure that a supply of protein is always available for your muscles.

• Keep your fat intake to a minimum. Large amounts of fat in your diet will add to your body fat and will cause you to lose minerals through frequent urination.

• Consume low-glycemic-index foods about two to three hours before workouts and matches. These foods help sustain the blood-sugar level.

• Drink plenty of water. Not only will this practice reduce your chances of becoming dehydrated, but every ounce of glycogen that is stored within the muscles needs 3 ounces of water stored along with it. Therefore, remaining properly hydrated will also help prevent weakened muscle contractions.

• Do not eat a new food just before a match. Different people often react differently to the same food. Before a match, eat just those foods that you know your body will handle well.

As a boxer, you should turn to Appendix C on page 345 for full discussions of the 15:30:55 and 20:20:60 dietary plans. Also presented are sample daily diets that use common, healthy foods to meet an athlete's energy and caloric needs. Use the directions on page 150 to estimate your average daily caloric requirement. Then use the directions in Chapter 13 or 14 to adjust your diet for off-season fat loss or muscle building, respectively.

Supplementation Guidelines

In addition to eating a proper diet, you should also take dietary supplements to make sure that any nutrients you lose due to sweating or training are replenished. The following tables will help guide you in selecting the supplements appropriate for you. The first table lists the nutrients recommended for boxers, as well as the range of intake for each nutrient. (For discussions of these nutrients, see Part One.) Note that within the ranges of intake, the lower amounts are for smaller individuals and lower-activity days, while the higher amounts are for larger individuals and higher-activity days.

RECOMMENDED NUTRIENTS AND RANGES OF INTAKE

For Boxers	
NUTRIENT	**RANGE OF INTAKE**
VITAMINS	
Vitamin A	8,000–16,000 IU
Beta-carotene	20,000–30,000 IU
Vitamin B_1 (thiamine)	30–120 mg
Vitamin B_2 (riboflavin)	30–120 mg
Vitamin B_3 (niacin)	40–80 mg
Vitamin B_5 (pantothenic acid)	20–100 mg
Vitamin B_6 (pyridoxine)	20–80 mg
Vitamin B_{12} (cobalamin)	12–120 mcg
Biotin	125–175 mcg
Folate	400–800 mcg
Vitamin C	800–2,000 mg
Vitamin D	400–800 IU
Vitamin E	200–600 IU
Vitamin K	60–160 mcg
MINERALS	
Boron	2–8 mg
Calcium	800–1,500 mg
Chromium	200–500 mcg
Copper	1–4 mg
Iodine	100–200 mcg

NUTRIENT	RANGE OF INTAKE
Iron	15–50 mg
Magnesium	250–650 mg
Manganese	12–35 mg
Molybdenum	100–200 mcg
Phosphorus	150–800 mg
Potassium	50–1,000 mg
Selenium	100–200 mcg
Zinc	15–50 mg
AMINO ACIDS	
L-glutamine	1,000–2,000 mg
FATTY ACIDS	
Alpha-linolenic acid	500–1,000 mg
Docosahexaenoic acid (DHA)	250–750 mg
Eiocosapentaenoic acid (EPA)	250–750 mg
Gamma linolenic acid (GLA)	100–400 mg
Linoleic acid	3,000–6,000 mg
METABOLITES	
Bioflavonoids	200–800 mg
Choline	100–600 mg
Creatine monohydrate	4,000–12,000 mg
Ferulic acid	50–100 mg
Glucosamine	750–1,500 mg
Inosine	500–1,000 mg
Inositol	100–600 mg
L-carnitine	750–2,000 mg
Octacosanol	1,000–3,000 mcg

IU = international units, mcg = micrograms, mg = milligrams.

The second table lists the different types of sport supplements available and indicates if their use by boxers is recommended in the preseason, during the season, or directly before a match. The list also includes a number of popular nutritional practices—bicarbonate loading, carbohydrate loading, creatine and/or inosine loading, and water loading. (For a discussion of any of these supplements or practices, see the appropriate section in Part One or Part Three.)

RECOMMENDED SPORTS SUPPLEMENTS AND NUTRITIONAL PRACTICES

For Boxers

	Intake Recommendation		
	PRESEASON	SEASON	PREMATCH
SUPPLEMENTS			
Multivitamins	Yes	Yes	No
Multiminerals	Yes	Yes	No

	Intake Recommendation		
	PRESEASON	SEASON	PREMATCH
Antioxidants	Yes	Yes	No
Fatty acids	Yes	Yes	No
Metabolites	Optional	Yes	Yes
Branched-chain amino acids	Yes	Yes	Yes
Herbs	Yes	Yes	No
Low-calorie protein drink (200–300 calories)	Yes	Yes	Yes
Carbohydrate drink	Yes	Yes	Yes
Fat-burning supplement	Yes	Optional	No
PRACTICES			
Bicarbonate loading	No	Optional	Yes
Carbohydrate loading	No	No	Optional
Creatine and/or inosine loading	Optional	Yes	Yes
Water loading	No	No	Optional

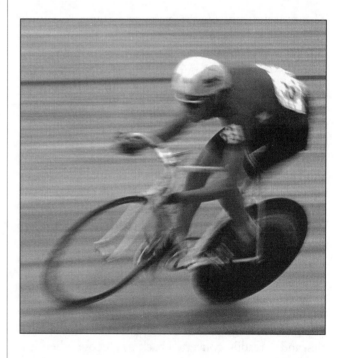

CYCLING

Also for Cyclocross and Mountain Biking

What kind of cyclist are you? If you are a combination power–middle-distance cyclist, your energy comes primarily from the immediate and glycolytic energy systems and you must eat and train accordingly. If you are an endurance cyclist, you need to focus the bulk of your nutrition and training efforts on building up your oxidative energy reserves. However, if you enjoy both kinds of cycling, you should combine your nutrition and training programs, stressing one only as a competition nears.

No matter what type of cyclist you are, you cannot completely ignore any facet of the sport. You must address each skill to some extent, whether you use it on a regular basis or not. All good cyclists are able to, for example, break away, climb hills, and sprint at the end of a race. Therefore, your training, both on and off your bicycle, should develop strength, anaerobic or aerobic endurance, and speed-strength equally. This calls for specialized training. Furthermore, the diverse energy output called for in cycling because of the variety of events requires the support of a carefully constructed nutrition program.

ENERGY SOURCES OF CYCLISTS

The muscles rely on three major systems to supply the energy they need—the immediate, glycolytic, and oxidative energy systems. For short-term energy for explosive-strength output, the muscles depend on the immediate energy systems. The immediate energy systems are nonoxidative—that is, they do not use oxygen. Instead, these systems generate energy through the use of adenosine triphosphate (ATP) and creatine phosphate (CP). CP is produced in the body and stored in the muscle fibers. It is broken down by enzymes to regenerate ATP, which is also stored in the muscle fibers. When the ATP is in turn broken down, the result is a spark of energy that triggers a muscle contraction.

For medium-term energy for repeated near-maximum exertion, the muscles turn to the glycolytic energy systems. In these systems, which are also nonoxidative, glycogen is used to produce energy. Glycogen is the storage form of glucose. It is stored in the liver and muscles, and is readily converted back to glucose when it is needed for energy.

For long-term energy for endurance activities, the muscles use the oxidative energy systems. In these systems, oxygen is used to oxidize long-chain fatty acids, protein, and glucose, which generates energy. For athletes, getting enough oxygen can mean a winning performance rather than a second-place showing.

Every sport involves a variety of skills, and each skill utilizes a unique combination of these three energy sources. The following table lists a number of major cycling events and shows how much your body relies on each of the energy sources when you compete in them. Percentages are also given for two similar sports.

WHERE YOUR ENERGY COMES FROM

For Cyclists		
Energy Systems		
IMMEDIATE	GLYCOLYTIC	OXIDATIVE
Criteria, 25 miles		

	IMMEDIATE	GLYCOLYTIC	OXIDATIVE
Criteria, 25 miles	0%	5%	95%
Criteria, 100 kilometers	0%	5%	95%
Kilometer	30%	50%	20%
Match sprint	30%	60%	10%
Pursuit, individual, 4,000 meters	10%	20%	70%
Pursuit, team, 4,000 meters	10%	20%	70%
Road race, 100 miles	0%	5%	95%
Time trial, team, 25 miles	0%	2%	98%
Time trial, team, 100 kilometers	0%	2%	98%
Track, 10 miles	5%	10%	85%

For Similar Sports			
Cyclocross	20%	30%	50%
Mountain biking	20%	30%	50%

When considering the type of nutritional support to give your training program, keep the following factors in mind:

☐ All athletes need to consume high-quality protein several times a day for effective recovery and adequate repair of damaged muscle tissue.

☐ Athletes whose muscles rely substantially on the immediate or glycolytic energy systems should keep their fat intake to a minimum because fat is not an efficient energy source for their intensive training, which is almost exclusively anaerobic in nature. Since the fat calories consumed by these athletes are not generally used for energy, they are stored as body fat.

☐ Athletes whose muscles rely substantially on the oxidative energy systems can eat more fat because their energy is manufactured through the oxidation of fatty acids. But even these athletes should watch their fat calories if they train aerobically (with oxygen) for less than half an hour at a time.

☐ All athletes should consume a carefully measured amount of high-quality carbohydrates several times a day to ensure an adequate supply of energy.

☐ The carbohydrates in all preworkout meals should consist of foods with low glycemic indexes to ensure that training intensity does not wane and that muscle tissue is not cannibalized for energy. (For the glycemic indexes of some common foods, see page 29.)

The aim of your nutrition program is to make your body healthy enough to accomplish recovery and tissue repair speedily and efficiently—without adding body fat. Your further aim is to do this while maintaining a high strength-to-weight ratio. These aims alone make diet very important for cyclists. You must eat just the right amount of food. Eat the wrong foods or the wrong amounts just a few times too often and you will sabotage your fitness efforts.

NUTRITION FOR CYCLISTS

Cyclists are either combination power–middle-distance athletes or endurance athletes. Depending on the type of cycling they specialize in, they obtain most of their energy from a combination of the immediate and glycolytic energy systems or from the oxidative energy systems. Therefore, as a cyclist, you need to plan your nutritional intake, from both food and supplement sources, to support the appropriate systems. In addition, if you are a combination power–middle-distance cyclist, your energy expenditure changes in the off-season and you need to adjust your caloric intake and macronutrient ratio to match. Following are dietary and supplementation guidelines for combination power–middle-distance cyclists to help you in planning your nutrition program. Dietary and supplementation guidelines for endurance cyclists can be found on page 223.

COMBINATION POWER–MIDDLE-DISTANCE CYCLISTS

Cyclists who compete in events that last less than about twenty minutes are combination power–middle-distance athletes. Among the typical events they participate in are the match sprint and 10-mile track.

Dietary Guidelines

The following pie charts illustrate how you should divide up your caloric intake to match the energy demands of power–middle-distance cycling during the preseason, season, and off-season. They show the target percentages of fat, protein, and carbohydrates that your five to six meals should supply each day.

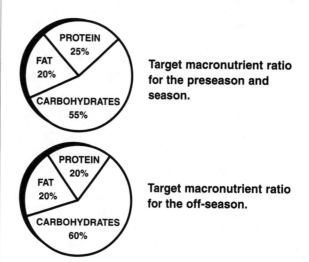

Target macronutrient ratio for the preseason and season.

Target macronutrient ratio for the off-season.

Note that fat has about 9 calories per gram, while protein and carbohydrates have only 4 calories per gram. Therefore, during the season, if you needed to consume a total of 2,500 calories per day, you would aim for 500 calories (20 percent of your total daily calories) from fat, 625 calories (25 percent of your total daily calories) from protein, and the remaining 1,375 calories (55 percent of your total daily calories) from carbohydrates.

Some other important considerations for combination power–middle-distance cyclists are:

☐ Carbohydrates are the major source of energy for short-term activities. Complex carbohydrates are the best source because they most effectively refill the glycogen stores in the muscles and liver. In addition, they elevate the blood sugar to a level sufficient for long sessions of intensive training.

☐ As a combination power–middle-distance athlete, you must make sure that you consume adequate amounts of both carbohydrates and protein. If your energy stores become drastically depleted or you experience lactic-acid buildup, you may suffer temporary muscle fatigue. If you do not refill your glycogen stores before your next workout or competition, your body may begin breaking down muscle tissue for the protein it needs for energy.

☐ Directly before workouts and competitions, consume carbohydrate drinks with high glycemic indexes to keep your blood sugar sustained at an appropriate level. This will allow you to train or compete intensively without having your explosiveness hindered by fatigue.

☐ As a combination power–middle-distance athlete, you need to stimulate the storage of glycogen in your muscles while promoting repair and growth of your muscle tissue and inhibiting buildup of body fat. To do this:

• Train anaerobically on a regular basis. Intensive training stimulates increased storage of glycogen in the muscles and liver, which provides additional energy for greater exercise capacity.

• Consume five to six meals a day. Eating several smaller meals rather than three larger ones will keep your blood-sugar level stable throughout the day and will ensure that a supply of protein is always available for your muscles.

• Keep your fat intake to a minimum. Large amounts of fat in your diet will add to your body fat and will cause you to lose minerals through frequent urination.

• Consume low-glycemic-index foods about two to three hours before workouts and competitions. These foods help sustain the blood-sugar level.

• Drink plenty of water. Not only will this practice reduce your chances of becoming dehydrated, but every ounce of glycogen that is stored within the muscles needs 3 ounces of water stored along with it. Therefore, remaining properly hydrated will also help prevent weakened muscle contractions.

• Do not eat a new food just before a competition. Different people often react differently to the same food. Before a competition, eat just those foods that you know your body will handle well.

As a combination power–middle-distance cyclist, you should turn to Appendix C on page 345 for full discussions of the 20:25:55 and 20:20:60 dietary plans. Also presented are sample daily diets that use common, healthy foods to meet an athlete's energy and caloric needs. Use the directions on page 150 to estimate your average daily caloric requirement. Then use the directions in Chapter 13 or 14 to

adjust your diet for off-season fat loss or muscle building, respectively.

Supplementation Guidelines

In addition to eating a proper diet, you should also take dietary supplements to make sure that any nutrients you lose due to sweating or training are replenished. The following tables will help guide you in selecting the supplements appropriate for you. The first table lists the nutrients recommended for combination power–middle-distance cyclists, as well as the range of intake for each nutrient. (For discussions of these nutrients, see Part One.) Note that within the ranges of intake, the lower amounts are for smaller individuals and lower-activity days, while the higher amounts are for larger individuals and higher-activity days.

RECOMMENDED NUTRIENTS AND RANGES OF INTAKE

For Combination Power–Middle-Distance Cyclists

NUTRIENT	RANGE OF INTAKE
VITAMINS	
Vitamin A	8,000–16,000 IU
Beta-carotene	25,000–35,000 IU
Vitamin B₁ (thiamine)	40–120 mg
Vitamin B₂ (riboflavin)	40–120 mg
Vitamin B₃ (niacin)	20–40 mg
Vitamin B₅ (pantothenic acid)	20–100 mg
Vitamin B₆ (pyridoxine)	20–80 mg
Vitamin B₁₂ (cobalamin)	12–120 mcg
Biotin	125–175 mcg
Folate	400–800 mcg
Vitamin C	800–2,000 mg
Vitamin D	400–800 IU
Vitamin E	200–800 IU
Vitamin K	60–160 mcg
MINERALS	
Boron	2–8 mg
Calcium	800–1,500 mg
Chromium	200–500 mcg
Copper	1–4 mg
Iodine	100–200 mcg
Iron	15–50 mg
Magnesium	250–650 mg
Manganese	12–35 mg

NUTRIENT	RANGE OF INTAKE
Molybdenum	100–200 mcg
Phosphorus	150–800 mg
Potassium	50–1,000 mg
Selenium	100–200 mcg
Zinc	15–50 mg
AMINO ACIDS	
L-glutamic acid	500–1,000 mg
L-glutamine	1,000–2,000 mg
FATTY ACIDS	
Alpha-linolenic acid	500–1,000 mg
Docosahexaenoic acid (DHA)	250–750 mg
Eiocosapentaenoic acid (EPA)	250–750 mg
Gamma linolenic acid (GLA)	100–400 mg
Linoleic acid	2,000–3,000 mg
METABOLITES	
Bioflavonoids	300–800 mg
Choline	200–600 mg
Creatine monohydrate	6,000–12,000 mg
Inosine	500–1,500 mg
Inositol	200–600 mg
L-carnitine	500–1,500 mg

IU = international units, mcg = micrograms, mg = milligrams.

The second table lists the different types of sports supplements available and indicates if their use by combination power–middle-distance cyclists is recommended in the preseason, during the season, or directly before a competition. The list also includes a number of popular nutritional practices—bicarbonate loading, carbohydrate loading, creatine and/or inosine loading, and water loading. (For a discussion of any of these supplements or practices, see the appropriate section in Part One or Part Three.)

RECOMMENDED SPORTS SUPPLEMENTS AND NUTRITIONAL PRACTICES

For Combination Power–Middle-Distance Cyclists

	Intake Recommendation		
	PRESEASON	SEASON	PRE-COMPETITION
SUPPLEMENTS			
Multivitamins	Yes	Yes	No
Multiminerals	Yes	Yes	No
Antioxidants	Yes	Yes	No
Fatty acids	Yes	Yes	No

Intake Recommendation

	PRESEASON	SEASON	PRE-COMPETITION
Metabolites	Optional	Yes	Yes
Branched-chain amino acids	Yes	Yes	Yes
Herbs	Yes	Yes	No
Medium-calorie protein drink (300–500 calories)	Yes	Yes	Yes
Carbohydrate drink	Yes	Yes	Yes
Fat-burning supplement	Yes	Optional	No
PRACTICES			
Bicarbonate loading	No	Optional	Optional
Carbohydrate loading	No	No	No
Creatine and/or inosine loading	No	Yes	Yes
Water loading	No	No	No

ENDURANCE CYCLISTS

Cyclists who compete in events that last longer than about twenty minutes are endurance athletes. Among the typical events they participate in are the 25-mile criteria, 4,000-meter pursuit, and 100-mile road race.

Dietary Guidelines

The following pie chart illustrates how you should divide up your caloric intake to match the energy demands of endurance cycling during the preseason, season, and off-season. It shows the target percentages of fat, protein, and carbohydrates that your five to six meals should supply each day.

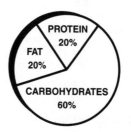

Target macronutrient ratio for the preseason, season, and off-season.

Note that fat has about 9 calories per gram, while protein and carbohydrates have only 4 calories per gram. Therefore, if you needed to consume a total of 2,500 calories per day, you would aim for 500 calories (20 percent of your total daily calories) from fat, 500 calories (20 percent of your total daily calories) from protein, and the remaining 1,500 calories (60 percent of your total daily calories) from carbohydrates.

Some other important considerations for endurance cyclists are:

☐ The energy source that is used during an aerobic activity depends upon the duration and intensity of the activity. During the first one and a half to two hours, both glycogen and body fat are the primary sources of energy. After one and a half to two hours, body fat alone becomes the primary source.

☐ While body fat is the primary source of energy during prolonged aerobic activities, it cannot be used efficiently unless some glycogen remains in the muscles and liver. Therefore, even ultra-endurance athletes must make sure to always keep their glycogen stores filled.

☐ As an endurance athlete, you need to encourage glycogen sparing in your body while stimulating the use of fat as your primary energy source. To do this:

• Train for endurance on a regular basis. Regular endurance training stimulates increased storage of both glycogen and fatty acids.

• Consume five to six meals a day. Eating several smaller meals rather than three larger ones will keep your blood-sugar level stable throughout the day.

• Do not load up on dietary fat. Consuming large amounts of fat was originally thought to benefit endurance athletes, whose primary source of energy is fat. However, fat loading can lead to frequent urination, which increases the loss of minerals essential to healthy heart action.

• Consume low-glycemic-index foods about two to three hours before workouts and competitions. These foods help sustain the blood-sugar level.

• Do not consume food or caloric beverages from two hours before an endurance activity to fifteen minutes before. Food and caloric beverages cause the insulin level to rise, which in turn can provoke transient hypoglycemia. Transient hypoglycemia interferes with the energy dynamics during exercise and can induce early onset of fatigue.

• Consume carbohydrates directly before and during endurance activities. Because exercise slows the release of insulin into the bloodstream, the ingestion of carbohydrates spares glycogen and allows the use of fat for energy. Carbohydrate drinks with high glycemic indexes help sustain the blood-sugar level, thereby preserving glycogen stores.

• During endurance activities, drink plenty of water.

Endurance activities cause profuse sweating, which results in loss of valuable fluids and minerals. Dehydration not only reduces performance but can seriously affect health.

• Drink electrolyte-containing beverages during endurance activities. These drinks help replace minerals that are lost through sweating.

• During endurance activities, drink 4 to 6 ounces of fluid every fifteen to thirty minutes. For every pound of body weight lost through sweating, 1 pint of fluid should be consumed. Chilled fluids are absorbed the quickest.

• Do not eat a new food just before a competition. Different people often react differently to the same food. Before a competition, eat just those foods that you know your body will handle well.

As an endurance cyclist, you should turn to Appendix C on page 345 for a full discussion of the 20:20:60 dietary plan. Also presented are sample daily diets that use common, healthy foods to meet an athlete's energy and caloric needs. Use the directions on page 150 to estimate your average daily caloric requirement. Then use the directions in Chapter 13 or 14 to adjust your diet for off-season fat loss or muscle building, respectively.

Supplementation Guidelines

In addition to eating a proper diet, you should also take dietary supplements to make sure that any nutrients you lose due to sweating or training are replenished. The following tables will help guide you in selecting the supplements appropriate for you. The first table lists the nutrients recommended for endurance cyclists, as well as the range of intake for each nutrient. (For discussions of these nutrients, see Part One.) Note that within the ranges of intake, the lower amounts are for smaller individuals and lower-activity days, while the higher amounts are for larger individuals and higher-activity days.

RECOMMENDED NUTRIENTS AND RANGES OF INTAKE

For Endurance Cyclists	
NUTRIENT	RANGE OF INTAKE
VITAMINS	
Vitamin A	8,000–16,000 IU
Beta-carotene	30,000–60,000 IU

NUTRIENT	RANGE OF INTAKE
Vitamin B₁ (thiamine)	100–250 mg
Vitamin B₂ (riboflavin)	100–200 mg
Vitamin B₃ (niacin)	10–20 mg
Vitamin B₅ (pantothenic acid)	100–200 mg
Vitamin B₆ (pyridoxine)	20–80 mg
Vitamin B₁₂ (cobalamin)	12–120 mcg
Biotin	125–200 mcg
Folate	400–800 mcg
Vitamin C	1,000–2,000 mg
Vitamin D	400–800 IU
Vitamin E	400–1,000 IU
Vitamin K	60–160 mcg
MINERALS	
Boron	2–8 mg
Calcium	800–1,500 mg
Chromium	200–500 mcg
Copper	1–4 mg
Iodine	100–200 mcg
Iron	15–50 mg
Magnesium	250–650 mg
Manganese	12–35 mg
Molybdenum	100–200 mcg
Phosphorus	150–800 mg
Potassium	50–1,000 mg
Selenium	100–200 mcg
Zinc	15–50 mg
AMINO ACIDS	
L-glutamic acid	1,000–1,500 mg
L-glutamine	1,000–2,000 mg
FATTY ACIDS	
Alpha-linolenic acid	500–1,000 mg
Docosahexaenoic acid (DHA)	400–1,000 mg
Eiocosapentaenoic acid (EPA)	400–1,000 mg
Gamma linolenic acid (GLA)	200–500 mg
Linoleic acid	500–1,000 mg
METABOLITES	
Bioflavonoids	500–1,000 mg
Choline	500–1,000 mg
Coenzyme Q₁₀	60–120 mg
Inositol	500–1,000 mg
L-carnitine	1,000–3,000 mg
Octacosanol	1,000–2,000 mcg
OTHER	
Caffeine*	200–400 mg

IU = international units, mcg = micrograms, mg = milligrams.

*Verify with your sports governing organization that caffeine consumption is permitted during competition.

The second table lists the different types of sports supplements available and indicates if their use by endurance cyclists is recommended in the preseason, during the season, or directly before a competition. The list also includes a number of popular nutritional practices—bicarbonate loading, carbohydrate loading, creatine and/or inosine loading, and water loading. (For a discussion of any of these supplements or practices, see the appropriate section in Part One or Part Three.)

RECOMMENDED SPORTS SUPPLEMENTS AND NUTRITIONAL PRACTICES

For Endurance Cyclists

	Intake Recommendation		
	PRESEASON	SEASON	PRE-COMPETITION
SUPPLEMENTS			
Multivitamins	Yes	Yes	No
Multiminerals	Yes	Yes	No
Antioxidants	Yes	Yes	Yes
Fatty acids	Yes	Yes	No
Metabolites	Optional	Yes	Yes
Branched-chain amino acids	Yes	Yes	Yes
Herbs	Yes	Yes	No
High-calorie protein drink (over 500 calories)	Yes	Yes	Yes
Carbohydrate drink with glycerol and electrolytes	Yes	Yes	Yes
Fat-burning supplement	Yes	No	No
PRACTICES			
Bicarbonate loading	No	No	No
Carbohydrate loading	No	No	Yes
Creatine and/or inosine loading	No	No	No
Water loading	No	No	Yes

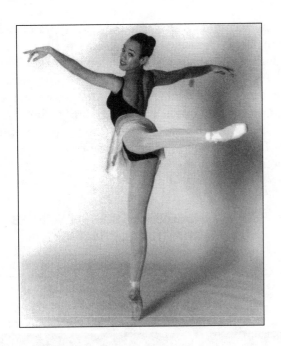

DANCING

Includes Ballet, Ballroom Dancing, Break Dancing, Fast Dancing, Ice Dancing, and Other Forms of Dancing

Since the beginning of time, men and women have danced. We dance together, and we dance alone. We dance to summon spirits, and we dance to thank them. We dance for social, sexual, and political reasons, and we dance just for the fun of it. It is said that we each, just like each individual culture in this world, dance to the beat of our own drummer.

So true is this old adage, in fact, that it is almost impossible to judge the energy expenditures of two people dancing even to the *same* drummer! These two people may be dancing with different verve or passion, they may be dancing with different kinds of steps, or they may simply be dancing to their individual rhythms.

Many people dance because it is their profession. Many more people dance just to have fun. Whether you dance for fun or for profit, if you take your dancing seriously enough to want to maximize your performance capabilities, you should apply the rules of performance nutrition and train like an athlete.

Almost all forms of dance require a variety of skills. A dancer must be a combination acrobat, leaper, and even weight lifter to execute the fundamental movements of the discipline. Dance conditioning, there-

fore, must take each of these areas into account.

Only the most rigorous training and nutrition program can prepare a dancer for a truly top-level performance. And although you probably will not be training for such a performance, you can still follow the routines practiced by the professionals to improve your skills and give your conditioning efforts a boost. Increased strength can make you a better dancer, even if you are strictly a social dancer.

Through the careful application of scientific training techniques, you can multiply your on-floor effectiveness in all areas of the discipline. You can improve your jumping ability, lifting ability, endurance, agility, and body control, dancing better even when you are fatigued. Furthermore, the incredible diversity of skills and energy demands of all forms of dance require the support of a carefully constructed nutrition program.

ENERGY SOURCES OF DANCERS

The muscles rely on three major systems to supply the energy they need—the immediate, glycolytic, and oxidative energy systems. For short-term energy for explosive-strength output, the muscles depend on the immediate energy systems. The immediate energy systems are nonoxidative—that is, they do not use oxygen. Instead, these systems generate energy through the use of adenosine triphosphate (ATP) and creatine phosphate (CP). CP is produced in the body and stored in the muscle fibers. It is broken down by enzymes to regenerate ATP, which is also stored in the muscle fibers. When the ATP is in turn broken down, the result is a spark of energy that triggers a muscle contraction.

For medium-term energy for repeated near-maximum exertion, the muscles turn to the glycolytic energy systems. In these systems, which are also nonoxidative, glycogen is used to produce energy. Glycogen is the storage form of glucose. It is stored in the liver and muscles, and is readily converted back to glucose when it is needed for energy.

For long-term energy for endurance activities, the muscles use the oxidative energy systems. In these systems, oxygen is used to oxidize long-chain fatty acids, protein, and glucose, which generates energy. For athletes, getting enough oxygen can mean a winning performance rather than a second-place showing.

Every activity involves a variety of skills, and each skill utilizes a unique combination of these three energy sources. The following table lists a number of major forms of dance and shows how much your body relies on each of the energy sources when you do them.

WHERE YOUR ENERGY COMES FROM

For Dancers

	Energy Systems		
	IMMEDIATE	GLYCOLYTIC	OXIDATIVE
Ballet	30%	50%	20%
Ballroom dancing	90%	10%	0%
Break dancing	90%	10%	0%
Fast dancing (such as bee-bop, hip-hop, and the jitterbug)	70%	30%	0%
Ice dancing	70%	30%	0%

When considering the type of nutritional support to give your training program, keep the following factors in mind:

☐ All athletes need to consume high-quality protein several times a day for effective recovery and adequate repair of damaged muscle tissue.

☐ Athletes whose muscles rely substantially on the immediate or glycolytic energy systems should keep their fat intake to a minimum because fat is not an efficient energy source for their intensive training, which is almost exclusively anaerobic in nature. Since the fat calories consumed by these athletes are not generally used for energy, they are stored as body fat.

☐ Athletes whose muscles rely substantially on the oxidative energy systems can eat more fat because their energy is manufactured through the oxidation of fatty acids. But even these athletes should watch their fat calories if they train aerobically (with oxygen) for less than half an hour at a time.

☐ All athletes should consume a carefully measured amount of high-quality carbohydrates several times a day to ensure an adequate supply of energy.

☐ The carbohydrates in all preworkout meals should consist of foods with low glycemic indexes to ensure that training intensity does not wane and that muscle tissue is not cannibalized for energy. (For the glycemic indexes of some common foods, see page 29.)

The aim of your nutrition program is to make your body healthy enough to accomplish recovery and tissue repair speedily and efficiently—without adding body fat. Your further aim is to do this while maintaining a high strength-to-weight ratio. These aims alone make diet very important for dancers.

You must eat just the right amount of food. Eat the wrong foods or the wrong amounts just a few times too often and you will sabotage your fitness efforts. Even more important, do not be in a hurry. It takes *years* to become a great dancer. Rush the nutrition and training processes and you will become fat, your recovery rate will decline, and your injury rate will rise.

NUTRITION FOR DANCERS

Dancers are either power or middle-distance athletes. Depending on the type of dancing they specialize in, they obtain most of their energy from the immediate energy systems or from the glycolytic energy systems. Therefore, as a dancer, you need to plan your nutritional intake, from both food and supplement sources, to support the appropriate systems. In addition, if you are a power dancer, your energy expenditure changes in the preseason and off-season, and you need to adjust your caloric intake and macronutrient ratio to match. Following are dietary and supplementation guidelines for power dancers to help you in planning your nutrition program. Dietary and supplementation guidelines for middle-distance dancers can be found on page 229.

POWER DANCERS

Dancers who perform for just minutes at a time are power athletes. Among the typical types of dancing they do are ballroom dancing and break dancing.

Dietary Guidelines

The following pie charts illustrate how you should divide up your caloric intake to match the energy demands of power dancing during the preseason, season, and off-season. They show the target percentages of fat, protein, and carbohydrates that your five to six meals should supply each day.

Note that fat has about 9 calories per gram, while protein and carbohydrates have only 4 calories per gram. Therefore, during the season, if you needed to consume a total of 2,500 calories per day, you would aim for 500 calories (20 percent of your total daily calories) from fat, 625 calories (25 percent of your total daily calories) from protein, and the remaining 1,375 calories (55 percent of your total daily calories) from carbohydrates.

227

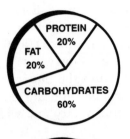

Target macronutrient ratio for the preseason and off-season.

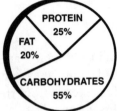

Target macronutrient ratio for the season.

Some other important considerations for power dancers are:

☐ Carbohydrates are the major source of energy for short-term activities. Complex carbohydrates are the best source because they most effectively refill the glycogen stores in the muscles and liver. In addition, they elevate the blood sugar to a level sufficient for long sessions of intensive training.

☐ As a power athlete, you must make sure that you consume adequate amounts of both carbohydrates and protein. If your energy stores become drastically depleted or you experience lactic-acid buildup, you may suffer temporary muscle fatigue. If you do not refill your glycogen stores before your next workout or performance, your body may begin breaking down muscle tissue for the protein it needs for energy.

☐ Directly before workouts and performances, consume carbohydrate drinks with high glycemic indexes to keep your blood sugar sustained at an appropriate level. This will allow you to train or perform intensively without having your explosiveness hindered by fatigue.

☐ As a power athlete, you need to stimulate the storage of glycogen in your muscles while promoting repair and growth of your muscle tissue and inhibiting buildup of body fat. To do this:

• Train anaerobically on a regular basis. Intensive training stimulates increased storage of glycogen in the muscles and liver, which provides additional energy for greater exercise capacity.

• Consume five to six meals a day. Eating several smaller meals rather than three larger ones will keep your blood-sugar level stable throughout the day and

will ensure that a supply of protein is always available for your muscles.

• Keep your fat intake to a minimum. Large amounts of fat in your diet will add to your body fat and will cause you to lose minerals through frequent urination.

• Consume low-glycemic-index foods about two to three hours before workouts and performances. These foods help sustain the blood-sugar level.

• Drink plenty of water. Not only will this practice reduce your chances of becoming dehydrated, but every ounce of glycogen that is stored within the muscles needs 3 ounces of water stored along with it. Therefore, remaining properly hydrated will also help prevent weakened muscle contractions.

As a power dancer, you should turn to Appendix C on page 345 for full discussions of the 20:20:60 and 20:25:55 dietary plans. Also presented are sample daily diets that use common, healthy foods to meet an athlete's energy and caloric needs. Use the directions on page 150 to estimate your average daily caloric requirement. Then use the directions in Chapter 13 or 14 to adjust your diet for off-season fat loss or muscle building, respectively.

Supplementation Guidelines

In addition to eating a proper diet, you should also take dietary supplements to make sure that any nutrients you lose due to sweating or training are replenished. The following tables will help guide you in selecting the supplements appropriate for you. The first table lists the nutrients recommended for power dancers, as well as the range of intake for each nutrient. (For discussions of these nutrients, see Part One.) Note that within the ranges of intake, the lower amounts are for smaller individuals and lower-activity days, while the higher amounts are for larger individuals and higher-activity days.

RECOMMENDED NUTRIENTS AND RANGES OF INTAKE

For Power Dancers	
NUTRIENT	**RANGE OF INTAKE**
VITAMINS	
Vitamin A	8,000–16,000 IU
Beta-carotene	15,000–25,000 IU
Vitamin B₁ (thiamine)	40–120 mg

NUTRIENT	RANGE OF INTAKE
Vitamin B$_2$ (riboflavin)	40–120 mg
Vitamin B$_3$ (niacin)	20–40 mg
Vitamin B$_5$ (pantothenic acid)	20–100 mg
Vitamin B$_6$ (pyridoxine)	20–80 mg
Vitamin B$_{12}$ (cobalamin)	12–120 mcg
Biotin	125–175 mcg
Folate	400–800 mcg
Vitamin C	800–2,000 mg
Vitamin D	400–800 IU
Vitamin E	200–800 IU
Vitamin K	60–160 mcg
MINERALS	
Boron	2–8 mg
Calcium	800–1,500 mg
Chromium	200–500 mcg
Copper	1–4 mg
Iodine	100–200 mcg
Iron	15–50 mg
Magnesium	250–650 mg
Manganese	12–35 mg
Molybdenum	100–200 mcg
Phosphorus	150–800 mg
Potassium	50–1,000 mg
Selenium	100–200 mcg
Zinc	15–50 mg
AMINO ACIDS	
L-glutamic acid	500–1,000 mg
L-glutamine	1,000–2,000 mg
FATTY ACIDS	
Alpha-linolenic acid	500–1,000 mg
Docosahexaenoic acid (DHA)	250–750 mg
Eiocosapentaenoic acid (EPA)	250–750 mg
Gamma linolenic acid (GLA)	100–400 mg
Linoleic acid	2,000–3,000 mg
METABOLITES	
Bioflavonoids	300–800 mg
Choline	200–600 mg
Inositol	200–600 mg
L-carnitine	500–1,500 mg
Octacosanol	1,000–2,000 mcg

IU = international units, mcg = micrograms, mg = milligrams.

The second table lists the different types of sports supplements available and indicates if their use by power dancers is recommended in the preseason, during the season, or directly before a performance. The list also includes a number of popular nutritional practices—bicarbonate loading, carbohydrate loading, creatine and/or inosine loading, and water loading. (For a discussion of any of these supplements or practices, see the appropriate section in Part One or Part Three.)

RECOMMENDED SPORTS SUPPLEMENTS AND NUTRITIONAL PRACTICES

For Power Dancers

	Intake Recommendation		
	PRESEASON	SEASON	PRE-PERFORMANCE
SUPPLEMENTS			
Multivitamins	Yes	Yes	No
Multiminerals	Yes	Yes	No
Antioxidants	Yes	Yes	No
Fatty acids	Yes	Yes	No
Metabolites	Optional	Yes	Yes
Branched-chain amino acids	Yes	Yes	Yes
Herbs	Yes	Yes	No
Low-calorie protein drink (200–300 calories)	Yes	Yes	Yes
Carbohydrate drink	Yes	Yes	Yes
Fat-burning supplement	Yes	Optional	No
PRACTICES			
Bicarbonate loading	No	No	No
Carbohydrate loading	No	No	Optional
Creatine and/or inosine loading	No	No	Optional
Water loading	No	No	Optional

MIDDLE-DISTANCE DANCERS

Dancers who perform for more than just minutes at a time are middle-distance athletes. Among the typical types of dancing they do are ballet and ice dancing.

Dietary Guidelines

The pie chart below illustrates how you should divide up your caloric intake to match the energy demands of middle-distance dancing during the preseason, season, and off-season. It shows the target percentages of fat, protein, and carbohydrates that your five to six meals should supply each day.

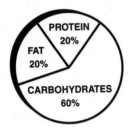

Target macronutrient ratio for the preseason, season, and off-season.

Note that fat has about 9 calories per gram, while protein and carbohydrates have only 4 calories per gram. Therefore, if you needed to consume a total of 2,500 calories per day, you would aim for 500 calories (20 percent of your total daily calories) from fat, 500 calories (20 percent of your total daily calories) from protein, and the remaining 1,500 calories (60 percent of your total daily calories) from carbohydrates.

Some other important considerations for middle-distance dancers are:

☐ Carbohydrates are the major source of energy for short-term activities. Complex carbohydrates are the best source because they most effectively refill the glycogen stores in the muscles and liver. In addition, they elevate the blood sugar to a level sufficient for long sessions of intensive training.

☐ As a middle-distance athlete, you must make sure that you consume adequate amounts of both carbohydrates and protein. If your energy stores become drastically depleted or you experience lactic-acid buildup, you may suffer temporary muscle fatigue. If you do not refill your glycogen stores before your next workout or performance, your body may begin breaking down muscle tissue for the protein it needs for energy.

☐ Directly before workouts and performances, consume carbohydrate drinks with high glycemic indexes to keep your blood sugar sustained at an appropriate level. This will allow you to train or perform intensively for longer periods of time.

☐ As a middle-distance athlete, you need to stimulate the storage of glycogen in your muscles while promoting repair and growth of your muscle tissue and inhibiting buildup of body fat. To do this:

• Train against your anaerobic threshold (to exhaus-

tion) on a regular basis. Intensive, exhaustive training stimulates increased storage of glycogen in the muscles and liver, which provides additional energy for greater exercise capacity.

• Consume five to six meals a day. Eating several smaller meals rather than three larger ones will keep your blood-sugar level stable throughout the day and will ensure that a supply of protein is always available for your muscles.

• Keep your fat intake to a minimum. Large amounts of fat in your diet will add to your body fat and will cause mineral loss through frequent urination.

• Consume low-glycemic-index foods about two to three hours before workouts and performances. These foods help sustain the blood-sugar level.

• Drink plenty of water. Not only will this practice reduce your chances of becoming dehydrated, but every ounce of glycogen that is stored within the muscles needs 3 ounces of water stored along with it. Therefore, remaining properly hydrated will also help prevent weakened muscle contractions and early onset of fatigue.

As a middle-distance dancer, you should turn to Appendix C on page 345 for a full discussion of the 20:20:60 dietary plan. Also presented are sample daily diets that use common, healthy foods to meet an athlete's energy and caloric needs. Use the directions on page 150 to estimate your average daily caloric requirement. Then use the directions in Chapter 13 or 14 to adjust your diet for off-season fat loss or muscle building, respectively.

Supplementation Guidelines

In addition to eating a proper diet, you should also take dietary supplements to make sure that any nutrients you lose due to sweating or training are replenished. The following tables will help guide you in selecting the supplements appropriate for you. The first table lists the nutrients recommended for middle-distance dancers, as well as the range of intake for each nutrient. (For discussions of these nutrients, see Part One.) Note that within the ranges of intake, the lower amounts are for smaller individuals and lower-activity days, while the higher amounts are for larger individuals and higher-activity days.

RECOMMENDED NUTRIENTS AND RANGES OF INTAKE

For Middle-Distance Dancers

NUTRIENT	RANGE OF INTAKE
VITAMINS	
Vitamin A	8,000–16,000 IU
Beta-carotene	25,000–40,000 IU
Vitamin B_1 (thiamine)	80–160 mg
Vitamin B_2 (riboflavin)	80–160 mg
Vitamin B_3 (niacin)	10–20 mg
Vitamin B_5 (pantothenic acid)	60–120 mg
Vitamin B_6 (pyridoxine)	20–80 mg
Vitamin B_{12} (cobalamin)	12–120 mcg
Biotin	125–175 mcg
Folate	400–800 mcg
Vitamin C	1,000–2,000 mg
Vitamin D	400–800 IU
Vitamin E	300–800 IU
Vitamin K	60–160 mcg
MINERALS	
Boron	2–8 mg
Calcium	800–1,500 mg
Chromium	200–500 mcg
Copper	1–4 mg
Iodine	100–200 mcg
Iron	15–50 mg
Magnesium	250–650 mg
Manganese	12–35 mg
Molybdenum	100–200 mcg
Phosphorus	150–800 mg
Potassium	50–1,000 mg
Selenium	100–200 mcg
Zinc	15–50 mg
AMINO ACIDS	
L-glutamic acid	500–1,000 mg
L-glutamine	1,000–2,000 mg
FATTY ACIDS	
Alpha-linolenic acid	500–1,000 mg
Docosahexaenoic acid (DHA)	350–750 mg
Eiocosapentaenoic acid (EPA)	350–750 mg
Gamma linolenic acid (GLA)	200–400 mg
Linoleic acid	1,000–2,000 mg
METABOLITES	
Bioflavonoids	400–900 mg
Choline	400–800 mg
Coenzyme Q_{10}	60–100 mg

NUTRIENT	RANGE OF INTAKE
Inositol	400–800 mg
L-carnitine	1,000–2,000 mg
Octacosanol	1,000–2,000 mcg

IU = international units, mcg = micrograms, mg = milligrams.

The second table lists the different types of sports supplements available and indicates if their use by middle-distance dancers is recommended in the preseason, during the season, or directly before a performance. The list also includes a number of popular nutritional practices—bicarbonate loading, carbohydrate loading, creatine and/or inosine loading, and water loading. (For a discussion of any of these supplements or practices, see the appropriate section in Part One or Part Three.)

RECOMMENDED SPORTS SUPPLEMENTS AND NUTRITIONAL PRACTICES

For Middle-Distance Dancers

	Intake Recommendation		
	PRESEASON	SEASON	PRE-PERFORMANCE
SUPPLEMENTS			
Multivitamins	Yes	Yes	No
Multiminerals	Yes	Yes	No
Antioxidants	Yes	Yes	No
Fatty acids	Yes	Yes	No
Metabolites	Yes	Yes	Yes
Branched-chain amino acids	Yes	Yes	Yes
Herbs	Yes	Yes	No
Medium-calorie protein drink (300–500 calories)	Yes	Yes	Yes
Carbohydrate drink with glycerol	Yes	Yes	Yes
Fat-burning supplement	Yes	Optional	No
PRACTICES			
Bicarbonate loading	No	No	No
Carbohydrate loading	No	No	Optional
Creatine and/or inosine loading	No	No	No
Water loading	No	No	Optional

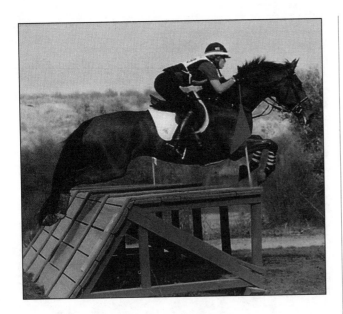

EQUESTRIAN

Also for Horseracing, Jousting, Polo, Quarter Horse Racing, and Rodeo

Taking a pony ride with your children on a lazy Sunday afternoon is fun, but riding a huge horse with a mind of its own at breakneck speeds with disaster looming at every step is downright draining. Equestrians require not only speed and strength in short, explosive bursts, but also a high level of anaerobic-strength endurance, as well as flexibility and agility. And in some equestrian events, a high energy level is critical for maintaining a focused, laserlike concentration while riding for prolonged periods of time under conditions that are exhausting for both rider and mount.

Every bit of your training and diet must reflect these elements. These elements are what define the equestrian sport. Nutritionally, this means emphasizing the efficient fulfillment of energy needs and maximizing the muscles' recovery and tissue-repair processes.

In most equestrian events, the energy output is anaerobic (without oxygen). This does not mean that training for or participating in equestrian competitions is easy, however. Training for all equestrian events is extremely intensive and grueling. At the highest levels, equestrian training forces you to operate at your anaerobic threshold (the point at which you must receive oxygen).

Muscles grow when they are stressed. In the equestrian sport, the aim is to make the muscles grow as strong and as quick as possible without putting on any unnecessary body weight, which would, of course, tend to slow down the animal. This calls for specialized training. Furthermore, the physical and mental demands of skillful riding also require the support of a carefully constructed nutrition program.

ENERGY SOURCES OF EQUESTRIANS

The muscles rely on three major systems to supply the energy they need—the immediate, glycolytic, and oxidative energy systems. For short-term energy for explosive-strength output, the muscles depend on the immediate energy systems. The immediate energy systems are nonoxidative—that is, they do not use oxygen. Instead, these systems generate energy through the use of adenosine triphosphate (ATP) and creatine phosphate (CP). CP is produced in the body and stored in the muscle fibers. It is broken down by enzymes to regenerate ATP, which is also stored in the muscle fibers. When the ATP is in turn broken down, the result is a spark of energy that triggers a muscle contraction.

For medium-term energy for repeated near-maximum exertion, the muscles turn to the glycolytic energy systems. In these systems, which are also nonoxidative, glycogen is used to produce energy. Glycogen is the storage form of glucose. It is stored in the liver and muscles, and is readily converted back to glucose when it is needed for energy.

For long-term energy for endurance activities, the muscles use the oxidative energy systems. In these systems, oxygen is used to oxidize long-chain fatty acids, protein, and glucose, which generates energy. For athletes, getting enough oxygen can mean a winning performance rather than a second-place showing.

Every sport involves a variety of skills, and each skill utilizes a unique combination of these three energy sources. The following table lists three major equestrian events and shows how much your body relies on each of the energy sources when you participate in them. Percentages are also given for the different legs of a modern pentathlon, as well as for a number of similar sports.

WHERE YOUR ENERGY COMES FROM

For Equestrians

	Energy Systems		
	IMMEDIATE	GLYCOLYTIC	OXIDATIVE
Events			
Dressage	100%	0%	0%
Jumping	100%	0%	0%
Three-day eventing	90%	10%	0%
Modern pentathlon			
Day 1—riding 600-meter course with 15 jumps	80%	20%	0%
Day 2—èpèe (round robin of one-touch duels)	100%	0%	0%
Day 3—shooting (with a pistol and rotating target)	75%	20%	5%
Day 4—300-meter freestyle swimming	40%	40%	20%
Day 5—4,000-meter cross-country run	5%	15%	80%

For Similar Sports

Horseracing	70%	30%	0%
Polo	80%	20%	0%
Quarter horse racing	80%	20%	0%
Rodeo	80%	20%	0%

When considering the type of nutritional support to give your training program, keep the following factors in mind:

☐ All athletes need to consume high-quality protein several times a day for effective recovery and adequate repair of damaged muscle tissue.

☐ Athletes whose muscles rely substantially on the immediate or glycolytic energy systems should keep their fat intake to a minimum because fat is not an efficient energy source for their intensive training, which is almost exclusively anaerobic in nature. Since the fat calories consumed by these athletes are not generally used for energy, they are stored as body fat.

☐ Athletes whose muscles rely substantially on the oxidative energy systems can eat more fat because their energy is manufactured through the oxidation of fatty acids. But even these athletes should watch their fat calories if they train aerobically (with oxygen) for less than half an hour at a time.

☐ All athletes should consume a carefully measured amount of high-quality carbohydrates several times a day to ensure an adequate supply of energy.

☐ The carbohydrates in all preworkout meals should consist of foods with low glycemic indexes to ensure that training intensity does not wane and that muscle tissue is not cannibalized for energy. (For the glycemic indexes of some common foods, see page 29.)

The aim of your nutrition program is to make your body healthy enough to accomplish recovery and tissue repair speedily and efficiently—without adding body fat. Your further aim is to do this while maintaining a high strength-to-weight ratio. These aims alone make diet very important for equestrians. You must eat just the right amount of food. Eat the wrong foods or the wrong amounts just a few times too often and you will sabotage your fitness efforts.

NUTRITION FOR EQUESTRIANS

Equestrians are either power or middle-distance athletes. Depending on the type of horsemanship they specialize in, their primary sources of energy are the immediate or the glycolytic energy systems. Therefore, as an equestrian, you need to plan your nutritional intake, from both food and supplement sources, to support the appropriate systems. In addition, if you are a power equestrian, your energy expenditure changes in the off-season, and you need to adjust your caloric intake and macronutrient ratio to match. Following are dietary and supplementation guidelines for power equestrians to help you in planning your nutrition program. Dietary and supplementation guidelines for middle-distance equestrians can be found on page 236.

POWER EQUESTRIANS

Equestrians who compete in events that last for just minutes are power athletes. Among the typical events they participate in are the dressage and jumping.

Dietary Guidelines

The following pie charts illustrate how you should divide up your caloric intake to match the energy demands of power equestrian events during the preseason, season, and off-season. They show the target percentages of fat, protein, and carbohydrates that your five to six meals should supply each day.

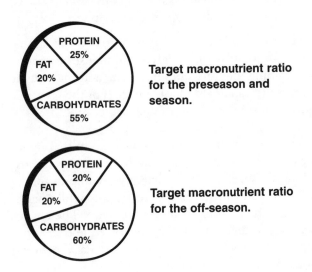

Target macronutrient ratio for the preseason and season.

Target macronutrient ratio for the off-season.

Note that fat has about 9 calories per gram, while protein and carbohydrates have only 4 calories per gram. Therefore, during the season, if you needed to consume a total of 2,500 calories per day, you would aim for 500 calories (20 percent of your total daily calories) from fat, 625 calories (25 percent of your total daily calories) from protein, and the remaining 1,375 calories (55 percent of your total daily calories) from carbohydrates.

Some other important considerations for power equestrians are:

☐ Carbohydrates are the major source of energy for short-term activities. Complex carbohydrates are the best source because they most effectively refill the glycogen stores in the muscles and liver. In addition, they elevate the blood sugar to a level sufficient for long sessions of intensive training.

☐ As a power athlete, you must make sure that you consume adequate amounts of both carbohydrates and protein. If your energy stores become drastically depleted or you experience lactic-acid buildup, you may suffer temporary muscle fatigue. If you do not refill your glycogen stores before your next workout or competiton, your body may begin breaking down

muscle tissue for the protein it needs for energy.

☐ Directly before workouts, consume carbohydrate drinks with high glycemic indexes to keep your blood sugar sustained at an appropriate level. This will allow you to train intensively without having your explosiveness hindered by fatigue.

☐ As a power athlete, you need to stimulate the storage of glycogen in your muscles while promoting repair and growth of your muscle tissue and inhibiting buildup of body fat. To do this:

• Train anaerobically on a regular basis. Intensive training stimulates increased storage of glycogen in the muscles and liver, which provides additional energy for greater exercise capacity.

• Consume five to six meals a day. Eating several smaller meals rather than three larger ones will keep your blood-sugar level stable throughout the day and will ensure that a supply of protein is always available for your muscles.

• Keep your fat intake to a minimum. Large amounts of fat in your diet will add to your body fat and will cause you to lose minerals through frequent urination.

• Consume low-glycemic-index foods about two to three hours before workouts and competitions. These foods help sustain the blood-sugar level.

• Drink plenty of water. Not only will this practice reduce your chances of becoming dehydrated, but every ounce of glycogen that is stored within the muscles needs 3 ounces of water stored along with it. Therefore, remaining properly hydrated will also help prevent weakened muscle contractions.

As a power equestrian, you should turn to Appendix C on page 345 for full discussions of the 20:25:55 and 20:20:60 dietary plans. Also presented are sample daily diets that use common, healthy foods to meet an athlete's energy and caloric needs. Use the directions on page 150 to estimate your average daily caloric requirement. Then use the directions in Chapter 13 or 14 to adjust your diet for off-season fat loss or muscle building, respectively.

Supplementation Guidelines

In addition to eating a proper diet, you should also take dietary supplements to make sure that any nutrients you lose due to sweating or training are replenished. The following tables will help guide you in selecting the supplements appropriate for you. The first table lists the nutrients recommended for power equestrians, as well as the range of intake for each nutrient. (For discussions of these nutrients, see Part One.) Note that within the ranges of intake, the lower amounts are for smaller individuals and lower-activity days, while the higher amounts are for larger individuals and higher-activity days.

RECOMMENDED NUTRIENTS AND RANGES OF INTAKE

For Power Equestrians

NUTRIENT	RANGE OF INTAKE
VITAMINS	
Vitamin A	8,000–16,000 IU
Beta-carotene	25,000–35,000 IU
Vitamin B$_1$ (thiamine)	40–120 mg
Vitamin B$_2$ (riboflavin)	40–120 mg
Vitamin B$_3$ (niacin)	20–40 mg
Vitamin B$_5$ (pantothenic acid)	20–100 mg
Vitamin B$_6$ (pyridoxine)	20–80 mg
Vitamin B$_{12}$ (cobalamin)	12–120 mcg
Biotin	125–175 mcg
Folate	400–800 mcg
Vitamin C	800–2,000 mg
Vitamin D	400–800 IU
Vitamin E	200–800 IU
Vitamin K	60–160 mcg
MINERALS	
Boron	2–8 mg
Calcium	800–1,500 mg
Chromium	200–500 mcg
Copper	1–4 mg
Iodine	100–200 mcg
Iron	15–50 mg
Magnesium	250–650 mg
Manganese	12–35 mg
Molybdenum	100–200 mcg
Phosphorus	150–800 mg
Potassium	50–1,000 mg
Selenium	100–200 mcg
Zinc	15–50 mg
AMINO ACIDS	
L-glutamic acid	500–1,000 mg
L-glutamine	1,000–2,000 mg

NUTRIENT	RANGE OF INTAKE
FATTY ACIDS	
Alpha-linolenic acid	500–1,000 mg
Docosahexaenoic acid (DHA)	250–750 mg
Eicosapentaenoic acid (EPA)	250–750 mg
Gamma linolenic acid (GLA)	100–400 mg
Linoleic acid	2,000–3,000 mg
METABOLITES	
Bioflavonoids	300–800 mg
Choline	200–600 mg
Creatine monohydrate	4,000–12,000 mg
Inosine	500–1,000 mg
Inositol	200–600 mg
L-carnitine	500–1,500 mg
Octacosanol	1,000–2,000 mcg

IU = international units, mcg = micrograms, mg = milligrams.

The second table lists the different types of sports supplements available and indicates if their use by power equestrians is recommended in the preseason, during the season, or directly before a competition. The list also includes a number of popular nutritional practices—bicarbonate loading, carbohydrate loading, creatine and/or inosine loading, and water loading. (For a discussion of any of these supplements or practices, see the appropriate section in Part One or Part Three.)

RECOMMENDED SPORTS SUPPLEMENTS AND NUTRITIONAL PRACTICES

For Power Equestrians

	Intake Recommendation		
	PRESEASON	SEASON	PRE-COMPETITION
SUPPLEMENTS			
Multivitamins	Yes	Yes	No
Multiminerals	Yes	Yes	No
Antioxidants	Yes	Yes	No
Fatty acids	Yes	Yes	No
Metabolites	Optional	Yes	Yes
Branched-chain amino acids	Yes	Yes	Yes
Herbs	Yes	Yes	No
Low-calorie protein drink (200–300 calories)	Yes	Yes	Yes
Carbohydrate drink	Yes	Yes	Yes
Fat-burning supplement	Yes	Optional	No

235

Intake Recommendation			
	PRESEASON	SEASON	PRE-COMPETITION
PRACTICES			
Bicarbonate loading	No	Optional	Yes
Carbohydrate loading	No	No	No
Creatine and/or inosine loading	No	Yes	Yes
Water loading	No	No	No

MIDDLE-DISTANCE EQUESTRIANS

Equestrians who compete in events that last longer than just minutes are middle-distrance athletes. Among the typical events they participate in are the modern pentathlon.

Dietary Guidelines

The following pie chart illustrates how you should divide up your caloric intake to match the energy demands of middle-distance equestrian events during the preseason, season, and off-season. It shows the target percentages of fat, protein, and carbohydrates that your five to six meals should supply each day.

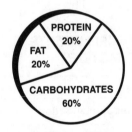

Target macronutrient ratio for the preseason, season, and off-season.

Note that fat has about 9 calories per gram, while protein and carbohydrates have only 4 calories per gram. Therefore, if you needed to consume a total of 2,500 calories per day, you would aim for 500 calories (20 percent of your total daily calories) from fat, 500 calories (20 percent of your total daily calories) from protein, and the remaining 1,500 calories (60 percent of your total daily calories) from carbohydrates.

Some other important considerations for middle-distance equestrians are:

☐ Carbohydrates are the major source of energy for short-term activities. Complex carbohydrates are the best source because they most effectively refill the glycogen stores in the muscles and liver. In addition, they elevate the blood sugar to a level sufficient for long sessions of intensive training.

☐ As a middle-distance athlete, you must make sure that you consume adequate amounts of both carbohydrates and protein. If your energy stores become drastically depleted or you experience lactic-acid buildup, you may suffer temporary muscle fatigue. If you do not refill your glycogen stores before your next workout or competition, your body may begin breaking down muscle tissue for the protein it needs for energy.

☐ Directly before workouts, consume carbohydrate drinks with high glycemic indexes to keep your blood sugar sustained at an appropriate level. This will allow you to train intensively for longer periods of time.

☐ As a middle-distance athlete, you need to stimulate the storage of glycogen in your muscles while promoting repair and growth of your muscle tissue and inhibiting buildup of body fat. To do this:

• Train against your anaerobic threshold (to exhaustion) on a regular basis. Intensive, exhaustive training stimulates increased storage of glycogen in the muscles and liver, which provides additional energy for greater exercise capacity.

• Consume five to six meals a day. Eating several smaller meals rather than three larger ones will keep your blood-sugar level stable throughout the day and will ensure that a supply of protein is always available for your muscles.

• Keep your fat intake to a minimum. Large amounts of fat in your diet will add to your body fat and will cause mineral loss through frequent urination.

• Consume low-glycemic-index foods two to three hours before workouts and competitions. These foods help sustain the blood-sugar level.

• Drink plenty of water. Not only will this practice reduce your chances of becoming dehydrated, but every ounce of glycogen that is stored within the muscles needs 3 ounces of water stored along with it. Therefore, remaining properly hydrated will also help prevent weakened muscle contractions and early onset of fatigue.

As a middle-distance equestrian, you should turn to Appendix C on page 345 for a full discussion of the 20:20:60 dietary plan. Also presented are sample daily diets that use common, healthy foods to meet an athlete's energy and caloric needs. Use the directions on page 150 to estimate your average daily caloric requirement. Then use the directions in Chapter 13 or 14 to adjust your diet for off-season fat loss or muscle building, respectively.

Supplementation Guidelines

In addition to eating a proper diet, you should also take dietary supplements to make sure that any nutrients you lose due to sweating or training are replenished. The following tables will help guide you in selecting the supplements appropriate for you. The first table lists the nutrients recommended for middle-distance equestrians, as well as the range of intake for each nutrient. (For discussions of these nutrients, see Part One.) Note that within the ranges of intake, the lower amounts are for smaller individuals and lower-activity days, while the higher amounts are for larger individuals and higher-activity days.

RECOMMENDED NUTRIENTS AND RANGES OF INTAKE

For Middle-Distance Equestrians

NUTRIENT	RANGE OF INTAKE
VITAMINS	
Vitamin A	8,000–16,000 IU
Beta-carotene	25,000–40,000 IU
Vitamin B$_1$ (thiamine)	80–160 mg
Vitamin B$_2$ (riboflavin)	80–160 mg
Vitamin B$_3$ (niacin)	10–20 mg
Vitamin B$_5$ (pantothenic acid)	60–120 mg
Vitamin B$_6$ (pyridoxine)	20–80 mg
Vitamin B$_{12}$ (cobalamin)	12–120 mcg
Biotin	125–175 mcg
Folate	400–800 mcg
Vitamin C	1,000–2,000 mg
Vitamin D	400–800 IU
Vitamin E	300–800 IU
Vitamin K	60–160 mcg
MINERALS	
Boron	2–8 mg
Calcium	800–1,500 mg
Chromium	200–500 mcg
Copper	1–4 mg
Iodine	100–200 mcg
Iron	15–50 mg

NUTRIENT	RANGE OF INTAKE
Magnesium	250–650 mg
Manganese	12–35 mg
Molybdenum	100–200 mcg
Phosphorus	150–800 mg
Potassium	50–1,000 mg
Selenium	100–200 mcg
Zinc	15–50 mg
AMINO ACIDS	
L-glutamic acid	500–1,000 mg
L-glutamine	1,000–2,000 mg
FATTY ACIDS	
Alpha-linolenic acid	500–1,000 mg
Docosahexaenoic acid (DHA)	350–750 mg
Eiocosapentaenoic acid (EPA)	350–750 mg
Gamma linolenic acid (GLA)	200–400 mg
Linoleic acid	1,000–2,000 mg
METABOLITES	
Bioflavonoids	400–900 mg
Choline	400–800 mg
Coenzyme Q$_{10}$	60–100 mg
Inositol	400–800 mg
L-carnitine	1,000–2,000 mg
Octacosanol	1,000–2,000 mcg

IU = international units, mcg = micrograms, mg = milligrams.

The second table lists the different types of sports supplements available and indicates if their use by middle-distance equestrians is recommended in the preseason, during the season, or directly before a competition. The list also includes a number of popular nutritional practices—bicarbonate loading, carbohydrate loading, creatine and/or inosine loading, and water loading. (For a discussion of any of these supplements or practices, see the appropriate section in Part One or Part Three.)

RECOMMENDED SPORTS SUPPLEMENTS AND NUTRITIONAL PRACTICES

For Middle-Distance Equestrians

	Intake Recommendation		
	PRESEASON	SEASON	PRE-COMPETITION
SUPPLEMENTS			
Multivitamins	Yes	Yes	No
Multiminerals	Yes	Yes	No
Antioxidants	Yes	Yes	No

	Intake Recommendation		
	PRESEASON	**SEASON**	**PRE-COMPETITION**
Fatty acids	Yes	Yes	No
Metabolites	No	Yes	Yes
Branched-chain amino acids	Yes	Yes	Yes
Herbs	Yes	Yes	No
Medium-calorie protein drink (300–500 calories)	Yes	Yes	Yes
Carbohydrate drink with glycerol	Yes	Yes	Yes
Fat-burning supplement	Yes	Optional	No
PRACTICES			
Bicarbonate loading	No	No	No
Carbohydrate loading	No	No	Optional
Creatine and/or inosine loading	No	No	No
Water loading	No	No	Yes

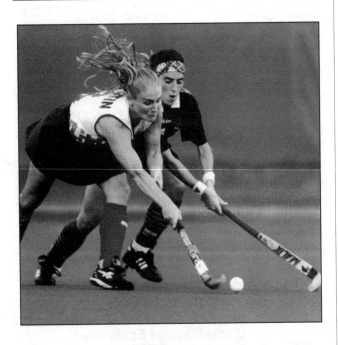

FIELD HOCKEY

Also for Lacrosse and Team Handball

Easily one of the most demanding sports in the world, field hockey is a game in which conditioning plays as big a role as skill. When you play field hockey, you are almost constantly on the run, making many sudden starts, stops, turns, jumps, pivots, and sprints. Therefore, it is essential that you have a solid nutritional foundation, an energy and recovery base to support your training and competition efforts.

Field hockey requires a variety of skills. A field-hockey player must be a combination sprinter, leaper, and even dancer to execute the fundamental movements of the game. Field-hockey conditioning, therefore, must take each of these areas into account.

Only the most rigorous nutrition and training program can prepare an athlete for the rigors of a field-hockey season. Increased strength can make you a better field-hockey player. Through the careful application of scientific training techniques, you can multiply your on-field effectiveness in all areas of the game. You can improve your jumping ability, sprinting ability, endurance, agility, and body control, playing better even when you are fatigued. Furthermore, the incredible diversity of skills and energy demands of field hockey require the support of a carefully constructed nutrition program.

ENERGY SOURCES OF FIELD-HOCKEY PLAYERS

The muscles rely on three major systems to supply the energy they need—the immediate, glycolytic, and oxidative energy systems. For short-term energy for explosive-strength output, the muscles depend on the immediate energy systems. The immediate energy systems are nonoxidative—that is, they do not use oxygen. Instead, these systems generate energy through the use of adenosine triphosphate (ATP) and creatine phosphate (CP). CP is produced in the body and stored in the muscle fibers. It is broken down by enzymes to regenerate ATP, which is also stored in the muscle fibers. When the ATP is in turn broken down, the result is a spark of energy that triggers a muscle contraction.

For medium-term energy for repeated near-maximum exertion, the muscles turn to the glycolytic energy systems. In these systems, which are also nonoxidative, glycogen is used to produce energy. Glycogen is the storage form of glucose. It is stored in the liver and muscles, and is readily converted back to glucose when it is needed for energy.

For long-term energy for endurance activities, the muscles use the oxidative energy systems. In these systems, oxygen is used to oxidize long-chain fatty acids, protein, and glucose, which generates energy. For athletes, getting enough oxygen can mean a winning performance rather than a second-place showing.

Every sport involves a variety of skills, and each skill utilizes a unique combination of these three energy sources. The following table lists the major field-hockey positions and shows how much your body relies on each of the energy sources when you play them.

WHERE YOUR ENERGY COMES FROM

For Field-Hockey Players			
	Energy Systems		
	IMMEDIATE	**GLYCOLYTIC**	**OXIDATIVE**
Forward	50%	30%	20%
Fullback	90%	10%	0%
Goalie	100%	0%	0%
Halfback	60%	20%	20%
Wing	50%	30%	20%

When considering the type of nutritional support to give your training program, keep the following factors in mind:

☐ All athletes need to consume high-quality protein several times a day for effective recovery and adequate repair of damaged muscle tissue.

☐ Athletes whose muscles rely substantially on the immediate or glycolytic energy systems should keep their fat intake to a minimum because fat is not an efficient energy source for their intensive training, which is almost exclusively anaerobic in nature. Since the fat calories consumed by these athletes are not generally used for energy, they are stored as body fat.

☐ Athletes whose muscles rely substantially on the oxidative energy systems can eat more fat because their energy is manufactured through the oxidation of fatty acids. But even these athletes should watch their fat calories if they train aerobically (with oxygen) for less than half an hour at a time.

☐ All athletes should consume a carefully measured amount of high-quality carbohydrates several times a day to ensure an adequate supply of energy.

☐ The carbohydrates in all preworkout meals should consist of foods with low glycemic indexes to ensure that training intensity does not wane and that muscle

tissue is not cannibalized for energy. (For the glycemic indexes of some common foods, see page 29.)

The aim of your nutrition program is to make your body healthy enough to accomplish recovery and tissue repair speedily and efficiently—without adding body fat. Your further aim is to do this while maintaining a high strength-to-weight ratio. These aims alone make diet very important for field-hockey players. You must eat just the right amount of food. Eat the wrong foods or the wrong amounts just a few times too often and you will sabotage your fitness efforts. Even more important, do not be in a hurry. It takes *years* to become a great field-hockey player. Rush the nutrition and training processes and you will become fat, your recovery rate will decline, and your injury rate will rise.

NUTRITION FOR FIELD-HOCKEY PLAYERS

Field-hockey players are either power or middle-distance athletes. Depending on the position they play, they need bursts of power, which are supported by energy from the immediate energy systems, or stamina, which is supported by energy from the glycolytic energy systems. Therefore, as a field-hockey player, you need to plan your nutritional intake, from both food and supplement sources, to support the appropriate systems. In addition, if you are a power field-hockey player, your energy expenditure changes in the off-season, and you need to adjust your caloric intake and macronutrient ratio to match. Following are dietary and supplementation guidelines for power field-hockey players to help you in planning your nutrition program. Dietary and supplementation guidelines for middle-distance field-hockey players can be found on page 242.

POWER FIELD-HOCKEY PLAYERS

The field-hockey players who usually play in spurts are power athletes. These players include the fullbacks and goalie.

Dietary Guidelines

The following pie charts illustrate how you should divide up your caloric intake to match the energy demands of your power field-hockey position during the preseason, season, and off-season. They show the target percentages of fat, protein, and carbohydrates that your five to six meals should supply each day.

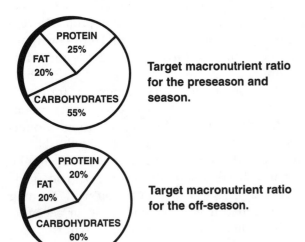

Target macronutrient ratio for the preseason and season.

Target macronutrient ratio for the off-season.

Note that fat has about 9 calories per gram, while protein and carbohydrates have only 4 calories per gram. Therefore, during the season, if you needed to consume a total of 2,500 calories per day, you would aim for 500 calories (20 percent of your total daily calories) from fat, 625 calories (25 percent of your total daily calories) from protein, and the remaining 1,375 calories (55 percent of your total daily calories) from carbohydrates.

Some other important considerations for power field-hockey players are:

☐ Carbohydrates are the major source of energy for short-term activities. Complex carbohydrates are the best source because they most effectively refill the glycogen stores in the muscles and liver. In addition, they elevate the blood sugar to a level sufficient for long sessions of intensive training.

☐ As a power athlete, you must make sure that you consume adequate amounts of both carbohydrates and protein. If your energy stores become drastically depleted or you experience lactic-acid buildup, you may suffer temporary muscle fatigue. If you do not refill your glycogen stores before your next workout or game, your body may begin breaking down muscle tissue for the protein it needs for energy.

☐ Directly before workouts and games, consume carbohydrate drinks with high glycemic indexes to keep your blood sugar sustained at an appropriate level. This will allow you to train or play intensively with-

out having your explosiveness hindered by fatigue.

☐ As a power athlete, you need to stimulate the storage of glycogen in your muscles while promoting repair and growth of your muscle tissue and inhibiting buildup of body fat. To do this:

• Train anaerobically on a regular basis. Intensive training stimulates increased storage of glycogen in the muscles and liver, which provides additional energy for greater exercise capacity.

• Consume five to six meals a day. Eating several smaller meals rather than three larger ones will keep your blood-sugar level stable throughout the day and will ensure that a supply of protein is always available for your muscles.

• Keep your fat intake to a minimum. Large amounts of fat in your diet will add to your body fat and will cause you to lose minerals through frequent urination.

• Consume low-glycemic-index foods about two to three hours before workouts and games. These foods help sustain the blood-sugar level.

• Drink plenty of water. Not only will this practice reduce your chances of becoming dehydrated, but every ounce of glycogen that is stored within the muscles needs 3 ounces of water stored along with it. Therefore, remaining properly hydrated will also help prevent weakened muscle contractions.

As a power field-hockey player, you should turn to Appendix C on page 345 for full discussions of the 20:25:55 and 20:20:60 dietary plans. Also presented are sample daily diets that use common, healthy foods to meet an athlete's energy and caloric needs. Use the directions on page 150 to estimate your average daily caloric requirement. Then use the directions in Chapter 13 or 14 to adjust your diet for off-season fat loss or muscle building, respectively.

Supplementation Guidelines

In addition to eating a proper diet, you should also take dietary supplements to make sure that any nutrients you lose due to sweating or training are replenished. The following tables will help guide you in selecting the supplements appropriate for you. The first table lists the nutrients recommended for power field-hockey players, as well as the range of intake for each nutrient. (For discussions of these nutrients, see Part One.) Note that within the ranges of intake, the lower amounts are for smaller individuals and lower-activity days, while the higher amounts are for larger individuals and higher-activity days.

RECOMMENDED NUTRIENTS AND RANGES OF INTAKE

For Power Field-Hockey Players

NUTRIENT	RANGE OF INTAKE
VITAMINS	
Vitamin A	8,000–16,000 IU
Beta-carotene	15,000–25,000 IU
Vitamin B$_1$ (thiamine)	40–120 mg
Vitamin B$_2$ (riboflavin)	40–120 mg
Vitamin B$_3$ (niacin)	20–40 mg
Vitamin B$_5$ (pantothenic acid)	20–100 mg
Vitamin B$_6$ (pyridoxine)	20–80 mg
Vitamin B$_{12}$ (cobalamin)	12–120 mcg
Biotin	125–175 mcg
Folate	400–800 mcg
Vitamin C	800–2,000 mg
Vitamin D	400–800 IU
Vitamin E	200–800 IU
Vitamin K	60–160 mcg
MINERALS	
Boron	2–8 mg
Calcium	800–1,500 mg
Chromium	200–500 mcg
Copper	1–4 mg
Iodine	100–200 mcg
Iron	15–50 mg
Magnesium	250–650 mg
Manganese	12–35 mg
Molybdenum	100–200 mcg
Phosphorus	150–800 mg
Potassium	50–1,000 mg
Selenium	100–200 mcg
Zinc	15–50 mg
AMINO ACIDS	
L-glutamic acid	500–1,000 mg
L-glutamine	1,000–2,000 mg
FATTY ACIDS	
Alpha-linolenic acid	500–1,000 mg
Docosahexaenoic acid (DHA)	250–750 mg
Eiocosapentaenoic acid (EPA)	250–750 mg
Gamma linolenic acid (GLA)	100–400 mg
Linoleic acid	2,000–3,000 mg

NUTRIENT	RANGE OF INTAKE
METABOLITES	
Bioflavonoids	300–800 mg
Choline	200–600 mg
Creatine monohydrate	4,000–8,000 mg
Inosine	500–1,500 mg
Inositol	200–600 mg
L-carnitine	500–1,500 mg
Octacosanol	1,000–2,000 mcg

IU = international units, mcg = micrograms, mg = milligrams.

The second table lists the different types of sports supplements available and indicates if their use by power field-hockey players is recommended in the preseason, during the season, or directly before a game. The list also includes a number of popular nutritional practices—bicarbonate loading, carbohydrate loading, creatine and/or inosine loading, and water loading. (For a discussion of any of these supplements or practices, see the appropriate section in Part One or Part Three.)

RECOMMENDED SPORTS SUPPLEMENTS AND NUTRITIONAL PRACTICES

For Power Field-Hockey Players

	Intake Recommendation		
	PRESEASON	SEASON	PREGAME
SUPPLEMENTS			
Multivitamins	Yes	Yes	No
Multiminerals	Yes	Yes	No
Antioxidants	Yes	Yes	No
Fatty acids	Yes	Yes	No
Metabolites	Optional	Yes	Yes
Branched-chain amino acids	Yes	Yes	Yes
Herbs	Yes	Yes	No
Low-calorie protein drink (200–300 calories)	Yes	Yes	Yes
Carbohydrate drink	Yes	Yes	Yes
Fat-burning supplement	Yes	Optional	No
PRACTICES			
Bicarbonate loading	No	No	Optional
Carbohydrate loading	No	No	Optional
Creatine and/or inosine loading	No	No	Yes
Water loading	No	No	Optional

MIDDLE-DISTANCE FIELD-HOCKEY PLAYERS

The field-hockey players who usually play for longer periods of time are middle-distance athletes. These players include the forwards, halfbacks, and wings.

Dietary Guidelines

The following pie chart illustrates how you should divide up your caloric intake to match the energy demands of your middle-distance field-hockey position during the preseason, season, and off-season. It shows the target percentages of fat, protein, and carbohydrates that your five to six meals should supply each day.

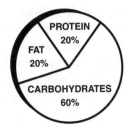

Target macronutrient ratio for the preseason, season, and off-season.

Note that fat has about 9 calories per gram, while protein and carbohydrates have only 4 calories per gram. Therefore, if you needed to consume a total of 2,500 calories per day, you would aim for 500 calories (20 percent of your total daily calories) from fat, 500 calories (20 percent of your total daily calories) from protein, and the remaining 1,500 calories (60 percent of your total daily calories) from carbohydrates.

Some other important considerations for middle-distance field-hockey players are:

☐ Carbohydrates are the major source of energy for short-term activities. Complex carbohydrates are the best source because they most effectively refill the glycogen stores in the muscles and liver. In addition, they elevate the blood sugar to a level sufficient for long sessions of intensive training.

☐ As a middle-distance athlete, you must make sure that you consume adequate amounts of both carbohydrates and protein. If your energy stores become drastically depleted or you experience lactic-acid buildup, you may suffer temporary muscle fatigue. If you do not refill your glycogen stores before your next workout or game, your body may begin breaking down muscle tissue for the protein it needs for energy.

☐ Directly before workouts and games, consume carbohydrate drinks with high glycemic indexes to keep your blood sugar sustained at an appropriate level. This will allow you to train or play intensively for longer periods of time.

☐ As a middle-distance athlete, you need to stimulate the storage of glycogen in your muscles while promoting repair and growth of your muscle tissue and inhibiting buildup of body fat. To do this:

• Train against your anaerobic threshold (to exhaustion) on a regular basis. Intensive, exhaustive training stimulates increased storage of glycogen in the muscles and liver, which provides additional energy for greater exercise capacity.

• Consume five to six meals a day. Eating several smaller meals rather than three larger ones will keep your blood-sugar level stable throughout the day and will ensure that a supply of protein is always available for your muscles.

• Keep your fat intake to a minimum. Large amounts of fat in your diet will add to your body fat and will cause mineral loss through frequent urination.

• Consume low-glycemic-index foods about two to three hours before workouts and games. These foods help sustain the blood-sugar level.

• Drink plenty of water. Not only will this practice reduce your chances of becoming dehydrated, but every ounce of glycogen that is stored within the muscles needs 3 ounces of water stored along with it. Therefore, remaining properly hydrated will also help prevent weakened muscle contractions and early onset of fatigue.

• Do not eat a new food just before a game. Different people often react differently to the same food. Before a game, eat just those foods that you know your body will handle well.

As a middle-distance field-hockey player, you should turn to Appendix C on page for a full discussion of the 20:20:60 dietary plan. Also presented are sample daily diets that use common, healthy foods to meet an athlete's energy and caloric needs. Use the directions on page 150 to estimate your average daily caloric requirement. Then use the directions in Chapter 13 or 14 to adjust your diet for off-season fat loss or muscle building, respectively.

Supplementation Guidelines

In addition to eating a proper diet, you should also take dietary supplements to make sure that any nutrients you lose due to sweating or training are replenished. The following tables will help guide you in selecting the supplements appropriate for you. The first table lists the nutrients recommended for middle-distance field-hockey players, as well as the range of intake for each nutrient. (For discussions of these nutrients, see Part One.) Note that within the ranges of intake, the lower amounts are for smaller individuals and lower-activity days, while the higher amounts are for larger individuals and higher-activity days.

RECOMMENDED NUTRIENTS AND RANGES OF INTAKE

For Middle-Distance Field-Hockey Players

NUTRIENT	RANGE OF INTAKE
VITAMINS	
Vitamin A	8,000–16,000 IU
Beta-carotene	25,000–35,000 IU
Vitamin B$_1$ (thiamine)	80–160 mg
Vitamin B$_2$ (riboflavin)	80–160 mg
Vitamin B$_3$ (niacin)	20–40 mg
Vitamin B$_5$ (pantothenic acid)	60–120 mg
Vitamin B$_6$ (pyridoxine)	20–80 mg
Vitamin B$_{12}$ (cobalamin)	12–120 mcg
Biotin	125–175 mcg
Folate	400–800 mcg
Vitamin C	1,000–2,000 mg
Vitamin D	400–800 IU
Vitamin E	300–800 IU
Vitamin K	60–160 mcg
MINERALS	
Boron	2–8 mg
Calcium	800–1,500 mg
Chromium	200–500 mcg
Copper	1–4 mg
Iodine	100–200 mcg
Iron	15–50 mg
Magnesium	250–650 mg
Manganese	12–35 mg
Molybdenum	100–200 mcg
Phosphorus	150–800 mg
Potassium	50–1,000 mg
Selenium	100–200 mcg
Zinc	15–50 mg
AMINO ACIDS	
L-glutamic acid	500–1,000 mg
L-glutamine	1,000–2,000 mg

NUTRIENT	RANGE OF INTAKE
FATTY ACIDS	
Alpha-linolenic acid	500–1,000 mg
Docosahexaenoic acid (DHA)	350–750 mg
Eiocosapentaenoic acid (EPA)	350–750 mg
Gamma linolenic acid (GLA)	200–400 mg
Linoleic acid	1,000–2,000 mg
METABOLITES	
Bioflavonoids	400–900 mg
Choline	400–800 mg
Coenzyme Q$_{10}$	60–100 mg
Inositol	400–800 mg
L-carnitine	1,000–2,000 mg
Octacosanol	1,000–2,000 mcg

IU = international units, mcg = micrograms, mg = milligrams.

The second table lists the different types of sports supplements available and indicates if their use by middle-distance field-hockey players is recommended in the preseason, during the season, or directly before a game. The list also includes a number of popular nutritional practices—bicarbonate loading, carbohydrate loading, creatine and/or inosine loading, and water loading. (For a discussion of any of these supplements or practices, see the appropriate section in Part One or Part Three.)

RECOMMENDED SPORTS SUPPLEMENTS AND NUTRITIONAL PRACTICES

For Middle-Distance Field-Hockey Players

	Intake Recommendation		
	PRESEASON	SEASON	PREGAME
SUPPLEMENTS			
Multivitamins	Yes	Yes	No
Multiminerals	Yes	Yes	No
Antioxidants	Yes	Yes	No
Fatty acids	Yes	Yes	No
Metabolites	Optional	Yes	Yes
Branched-chain amino acids	Yes	Yes	Yes
Herbs	Yes	Yes	No
Medium-calorie protein drink (300–500 calories)	Yes	Yes	Yes
Carbohydrate drink with glycerol	Yes	Yes	Yes

	Intake Recommendation		
	PRESEASON	SEASON	PREGAME
Fat-burning supplement	Yes	Optional	No
PRACTICES			
Bicarbonate loading	No	No	No
Carbohydrate loading	No	No	Optional
Creatine and/or inosine loading	No	No	No
Water loading	No	No	Yes

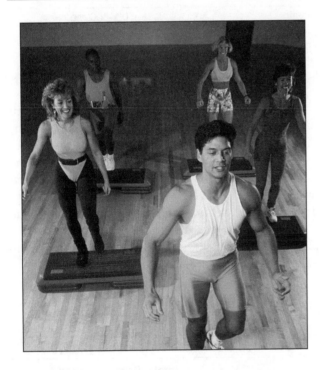

FITNESS ACTIVITIES

Includes All Recreational Activities

Millions of people play sports for fitness and fun alone. Sure, winning is enjoyable, and it is human nature to want to win, but for these people, fitness is the objective.

Another large group of people enjoys a number of activities that, while not sports in the formal sense of the word, nonetheless involve sport movements or resemble a sport. These activities are noncompetitive, but their participants find it just as gratifying to work to improve their skills and beat their own personal best.

In fitness, what works for one person in terms of results and fun does not necessarily work for another. In

addition, what is considered an adequate level of fitness by one person is not necessarily considered as such by others. For example, construction workers need to maintain a different level of fitness than secretaries do because the demands of their lifestyles are different. Coaches do not need the same level of fitness as the athletes they train, and generals do not need the same level of fitness as the soldiers they command.

Regardless of what level of fitness your lifestyle demands and the activities that you enjoy to maintain it, you should consider organizing your fitness training to at least some degree to maximize the results you achieve in the time you have available. Furthermore, whether your training program is organized or haphazard, the specialized energy output of your particular fitness activity requires the support of a carefully constructed nutrition program.

ENERGY SOURCES OF FITNESS EXERCISERS

The muscles rely on three major systems to supply the energy they need—the immediate, glycolytic, and oxidative energy systems. For short-term energy for explosive-strength output, the muscles depend on the immediate energy systems. The immediate energy systems are nonoxidative—that is, they do not use oxygen. Instead, these systems generate energy through the use of adenosine triphosphate (ATP) and creatine phosphate (CP). CP is produced in the body and stored in the muscle fibers. It is broken down by enzymes to regenerate ATP, which is also stored in the muscle fibers. When the ATP is in turn broken down, the result is a spark of energy that triggers a muscle contraction.

For medium-term energy for repeated near-maximum exertion, the muscles turn to the glycolytic energy systems. In these systems, which are also nonoxidative, glycogen is used to produce energy. Glycogen is the storage form of glucose. It is stored in the liver and muscles, and is readily converted back to glucose when it is needed for energy.

For long-term energy for endurance activities, the muscles use the oxidative energy systems. In these systems, oxygen is used to oxidize long-chain fatty acids, protein, and glucose, which generates energy. For athletes, getting enough oxygen can mean a winning performance rather than a second-place showing.

Every activity involves a variety of skills, and each skill utilizes a unique combination of these three energy sources. The table following lists a number of popular fitness activities, including wheelchair fitness activities, and shows how much your body relies on each of the energy sources when you participate in them. Percentages are also given for general categories of fitness activities and different lengths of aerobic activities.

WHERE YOUR ENERGY COMES FROM

For Fitness Exercisers

	Energy Systems		
	IMMEDIATE	GLYCOLYTIC	OXIDATIVE
Fitness categories			
Activities that involve walking, jogging, or cycling slowly for long distances	0%	5%	95%
Traditional weight-loss activities (such as running on a treadmill, stationary cycling, and swimming laps)	0%	5%	95%
Activities with an aerobic orientation	10%	30%	60%
Activities with a middle-distance orientation	20%	60%	20%
Activities with a cross-training orientation	34%	33%	33%
Weight-training activities	40%	50%	10%
Activities with a power orientation	90%	10%	0%
Aerobic activities			
1-mile run or 6–9 minutes of exercise	5%	50%	45%
1-mile power walk or 9–12 minutes of exercise	5%	40%	55%
5-mile power walk or 70–90 minutes of exercise	0%	25%	75%
5-mile run or 50–70 minutes of exercise	0%	10%	90%
10-mile run or 90–120 minutes of exercise	0%	5%	95%
Marathon run or 3–4 hours of exercise	0%	3%	97%

	Energy Systems		
	IMMEDIATE	GLYCOLYTIC	OXIDATIVE
Fitness activities			
Arm/wrist wrestling	90%	10%	0%
Ballooning	90%	10%	0%
Baton twirling	80%	20%	0%
Billiards/pool	80%	20%	0%
Cheerleading	80%	20%	0%
Croquet	100%	0%	0%
Épée/fencing/foil	90%	10%	0%
Frisbee	100%	0%	0%
Hang gliding	60%	40%	0%
Horseshoes	90%	10%	0%
Parachuting	90%	10%	0%
Scuba diving	50%	30%	20%
Skateboarding	80%	15%	5%
Soaring	80%	20%	0%
Surfing	40%	50%	10%
Table tennis (ping pong)	100%	0%	0%
Tug of war	60%	30%	10%
Water skiing	70%	20%	10%
Yachting	40%	40%	20%
Wheelchair fitness activities			
Basketball	40%	40%	20%
Road racing (for endurance)	10%	40%	50%
Road racing (for speed)	80%	20%	0%
Tennis	80%	20%	0%

When considering the type of nutritional support to give your fitness activity, keep the following factors in mind:

☐ All athletes need to consume high-quality protein several times a day for effective recovery and adequate repair of damaged muscle tissue.

☐ Athletes whose muscles rely substantially on the immediate or glycolytic energy systems should keep their fat intake to a minimum because fat is not an efficient energy source for their intensive training, which is almost exclusively anaerobic in nature. Since the fat calories consumed by these athletes are not generally used for energy, they are stored as body fat.

☐ Athletes whose muscles rely substantially on the oxidative energy systems can eat more fat because their energy is manufactured through the oxidation of fatty acids. But even these athletes should watch their fat calories if they train aerobically (with oxygen) for less than half an hour at a time.

☐ All athletes should consume a carefully measured amount of high-quality carbohydrates several times a day to ensure an aequate supply of energy.

☐ The carbohydrates in all preworkout meals should consist of foods with low glycemic indexes to ensure that training intensity does not wane and that muscle tissue is not cannibalized for energy. (For the glycemic indexes of some common foods, see page 29.)

The aim of your nutrition program is to make your body healthy enough to accomplish recovery and tissue repair speedily and efficiently—without adding body fat. This aim alone makes diet very important for fitness exercisers. You must eat just the right amount of food. Eat the wrong foods or the wrong amounts just a few times too often and you will sabotage your fitness efforts.

NUTRITION FOR FITNESS EXERCISERS

Fitness exercisers are either power, middle-distance, or endurance athletes. Their primary source of energy is determined by the specific activity they participate in. Some activities require bursts of power, which are supported by energy from the immediate energy systems. Some activities require stamina, which is supported by energy from the glycolytic energy systems. Still other activities require endurance, which is supported by energy from the oxidative energy systems. Therefore, as a fitness exerciser, you need to plan your nutritional intake, from both food and supplement sources, to support the appropriate systems. In addition, if you are a power fitness exerciser, your energy expenditure changes in the preseason and off-season, and you need to adjust your caloric intake and macronutrient ratio to match. Following are dietary and supplementation guidelines for power fitness exercisers to help you in planning your nutrition program. Dietary and supplementation guidelines for middle-distance fitness exercisers can be found on page 248, and guidelines for endurance fitness exercisers can be found on page 250.

POWER FITNESS EXERCISERS

Fitness exercisers who participate in activities that require spurts of energy are power athletes. Among the typical activities they enjoy are arm wrestling, croquet, and table tennis.

Dietary Guidelines

The following pie charts illustrate how you should divide up your caloric intake to match the energy demands of your power fitness activity during the preseason, season, and off-season. They show the target percentages of fat, protein, and carbohydrates that your five to six meals should supply each day.

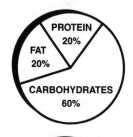

Target macronutrient ratio for the preseason and off-season.

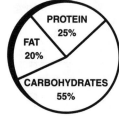

Target macronutrient ratio for the season.

Note that fat has about 9 calories per gram, while protein and carbohydrates have only 4 calories per gram. Therefore, during the season, if you needed to consume a total of 2,500 calories per day, you would aim for 500 calories (20 percent of your total daily calories) from fat, 625 calories (25 percent of your total daily calories) from protein, and the remaining 1,375 calories (55 percent of your total daily calories) from carbohydrates.

Some other important considerations for power fitness exercisers are:

☐ Carbohydrates are the major source of energy for short-term activities. Complex carbohydrates are the best source because they most effectively refill the glycogen stores in the muscles and liver. In addition, they elevate the blood sugar to a level sufficient for long sessions of intensive training.

☐ As a power athlete, you must make sure that you consume adequate amounts of both carbohydrates and protein. If your energy stores become drastically depleted or you experience lactic-acid buildup, you may suffer temporary muscle fatigue. If you do not refill your glycogen stores before your next workout or fitness-activity session, your body may begin breaking down muscle tissue for the protein it needs for energy.

☐ Directly before workouts and fitness-activity sessions, consume carbohydrate drinks with high glycemic indexes to keep your blood sugar sustained at an appropriate level. This will allow you to train or play intensively without having your explosiveness hindered by fatigue.

☐ As a power athlete, you need to stimulate the storage of glycogen in your muscles while promoting repair and growth of your muscle tissue and inhibiting buildup of body fat. To do this:

• Train anaerobically on a regular basis. Intensive training stimulates increased storage of glycogen in the muscles and liver, which provides additional energy for greater exercise capacity.

• Consume five to six meals a day. Eating several smaller meals rather than three larger ones will keep your blood-sugar level stable throughout the day and will ensure that a supply of protein is always available for your muscles.

• Keep your fat intake to a minimum. Large amounts of fat in your diet will add to your body fat and will cause you to lose minerals through frequent urination.

• Consume low-glycemic-index foods about two to three hours before workouts and fitness-activity sessions. These foods help sustain the blood-sugar level.

• Drink plenty of water. Not only will this practice reduce your chances of becoming dehydrated, but every ounce of glycogen that is stored within the muscles needs 3 ounces of water stored along with it. Therefore, remaining properly hydrated will also help prevent weakened muscle contractions.

As a power fitness exerciser, you should turn to Appendix C on page 345 for full discussions of the 20:25:55 and 20:20:60 dietary plans. Also presented are sample daily diets that use common, healthy foods to meet an athlete's energy and caloric needs. Use the directions on page 150 to estimate your average daily caloric requirement. Then use the directions in Chapter 14 or 15 to adjust your diet for off-season fat loss or muscle building, respectively.

Supplementation Guidelines

In addition to eating a proper diet, you should also take dietary supplements to make sure that any nutrients you lose due to sweating or training are replenished. The following tables will help guide you in selecting the supplements appropriate for you. The first table lists the nutrients recommended for power fitness exercisers, as well as the range of intake for each nutrient. (For discussions of these nutrients, see Part One.) Note that within the ranges of intake, the lower amounts are for smaller individuals and lower-activity days, while the higher amounts are for larger individuals and higher-activity days.

RECOMMENDED NUTRIENTS AND RANGES OF INTAKE

For Power Fitness Exercisers

NUTRIENT	RANGE OF INTAKE
VITAMINS	
Vitamin A	8,000–16,000 IU
Beta-carotene	15,000–30,000 IU
Vitamin B$_1$ (thiamine)	30–80 mg
Vitamin B$_2$ (riboflavin)	30–80 mg
Vitamin B3 (niacin)	20–60 mg
Vitamin B$_5$ (pantothenic acid)	20–70 mg
Vitamin B$_6$ (pyridoxine)	20–60 mg
Vitamin B$_{12}$ (cobalamin)	12–100 mcg
Biotin	125–175 mcg
Folate	400–800 mcg
Vitamin C	800–1,500 mg
Vitamin D	400–800 IU
Vitamin E	200–600 IU
Vitamin K	60–160 mcg
MINERALS	
Boron	2–8 mg
Calcium	800–1,500 mg
Chromium	200–500 mcg
Copper	1–4 mg
Iodine	100–200 mcg
Iron	15–50 mg
Magnesium	250–650 mg
Manganese	12–35 mg
Molybdenum	100–200 mcg

NUTRIENT	RANGE OF INTAKE
Phosphorus	150–800 mg
Potassium	50–1,000 mg
Selenium	100–200 mcg
Zinc	15–50 mg
AMINO ACIDS	
L-glutamine	1,000–2,000 mg
FATTY ACIDS	
Alpha-linolenic acid	1,000–2,000 mg
Docosahexaenoic acid (DHA)	250–750 mg
Eiocosapentaenoic acid (EPA)	250–750 mg
Gamma linolenic acid (GLA)	100–400 mg
Linoleic acid	2,000–4,000 mg
METABOLITES	
Bioflavonoids	100–600 mg
Choline	100–600 mg
Creatine monohydrate	4,000–8,000 mg
Ferulic acid	50–100 mg
Inosine	500–1,000 mg
Inositol	100–600 mg
L-carnitine	750–2,000 mg
Octacosanol	1,000–3,000 mcg

IU = international units, mcg = micrograms, mg = milligrams.

The second table lists the different types of sports supplements available and indicates if their use by power fitness exercisers is recommended in the preseason, during the season, or directly before a fitness-activity session. The list also includes a number of popular nutritional practices—bicarbonate loading, carbohydrate loading, creatine and/or inosine loading, and water loading. (For a discussion of any of these supplements or practices, see the appropriate section in Part One or Part Three.)

RECOMMENDED SPORTS SUPPLEMENTS AND NUTRITIONAL PRACTICES

For Power Fitness Exercisers

	Intake Recommendation		
	PRESEASON	**SEASON**	**PREACTIVITY**
SUPPLEMENTS			
Multivitamins	Yes	Yes	Yes
Multiminerals	Yes	Yes	Yes
Antioxidants	Yes	Yes	Yes
Fatty acids	Yes	Yes	Yes

Intake Recommendation			
	PRESEASON	**SEASON**	**PREACTIVITY**
Metabolites	Optional	Yes	Yes
Branched-chain amino acids	Yes	Yes	Yes
Herbs	Yes	Yes	No
Low-calorie protein drink (200–300 calories)	Yes	Yes	Yes
Carbohydrate drink	Yes	Yes	Yes
Fat-burning supplement	Yes	Optional	No
PRACTICES			
Bicarbonate loading	No	Optional	Optional
Carbohydrate loading	No	No	No
Creatine and/or inosine loading	Optional	Optional	Optional
Water loading	No	No	Optional

MIDDLE-DISTANCE FITNESS EXERCISERS

Fitness exercisers who participate in activities that require a steady supply of energy for up to about one and a half hours are middle-distance athletes. Among the typical activities they enjoy are hang gliding, surfing, and wheelchair basketball.

Dietary Guidelines

The following pie chart illustrates how you should divide up your caloric intake to match the energy demands of your middle-distance fitness activity during the preseason, season, and off-season. It shows the target percentages of fat, protein, and carbohydrates that your five to six meals should supply each day.

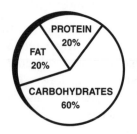

Target macronutrient ratio for the preseason, season, and off-season.

Note that fat has about 9 calories per gram, while protein and carbohydrates have only 4 calories per gram. Therefore, if you needed to consume a total of 2,500 calories per day, you would aim for 500 calories (20 percent of your total daily calories) from fat, 500 calories (20 percent of your total daily calories) from protein, and the remaining 1,500 calories (60 percent of your total daily calories) from carbohydrates.

Some other important considerations for middle-distance fitness exercisers are:

□ Carbohydrates are the major source of energy for short-term activities. Complex carbohydrates are the best source because they most effectively refill the glycogen stores in the muscles and liver. In addition, they elevate the blood sugar to a level sufficient for long sessions of intensive training.

□ As a middle-distance athlete, you must make sure that you consume adequate amounts of both carbohydrates and protein. If your energy stores become drastically depleted or you experience lactic-acid buildup, you may suffer temporary muscle fatigue. If you do not refill your glycogen stores before your next workout or fitness-activity session, your body may begin breaking down muscle tissue for the protein it needs for energy.

□ Directly before workouts and fitness-activity sessions, consume carbohydrate drinks with high glycemic indexes to keep your blood sugar sustained at an appropriate level. This will allow you to train or play intensively for longer periods of time.

□ As a middle-distance athlete, you need to stimulate the storage of glycogen in your muscles while promoting repair and growth of your muscle tissue and inhibiting buildup of body fat. To do this:

• Train against your anaerobic threshold (to exhaustion) on a regular basis. Intensive, exhaustive training stimulates increased storage of glycogen in the muscles and liver, which provides additional energy for greater exercise capacity.

• Consume five to six meals a day. Eating several smaller meals rather than three larger ones will keep your blood-sugar level stable throughout the day and will ensure that a supply of protein is always available for your muscles.

• Keep your fat intake to a minimum. Large amounts of fat in your diet will add to your body fat and will cause mineral loss through frequent urination.

• Consume low-glycemic-index foods about two to three hours before workouts and fitness-activity sessions. These foods help sustain the blood-sugar level.

• Drink plenty of water. Not only will this practice reduce your chances of becoming dehydrated, but every ounce of glycogen that is stored within the muscles needs 3 ounces of water stored along with it. Therefore, remaining properly hydrated will also help prevent weakened muscle contractions and early onset of fatigue.

As a middle-distance fitness exerciser, you should turn to Appendix C on page 345 for a full discussion of the 20:20:60 dietary plan. Also presented are sample daily diets that use common, healthy foods to meet an athlete's energy and caloric needs. Use the directions on page 150 to estimate your average daily caloric requirement. Then use the directions in Chapter 13 or 14 to adjust your diet for off-season fat loss or muscle building, respectively.

Supplementation Guidelines

In addition to eating a proper diet, you should also take dietary supplements to make sure that any nutrients you lose due to sweating or training are replenished. The following tables will help guide you in selecting the supplements appropriate for you. The first table lists the nutrients recommended for middle-distance fitness exercisers, as well as the range of intake for each nutrient. (For discussions of these nutrients, see Part One.) Note that within the ranges of intake, the lower amounts are for smaller individuals and lower-activity days, while the higher amounts are for larger individuals and higher-activity days.

RECOMMENDED NUTRIENTS AND RANGES OF INTAKE

For Middle-Distance Fitness Exercisers

NUTRIENT	RANGE OF INTAKE
VITAMINS	
Vitamin A	8,000–16,000 IU
Beta-carotene	15,000–30,000 IU
Vitamin B_1 (thiamine)	40–90 mg
Vitamin B_2 (riboflavin)	40–90 mg
Vitamin B_3 (niacin)	20–40 mg
Vitamin B_5 (pantothenic acid)	20–60 mg
Vitamin B_6 (pyridoxine)	20–50 mg
Vitamin B_{12} (cobalamin)	12–80 mcg
Biotin	125–175 mcg
Folate	400–800 mcg

NUTRIENT	RANGE OF INTAKE
Vitamin C	800–1,200 mg
Vitamin D	400–800 IU
Vitamin E	200–800 IU
Vitamin K	60–160 mcg
MINERALS	
Boron	2–8 mg
Calcium	800–1,500 mg
Chromium	200–500 mcg
Copper	1–4 mg
Iodine	100–200 mcg
Iron	15–50 mg
Magnesium	250–650 mg
Manganese	12–35 mg
Molybdenum	100–200 mcg
Phosphorus	150–800 mg
Potassium	50–1,000 mg
Selenium	100–200 mcg
Zinc	15–50 mg
AMINO ACIDS	
L-glutamic acid	500–1,000 mg
L-glutamine	1,000–2,000 mg
FATTY ACIDS	
Alpha-linolenic acid	500–1,500 mg
Docosahexaenoic acid (DHA)	250–750 mg
Eiocosapentaenoic acid (EPA)	250–750 mg
Gamma linolenic acid (GLA)	100–400 mg
Linoleic acid	1,000–2,000 mg
METABOLITES	
Bioflavonoids	300–800 mg
Choline	200–600 mg
Inositol	200–600 mg
L-carnitine	500–1,500 mg
Octacosanol	1,000–2,000 mcg

IU = international units, mcg = micrograms, mg = milligrams.

The second table lists the different types of sports supplements available and indicates if their use by middle-distance fitness exercisers is recommended in the preseason, during the season, or directly before a fitness-activity session. The list also includes a number of popular nutritional practices—bicarbonate loading, carbohydrate loading, creatine and/or inosine loading, and water loading. (For a discussion of any of these supplements or practices, see the appropriate section in Part One or Part Three.)

RECOMMENDED SPORTS SUPPLEMENTS AND NUTRITIONAL PRACTICES

For Middle-Distance Fitness Exercisers

	Intake Recommendation		
	PRESEASON	SEASON	PREACTIVITY
SUPPLEMENTS			
Multivitamins	Yes	Yes	Yes
Multiminerals	Yes	Yes	Yes
Antioxidants	Yes	Yes	Yes
Fatty acids	Yes	Yes	Yes
Metabolites	Optional	Yes	Yes
Branched-chain amino acids	Yes	Yes	Yes
Herbs	Yes	Yes	No
Medium-calorie protein drink (300–500 calories)	Yes	Yes	Yes
Carbohydrate drink	Yes	Yes	Yes
Fat-burning supplement	Yes	Optional	No
PRACTICES			
Bicarbonate loading	No	No	No
Carbohydrate loading	No	No	Optional
Creatine and/or inosine loading	No	No	No
Water loading	No	No	Optional

ENDURANCE FITNESS EXERCISERS

Fitness exercisers who participate in activities that require a steady supply of energy for more than about one and a half hours are endurance athletes. Among the typical activities they enjoy are 5-mile power walks, marathon running, and aerobic dance.

Dietary Guidelines

The following pie chart illustrates how you should divide up your caloric intake to match the energy demands of your endurance fitness activity during the preseason, season, and off-season. It shows the target percentages of fat, protein, and carbohydrates that your five to six meals should supply each day.

Note fat has about 9 calories per gram, while protein and carbohydrates have only 4 calories per gram. Therefore, if you needed to consume a total of 2,500

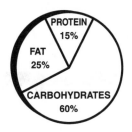

Target macronutrient ratio for the preseason, season, and off-season.

calories per day, you would aim for 625 calories (25 percent of your total daily calories) from fat, 375 calories (15 percent of your total daily calories) from protein, and the remaining 1,500 calories (60 percent of your total daily calories) from carbohydrates.

Some other important considerations for endurance fitness exercisers are:

☐ The energy source that is used during an aerobic activity depends upon the duration and intensity of the activity. During the first one and a half to two hours, both glycogen and body fat are the primary sources of energy. After one and a half to two hours, body fat alone becomes the primary source.

☐ While body fat is the primary source of energy during prolonged aerobic activities, it cannot be used efficiently unless some glycogen remains in the muscles and liver. Therefore, even ultra-endurance athletes must make sure to always keep their glycogen stores filled.

☐ As an endurance athlete, you need to encourage glycogen sparing in your body while stimulating the use of fat as your primary energy source. To do this:

• Train for endurance on a regular basis. Regular endurance training stimulates increased storage of both glycogen and fatty acids.

• Consume five to six meals a day. Eating several smaller meals rather than three larger ones will keep your blood-sugar level stable throughout the day.

• Do not load up on dietary fat. Consuming large amounts of fat was originally thought to benefit endurance athletes, whose primary source of energy is fat. However, fat loading can lead to frequent urination, which increases the loss of minerals essential to healthy heart action.

• Consume low-glycemic-index foods about two to three hours before workouts and fitness-activvity sessions. These foods help sustain the blood-sugar level.

• Do not consume food or caloric beverages from two hours before an endurance activity to fifteen minutes before. Food and caloric beverages cause the

insulin level to rise, which in turn can provoke transient hypoglycemia. Transient hypoglycemia interferes with the energy dynamics during exercise and can induce early onset of fatigue.

• Consume carbohydrates directly before and during endurance activities. Because exercise slows the release of insulin into the bloodstream, the ingestion of carbohydrates spares glycogen and allows the use of fat for energy. Carbohydrate drinks with high glycemic indexes help sustain the blood-sugar level, thereby preserving glycogen stores.

• During endurance activities, drink plenty of water. Endurance activities cause profuse sweating, which results in loss of valuable fluids and minerals. Dehydration not only reduces performance but can seriously affect health.

• Drink electrolyte-containing beverages during endurance activities. These drinks help replace minerals that are lost through sweating.

• During endurance activities, drink 4 to 6 ounces of fluid every fifteen to thirty minutes. For every pound of body weight lost through sweating, 1 pint of fluid should be consumed. Chilled fluids are absorbed the quickest.

As an endurance fitness exerciser, you should turn to Appendix C on page 345 for a full discussion of the 25:15:60 dietary plan. Also presented are sample daily diets that use common, healthy foods to meet an athlete's energy and caloric needs. Use the directions on page 150 to estimate your average daily caloric requirement. Then use the directions in Chapter 13 or 14 to adjust your diet for off-season fat loss or muscle building, respectively.

Supplementation Guidelines

In addition to eating a proper diet, you should also take dietary supplements to make sure that any nutrients you lose due to sweating or training are replenished. The following tables will help guide you in selecting the supplements appropriate for you. The first table lists the nutrients recommended for endurance fitness exercisers, as well as the range of intake for each nutrient. (For discussions of these nutrients, see Part One.) Note that within the ranges of intake, the lower amounts are for smaller individuals and lower-activity days, while the higher amounts are for larger individuals and higher-activity days.

RECOMMENDED NUTRIENTS AND RANGES OF INTAKE

For Endurance Fitness Exercisers

NUTRIENT	RANGE OF INTAKE
VITAMINS	
Vitamin A	8,000–16,000 IU
Beta-carotene	15,000–40,000 IU
Vitamin B_1 (thiamine)	60–120 mg
Vitamin B_2 (riboflavin)	60–120 mg
Vitamin B_3 (niacin)	10–20 mg
Vitamin B_5 (pantothenic acid)	60–120 mg
Vitamin B_6 (pyridoxine)	20–60 mg
Vitamin B_{12} (cobalamin)	12–120 mcg
Biotin	125–200 mcg
Folate	400–800 mcg
Vitamin C	1,000–2,000 mg
Vitamin D	400–800 IU
Vitamin E	400–1,000 IU
Vitamin K	60–160 mcg
MINERALS	
Boron	2–8 mg
Calcium	800–1,500 mg
Chromium	200–500 mcg
Copper	1–4 mg
Iodine	100–200 mcg
Iron	15–50 mg
Magnesium	250–650 mg
Manganese	12–35 mg
Molybdenum	100–200 mcg
Phosphorus	150–800 mg
Potassium	50–1,000 mg
Selenium	100–200 mcg
Zinc	15–50 mg
AMINO ACIDS	
L-glutamic acid	1,000–1,500 mg
L-glutamine	1,000–2,000 mg
FATTY ACIDS	
Alpha-linolenic acid	500–1,000 mg
Docosahexaenoic acid (DHA)	400–1,000 mg
Eiocosapentaenoic acid (EPA)	400–1,000 mg
Gamma linolenic acid (GLA)	200–500 mg
Linoleic acid	500–1,000 mg
METABOLITES	
Bioflavonoids	500–1,000 mg
Choline	500–1,000 mg
Coenzyme Q_{10}	30–80 mg
Inositol	500–1,000 mg

NUTRIENT	RANGE OF INTAKE
L-carnitine	1,000–3,000 mg
Octacosanol	1,000–2,000 mcg
OTHER	
Caffeine*	200–400 mg

IU = international units, mcg = micrograms, mg = milligrams.
*Verify with your sports governing organization that caffeine consumption is permitted during competition.

The second table lists the different types of sports supplements available and indicates if their use by endurance fitness exercisers is recommended in the preseason, during the season, or directly before a fitness-activity session. The list also includes a number of popular nutritional practices—bicarbonate loading, carbohydrate loading, creatine and/or inosine loading, and water loading. (For a discussion of any of these supplements or practices, see the appropriate section in Part One or Part Three.)

RECOMMENDED SPORTS SUPPLEMENTS AND NUTRITIONAL PRACTICES

For Endurance Fitness Exercisers

	Intake Recommendation		
	PRESEASON	SEASON	PREACTIVITY
SUPPLEMENTS			
Multivitamins	Yes	Yes	Yes
Multiminerals	Yes	Yes	Yes
Antioxidants	Yes	Yes	No
Fatty acids	Yes	Yes	Yes
Metabolites	Optional	Yes	Yes
Branched-chain amino acids	Yes	Yes	Yes
Herbs	Yes	Yes	No
High-calorie protein drink (over 500 calories)	Yes	Yes	Yes
Carbohydrate drink with glycerol and electrolytes	Yes	Yes	Yes
Fat-burning supplement	Yes	Yes	No
PRACTICES			
Bicarbonate loading	No	No	No
Carbohydrate loading	No	Optional	Yes
Creatine and/or inosine loading	No	No	No
Water loading	No	Optional	Yes

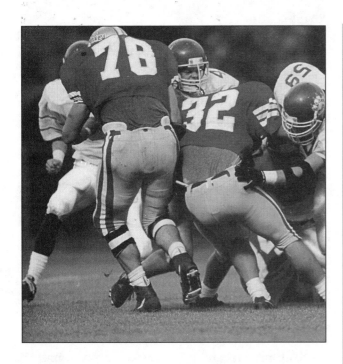

FOOTBALL

Includes American, Australian, and Canadian Football

Also for Rugby and Speedskating

Football is a game of blocks, tackles, leaps, bounds, and a multitude of other potentially crippling, body-contorting movements. Whether the American, Canadian, or Australian version, it is a multifaceted game that involves a wide range of skills and movements. It requires not only speed and strength in short, explosive bursts, but also a high level of anaerobic-strength endurance, as well as flexibility and agility. Running with the ball is a prime example. The more explosive strength as well as starting strength you possess to put into your forward movement, the tougher it is for an opponent to bring you down. At the same time, the quicker and more agile you are, the better you are able to weave your way to a touchdown. Kicking is another example. Kicking also requires starting strength, for a strong kick, as well as flexibility and agility, for the proper follow-through.

Every bit of your training and diet must reflect these elements. These elements are what make football "ballistic" in nature. In fact, football is very "ballistic," so improved recovery and tissue repair plus increased speed and strength are your training and dietary goals, especially during the preseason and sea-

son. Nutritionally, this means emphasizing short-term energy needs and maximizing the muscles' recovery and tissue-repair processes.

In football, the energy output is primarily anaerobic (without oxygen). This does not mean that training for or playing the game is easy, however. You must hit, grapple, throw, and perform other lightning-quick reflexive movements over and over again, repeatedly testing your tolerance to pain and fatigue, caused by lactic-acid buildup in your muscles. Football training is extremely intensive and grueling. At the highest levels, football speed training forces you to operate at your anaerobic threshold (the point at which you must receive oxygen).

Muscles grow when they are stressed. In football, the aim is to make the muscles grow as strong and as quick as possible. This calls for specialized training. Furthermore, the incredible force output of football, especially coupled with the ballistic aspects of the game, requires the support of a carefully constructed nutrition program.

ENERGY SOURCES OF FOOTBALL PLAYERS

The muscles rely on three major systems to supply the energy they need—the immediate, glycolytic, and oxidative energy systems. For short-term energy for explosive-strength output, the muscles depend on the immediate energy systems. The immediate energy systems are nonoxidative—that is, they do not use oxygen. Instead, these systems generate energy through the use of adenosine triphosphate (ATP) and creatine phosphate (CP). CP is produced in the body and stored in the muscle fibers. It is broken down by enzymes to regenerate ATP, which is also stored in the muscle fibers. When the ATP is in turn broken down, the result is a spark of energy that triggers a muscle contraction.

For medium-term energy for repeated near-maximum exertion, the muscles turn to the glycolytic energy systems. In these systems, which are also nonoxidative, glycogen is used to produce energy. Glycogen is the storage form of glucose. It is stored in the liver and muscles, and is readily converted back to glucose when it is needed for energy.

For long-term energy for endurance activities, the muscles use the oxidative energy systems. In these systems, which are also nonoxidative, oxygen is used to oxidize long-chain fatty acids, protein, and glucose, which generates energy. For athletes, getting enough oxygen can mean a winning performance rather than a second-place showing.

Every sport involves a variety of skills, and each skill utilizes a unique combination of these three energy sources. The following table lists the major football positions and shows how much your body relies on each of the energy sources when you play them. Percentages are also given for an average workout.

WHERE YOUR ENERGY COMES FROM

For Football Players

	Energy Systems		
	IMMEDIATE	GLYCOLYTIC	OXIDATIVE
Positions*			
Defensive lineman	70%	30%	0%
Linebacker	70%	30%	0%
Offensive lineman	70%	30%	0%
Punter	100%	0%	0%
Quarterback	80%	20%	0%
Running back	80%	20%	0%
Special team	70%	30%	0%
Tight end	80%	20%	0%
Wide receiver	80%	20%	0%
Average workout	60%	30%	10%

*Percentages given are for games and workouts.

When considering the type of nutritional support to give your training program, keep the following factors in mind:

☐ All athletes need to consume high-quality protein several times a day for effective recovery and adequate repair of damaged muscle tissue.

☐ Athletes whose muscles rely substantially on the immediate or glycolytic energy systems should keep their fat intake to a minimum because fat is not an efficient energy source for their intensive training, which is almost exclusively anaerobic in nature. Since the fat calories consumed by these athletes are not generally used for energy, they are stored as body fat.

☐ All athletes should consume a carefully measured amount of high-quality carbohydrates several times a day to ensure an adequate supply of energy.

☐ The carbohydrates in all preworkout meals should consist of foods with low glycemic indexes to ensure that training intensity does not wane and that muscle

tissue is not cannibalized for energy. (For the glycemic indexes of some common foods, see page 29.)

The aim of your nutrition program is to make your body healthy enough to accomplish recovery and tissue repair speedily and efficiently—without adding body fat. Your further aim is to do this while maintaining a high strength-to-weight ratio. These aims alone make diet as critical as training for football players. You must eat just the right amount of food. Eat the wrong foods or the wrong amounts just a few times too often and you will sabotage your fitness efforts. Even more important, do not be in a hurry. It takes *years* to become a great football player. Rush the nutrition and training processes and you will become fat, your recovery rate will decline, and your injury rate will rise.

NUTRITION FOR FOOTBALL PLAYERS

Football players are combination power–middle-distance athletes. They obtain most of their energy from a combination of the immediate and glycolytic energy systems. Therefore, as a football player, you need to plan your nutritional intake, from both food and supplement sources, to support these nonoxidative systems. In addition, since your energy expenditure changes in the off-season, you need to adjust your caloric intake and macronutrient ratio to match. Following are dietary guidelines for football players to help you in planning your nutrition program. Supplementation guidelines for football players can be found on page 225.

Dietary Guidelines

The following pie charts illustrate how you should divide up your caloric intake to match the energy demands of football during the preseason, season, and off-season. They show the target percentages of fat, protein, and carbohydrates that your five to six meals should supply each day.

Note that fat has about 9 calories per gram, while protein and carbohydrates have only 4 calories per gram. Therefore, during the season, if you needed to consume a total of 2,500 calories per day, you would aim for 375 calories (15 percent of your total daily calories) from fat, 750 calories (30 percent of your total daily calories) from protein, and the remaining 1,375 calories (55 percent of your total daily calories) from carbohydrates.

Some other important considerations for football players are:

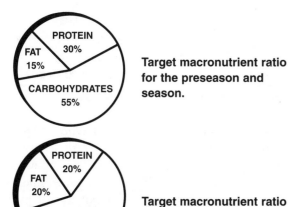

Target macronutrient ratio for the preseason and season.

PROTEIN 30%
FAT 15%
CARBOHYDRATES 55%

Target macronutrient ratio for the off-season.

PROTEIN 20%
FAT 20%
CARBOHYDRATES 60%

☐ Carbohydrates are the major source of energy for short-term activities. Complex carbohydrates are the best source because they most effectively refill the glycogen stores in the muscles and liver. In addition, they elevate the blood sugar to a level sufficient for long sessions of intensive training.

☐ As a combination power–middle-distance athlete, you must make sure that you consume adequate amounts of both carbohydrates and protein. If your energy stores become drastically depleted or you experience lactic-acid buildup, you may suffer temporary muscle fatigue. If you do not refill your glycogen stores before your next workout or game, your body may begin breaking down muscle tissue for the protein it needs for energy.

☐ Directly before workouts and games, consume carbohydrate drinks with high glycemic indexes to keep your blood sugar sustained at an appropriate level. This will allow you to train or play intensively for longer periods of time.

☐ As a combination power–middle-distance athlete, you need to stimulate the storage of glycogen in your muscles while promoting repair and growth of your muscle tissue and inhibiting buildup of body fat. To do this:

• Train against your anaerobic threshold (to exhaustion) on a regular basis. Intensive, exhaustive training stimulates increased storage of glycogen in the muscles and liver, which provides additional energy for greater exercise capacity.

• Consume five to six meals a day. Eating several smaller meals rather than three larger ones will keep your blood-sugar level stable throughout the day and will ensure that a supply of protein is always available for your muscles.

• Keep your fat intake to a minimum. Large amounts of fat in your diet will add to your body fat and will cause mineral loss through frequent urination.

• Consume low-glycemic-index foods about two to three hours before workouts and games. These foods help sustain the blood-sugar level.

• Drink plenty of water. Not only will this practice reduce your chances of becoming dehydrated, but every ounce of glycogen that is stored within the muscles needs 3 ounces of water stored along with it. Therefore, remaining properly hydrated will also help prevent weakened muscle contractions and early onset of fatigue.

• Do not eat a new food just before a game. Different people often react differently to the same food. Before a game, eat just those foods that you know your body will handle well.

As a football player, you should turn to Appendix C on page 345 for full discussions of the 15:30:55 and 20:20:60 dietary plans. Also presented are sample daily diets that use common, healthy foods to meet an athlete's energy and caloric needs. Use the directions on page 150 to estimate your average daily caloric requirement. Then use the directions in Chapter 13 or 14 to adjust your diet for off-season fat loss or muscle building, respectively.

Supplementation Guidelines

In addition to eating a proper diet, you should also take dietary supplements to make sure that any nutrients you lose due to sweating or training are replenished. The following tables will help guide you in selecting the supplements appropriate for you. The first table lists the nutrients recommended for football players, as well as the range of intake for each nutrient. (For discussions of these nutrients, see Part One.) Note that within the ranges of intake, the lower amounts are for smaller individuals and lower-activity days, while the higher amounts are for larger individuals and higher-activity days.

RECOMMENDED NUTRIENTS AND RANGES OF INTAKE

For Football Players

NUTRIENT	RANGE OF INTAKE
VITAMINS	
Vitamin A	8,000–16,000 IU
Beta-carotene	15,000–25,000 IU
Vitamin B_1 (thiamine)	30–120 mg
Vitamin B_2 (riboflavin)	30–120 mg
Vitamin B_3 (niacin)	40–80 mg
Vitamin B_5 (pantothenic acid)	20–100 mg
Vitamin B_6 (pyridoxine)	20–80 mg
Vitamin B_{12} (cobalamin)	12–120 mcg
Biotin	125–175 mcg
Folate	400–800 mcg
Vitamin C	800–2,000 mg
Vitamin D	400–800 IU
Vitamin E	200–600 IU
Vitamin K	60–160 mcg
MINERALS	
Boron	2–8 mg
Calcium	800–1,500 mg
Chromium	200–500 mcg
Copper	1–4 mg
Iodine	100–200 mcg
Iron	15–50 mg
Magnesium	250–650 mg
Manganese	12–35 mg
Molybdenum	100–200 mcg
Phosphorus	150–800 mg
Potassium	50–1,000 mg
Selenium	100–200 mcg
Zinc	15–50 mg
AMINO ACIDS	
L-glutamine	1,000–2,000 mg
FATTY ACIDS	
Alpha-linolenic acid	1,500–3,000 mg
Docosahexaenoic acid (DHA)	250–750 mg
Eiocosapentaenoic acid (EPA)	250–750 mg
Gamma linolenic acid (GLA)	100–400 mg
Linoleic acid	3,000–6,000 mg
METABOLITES	
Bioflavonoids	200–800 mg
Choline	100–600 mg
Creatine monohydrate	8,000–20,000 mg

NUTRIENT	RANGE OF INTAKE
Ferulic acid	50–100 mg
Inosine	500–1,000 mg
Inositol	100–600 mg
L-carnitine	750–2,000 mg
Octacosanol	3,000–6,000 mcg

IU = international units, mcg = micrograms, mg = milligrams.

The second table lists the different types of sports supplements available and indicates if their use by football players is recommended in the preseason, during the season, or directly before a game. The list also includes a number of popular nutritional practices—bicarbonate loading, carbohydrate loading, creatine and/or inosine loading, and water loading. (For a discussion of any of these supplements or practices, see the appropriate section in Part One or Part Three.)

RECOMMENDED SPORTS SUPPLEMENTS AND NUTRITIONAL PRACTICES

For Football Players

	Intake Recommendation		
	PRESEASON	SEASON	PREGAME
SUPPLEMENTS			
Multivitamins	Yes	Yes	Yes
Multiminerals	Yes	Yes	Yes
Antioxidants	Yes	Yes	Yes
Fatty acids	Yes	Yes	Yes
Metabolites	No	Yes	Yes
Branched-chain amino acids	Yes	Yes	Yes
Herbs	Yes	Yes	No
Medium-calorie protein drink (300–500 calories)	Yes	Yes	Yes
Carbohydrate drink	Yes	Yes	Yes
Fat-burning supplement	Yes	Optional	No
PRACTICES			
Bicarbonate loading	No	Optional	Optional
Carbohydrate loading	No	No	Optional
Creatine and/or inosine loading	Optional	Yes	Yes
Water loading	No	No	Optional

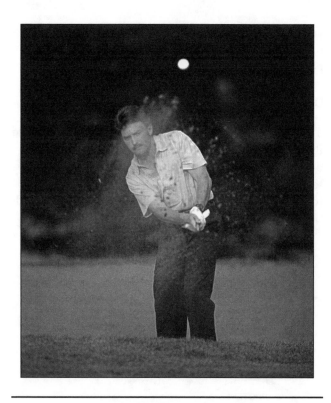

GOLF

Also for Disc Golf

In golf, the energy output is primarily anaerobic (without oxygen). Playing eighteen holes for a bit of fresh air is fun, but for serious golfers, it can be downright draining due to the mental focus, skill, and conditioning required to ensure victory at each hole. The muscles in your hands slowly become fatigued and you begin to lose fine motor control over the club. Your wrist and forearm muscles tire similarly. Training for golf tournaments is not easy either. It is grueling and mind-numbing. At the highest levels, golf forces you to train like an elite athlete, pushing your threshold of both physical and mental fatigue.

While it is not yet the norm for golfers to follow a specialized training program, it will become so. It is inevitable, since it is part of the quest to become number one in most sports. Furthermore, the energy output of tournament golf requires the support of a carefully constructed nutrition program.

ENERGY SOURCES OF GOLFERS

The muscles rely on three major systems to supply the energy they need—the immediate, glycolytic, and oxidative energy systems. For short-term energy for explosive-strength output, the muscles depend on the immediate energy systems. The immediate energy systems are nonoxidative—that is, they do not use oxygen. Instead, these systems generate energy through the use of adenosine triphosphate (ATP) and creatine phosphate (CP). CP is produced in the body and stored in the muscle fibers. It is broken down by enzymes to regenerate ATP, which is also stored in the muscle fibers. When the ATP is in turn broken down, the result is a spark of energy that triggers a muscle contraction.

For medium-term energy for repeated near-maximum exertion, the muscles turn to the glycolytic energy systems. In these systems, which are also nonoxidative, glycogen is used to produce energy. Glycogen is the storage form of glucose. It is stored in the liver and muscles, and is readily converted back to glucose when it is needed for energy.

For long-term energy for endurance activities, the muscles use the oxidative energy systems. In these systems, oxygen is used to oxidize long-chain fatty acids, protein, and glucose, which generates energy. For athletes, getting enough oxygen can mean a winning performance rather than a second-place showing.

Every sport involves a variety of skills, and each skill utilizes a unique combination of these three energy sources. The following table shows how much your body relies on each of the energy sources during an average golf game and an average golf tournament. Percentages are also given for the third day of sudden-death play.

WHERE YOUR ENERGY COMES FROM

For Golfers		
Energy Systems		
IMMEDIATE	GLYCOLYTIC	OXIDATIVE
Average game (18 holes)		
40%	50%	10%
Average tournament (36 holes)		
50%	40%	10%
Third day of sudden death		
60%	30%	10%

When considering the type of nutritional support to give your training program, keep the following factors in mind:

☐ All athletes need to consume high-quality protein

several times a day for effective recovery and adequate repair of damaged muscle tissue.

☐ Athletes whose muscles rely substantially on the immediate or glycolytic energy systems should keep their fat intake to a minimum because fat is not an efficient energy source for their intensive training, which is almost exclusively anaerobic in nature. Since the fat calories consumed by these athletes are not generally used for energy, they are stored as body fat.

☐ All athletes should consume a carefully measured amount of high-quality carbohydrates several times a day to ensure an adequate supply of energy.

☐ Athletes who need to remain mentally focused for prolonged periods of time must keep their liver glycogen stores filled. Liver glycogen is the primary fuel that the brain burns for energy, and when the stores become depleted, focus and timing begin to suffer.

☐ The carbohydrates in all preworkout meals should consist of foods with low glycemic indexes to ensure that training intensity does not wane and that muscle tissue is not cannibalized for energy. (For the glycemic indexes of some common foods, see page 29).

The aim of your nutrition program is to make your body healthy enough to accomplish recovery and tissue repair speedily and efficiently—without adding body fat. Your further aim is to do this while maintaining a high strength-to-weight ratio. These aims alone make diet as critical as training for golfers. You must eat just the right amount of food. Eat the wrong foods or the wrong amounts just a few times too often and you will sabotage your fitness efforts. Even more important, do not be in a hurry. It takes *years* to become a great golfer. Rush the nutrition and training processes and you will become fat, you may become overtrained, and your handicap will suffer.

NUTRITION FOR GOLFERS

Golfers are combination power–middle-distance athletes. They obtain most of their energy from a combination of the immediate and glycolytic energy systems. Therefore, as a golfer, you need to plan your nutritional intake, from both food and supplement sources, to support these nonoxidative systems. In addition, since your energy expenditure changes in the preseason and off-season, you need to adjust your caloric intake and macronutrient ratio to match. Following are dietary guidelines for golfers to help

you in planning your nutrition program. Supplementation guidelines for golfers can be found on page 259.

Dietary Guidelines

The following pie charts illustrate how you should divide up your caloric intake to match the energy demands of golf during the preseason, season, and off-season. They show the target percentages of fat, protein, and carbohydrates that your five to six meals should supply each day.

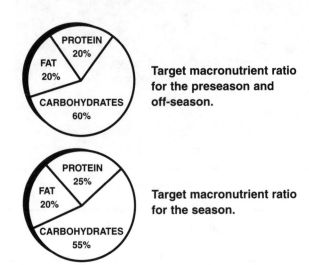

Target macronutrient ratio for the preseason and off-season.

Target macronutrient ratio for the season.

Note that fat has about 9 calories per gram, while protein and carbohydrates have only 4 calories per gram. Therefore, during the season, if you needed to consume a total of 2,500 calories per day, you would aim for 500 calories (20 percent of your total daily calories) from fat, 625 calories (25 percent of your total daily calories) from protein, and the remaining 1,375 calories (55 percent of your total daily calories) from carbohydrates.

Some other important considerations for golfers are:

☐ Carbohydrates are the major source of energy for short-term activities. Complex carbohydrates are the best source because they most effectively refill the glycogen stores in the muscles and liver. In addition, they elevate the blood sugar to a level sufficient for long sessions of intensive training.

☐ As a combination power–middle-distance athlete, you must make sure that you consume adequate amounts of both carbohydrates and protein. If your energy stores become drastically depleted or you experience lactic-acid buildup, you may suffer temporary muscle fatigue. If you do not refill your glycogen stores before your next workout or game, your body may begin breaking down muscle tissue for the protein it needs for energy.

☐ Directly before workouts and games, consume carbohydrate drinks with high glycemic indexes to keep your blood sugar sustained at an appropriate level. This will allow you to train or play intensively for longer periods of time.

☐ As a combination power–middle-distance athlete, you need to stimulate the storage of glycogen in your muscles while promoting repair and growth of your muscle tissue and inhibiting buildup of body fat. To do this:

• Train against your anaerobic threshold (to exhaustion) on a regular basis. Intensive, exhaustive training stimulates increased storage of glycogen in the muscles and liver, which provides additional energy for greater exercise capacity.

• Consume five to six meals a day. Eating several smaller meals rather than three larger ones will keep your blood-sugar level stable throughout the day and will ensure that a supply of protein is always available for your muscles.

• Keep your fat intake to a minimum. Large amounts of fat in your diet will add to your body fat and will cause mineral loss through frequent urination.

• Consume low-glycemic-index foods about two to three hours before workouts and games. These foods help sustain the blood-sugar level.

• Drink plenty of water. Not only will this practice reduce your chances of becoming dehydrated, but every ounce of glycogen that is stored within the muscles needs 3 ounces of water stored along with it. Therefore, remaining properly hydrated will also help prevent weakened muscle contractions and early onset of fatigue.

As a golfer, you should turn to Appendix C on page 345 for full discussions of the 20:20:60 and 20:25:55 dietary plans. Also presented are sample daily diets that use common, healthy foods to meet an athlete's energy and caloric needs. Use the directions on page 150 to estimate your average daily caloric requirement. Then use the directions in Chapter 13 or 14 to adjust your diet for off-season fat loss or muscle building, respectively.

Supplementation Guidelines

In addition to eating a proper diet, you should also take dietary supplements to make sure that any nutrients you lose due to sweating or training are replenished. The following tables will help guide you in selecting the supplements appropriate for you. The first table lists the nutrients recommended for golfers, as well as the range of intake for each nutrient. (For discussions of these nutrients, see Part One.) Note that within the ranges of intake, the lower amounts are for smaller individuals and lower-activity days, while the higher amounts are for larger individuals and higher-activity days.

RECOMMENDED NUTRIENTS AND RANGES OF INTAKE

For Golfers

NUTRIENT	RANGE OF INTAKE
VITAMINS	
Vitamin A	8,000–16,000 IU
Beta-carotene	15,000–30,000 IU
Vitamin B₁ (thiamine)	40–120 mg
Vitamin B₂ (riboflavin)	40–120 mg
Vitamin B₃ (niacin)	20–40 mg
Vitamin B₅ (pantothenic acid)	20–100 mg
Vitamin B₆ (pyridoxine)	20–80 mg
Vitamin B₁₂ (cobalamin)	12–120 mcg
Biotin	125–175 mcg
Folate	400–800 mcg
Vitamin C	800–2,000 mg
Vitamin D	400–800 IU
Vitamin E	200–800 IU
Vitamin K	60–160 mcg
MINERALS	
Boron	2–8 mg
Calcium	800–1,500 mg
Chromium	200–500 mcg
Copper	1–4 mg
Iodine	100–200 mcg
Iron	15–50 mg
Magnesium	250–650 mg
Manganese	12–35 mg
Molybdenum	100–200 mcg
Phosphorus	150–800 mg
Potassium	50–1,000 mg
Selenium	100–200 mcg
Zinc	15–50 mg

NUTRIENT	RANGE OF INTAKE
AMINO ACIDS	
L-glutamic acid	500–1,000 mg
L-glutamine	1,000–2,000 mg
FATTY ACIDS	
Alpha-linolenic acid	500–1,000 mg
Docosahexaenoic acid (DHA)	250–750 mg
Eiocosapentaenoic acid (EPA)	250–750 mg
Gamma linolenic acid (GLA)	100–400 mg
Linoleic acid	2,000–3,000 mg
METABOLITES	
Bioflavonoids	300–800 mg
Choline	200–600 mg
Creatine monohydrate	4,000–8,000 mg
Inositol	200–600 mg
L-carnitine	500–1,000 mg
Octacosanol	6,000–12,000 mcg

IU = international units, mcg = micrograms, mg = milligrams.

The second table lists the different kinds of sports supplements available and indicates if their use by golfers is recommended in the preseason, during the season, or directly before a game. The list also includes a number of popular nutritional practices—bicarbonate loading, carbohydrate loading, creatine and/or inosine loading, and water loading. (For a discussion of any of these supplements or practices, see the appropriate section in Part One or Part Three.)

RECOMMENDED SPORTS SUPPLEMENTS AND NUTRITIONAL PRACTICES

For Golfers

	Intake Recommendation		
	PRESEASON	SEASON	PREGAME
SUPPLEMENTS			
Multivitamins	Yes	Yes	Yes
Multiminerals	Yes	Yes	Yes
Antioxidants	Yes	Yes	Yes
Fatty acids	Yes	Yes	Yes
Metabolites	Optional	Yes	Yes
Branched-chain amino acids	Yes	Yes	Yes
Herbs	Yes	Yes	No
Low-calorie protein drink (200–300 calories)	Yes	Yes	Yes
Carbohydrate drink	Yes	Yes	Yes

	Intake Recommendation		
	PRESEASON	SEASON	PREGAME
Fat-burning supplement	Yes	Optional	No
PRACTICES			
Bicarbonate loading	No	No	No
Carbohydrate loading	No	No	Optional
Creatine and/or inosine loading	No	No	Optional
Water loading	No	No	Optional

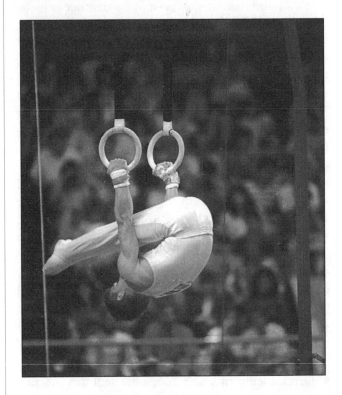

GYMNASTICS

Includes Acrobatics, Balance Beam, Floor Exercise, Horizontal Bar, Parallel Bars, Side Horse, Still Rings, Uneven Parallel Bars, and Vaulting

Also for Circus Acrobatics, Diving, and Trampoline

Gymnastics is a sport of jumps, twirls, somersaults, and a multitude of other movements that require lightning-fast reflexes. It is a multifaceted sport that involves a wide range of skills and force output. Both the men's and women's events require not only speed and strength in short, explosive bursts, but also a high level of anaerobic-strength endurance, flexibility, agility, and tolerance to pain and fatigue caused by lactic-acid buildup in the muscles.

Every bit of your training and diet must reflect these elements. These elements are what make gymnastics explosive in nature. In fact, gymnastics is very explosive, so improved recovery and tissue repair plus increased speed and strength are your year-round training and dietary goals. Nutritionally, this means emphasizing short-term energy needs and maximizing the muscles' recovery and tissue-repair processes.

In gymnastics, the energy output is primarily anaerobic (without oxygen). This does not mean that training for or competing in gymnastics is easy, however. Gymnastics training is extremely intensive and grueling. At the highest levels, gymnastics training forces you to operate at your anaerobic threshold (the point at which you must receive oxygen).

Muscles grow when they are stressed. In gymnastics, the aim is to make the muscles grow as strong and as quick as possible. This calls for specialized training. Furthermore, the incredible force output of gymnastics, especially coupled with the explosive aspects of the sport, requires the support of a carefully contructed nutrition program.

ENERGY SOURCES OF GYMNASTS

The muscles rely on three major systems to supply the energy they need—the immediate, glycolytic, and oxidative energy systems. For short-term energy for explosive-strength output, the muscles depend on the immediate energy systems. The immediate energy systems are nonoxidative—that is, they do not use oxygen. Instead, these systems generate energy through the use of adenosine triphosphate (ATP) and creatine phosphate (CP). CP is produced in the body and stored in the muscle fibers. It is broken down by enzymes to regenerate ATP, which is also stored in the muscle fibers. When the ATP is in turn broken down, the result is a spark of energy that triggers a muscle contraction.

For medium-term energy for repeated near-maximum exertion, the muscles turn to the glycolytic energy systems. In these systems, which are also non-oxidative, glycogen is used to produce energy. Glycogen is the storage form of glucose. It is stored in the liver and muscles, and is readily converted back to glucose when it is needed for energy.

For long-term energy for endurance activities, the muscles use the oxidative energy systems. In these systems, oxygen is used to oxidize long-chain fatty acids, protein, and glucose, which generates energy. For athletes, getting enough oxygen can mean a winning performance rather than a second-place showing.

Every sport involves a variety of skills, and each skill utilizes a unique combination of these three energy sources. The following table lists the major gymnastics events and shows how much your body relies on each of the energy sources when you participate in them. Percentages are also given for three similar sports.

WHERE YOUR ENERGY COMES FROM

For Gymnasts		
Energy Systems		
IMMEDIATE	GLYCOLYTIC	OXIDATIVE
Balance beam (women)		
70%	30%	0%
Floor exercise (men and women)		
60%	40%	0%
Horizontal bar (men)		
70%	30%	0%
Parallel bars (men)		
70%	30%	0%
Side horse (men)		
60%	40%	0%
Still rings (men)		
70%	30%	0%
Uneven parallel bars (men and women)		
70%	30%	0%
Vaulting (men and women)		
100%	0%	0%

For Similar Sports		
Acrobatics (circus)	80%	20%	0%
Diving	100%	0%	0%
Trampoline	80%	20%	0%

When considering the type of nutritional support to give your training program, keep the following factors in mind:

☐ All athletes need to consume high-quality protein several times a day for effective recovery and adequate repair of damaged muscle tissue.

☐ Athletes whose muscles rely substantially on the immediate or glycolytic energy systems should keep their fat intake to a minimum because fat is not an efficient energy source for their intensive training, which is almost exclusively anaerobic in nature. Since the fat calories consumed by these athletes are not generally used for energy, they are stored as body fat.

☐ All athletes should consume a carefully measured amount of high-quality carbohydrates several times a day to ensure an adequate supply of energy.

☐ The carbohydrates in all preworkout meals should consist of foods with low glycemic indexes to ensure that training intensity does not wane and that muscle tissue is not cannibalized for energy. (For the glycemic indexes of some common foods, see page 29.)

The aim of your nutrition program is to make your body healthy enough to accomplish recovery and tissue repair speedily and efficiently—without adding body fat. Your further aim is to do this while maintaining a high strength-to-weight ratio. These aims alone make diet as critical as training for gymnasts. You must eat just the right amount of food. Eat the wrong foods or the wrong amounts just a few times too often and you will sabotage your fitness efforts.

NUTRITION FOR GYMNASTS

Gymnasts are power athletes. They obtain most of their energy from a combination of the immediate and glycolytic energy systems. Therefore, as a gymnast, you need to plan your nutritional intake, from both food and supplement sources, to support these nonoxidative systems. In addition, since your energy expenditure changes in the preseason and off-season, you need to adjust your caloric intake and macronutrient ratio to match. Following are dietary guidelines for gymnasts to help you in planning your nutrition program. Supplementation guidelines for gymnasts can be found on page 263.

Dietary Guidelines

The following pie charts illustrate how you should divide up your caloric intake to match the energy demands of gymnastics during the preseason, season, and off-season. They show the target percentages of fat, protein, and carbohydrates that your five to six meals should supply each day.

Note that fat has about 9 calories per gram, while protein and carbohydrates have only 4 calories per gram. Therefore, during the season, if you needed to consume a total of 2,500 calories per day, you would aim for 375 calories (15 percent of your total daily calories) from fat, 750 calories (30 percent of your total daily calories) from protein, and the remaining 1,375 calories (55 percent of your total daily calories) from carbohydrates.

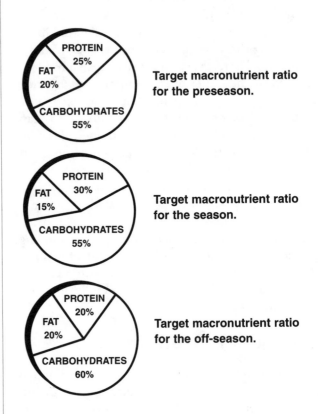

Target macronutrient ratio for the preseason.

Target macronutrient ratio for the season.

Target macronutrient ratio for the off-season.

Some other important considerations for gymnasts are:

☐ Carbohydrates are the major source of energy for short-term activities. Complex carbohydrates are the best source because they most effectively refill the glycogen stores in the muscles and liver. In addition, they elevate the blood sugar to a level sufficient for long sessions of intensive training.

☐ As a power athlete, you must make sure that you consume adequate amounts of both carbohydrates and protein. If your energy stores become drastically depleted or you experience lactic-acid buildup, you may suffer temporary muscle fatigue. If you do not refill your glycogen stores before your next workout or competition, your body may begin breaking down muscle tissue for the protein it needs for energy.

☐ Directly before workouts and competitions, consume

carbohydrate drinks with high glycemic indexes to keep your blood sugar sustained at an appropriate level. This will allow you to train or compete intensively without having your explosiveness hindered by fatigue.

☐ As a power athlete, you need to stimulate the storage of glycogen in your muscles while promoting repair and growth of your muscle tissue and inhibiting buildup of body fat. To do this:

• Train anaerobically on a regular basis. Intensive training stimulates increased storage of glycogen in the muscles and liver, which provides additional energy for greater exercise capacity.

• Consume five to six meals a day. Eating several smaller meals rather than three larger ones will keep your blood-sugar level stable throughout the day and will ensure that a supply of protein is always available for your muscles.

• Keep your fat intake to a minimum. Large amounts of fat in your diet will add to your body fat and will cause you to lose minerals through frequent urination.

• Consume low-glycemic-index foods about two to three hours before workouts and competitions. These foods help sustain the blood-sugar level.

• Drink plenty of water. Not only will this practice reduce your chances of becoming dehydrated, but every ounce of glycogen that is stored within the muscles needs 3 ounces of water stored along with it. Therefore, remaining properly hydrated will also help prevent weakened muscle contractions.

• Do not eat a new food just before a competition. Different people often react differently to the same food. Before a competition, eat just those foods that you know your body will handle well.

As a gymnast, you should turn to Appendix C on page 345 for full discussions of the 20:25:55, 15:30:55, and 20:20:60 dietary plans. Also presented are sample daily diets that use common, healthy foods to meet an athlete's energy and caloric needs. Use the directions on page 150 to estimate your average daily caloric requirement. Then use the directions in Chapter 13 or 14 to adjust your diet for off-season fat loss or muscle building, respectively.

Supplementation Guidelines

In addition to eating a proper diet, you should also take dietary supplements to make sure that any nutri-

ents you lose due to sweating or training are replenished. The following tables will help guide you in selecting the supplements appropriate for you. The first table lists the nutrients recommended for gymnasts, as well as the range of intake for each nutrient. (For discussions of these nutrients, see Part One.) Note that within the ranges of intake, the lower amounts are for smaller individuals and lower-activity days, while the higher amounts are for larger individuals and higher-activity days.

RECOMMENDED NUTRIENTS AND RANGES OF INTAKE

For Gymnasts

NUTRIENT	RANGE OF INTAKE
VITAMINS	
Vitamin A	8,000–16,000 IU
Beta-carotene	15,000–30,000 IU
Vitamin B_1 (thiamine)	30–120 mg
Vitamin B_2 (riboflavin)	30–120 mg
Vitamin B_3 (niacin)	40–80 mg
Vitamin B_5 (pantothenic acid)	20–100 mg
Vitamin B_6 (pyridoxine)	20–80 mg
Vitamin B_{12} (cobalamin)	12–120 mcg
Biotin	125–175 mcg
Folate	400–800 mcg
Vitamin C	800–2,000 mg
Vitamin D	400–800 IU
Vitamin E	200–600 IU
Vitamin K	60–160 mcg
MINERALS	
Boron	2–8 mg
Calcium	800–1,500 mg
Chromium	200–500 mcg
Copper	1–4 mg
Iodine	100–200 mcg
Iron	15–50 mg
Magnesium	250–650 mg
Manganese	12–35 mg
Molybdenum	100–200 mcg
Phosphorus	150–800 mg
Potassium	50–1,000 mg
Selenium	100–200 mcg
Zinc	15–50 mg
AMINO ACIDS	
L-glutamine	1,000–2,000 mg

NUTRIENT	RANGE OF INTAKE
FATTY ACIDS	
Alpha-linolenic acid	1,500–3,000 mg
Docosahexaenoic acid (DHA)	250–750 mg
Eiocosapentaenoic acid (EPA)	250–750 mg
Gamma linolenic acid (GLA)	100–400 mg
Linoleic acid	3,000–6,000 mg
METABOLITES	
Bioflavonoids	200–800 mg
Choline	200–600 mg
Creatine monohydrate	4,000–12,000 mg
Ferulic acid	50–100 mg
Inosine	500–1,000 mg
Inositol	200–600 mg
L-carnitine	1,000–2,000 mg
Octacosanol	3,000–6,000 mcg

IU = international units, mcg = micrograms, mg = milligrams.

The second table lists the different types of sports supplements available and indicates if their use by gymnasts is recommended in the preseason, during the season, or directly before a competition. The list also includes a number of popular nutritional practices—bicarbonate loading, carbohydrate loading, creatine and/or inosine loading, and water loading. (For a discussion of any of these supplements or practices, see the appropriate section in Part One or Part Three.)

RECOMMENDED SPORTS SUPPLEMENTS AND NUTRITIONAL PRACTICES

For Gymnasts

	Intake Recommendation		
	PRESEASON	SEASON	PRE-COMPETITION
SUPPLEMENTS			
Multivitamins	Yes	Yes	No
Multiminerals	Yes	Yes	No
Antioxidants	Yes	Yes	No
Fatty acids	Yes	Yes	No
Metabolites	Optional	Yes	Yes
Branched-chain amino acids	Yes	Yes	Yes
Herbs	Yes	Yes	No
Low-calorie protein drink (200–300 calories)	Yes	Yes	Yes
Carbohydrate drink	Yes	Yes	Yes
Fat-burning supplement	Yes	Optional	No

	Intake Recommendation		
	PRESEASON	SEASON	PRE-COMPETITION
PRACTICES			
Bicarbonate loading	No	Optional	Optional
Carbohydrate loading	No	No	No
Creatine and/or inosine loading	Optional	Yes	Yes
Water loading	No	No	No

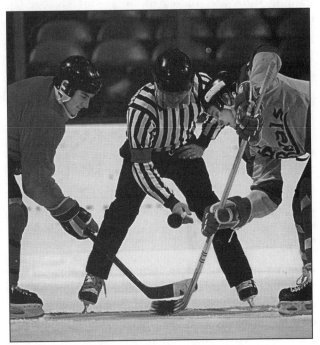

HOCKEY

Hockey is a game that places tough physical demands on its players. For one thing, the playing surface is slippery. For another, the skating speeds reached are often around thirty to forty miles per hour. Hockey players must cut, turn, maneuver, and race for the puck, all while fending off opponents' body checks. To be successful, a hockey player must have a superior level of strength endurance, as well as agility and exceptional balance.

Every bit of your training and diet must reflect these elements. These elements are what make hockey explosive in nature. In fact, hockey is very explosive, so improved recovery and tissue repair plus increased speed and strength are your year-round training and dietary goals. Nutritionally, this means emphasizing short-term energy needs and maximizing the muscles' recovery and tissue-repair processes.

In hockey, the energy output is primarily anaerobic (without oxygen). This does not mean that training for or playing the game is easy, however. You must body check, speed to the puck, push, defend against your opponents, and perform other lightning-quick reflexive movements over and over again, repeatedly testing your tolerance to pain and fatigue, caused by lactic-acid buildup in your muscles. Hockey training is extremely intensive and grueling. At the highest levels, hockey training forces you to operate at your anaerobic threshold (the point at which you must receive oxygen).

Muscles grow when they are stressed. In hockey, the aim is to make the muscles grow as strong and as quick as possible. This calls for specialized training. Furthermore, the incredible energy output of hockey, especially coupled with the explosive aspects of the game, requires the support of a carefully constructed nutrition program.

ENERGY SOURCES OF HOCKEY PLAYERS

The muscles rely on three major systems to supply the energy they need—the immediate, glycolytic, and oxidative energy systems. For short-term energy for explosive-strength output, the muscles depend on the immediate energy systems. The immediate energy systems are nonoxidative—that is, they do not use oxygen. Instead, these systems generate energy through the use of adenosine triphosphate (ATP) and creatine phosphate (CP). CP is produced in the body and stored in the muscle fibers. It is broken down by enzymes to regenerate ATP, which is also stored in the muscle fibers. When the ATP is in turn broken down, the result is a spark of energy that triggers a muscle contraction.

For medium-term energy for repeated near-maximum exertion, the muscles turn to the glycolytic energy systems. In these systems, which are also nonoxidative, glycogen is used to produce energy. Glycogen is the storage form of glucose. It is stored in the liver and muscles, and is readily converted back to glucose when it is needed for energy.

For long-term energy for endurance activities, the muscles use the oxidative energy systems. In these systems, oxygen is used to oxidize long-chain fatty acids, protein, and glucose, which generates energy. For athletes, getting enough oxygen can mean a winning performance rather than a second-place showing.

Every sport involves a variety of skills, and each skill utilizes a unique combination of these three energy sources. The following table shows how much your body relies on each of the energy sources during an average hockey game. It also gives percentages for two kinds of average workouts.

WHERE YOUR ENERGY COMES FROM

For Hockey Players		
Energy Systems		
IMMEDIATE	GLYCOLYTIC	OXIDATIVE
Average game		
50%	40%	10%
Average workouts		
Off-season 60%	30%	10%
Pregame 50%	40%	10%

When considering the type of nutritional support to give your training program, keep the following factors in mind:

☐ All athletes need to consume high-quality protein several times a day for effective recovery and adequate repair of damaged muscle tissue.

☐ Athletes whose muscles rely substantially on the immediate or glycolytic energy systems should keep their fat intake to a minimum because fat is not an efficient energy source for their intensive training, which is almost exclusively anaerobic in nature. Since the fat calories consumed by these athletes are not generally used for energy, they are stored as body fat.

☐ All athletes should consume a carefully measured amount of high-quality carbohydrates several times a day to ensure an adequate supply of energy.

☐ The carbohydrates in all preworkout meals should consist of foods with low glycemic indexes to ensure that training intensity does not wane and that muscle tissue is not cannibalized for energy. (For the glycemic indexes of some common foods, see page 29.)

The aim of your nutrition program is to make your body healthy enough to accomplish recovery and tissue repair speedily and efficiently—without adding body fat. These aims alone make diet as critical as training for hockey players. You must eat just the right amount of food. Eat the wrong foods or the wrong amounts just a few times too often and you will sabotage your fitness efforts. Even more important, do not be in a hurry. It takes *years* to become a great hockey player. Rush the nutrition and training processes and you will become fat, your recovery rate will decline, and your injury rate will rise.

NUTRITION FOR HOCKEY PLAYERS

Hockey players are middle-distance athletes. No matter what position they play, they need stamina, which is supported by energy from the glycolytic energy systems. Therefore, as a hockey player, you need to plan your nutritional intake, from both food and supplement sources, to support the glycolytic systems. In addition, since your energy expenditure changes in the preseason and off-season, you need to adjust your caloric intake and macronutrient ratio to match. Following are dietary guidelines for hockey players to help you in planning your nutrition program. Supplementation guidelines for hockey players can be found on page 267.

Dietary Guidelines

The following pie charts illustrate how you should divide up your caloric intake to match the energy demands of hockey during the preseason, season, and off-season. They show the target percentages of fat, protein, and carbohydrates that your five to six meals should supply each day.

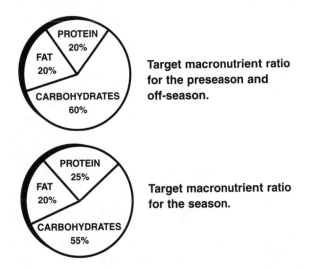

Target macronutrient ratio for the preseason and off-season.

Target macronutrient ratio for the season.

Note that fat has about 9 calories per gram, while protein and carbohydrates have only 4 calories per gram. Therefore, during the season, if you needed to

consume a total of 2,500 calories per day, you would aim for 500 calories (20 percent of your total daily calories) from fat, 625 calories (25 percent of your total daily calories) from protein, and the remaining 1,375 calories (55 percent of your total daily calories) from carbohydrates.

Some other important considerations for hockey players are:

☐ Carbohydrates are the major source of energy for short-term activities. Complex carbohydrates are the best source because they most effectively refill the glycogen stores in the muscles and liver. In addition, they elevate the blood sugar to a level sufficient for long sessions of intensive training.

☐ As a middle-distance athlete, you must make sure that you consume adequate amounts of both carbohydrates and protein. If your energy stores become drastically depleted or you experience lactic-acid buildup, you may suffer temporary muscle fatigue. If you do not refill your glycogen stores before your next workout or game, your body may begin breaking down muscle tissue for the protein it needs for energy.

☐ Directly before workouts and games, consume carbohydrate drinks with high glycemic indexes to keep your blood sugar sustained at an appropriate level. This will allow you to train or play intensively for longer periods of time.

☐ As a middle-distance athlete, you need to stimulate the storage of glycogen in your muscles while promoting repair and growth of your muscle tissue and inhibiting buildup of body fat. To do this:

• Train against your anaerobic threshold (to exhaustion) on a regular basis. Intensive, exhaustive training stimulates increased storage of glycogen in the muscles and liver, which provides additional energy for greater exercise capacity.

• Consume five to six meals a day. Eating several smaller meals rather than three larger ones will keep your blood-sugar level stable throughout the day and will ensure that a supply of protein is always available for your muscles.

• Keep your fat intake to a minimum. Large amounts of fat in your diet will add to your body fat and will cause mineral loss through frequent urination.

• Consume low-glycemic-index foods about two to three hours before workouts and games. These foods help sustain the blood-sugar level.

• Drink plenty of water. Not only will this practice reduce your chances of becoming dehydrated, but every ounce of glycogen that is stored within the muscles needs 3 ounces of water stored along with it. Therefore, remaining properly hydrated will also help prevent weakened muscle contractions and early onset of fatigue.

As a hockey player, you should turn to Appendix C on page 345 for full discussions of the 20:20:60 and 20:25:55 dietary plans. Also presented are sample daily diets that use common, healthy foods to meet an athlete's energy and caloric needs. Use the directions on page 150 to estimate your average daily caloric requirement. Then use the directions in Chapter 13 or 14 to adjust your diet for off-season fat loss or muscle building, respectively.

Supplementation Guidelines

In addition to eating a proper diet, you should also take dietary supplements to make sure that any nutrients you lose due to sweating or training are replenished. The following tables will help guide you in selecting the supplements appropriate for you. The first table lists the nutrients recommended for hockey players, as well as the range of intake for each nutrient. (For discussions of these nutrients, see Part One.) Note that within the ranges of intake, the lower amounts are for smaller individuals and lower-activity days, while the higher amounts are for larger individuals and higher-activity days.

RECOMMENDED NUTRIENTS AND RANGES OF INTAKE

For Hockey Players

NUTRIENT	RANGE OF INTAKE
VITAMINS	
Vitamin A	8,000–16,000 IU
Beta-carotene	15,000–30,000 IU
Vitamin B$_1$ (thiamine)	40–120 mg
Vitamin B$_2$ (riboflavin)	40–120 mg
Vitamin B$_3$ (niacin)	20–40 mg
Vitamin B$_5$ (pantothenic acid)	20–100 mg
Vitamin B$_6$ (pyridoxine)	20–80 mg
Vitamin B$_{12}$ (cobalamin)	12–120 mcg
Biotin	125–175 mcg

NUTRIENT	RANGE OF INTAKE
Folate	400–800 mcg
Vitamin C	800–2,000 mg
Vitamin D	400–800 IU
Vitamin E	200–800 IU
Vitamin K	60–160 mcg
MINERALS	
Boron	2–8 mg
Calcium	800–1,500 mg
Chromium	200–500 mcg
Copper	1–4 mg
Iodine	100–200 mcg
Iron	15–50 mg
Magnesium	250–650 mg
Manganese	12–35 mg
Molybdenum	100–200 mcg
Phosphorus	150–800 mg
Potassium	50–1,000 mg
Selenium	100–200 mcg
Zinc	15–50 mg
AMINO ACIDS	
L-glutamic acid	1,000–2,000 mg
L-glutamine	1,000–2,000 mg
FATTY ACIDS	
Alpha-linolenic acid	500–1,000 mg
Docosahexaenoic acid (DHA)	250–750 mg
Eiocosapentaenoic acid (EPA)	250–750 mg
Gamma linolenic acid (GLA)	100–400 mg
Linoleic acid	2,000–3,000 mg
METABOLITES	
Bioflavonoids	300–800 mg
Choline	200–600 mg
Inositol	200–600 mg
L-carnitine	1,000–1,500 mg
Octacosanol	6,000–12,000 mcg

IU = international units, mcg = micrograms, mg = milligrams.

The second table lists the different types of sports supplements available and indicates if their use by hockey players is recommended in the preseason, during the season, or directly before a game. The list also includes a number of popular nutritional practices—bicarbonate loading, carbohydrate loading, creatine and/or inosine loading, and water loading. (For a discussion of any of these supplements or practices, see the appropriate section in Part One or Part Three.)

RECOMMENDED SPORTS SUPPLEMENTS AND NUTRITIONAL PRACTICES

For Hockey Players

Intake Recommendation

	PRESEASON	SEASON	PRE-COMPETITION
SUPPLEMENTS			
Multivitamins	Yes	Yes	Yes
Multiminerals	Yes	Yes	Yes
Antioxidants	Yes	Yes	Yes
Fatty acids	Yes	Yes	Yes
Metabolites	Optional	Yes	Yes
Branched-chain amino acids	Yes	Yes	Yes
Herbs	Yes	Yes	No
Low-calorie protein drink (200–300 calories)	Yes	Yes	Yes
Carbohydrate drink	Yes	Yes	Yes
Fat-burning supplement	Yes	Optional	No
PRACTICES			
Bicarbonate loading	No	No	No
Carbohydrate loading	No	No	Optional
Creatine and/or inosine loading	No	No	No
Water loading	No	No	Optional

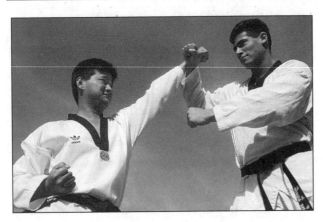

MARTIAL ARTS

Includes Judo, Karate, Kickboxing,
Tae Kwon Do, and Other Martial Arts

The martial arts—including judo, karate, kickboxing, and tae kwon do—are all multifaceted disciplines that involve a wide range of skills and movements. They require not only speed and strength in short, explosive bursts, but also a high level of anaerobic-strength endurance, as well as flexibility and agility.

Every bit of your training and diet must reflect these elements. These elements are what make the martial arts explosive in nature. In fact, the martial arts are very explosive, so improved recovery and tissue repair plus increased speed and strength are your year-round training and dietary goals. Nutritionally, this means emphasizing short-term energy needs and maximizing the muscles' recovery and tissue-repair processes.

In the martial arts, the energy output is primarily anaerobic (without oxygen). This does not mean that training for or competing in any of the martial arts is easy, however. You must kick, grapple, throw, deliver blows, and perform other lightning-quick reflexive movements over and over again, repeatedly testing your tolerance to pain and fatigue, caused by lactic-acid buildup in your muscles. The training for each of the disciplines is extremely intensive and grueling. At the highest levels, martial-arts training forces you to operate at your anaerobic threshold (the point at which you must receive oxygen).

Muscles grow when they are stressed. In the martial arts, the aim is to make the muscles grow as strong and as quick as possible. This calls for specialized training. Furthermore, the incredible force output of each of the martial arts, especially coupled with the explosive aspects of the disciplines, requires the support of a carefully contructed nutrition program.

ENERGY SOURCES OF MARTIAL ARTISTS

The muscles rely on three major systems to supply the energy they need—the immediate, glycolytic, and oxidative energy systems. For short-term energy for explosive-strength output, the muscles depend on the immediate energy systems. The immediate energy systems are nonoxidative—that is, they do not use oxygen. Instead, these systems generate energy through the use of adenosine triphosphate (ATP) and creatine phosphate (CP). CP is produced in the body and stored in the muscle fibers. It is broken down by enzymes to regenerate ATP, which is also stored in the muscle fibers. When the ATP is in turn broken down, the result is a spark of energy that triggers a muscle contraction.

For medium-term energy for repeated near-maximum exertion, the muscles turn to the glycolytic energy systems. In these systems, which are also nonoxidative, glycogen is used to produce energy. Glycogen is the storage form of glucose. It is stored in the liver and muscles, and is readily converted back to glucose when it is needed for energy.

For long-term energy for endurance activities, the muscles use the oxidative energy systems. In these systems, oxygen is used to oxidize long-chain fatty acids, protein, and glucose, which generates energy. For athletes, getting enough oxygen can mean a winning performance rather than a second-place showing.

Every sport involves a variety of skills, and each skill utilizes a unique combination of these three energy sources. The following table shows how much your body relies on each of the energy sources during an average match in four of the martial arts. Percentages are also given for two kinds of average workouts.

WHERE YOUR ENERGY COMES FROM

For Martial Artists			
	Energy Systems		
	IMMEDIATE	GLYCOLYTIC	OXIDATIVE
Average matches			
Judo	50%	40%	10%
Karate	50%	40%	10%
Kickboxing	50%	40%	10%
Tae kwon do	50%	40%	10%
Average workouts			
Off-season	60%	30%	10%
Prematch	50%	40%	10%

When considering the type of nutritional support to give your training program, keep the following factors in mind:

□ All athletes need to consume high-quality protein several times a day for effective recovery and adequate repair of damaged muscle tissue.

□ Athletes whose muscles rely substantially on the immediate or glycolytic energy systems should keep their fat intake to a minimum because fat is not an efficient energy source for their intensive training, which is almost exclusively anaerobic in nature. Since the fat calories consumed by these athletes are not generally used for energy, they are stored as body fat.

□ All athletes should consume a carefully measured amount of high-quality carbohydrates several times a day to ensure an adequate supply of energy.

□ The carbohydrates in all preworkout meals should consist of foods with low glycemic indexes to ensure that training intensity does not wane and that muscle tissue is not cannibalized for energy. (For the glycemic indexes of some common foods, see page 29.)

The aim of your nutrition program is to make your body healthy enough to accomplish recovery and tissue repair speedily and efficiently—without adding body fat. Your further aims are to do this while maintaining a high strength-to-weight ratio plus remaining within 3 to 4 percent of your competition body weight. These aims alone make diet as critical as training for martial artists. You must eat just the right amount of food. Eat the wrong foods or the wrong amounts just a few times too often and you will sabotage your fitness efforts. Even more important, do not be in a hurry. It takes *years* to become a great martial artist. Rush the training and nutritional processes and you will become fat, your recovery rate will decline, and your injury rate will rise.

NUTRITION FOR MARTIAL ARTISTS

Martial artists are power athletes. No matter which discipline they practice, they obtain most of their energy from a combination of the immediate and glycolytic energy systems. Therefore, as a martial artist, you need to plan your nutritional intake, from both food and supplement sources, to support these nonoxidative systems. In addition, since your energy expenditure changes in the preseason and off-season, you need to adjust your caloric intake and macronutrient ratio to match. Following are dietary guidelines for martial artists to help you in planning your nutrition program. Supplementation guidelines for martial artists can be found on page 270.

Dietary Guidelines

The following pie charts illustrate how you should divide up your caloric intake to match the energy demands of the martial arts during the preseason, season, and off-season. They show the target percentages of fat, protein, and carbohydrates that your five to six meals should supply each day.

Note that fat has about 9 calories per gram, while protein and carbohydrates have only 4 calories per gram. Therefore, during the season, if you needed to consume a total of 2,500 calories per day, you would

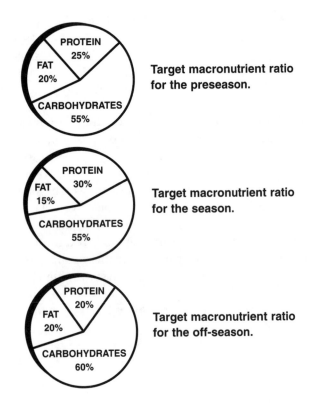

Target macronutrient ratio for the preseason.

Target macronutrient ratio for the season.

Target macronutrient ratio for the off-season.

aim for 375 calories (15 percent of your total daily calories) from fat, 750 calories (30 percent of your total daily calories) from protein, and the remaining 1,375 calories (55 percent of your total daily calories) from carbohydrates.

Some other important considerations for martial artists are:

☐ Carbohydrates are the major source of energy for short-term activities. Complex carbohydrates are the best source because they most effectively refill the glycogen stores in the muscles and liver. In addition, they elevate the blood sugar to a level sufficient for long sessions of intensive training.

☐ As a power athlete, you must make sure that you consume adequate amounts of both carbohydrates and protein. If your energy stores become drastically depleted or you experience lactic-acid buildup, you may suffer temporary muscle fatigue. If you do not refill your glycogen stores before your next workout or match, your body may begin breaking down muscle tissue for the protein it needs for energy.

☐ Directly before workouts, consume carbohydrate drinks with high glycemic indexes to keep your blood sugar sustained at an appropriate level. This will allow you to train intensively without having your explosiveness hindered by fatigue.

☐ As a power athlete, you need to stimulate the storage of glycogen in your muscles while promoting repair and growth of your muscle tissue and inhibiting buildup of body fat. To do this:

• Train anaerobically on a regular basis. Intensive training stimulates increased storage of glycogen in the muscles and liver, which provides additional energy for greater exercise capacity.

• Consume five to six meals a day. Eating several smaller meals rather than three larger ones will keep your blood-sugar level stable throughout the day and will ensure that a supply of protein is always available for your muscles.

• Keep your fat intake to a minimum. Large amounts of fat in your diet will add to your body fat and will cause you to lose minerals through frequent urination.

• Consume low-glycemic-index foods about two to three hours before workouts and matches. These foods help sustain the blood-sugar level.

• Drink plenty of water. Not only will this practice reduce your chances of becoming dehydrated, but every ounce of glycogen that is stored within the muscles needs 3 ounces of water stored along with it. Therefore, remaining properly hydrated will also help prevent weakened muscle contractions.

• Do not eat a new food just before a match. Different people often react differently to the same food. Before a match, eat just those foods that you know your body will handle well.

As a martial artist, you should turn to Appendix C on page 345 for full discussions of the 20:25:55, 15:30:55, and 20:20:60 dietary plans. Also presented are sample daily diets that use common, healthy foods to meet an athlete's energy and caloric needs. Use the directions on page 150 to estimate your average daily caloric requirement. Then use the directions in Chapter 13 or 14 to adjust your diet for off-season fat loss or muscle building, respectively.

Supplementation Guidelines

In addition to eating a proper diet, you should also take dietary supplements to make sure that any nutrients you lose due to sweating or training are replenished. The following tables will help guide you in selecting the supplements appropriate for you. The first table lists the nutrients recommended for martial artists, as well as the range of intake for each nutrient. (For discussions of these nutrients, see Part One.) Note that within the ranges of intake, the lower amounts are for smaller individuals and lower-activity days, while the higher amounts are for larger individuals and higher-activity days.

RECOMMENDED NUTRIENTS AND RANGES OF INTAKE

For Martial Artists

NUTRIENT	RANGE OF INTAKE
VITAMINS	
Vitamin A	8,000–16,000 IU
Beta-carotene	15,000–30,000 IU
Vitamin B_1 (thiamine)	30–120 mg
Vitamin B_2 (riboflavin)	30–120 mg
Vitamin B_3 (niacin)	40–80 mg
Vitamin B_5 (pantothenic acid)	20–100 mg
Vitamin B_6 (pyridoxine)	20–80 mg
Vitamin B_{12} (cobalamin)	12–120 mcg
Biotin	125–175 mcg
Folate	400–800 mcg
Vitamin C	800–2,000 mg
Vitamin D	400–800 IU
Vitamin E	200–600 IU
Vitamin K	60–160 mcg
MINERALS	
Boron	2–8 mg
Calcium	800–1,500 mg
Chromium	200–500 mcg
Copper	1–4 mg
Iodine	100–200 mcg
Iron	15–50 mg
Magnesium	250–650 mg
Manganese	12–35 mg
Molybdenum	100–200 mcg
Phosphorus	150–800 mg
Potassium	50–1,000 mg
Selenium	100–200 mcg
Zinc	15–50 mg
AMINO ACIDS	
L-glutamine	1,000–2,000 mg
FATTY ACIDS	
Alpha-linolenic acid	1,500–3,000 mg

NUTRIENT	RANGE OF INTAKE
Docosahexaenoic acid (DHA)	250–750 mg
Eiocosapentaenoic acid (EPA)	250–750 mg
Gamma linolenic acid (GLA)	100–400 mg
Linoleic acid	3,000–6,000 mg
METABOLITES	
Bioflavonoids	200–800 mg
Choline	100–600 mg
Creatine monohydrate	8,000–18,000 mg
Ferulic acid	50–100 mg
Inositol	100–600 mg
L-carnitine	750–2,000 mg
Octacosanol	6,000–12,000 mcg
HERBS	
Ginseng	1,000–2,000 mg

IU = international units, mcg = micrograms, mg = milligrams.

The second table lists the different types of sports supplements available and indicates if their use by martial artists is recommended in the preseason, during the season, or directly before a match. The list also includes a number of popular nutritional practices—bicarbonate loading, carbohydrate loading, creatine and/or inosine loading, and water loading. (For a discussion of any of these supplements or practices, see the appropriate section in Part One or Part Three.)

RECOMMENDED SPORTS SUPPLEMENTS AND NUTRITIONAL PRACTICES

For Martial Artists

	Intake Recommendation		
	PRESEASON	SEASON	PREMATCH
SUPPLEMENTS			
Multivitamins	Yes	Yes	No
Multiminerals	Yes	Yes	No
Antioxidants	Yes	Yes	No
Fatty acids	Yes	Yes	No
Metabolites	Yes	Yes	Yes
Branched-chain amino acids	Yes	Yes	Yes
Herbs	Yes	Yes	Yes
Low-calorie protein drink (200–300 calories)	Yes	Yes	Yes
Carbohydrate drink	Yes	Yes	Yes
Fat-burning supplement	Yes	Optional	No

Intake Recommendation			
	PRESEASON	SEASON	PREMATCH
PRACTICES			
Bicarbonate loading	No	Optional	Optional
Carbohydrate loading	No	No	No
Creatine and/or inosine loading	No	Optional	Optional
Water loading	No	No	No

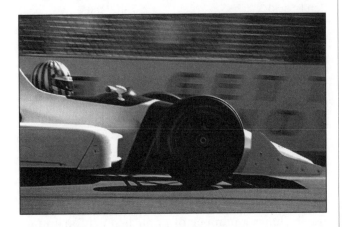

MOTOR SPORTS

Includes Demolition Derby, Drag Racing, Driving, Formula I Racing, Hydroplaning, Motocross, Motorcycling, Rallye, Snowmobiling, Sports-Car Racing, and Other Motor Sports

Taking a ride on a Sunday afternoon for a little bit of fresh air and a change of scenery is fun, but driving a mega-horsepower monster at blistering speeds with disaster looming around every turn is downright draining. Motor-sport drivers require not only speed and strength in short, explosive bursts, but also a high level of anaerobic-strength endurance, as well as flexibility and agility. And in the longer competitions, a high energy level is critical for maintaining a focused, laserlike concentration while driving for hours under exhausting conditions including a cockpit temperature that may exceed 150°F!

Every bit of your training and diet must reflect these elements. These elements are what define the motor sports. Nutritionally, this means emphasizing the efficient fulfillment of energy requirements and maximizing the muscles' recovery and tissue-repair processes.

In most of the motor sports, the energy output is anaerobic (without oxygen). This does not mean that training for or competing in a motor sport is easy, however. Training for all the motor sports is extremely intensive and grueling. At the highest levels, motor-sport training forces you to operate at your anaerobic threshold (the point at which you must receive oxygen).

Muscles grow when they are stressed. In the motor sports, the aim is to make the muscles grow as strong and as quick as possible. This calls for specialized training. Furthermore, the physical and mental demands of skillful driving also require the support of a carefully constructed nutrition program.

ENERGY SOURCES OF MOTOR-SPORT DRIVERS

The muscles rely on three major systems to supply the energy they need—the immediate, glycolytic, and oxidative energy systems. For short-term energy for explosive-strength output, the muscles depend on the immediate energy systems. The immediate energy systems are nonoxidative—that is, they do not use oxygen. Instead, these systems generate energy through the use of adenosine triphosphate (ATP) and creatine phosphate (CP). CP is produced in the body and stored in the muscle fibers. It is broken down by enzymes to regenerate ATP, which is also stored in the muscle fibers. When the ATP is in turn broken down, the result is a spark of energy that triggers a muscle contraction.

For medium-term energy for repeated near-maximum exertion, the muscles turn to the glycolytic energy systems. In these systems, which are also nonoxidative, glycogen is used to produce energy. Glycogen is the storage form of glucose. It is stored in the liver and muscles, and is readily converted back to glucose when it is needed for energy.

For long-term energy for endurance activities, the muscles use the oxidative energy systems. In these systems, oxygen is used to oxidize long-chain fatty acids, protein, and glucose, which generates energy. For athletes, getting enough oxygen can mean a winning performance rather than a second-place showing.

Every sport involves a variety of skills, and each skill utilizes a unique combination of these three energy sources. The following table lists a number of the major motor sports and shows how much your body relies on each of the energy sources when you participate in them.

WHERE YOUR ENERGY COMES FROM

For Motor-Sport Drivers

	Energy Systems		
	IMMEDIATE	GLYCOLYTIC	OXIDATIVE
Demolition derby	50%	40%	10%
Drag racing	100%	0%	0%
Formula I racing	20%	70%	10%
Hydroplaning	50%	40%	10%
Motocross	50%	40%	10%
Rallye	20%	70%	10%
Sports-car racing	20%	70%	10%

When considering the type of nutritional support to give your training program, keep the following factors in mind:

☐ All athletes need to consume high-quality protein several times a day for effective recovery and adequate repair of damaged muscle tissue.

☐ Athletes whose muscles rely substantially on the immediate or glycolytic energy systems should keep their fat intake to a minimum because fat is not an efficient energy source for their intensive training, which is almost exclusively anaerobic in nature. Since the fat calories consumed by these athletes are not generally used for energy, they are stored as body fat.

☐ All athletes should consume a carefully measured amount of high-quality carbohydrates several times a day to ensure an adequate supply of energy.

☐ Athletes who need to remain mentally focused for prolonged periods of time must keep their liver glycogen stores filled. Liver glycogen is the primary fuel that the brain burns for energy, and when the stores become depleted, focus and timing begin to suffer.

☐ The carbohydrates in all preworkout meals should consist of foods with low glycemic indexes to ensure that training intensity does not wane and that muscle tissue is not cannibalized for energy. (For the glycemic indexes of some common foods, see page 29.)

The aim of your nutrition program is to make your body healthy enough to accomplish recovery and tissue repair speedily and efficiently—without adding body fat. Your further aim is to do this while maintaining a high strength-to-weight ratio. These aims alone make diet as critical as training in the motor sports. You must eat just the right amount of food. Eat the wrong foods or the wrong amounts just a few

times too often and you will sabotage your fitness efforts. With the thousands of dollars spent designing light machines, it does not make sense for a driver to carry excess body weight.

NUTRITION FOR MOTOR-SPORT DRIVERS

Motor-sport drivers are middle-distance athletes. No matter what motor sport they specialize in, they need stamina, which is supported by energy from the glycolytic energy systems. Therefore, as a motor-sport driver, you need to plan your nutritional intake, from both food and supplement sources, to support the glycolytic systems. In addition, since your energy expenditure changes in the preseason and off-season, you need to adjust your caloric intake and macronutrient ratio to match. Following are dietary guidelines for motor-sport drivers to help you in planning your nutrition program. Supplementation guidelines for motor-sport drivers can be found on page 274.

Dietary Guidelines

The following pie charts illustrate how you should divide up your caloric intake to match the energy demands of the motor sports during the preseason, season, and off-season. They show the target percentages of fat, protein, and carbohydrates that your five to six meals should supply each day.

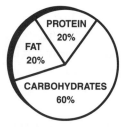

Target macronutrient ratio for the preseason and off-season.

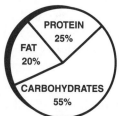

Target macronutrient ratio for the season.

Note that fat has about 9 calories per gram, while protein and carbohydrates have only 4 calories per gram. Therefore, during the season, if you needed to consume a total of 2,500 calories per day, you would aim for 500 calories (20 percent of your total daily calories) from fat, 625 calories (25 percent of your total daily calories) from protein, and the remaining 1,375 calories (55 percent of your total daily calories) from carbohydrates.

Some other important considerations for motor-sport drivers are:

☐ Carbohydrates are the major source of energy for short-term activities. Complex carbohydrates are the best source because they most effectively refill the glycogen stores in the muscles and liver. In addition, they elevate the blood sugar to a level sufficient for long sessions of intensive training.

☐ As a middle-distance athlete, you must make sure that you consume adequate amounts of both carbohydrates and protein. If your energy stores become drastically depleted or you experience lactic-acid buildup, you may suffer temporary muscle fatigue. If you do not refill your glycogen stores before your next workout or competition, your body may begin breaking down muscle tissue for the protein it needs for energy.

☐ Directly before workouts and competitions, consume carbohydrate drinks with high glycemic indexes to keep your blood sugar sustained at an appropriate level. This will allow you to train or compete intensively for longer periods of time.

☐ As a middle-distance athlete, you need to stimulate the storage of glycogen in your muscles while promoting repair and growth of your muscle tissue and inhibiting buildup of body fat. To do this:

• Train against your anaerobic threshold (to exhaustion) on a regular basis. Intensive, exhaustive training stimulates increased storage of glycogen in the muscles and liver, which provides additional energy for greater exercise capacity.

• Consume five to six meals a day. Eating several smaller meals rather than three larger ones will keep your blood-sugar level stable throughout the day and will ensure that a supply of protein is always available for your muscles.

• Keep your fat intake to a minimum. Large amounts of fat in your diet will add to your body fat and will cause mineral loss through frequent urination.

• Consume low-glycemic-index foods about two to three hours before workouts and competitions. These foods help sustain the blood-sugar level.

• Drink plenty of water. Not only will this practice reduce your chances of becoming dehydrated, but every ounce of glycogen that is stored within the

muscles needs 3 ounces of water stored along with it. Therefore, remaining properly hydrated will also help prevent weakened muscle contractions and early onset of fatigue.

• Do not eat a new food just before a competition. Different people often react differently to the same food. Before a competition, eat just those foods that you know your body will handle well.

As a motor-sport driver, you should turn to Appendix C on page 345 for full discussions of the 20:20:60 and 20:25:55 dietary plans. Also presented are sample daily diets that use common, healthy foods to meet an athlete's energy and caloric needs. Use the directions on page 150 to estimate your average daily caloric requirement. Then use the directions in Chapter 13 or 14 to adjust your diet for off-season fat loss or muscle building, respectively.

Supplementation Guidelines

In addition to eating a proper diet, you should also take dietary supplements to make sure that any nutrients you lose due to sweating or training are replenished. The following tables will help guide you in selecting the supplements appropriate for you. The first table lists the nutrients recommended for motor-sport drivers, as well as the range of intake for each nutrient. (For discussions of these nutrients, see Part One.) Note that within the ranges of intake, the lower amounts are for smaller individuals and lower-activity days, while the higher amounts are for larger individuals and higher-activity days.

RECOMMENDED NUTRIENTS AND RANGES OF INTAKE

For Motor-Sport Drivers	
NUTRIENT	RANGE OF INTAKE
VITAMINS	
Vitamin A	8,000–16,000 IU
Beta-carotene	20,000–40,000 IU
Vitamin B₁ (thiamine)	40–120 mg
Vitamin B₂ (riboflavin)	40–120 mg
Vitamin B₃ (niacin)	20–40 mg
Vitamin B₅ (pantothenic acid)	20–100 mg
Vitamin B₆ (pyridoxine)	20–80 mg
Vitamin B₁₂ (cobalamin)	12–120 mcg
Biotin	125–175 mcg
Folate	400–800 mcg

NUTRIENT	RANGE OF INTAKE
Vitamin C	800–2,000 mg
Vitamin D	400–800 IU
Vitamin E	200–800 IU
Vitamin K	60–160 mcg
MINERALS	
Boron	2–8 mg
Calcium	800–1,500 mg
Chromium	200–500 mcg
Copper	1–4 mg
Iodine	100–200 mcg
Iron	15–50 mg
Magnesium	250–650 mg
Manganese	12–35 mg
Molybdenum	100–200 mcg
Phosphorus	150–800 mg
Potassium	50–1,000 mg
Selenium	100–200 mcg
Zinc	15–50 mg
AMINO ACIDS	
L-glutamic acid	500–1,000 mg
L-glutamine	1,000–2,000 mg
FATTY ACIDS	
Alpha-linolenic acid	500–1,000 mg
Docosahexaenoic acid (DHA)	250–750 mg
Eiocosapentaenoic acid (EPA)	250–750 mg
Gamma linolenic acid (GLA)	100–400 mg
Linoleic acid	2,000–3,000 mg
METABOLITES	
Bioflavonoids	300–800 mg
Choline	200–600 mg
Inositol	200–600 mg
L-carnitine	500–1,000 mg
Octacosanol	6,000–12,000 mcg

IU = international units, mcg = micrograms, mg = milligrams.

RECOMMENDED SPORTS SUPPLEMENTS AND NUTRITIONAL PRACTICES

For Motor-Sport Drivers

	Intake Recommendation		
	PRESEASON	SEASON	PRE-COMPETITION
SUPPLEMENTS			
Multivitamins	Yes	Yes	Yes
Multiminerals	Yes	Yes	Yes
Antioxidants	Yes	Yes	No
Fatty acids	Yes	Yes	Yes
Metabolites	Optional	Yes	Yes
Branched-chain amino acids	Yes	Yes	Yes
Herbs	Yes	Yes	No
Medium-calorie protein drink (300–500 calories)	Yes	Yes	Yes
Carbohydrate drink	Yes	Yes	Yes
Fat-burning supplement	Yes	Optional	No
PRACTICES			
Bicarbonate loading	No	No	No
Carbohydrate loading	No	No	Optional
Creatine and/or inosine loading	No	No	No
Water loading	No	No	Optional

The second table lists the different types of sports supplements available and indicates if their use by motor-sport drivers is recommended in the preseason, during the season, or directly before a competition. The list also includes a number of popular nutritional practices—bicarbonate loading, carbohydrate loading, creatine and/or inosine loading, and water loading. (For a discussion of any of these supplements or practices, see the appropriate section in Part One or Part Three.)

275

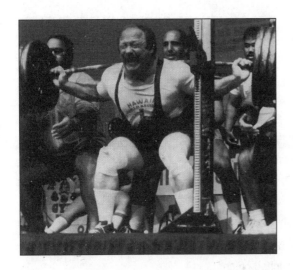

POWERLIFTING

Powerlifting is the premier sport in the world that tests limit (maximum) strength. Other sports do not even come close. This is because in powerlifting, the resistance (barbell) is too heavy to be moved very quickly. As a result, there is ample time to activate as many muscle fibers as necessary to complete a limit lift (the lifting of maximum weight). In sports such as weightlifting and shot-putting, the movement is completed within milliseconds, which is not enough time to reach maximum capacity. This is not to say, however, that power lifters should not *try* to move the weight as quickly as possible. If you ever want to become great at the sport, you *must* try.

In powerlifting, the energy output is primarily anaerobic (without oxygen). This does not mean that training for or competing in powerlifting is easy, however. Powerlifting contests generally require the performance of nine limit lifts, with perhaps five times as many near-limit lifts done to warm up. On top of this, most contests last five hours or more. Training as a power lifter is also intensive and grueling. At the highest levels, training for powerlifting forces you to operate at your anaerobic threshold (the point at which you must receive oxygen) for up to an hour and a half.

In powerlifting, the aim is to make the muscles as strong and as quick as possible. This calls for specialized training. Furthermore, the unique energy output of powerlifting requires the support of a carefully constructed nutrition program.

ENERGY SOURCES OF POWER LIFTERS

The muscles rely on three major systems to supply the energy they need—the immediate, glycolytic, and oxidative energy systems. For short-term energy for explosive-strength output, the muscles depend on the immediate energy systems. The immediate energy systems are nonoxidative—that is, they do not use oxygen. Instead, these systems generate energy through the use of adenosine triphosphate (ATP) and creatine phosphate (CP). CP is produced in the body and stored in the muscle fibers. It is broken down by enzymes to regenerate ATP, which is also stored in the muscle fibers. When the ATP is in turn broken down, the result is a spark of energy that triggers a muscle contraction.

For medium-term energy for repeated near-maximum exertion, the muscles turn to the glycolytic energy systems. In these systems, which are also nonoxidative, glycogen is used to produce energy. Glycogen is the storage form of glucose. It is stored in the liver and muscles, and is readily converted back to glucose when it is needed for energy.

For long-term energy for endurance activities, the muscles use the oxidative energy systems. In these systems, oxygen is used to oxidize long-chain fatty acids, protein, and glucose, which generates energy. For athletes, getting enough oxygen can mean a winning performance rather than a second-place showing.

Every sport involves a variety of skills, and each skill utilizes a unique combination of these three energy sources. The following table shows how much your body relies on each of the energy sources during an average powerlifting contest. Percentages are also given for an average warm-up and an average workout.

WHERE YOUR ENERGY COMES FROM

For Power Lifters		
Energy Systems		
IMMEDIATE	GLYCOLYTIC	OXIDATIVE
Average contest		
100%	0%	0%
Average precontest warm-up (1–4 reps per set)		
100%	0%	0%
Average off-season workout (5–10 reps per set)		
80%	20%	0%

When considering the type of nutritional support

to give your training program, keep the following factors in mind:

☐ All athletes need to consume high-quality protein several times a day for effective recovery and adequate repair of damaged muscle tissue.

☐ Athletes whose muscles rely substantially on the immediate energy systems should keep their fat intake to a minimum because fat is not an efficient energy source for their intensive training, which is almost exclusively anaerobic in nature. Since the fat calories consumed by these athletes are not generally used for energy, they are stored as body fat.

☐ All athletes should consume a carefully measured amount of high-quality carbohydrates several times a day to ensure an adequate supply of energy.

☐ The carbohydrates in all preworkout meals should consist of foods with low glycemic indexes to ensure that training intensity does not wane and that muscle tissue is not cannibalized for energy. (For the glycemic indexes of some common foods, see page 29.)

The aim of your nutrition program is to make your body healthy enough to accomplish recovery and tissue repair speedily and efficiently—without adding body fat. Your further aims are to do this while maintaining a high strength-to-weight ratio plus remaining within 3 to 4 percent of your competition body weight. These aims alone make diet as critical as training for power lifters. You must eat just the right amount of food. Eat the wrong foods or the wrong amounts just a few times too often and you will sabotage your fitness efforts. Even more important, do not be in a hurry. It takes *years* to become a great power lifter. Rush the nutrition and training processes and you will become injured, not strong.

NUTRITION FOR POWER LIFTERS

Power lifters are power athletes. Their primary energy sources are the immediate energy systems. Therefore, as a power lifter, you need to plan your nutritional intake, from both food and supplement sources, to support the immediate systems. In addition, since your energy expenditure changes in the off-season, you need to adjust your caloric intake and macronutrient ratio to match. Following are dietary guidelines for power lifters to help you in planning your nutrition program. Supplementation guidelines for power lifters can be found on page 278.

Dietary Guidelines

The following pie charts illustrate how you should divide up your caloric intake to match the energy demands of powerlifting during the preseason, season, and off-season. They show the target percentages of fat, protein, and carbohydrates that your five to six meals should supply each day.

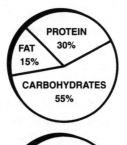

Target macronutrient ratio for the preseason and season.

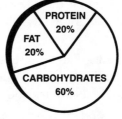

Target macronutrient ratio for the off-season.

Note that fat has about 9 calories per gram, while protein and carbohydrates have only 4 calories per gram. Therefore, during the season, if you needed to consume a total of 2,500 calories per day, you would aim for 375 calories (15 percent of your total daily calories) from fat, 750 calories (30 percent of your total daily calories) from protein, and the remaining 1,375 calories (55 percent of your total daily calories) from carbohydrates.

Some other important considerations for power lifters are:

☐ Carbohydrates are the major source of energy for short-term activities. Complex carbohydrates are the best source because they most effectively refill the glycogen stores in the muscles and liver. In addition, they elevate the blood sugar to a level sufficient for long sessions of intensive training.

☐ As a power athlete, you must make sure that you consume adequate amounts of both carbohydrates and protein. If your energy stores become drastically depleted or you experience lactic-acid buildup, you may suffer temporary muscle fatigue. If you do not refill your glycogen stores before your next workout or contest, your body may begin breaking down muscle tissue for the protein it needs for energy.

☐ Directly before workouts, consume carbohydrate drinks with high glycemic indexes to keep your blood sugar sustained at an appropriate level. This will allow you to train intensively without having your explosiveness hindered by fatigue.

☐ As a power athlete, you need to stimulate the storage of glycogen in your muscles while promoting repair and growth of your muscle tissue and inhibiting buildup of body fat. To do this:

• Train anaerobically on a regular basis. Intensive training stimulates increased storage of glycogen in the muscles and liver, which provides additional energy for greater exercise capacity.

• Consume five to six meals a day. Eating several smaller meals rather than three larger ones will keep your blood-sugar level stable throughout the day and will ensure that a supply of protein is always available for your muscles.

• Keep your fat intake to a minimum. Large amounts of fat in your diet will add to your body fat and will cause you to lose minerals through frequent urination.

• Consume low-glycemic-index foods about two to three hours before workouts and contests. These foods help sustain the blood-sugar level.

• Drink plenty of water. Not only will this practice reduce your chances of becoming dehydrated, but every ounce of glycogen that is stored within the muscles needs 3 ounces of water stored along with it. Therefore, remaining properly hydrated will also help prevent weakened muscle contractions.

• Do not eat a new food just before a contest. Different people often react differently to the same food. Before a contest, eat just those foods that you know your body will handle well.

As a power lifter, you should turn to Appendix C on page 345 for full discussions of the 15:30:55 and 20:20:60 dietary plans. Also presented are sample daily diets that use common, healthy foods to meet an athlete's energy and caloric needs. Use the directions on page 150 to estimate your average daily caloric requirement. Then use the directions in Chapter 13 or 14 to adjust your diet for off-season fat loss or muscle building, respectively.

Supplementation Guidelines

In addition to eating a proper diet, you should also take dietary supplements to make sure that any nutrients you lose due to sweating or training are replenished. The following tables will help guide you in selecting the supplements appropriate for you. The first table lists the nutrients recommended for power lifters, as well as the range of intake for each nutrient. (For discussions of these nutrients, see Part One.) Note that within the ranges of intake, the lower amounts are for smaller individuals and lower-activity days, while the higher amounts are for larger individuals and higher-activity days.

RECOMMENDED NUTRIENTS AND RANGES OF INTAKE

For Power Lifters

NUTRIENT	RANGE OF INTAKE
VITAMINS	
Vitamin A	8,000–16,000 IU
Beta-carotene	20,000–35,000 IU
Vitamin B$_1$ (thiamine)	30–120 mg
Vitamin B$_2$ (riboflavin)	30–120 mg
Vitamin B$_3$ (niacin)	40–80 mg
Vitamin B$_5$ (pantothenic acid)	20–100 mg
Vitamin B$_6$ (pyridoxine)	20–80 mg
Vitamin B$_{12}$ (cobalamin)	12–120 mcg
Biotin	125–175 mcg
Folate	400–800 mcg
Vitamin C	800–2,000 mg
Vitamin D	400–800 IU
Vitamin E	200–600 IU
Vitamin K	60–160 mcg
MINERALS	
Boron	2–8 mg
Calcium	800–1,500 mg
Chromium	200–500 mcg
Copper	1–4 mg
Iodine	100–200 mcg
Iron	15–50 mg
Magnesium	250–650 mg
Manganese	12–35 mg
Molybdenum	100–200 mcg
Phosphorus	150–800 mg
Potassium	50–1,000 mg
Selenium	100–200 mcg
Zinc	15–50 mg
AMINO ACIDS	
L-arginine	1,000–4,000 mg

NUTRIENT	RANGE OF INTAKE
L-glutamine	1,000–3,000 mg
L-ornithine	1,000–4,000 mg
FATTY ACIDS	
Alpha-linolenic acid	2,000–4,000 mg
Docosahexaenoic acid (DHA)	250–750 mg
Eiocosapentaenoic acid (EPA)	250–750 mg
Gamma linolenic acid (GLA)	300–600 mg
Linoleic acid	3,000–6,000 mg
METABOLITES	
Beta-hydroxy beta-methylbutyrate	2,000–4,000 mg
Bioflavonoids	200–800 mg
Choline	100–600 mg
Creatine monohydrate	8,000–20,000 mg
Ferulic acid	50–100 mg
Inosine	1,000–2,000 mg
Inositol	100–600 mg
L-carnitine	1,500–3,000 mg

IU = international units, mcg = micrograms, mg = milligrams.

The second table lists the different types of sports supplements available and indicates if their use by power lifters is recommended in the preseason, during the season, or directly before a contest. The list also includes a number of popular nutritional practices—bicarbonate loading, carbohydrate loading, creatine and/or inosine loading, and water loading. (For a discussion of any of these supplements or practices, see the appropriate section in Part One or Part Three.)

RECOMMENDED SPORTS SUPPLEMENTS AND NUTRITIONAL PRACTICES

For Power Lifters

	Intake Recommendation		
	PRESEASON	SEASON	PRECONTEST
SUPPLEMENTS			
Multivitamins	Yes	Yes	No
Multiminerals	Yes	Yes	No
Antioxidants	Yes	Yes	No
Fatty acids	Yes	Yes	No
Metabolites	Optional	Yes	Yes
Branched-chain amino acids	Yes	Yes	Yes
Herbs	Yes	Yes	No
Low-calorie protein drink (200–300 calories)	Yes	Yes	Yes

	Intake Recommendation		
	PRESEASON	SEASON	PRECONTEST
Carbohydrate drink	Yes	Yes	Yes
Fat-burning supplement	Yes	Optional	No
PRACTICES			
Bicarbonate loading	No	Optional	Optional
Carbohydrate loading	No	No	Optional
Creatine and/or inosine loading	Optional	Yes	Yes
Water loading	No	No	No

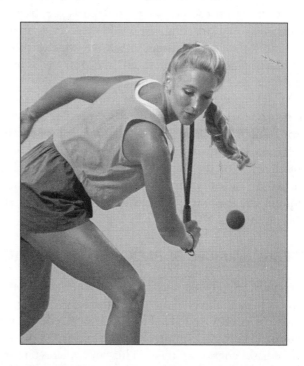

RACKET SPORTS

Includes Badminton, Handball, Jai Alai, Platform Tennis, Racquetball, Squash, and Other Racket Sports

The racket sports—including badminton, jai alai, platform tennis, racquetball, and squash—are all games that involve a wide range of skills and movements. They require not only speed and strength in short, explosive bursts, but also a high level of anaerobic-strength endurance, as well as flexibility and agility.

Every bit of your training and diet must reflect these elements. These elements are what make most of the racket sports explosive in nature. In fact, the racket sports tend to be very explosive, so improved recovery and tissue repair plus increased speed and strength are your year-round training and dietary goals. Nutritionally, this means emphasizing short-term energy needs and maximizing the muscles' recovery and tissue-repair processes.

In the racket sports, the energy output is primarily anaerobic (without oxygen). This does not mean that training for or playing any of the racket sports is easy, however. Serving, returning, and volleying the ball all require not only "touch" and finesse but also lightning-quick reflexes and a high tolerance to pain and fatigue from lactic-acid buildup in the muscles. The training for each of the racket sports is extremely intensive and grueling. At the highest levels, speed training for successful court play forces you to operate at your anaerobic threshold (the point at which you must receive oxygen).

Muscles grow when they are stressed. In the racket sports, the aim is to make the muscles grow as strong and as quick as possible. This calls for specialized training. Furthermore, the incredible energy output of each of the racket sports, especially coupled with the fast, often explosive aspects of the games, requires the support of a carefully constructed nutrition program.

ENERGY SOURCES OF RACKET-SPORT PLAYERS

The muscles rely on three major systems to supply the energy they need—the immediate, glycolytic, and oxidative energy systems. For short-term energy for explosive-strength output, the muscles depend on the immediate energy systems. The immediate energy systems are nonoxidative—that is, they do not use oxygen. Instead, these systems generate energy through the use of adenosine triphosphate (ATP) and creatine phosphate (CP). CP is produced in the body and stored in the muscle fibers. It is broken down by enzymes to regenerate ATP, which is also stored in the muscle fibers. When the ATP is in turn broken down, the result is a spark of energy that triggers a muscle contraction.

For medium-term energy for repeated near-maximum exertion, the muscles turn to the glycolytic energy systems. In these systems, which are also nonoxidative, glycogen is used to produce energy. Glycogen is the storage form of glucose. It is stored in the liver and muscles, and is readily converted back to glucose when it is needed for energy.

For long-term energy for endurance activities, the muscles use the oxidative energy systems. In these systems, oxygen is used to oxidize long-chain fatty acids, protein, and glucose, which generates energy. For athletes, getting enough oxygen can mean a winning performance rather than a second-place showing.

Every sport involves a variety of skills, and each skill utilizes a unique combination of these three energy sources. The following table lists a number of the major racket sports and shows how much your body relies on each of the energy sources when you participate in an average game of each.

WHERE YOUR ENERGY COMES FROM

For Racket-Sport Players		
Energy Systems		
IMMEDIATE	GLYCOLYTIC	OXIDATIVE
Badminton 90%	10%	0%
Handball 80%	15%	5%
Jai alai 80%	15%	5%
Platform tennis 50%	40%	10%
Racquetball 80%	15%	5%
Squash 80%	15%	5%

When considering the type of nutritional support to give your training program, keep the following factors in mind:

☐ All athletes need to consume high-quality protein several times a day for effective recovery and adequate repair of damaged muscle tissue.

☐ Athletes whose muscles rely substantially on the immediate or glycolytic energy systems should keep their fat intake to a minimum because fat is not an efficient energy source for their intensive training, which is almost exclusively anaerobic in nature. Since the fat calories consumed by these athletes are not generally used for energy, they are stored as body fat.

☐ All athletes should consume a carefully measured amount of high-quality carbohydrates several times a day to ensure an adequate supply of energy.

☐ The carbohydrates in all preworkout meals should consist of foods with low glycemic indexes to ensure that training intensity does not wane and that muscle tissue is not cannibalized for energy. (For the glycemic indexes of some common foods, see page 29.)

The aim of your nutrition program is to make your

body healthy enough to accomplish recovery and tissue repair speedily and efficiently—without adding body fat. Your further aim is to do this while maintaining a high strength-to-weight ratio. These aims alone make diet as critical as training for racket-sport players. You must eat just the right amount of food. Eat the wrong foods or the wrong amounts just a few times too often and you will sabotage your fitness efforts.

NUTRITION FOR RACKET-SPORT PLAYERS

Racket-sport players are middle-distance athletes. No matter what racket sport they play, they need stamina, which is supported by energy from the glycolytic energy systems. Therefore, as a racket-sport player, you need to plan your nutritional intake, from both food and supplement sources, to support the glycolytic systems. In addition, since your energy expenditure changes in the off-season, you need to adjust your caloric intake and macronutrient ratio to match. Following are dietary guidelines for racket-sport players to help you in planning your nutrition program. Supplementation guidelines for racket-sport players can be found on page 282.

Dietary Guidelines

The following pie charts illustrate how you should divide up your caloric intake to match the energy demands of the racket sports during the preseason, season, and off-season. They show the target percentages of fat, protein, and carbohydrates that your five to six meals should supply each day.

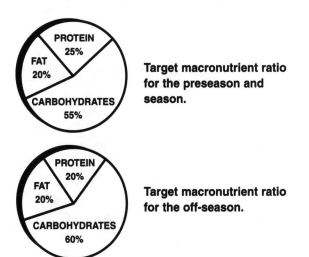

Target macronutrient ratio for the preseason and season.

Target macronutrient ratio for the off-season.

Note that fat has about 9 calories per gram, while protein and carbohydrates have only 4 calories per gram. Therefore, during the season, if you needed to consume a total of 2,500 calories per day, you would aim for 500 calories (20 percent of your total daily calories) from fat, 625 calories (25 percent of your total daily calories) from protein, and the remaining 1,375 calories (55 percent of your total daily calories) from carbohydrates.

Some other important considerations for racket-sport players are:

☐ Carbohydrates are the major source of energy for short-term activities. Complex carbohydrates are the best source because they most effectively refill the glycogen stores in the muscles and liver. In addition, they elevate the blood sugar to a level sufficient for long sessions of intensive training.

☐ As a middle-distance athlete, you must make sure that you consume adequate amounts of both carbohydrates and protein. If your energy stores become drastically depleted or you experience lactic-acid buildup, you may suffer temporary muscle fatigue. If you do not refill your glycogen stores before your next workout or game, your body may begin breaking down muscle tissue for the protein it needs for energy.

☐ Directly before workouts and games, consume carbohydrate drinks with high glycemic indexes to keep your blood sugar sustained at an appropriate level. This will allow you to train or play intensively for longer periods of time.

☐ As a middle-distance athlete, you need to stimulate the storage of glycogen in your muscles while promoting repair and growth of your muscle tissue and inhibiting buildup of body fat. To do this:

• Train against your anaerobic threshold (to exhaustion) on a regular basis. Intensive, exhaustive training stimulates increased storage of glycogen in the muscles and liver, which provides additional energy for greater exercise capacity.

• Consume five to six meals a day. Eating several smaller meals rather than three larger ones will keep your blood-sugar level stable throughout the day and will ensure that a supply of protein is always available for your muscles.

• Keep your fat intake to a minimum. Large amounts of fat in your diet will add to your body fat and will cause mineral loss through frequent urination.

- Consume low-glycemic-index foods about two to three hours before workouts and games. These foods help sustain the blood-sugar level.

- Drink plenty of water. Not only will this practice reduce your chances of becoming dehydrated, but every ounce of glycogen that is stored within the muscles needs 3 ounces of water stored along with it. Therefore, remaining properly hydrated will also help prevent weakened muscle contractions and early onset of fatigue.

- Do not eat a new food just before a game. Different people often react differently to the same food. Before a game, eat just those foods that you know your body will handle well.

As a racket-sport player, you should turn to Appendix C on page 345 for full discussions of the 20:25:55 and 20:20:60 dietary plans. Also presented are sample daily diets that use common, healthy foods to meet an athlete's energy and caloric needs. Use the directions on page 150 to estimate your average daily caloric requirement. Then use the directions in Chapter 13 or 14 to adjust your diet for off-season fat loss or muscle building, respectively.

Supplementation Guidelines

In addition to eating a proper diet, you should also take dietary supplements to make sure that any nutrients you lose due to sweating or training are replenished. The following tables will help guide you in selecting the supplements appropriate for you. The first table lists the nutrients recommended for racket-sport players, as well as the range of intake for each nutrient. (For discussions of these nutrients, see Part One.) Note that within the ranges of intake, the lower amounts are for smaller individuals and lower-activity days, while the higher amounts are for larger individuals and higher-activity days.

RECOMMENDED NUTRIENTS AND RANGES OF INTAKE

For Racket-Sport Players

NUTRIENT	RANGE OF INTAKE
VITAMINS	
Vitamin A	8,000–16,000 IU
Beta-carotene	20,000–40,000 IU
Vitamin B$_1$ (thiamine)	30–120 mg

NUTRIENT	RANGE OF INTAKE
Vitamin B$_2$ (riboflavin)	30–120 mg
Vitamin B$_3$ (niacin)	40–80 mg
Vitamin B$_5$ (pantothenic acid)	20–100 mg
Vitamin B$_6$ (pyridoxine)	20–80 mg
Vitamin B$_{12}$ (cobalamin)	12–120 mcg
Biotin	125–175 mcg
Folate	400–800 mcg
Vitamin C	800–2,000 mg
Vitamin D	400–800 IU
Vitamin E	200–600 IU
Vitamin K	60–160 mcg
MINERALS	
Boron	2–8 mg
Calcium	800–1,500 mg
Chromium	200–500 mcg
Copper	1–4 mg
Iodine	100–200 mcg
Iron	15–50 mg
Magnesium	250–650 mg
Manganese	12–35 mg
Molybdenum	100–200 mcg
Phosphorus	150–800 mg
Potassium	50–1,000 mg
Selenium	100–200 mcg
Zinc	15–50 mg
AMINO ACIDS	
L-glutamine	1,000–2,000 mg
FATTY ACIDS	
Alpha-linolenic acid	500–1,000 mg
Docosahexaenoic acid (DHA)	250–750 mg
Eiocosapentaenoic acid (EPA)	250–750 mg
Gamma linolenic acid (GLA)	100–400 mg
Linoleic acid	2,000–3,000 mg
METABOLITES	
Bioflavonoids	200–800 mg
Choline	100–600 mg
Creatine monohydrate	4,000–8,000 mg
Ferulic acid	20–40 mg
Inosine	500–1,000 mg
Inositol	100–600 mg
L-carnitine	1,000–2,000 mg
Octacosanol	6,000–12,000 mcg

IU = international units, mcg = micrograms, mg = milligrams.

The second table lists the different types of sports supplements available and indicates if their use by racket-sport players is recommended in the preseason, during the season, or directly before a game. The list also includes a number of popular nutritional practices—bicarbonate loading, carbohydrate loading, creatine and/or inosine loading, and water loading. (For a discussion of any of these supplements or practices, see the appropriate section in Part One or Part Three.)

RECOMMENDED SPORTS SUPPLEMENTS AND NUTRITIONAL PRACTICES

For Racket-Sport Players

	Intake Recommendation		
	PRESEASON	SEASON	PREGAME
SUPPLEMENTS			
Multivitamins	Yes	Yes	No
Multiminerals	Yes	Yes	No
Antioxidants	Yes	Yes	No
Fatty acids	Yes	Yes	No
Metabolites	Optional	Yes	Yes
Branched-chain amino acids	Yes	Yes	Yes
Herbs	Yes	Yes	No
Low-calorie protein drink (200–300 calories)	Yes	Yes	Yes
Carbohydrate drink	Yes	Yes	Yes
Fat-burning supplement	Yes	Optional	No
PRACTICES			
Bicarbonate loading	No	No	No
Carbohydrate loading	No	No	Optional
Creatine and/or inosine loading	Optional	Yes	Yes
Water loading	No	No	Yes

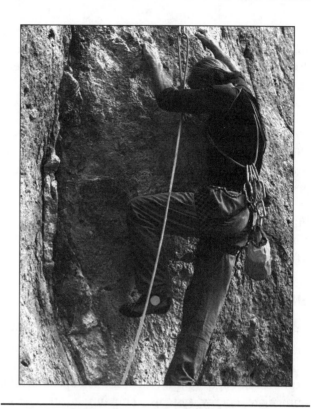

ROCK CLIMBING

Also for Climbing

Rock climbing is a multifaceted sport that involves a wide range of skills and movements. There are several different forms of rock climbing—such as free climbing, solo climbing, and aided climbing—and they each require not only speed and strength in short, explosive bursts, but also a high level of anaerobic-strength endurance, flexibility, agility, and tolerance to pain and fatigue caused by lactic-acid buildup in the muscles.

Every bit of your training and diet must reflect these elements. These elements are what make rock climbing explosive in nature. At the same time, however, rock climbing constantly forces you to push your anaerobic threshold (the point at which you must receive oxygen). You must push, pull, grip, and perform a number of movements requiring sheer strength over and over again, repeatedly testing your tolerance to pain and fatigue. Because of these factors, improved recovery and tissue repair plus increased speed and strength are your year-round training and dietary goals. Nutritionally, this means emphasizing short-term energy needs and maximizing the muscles' recovery and tissue-repair processes.

In rock climbing, the energy output is primarily anaerobic (without oxygen). This does not mean that training for or doing a rock climb is easy, however. Training for rock climbing is extremely intensive and grueling. At the highest levels, it forces you to operate at your anaerobic threshold.

Muscles grow when they are stressed. In rock climbing, the aim is to make the muscles grow as strong and as quick as possible—but only to the point at which your strength-to-weight ratio is maximized. This calls for specialized training. Furthermore, the incredible force output of rock climbing requires the support of a carefully constructed nutrition program.

ENERGY SOURCES OF ROCK CLIMBERS

The muscles rely on three major systems to supply the energy they need—the immediate, glycolytic, and oxidative energy systems. For short-term energy for explosive-strength output, the muscles depend on the immediate energy systems. The immediate energy systems are nonoxidative—that is, they do not use oxygen. Instead, these systems generate energy through the use of adenosine triphosphate (ATP) and creatine phosphate (CP). CP is produced in the body and stored in the muscle fibers. It is broken down by enzymes to regenerate ATP, which is also stored in the muscle fibers. When the ATP is in turn broken down, the result is a spark of energy that triggers a muscle contraction.

For medium-term energy for repeated near-maximum exertion, the muscles turn to the glycolytic energy systems. In these systems, which are also nonoxidative, glycogen is used to produce energy. Glycogen is the storage form of glucose. It is stored in the liver and muscles, and is readily converted back to glucose when it is needed for energy.

For long-term energy for endurance activities, the muscles use the oxidative energy systems. In these systems, oxygen is used to oxidize long-chain fatty acids, protein, and glucose, which generates energy. For athletes, getting enough oxygen can mean a winning performance rather than a second-place showing.

Every sport involves a variety of skills, and each skill utilizes a unique combination of these three energy sources. The following table shows how much your body relies on each of the energy sources during an average rock climb. Percentages are also given for two kinds of average workouts.

WHERE YOUR ENERGY COMES FROM

For Rock Climbers

	Energy Systems		
	IMMEDIATE	GLYCOLYTIC	OXIDATIVE
Average climb	40%	50%	10%
Average workouts			
In-season	50%	40%	10%
Off-season	60%	30%	10%

When considering the type of nutritional support to give your training program, keep the following factors in mind:

☐ All athletes need to consume high-quality protein several times a day for effective recovery and adequate repair of damaged muscle tissue.

☐ Athletes whose muscles rely substantially on the immediate or glycolytic energy systems should keep their fat intake to a minimum because fat is not an efficient energy source for their intensive training, which is almost exclusively anaerobic in nature. Since the fat calories consumed by these athletes are not generally used for energy, they are stored as body fat.

☐ All athletes should consume a carefully measured amount of high-quality carbohydrates several times a day to ensure an adequate supply of energy.

☐ The carbohydrates in all preworkout meals should consist of foods with low glycemic indexes to ensure that training intensity does not wane and that muscle tissue is not cannibalized for energy. (For the glycemic indexes of some common foods, see page 29.)

The aim of your nutrition program is to make your body healthy enough to accomplish recovery and tissue repair speedily and efficiently—without adding body fat. Your further aims are to do this while maintaining a high strength-to-weight ratio plus remaining within 3 to 4 percent of your competition body weight. These aims alone make diet as critical as training for rock climbers. You must eat just the right amount of food. Eat the wrong foods or the wrong amounts just a few times too often and you will sabotage your fitness efforts. Even more important, do not be in a hurry. It takes *years* to become a great rock climber. Rush the nutrition and training processes and you will become fat, your recovery rate will decline, and your injury rate will rise.

NUTRITION FOR ROCK CLIMBERS

Rock climbers are combination power–middle-distance athletes. They obtain most of their energy from a combination of the immediate and glycolytic energy systems. Therefore, as a rock climber, you need to plan your nutritional intake, from both food and supplement sources, to support these nonoxidative systems. In addition, since your energy expenditure changes in the off-season, you need to adjust your caloric intake and macronutrient ratio to match. Following are dietary guidelines for rock climbers to help you in planning your nutrition program. Supplementation guidelines for rock climbers can be found on page 286.

Dietary Guidelines

The following pie charts illustrate how you should divide up your caloric intake to match the energy demands of rock climbing during the preseason, season, and off-season. They show the target percentages of fat, protein, and carbohydrates that your five to six meals should supply each day.

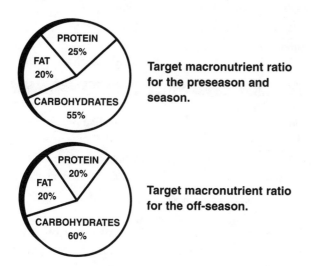

Target macronutrient ratio for the preseason and season.

Target macronutrient ratio for the off-season.

Note that fat has about 9 calories per gram, while protein and carbohydrates have only 4 calories per gram. Therefore, during the season, if you needed to consume a total of 2,500 calories per day, you would aim for 500 calories (20 percent of your total daily calories) from fat, 625 calories (25 percent of your total daily calories) from protein, and the remaining 1,375 calories (55 percent of your total daily calories) from carbohydrates.

Some other important considerations for rock climbers are:

☐ Carbohydrates are the major source of energy for short-term activities. Complex carbohydrates are the best source because they most effectively refill the glycogen stores in the muscles and liver. In addition, they elevate the blood sugar to a level sufficient for long sessions of intensive training.

☐ As a combination power–middle-distance athlete, you must make sure that you consume adequate amounts of both carbohydrates and protein. If your energy stores become drastically depleted or you experience lactic-acid buildup, you may suffer temporary muscle fatigue. If you do not refill your glycogen stores before your next workout or climb, your body may begin breaking down muscle tissue for the protein it needs for energy.

☐ Directly before workouts and climbs, consume carbohydrate drinks with high glycemic indexes to keep your blood sugar sustained at an appropriate level. This will allow you to train or climb intensively for longer periods of time.

☐ As a combination power–middle-distance athlete, you need to stimulate the storage of glycogen in your muscles while promoting repair and growth of your muscle tissue and inhibiting buildup of body fat. To do this:

• Train against your anaerobic threshold (to exhaustion) on a regular basis. Intensive, exhaustive training stimulates increased storage of glycogen in the muscles and liver, which provides additional energy for greater exercise capacity.

• Consume five to six meals a day. Eating several smaller meals rather than three larger ones will keep your blood-sugar level stable throughout the day and will ensure that a supply of protein is always available for your muscles.

• Keep your fat intake to a minimum. Large amounts of fat in your diet will add to your body fat and will cause mineral loss through frequent urination.

• Consume low-glycemic-index foods about two to three hours before workouts and climbs. These foods help sustain the blood-sugar level.

• Drink plenty of water. Not only will this practice reduce your chances of becoming dehydrated, but every ounce of glycogen that is stored within the muscles needs 3 ounces of water stored along with it. Therefore, remaining properly hydrated will also help prevent weakened muscle contractions and early onset of fatigue.

• Do not eat a new food just before a climb. Different people often react differently to the same food. Before a climb, eat just those foods that you know your body will handle well.

As a rock climber, you should turn to Appendix C on page 345 for full discussions of the 20:25:55 and 20:20:60 dietary plans. Also presented are sample daily diets that use common, healthy foods to meet an athlete's energy and caloric needs. Use the directions on page 150 to estimate your average daily caloric requirement. Then use the directions in Chapter 13 or 14 to adjust your diet for off-season fat loss or muscle building, respectively.

Supplementation Guidelines

In addition to eating a proper diet, you should also take dietary supplements to make sure that any nutrients you lose due to sweating or training are replenished. The following tables will help guide you in selecting the supplements appropriate for you. The first table lists the nutrients recommended for rock climbers, as well as the range of intake for each nutrient. (For discussions of these nutrients, see Part One.) Note that within the ranges of intake, the lower amounts are for smaller individuals and lower-activity days, while the higher amounts are for larger individuals and higher-activity days.

RECOMMENDED NUTRIENTS AND RANGES OF INTAKE

For Rock Climbers

NUTRIENT	RANGE OF INTAKE
VITAMINS	
Vitamin A	8,000–16,000 IU
Beta-carotene	15,000–30,000 IU
Vitamin B₁ (thiamine)	40–120 mg
Vitamin B₂ (riboflavin)	40–120 mg
Vitamin B₃ (niacin)	20–40 mg
Vitamin B₅ (pantothenic acid)	20–100 mg
Vitamin B₆ (pyridoxine)	20–80 mg
Vitamin B₁₂ (cobalamin)	12–120 mcg
Biotin	125–175 mcg
Folate	400–800 mcg
Vitamin C	800–2,000 mg
Vitamin D	400–800 IU

NUTRIENT	RANGE OF INTAKE
Vitamin E	200–800 IU
Vitamin K	60–160 mcg
Boron	2–8 mg
MINERALS	
Calcium	800–1,500 mg
Chromium	200–500 mcg
Copper	1–4 mg
Iodine	100–200 mcg
Iron	15–50 mg
Magnesium	250–650 mg
Manganese	12–35 mg
Molybdenum	100–200 mcg
Phosphorus	150–800 mg
Potassium	50–1,000 mg
Selenium	100–200 mcg
Zinc	15–50 mg
AMINO ACIDS	
L-glutamic acid	1,000–2,000 mg
L-glutamine	1,000–2,000 mg
FATTY ACIDS	
Alpha-linolenic acid	500–1,000 mg
Docosahexaenoic acid (DHA)	250–750 mg
Eiocosapentaenoic acid (EPA)	250–750 mg
Gamma linolenic acid (GLA)	100–400 mg
Linoleic acid	2,000–3,000 mg
METABOLITES	
Bioflavonoids	300–800 mg
Choline	200–600 mg
Inositol	200–600 mg
L-carnitine	1,000–2,000 mg
Octacosanol	1,000–2,000 mcg

IU = international units, mcg = micrograms, mg = milligrams.

The second table lists the different types of sports supplements available and indicates if their use by rock climbers is recommended in the preseason, during the season, or directly before a climb. The list also includes a number of popular nutritional practices—bicarbonate loading, carbohydrate loading, creatine and/or inosine loading, and water loading. (For a discussion of any of these supplements or practices, see the appropriate section in Part One or Part Three.)

RECOMMENDED SPORTS SUPPLEMENTS AND NUTRITIONAL PRACTICES

For Rock Climbers

	Intake Recommendation		
	PRESEASON	SEASON	PRECLIMB
SUPPLEMENTS			
Multivitamins	Yes	Yes	No
Multiminerals	Yes	Yes	No
Antioxidants	Yes	Yes	No
Fatty acids	Yes	Yes	No
Metabolites	Optional	Yes	Yes
Branched-chain amino acids	Yes	Yes	Yes
Herbs	Yes	Yes	No
Medium-calorie protein drink (300–500 calories)	Yes	Yes	Yes
Carbohydrate drink	Yes	Yes	Yes
Fat-burning supplement	Yes	Optional	No
PRACTICES			
Bicarbonate loading	No	No	No
Carbohydrate loading	No	No	Optional
Creatine and/or inosine loading	No	No	No
Water loading	No	No	Optional

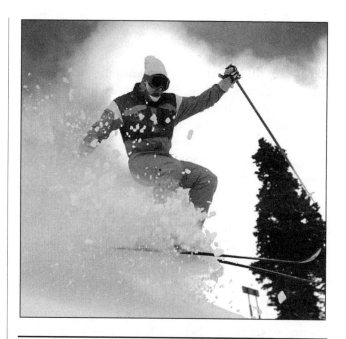

SKIING

Includes Alpine (Downhill), Cross-Country, Freestyle, and Nordic Skiing, and Ski Jumping

Also for Biathlon, Bobsledding, Grass Skiing, Luge, Snowboarding, Snowshoe Racing, and Tobogganing

What kind of skier are you? If you are a downhill skier, your energy comes primarily from the immediate energy systems and you must eat and train accordingly. If you are a biathlon skier, you need to focus the bulk of your nutrition and training efforts on building up your glycolytic and oxidative energy reserves. If you are a cross-country skier, you need to concentrate on your oxidative energy systems. However, if you enjoy two or all three kinds of skiing, you should combine your nutrition and training programs, stressing one only as a competition nears.

No matter what type of skier you are, you cannot completely ignore any facet of the sport. You must address each skill to some extent, whether you use it on a regular basis or not. Therefore, your training, both on and off the slopes, should develop strength, anaerobic or aerobic endurance, and speed–strength equally. This calls for specialized training. Furthermore, the unique energy output called for by each type of skiing requires the support of a carefully constructed nutrition program.

287

ENERGY SOURCES OF SKIERS

The muscles rely on three major systems to supply the energy they need—the immediate, glycolytic, and oxidative energy systems. For short-term energy for explosive-strength output, the muscles depend on the immediate energy systems. The immediate energy systems are nonoxidative—that is, they do not use oxygen. Instead, these systems generate energy through the use of adenosine triphosphate (ATP) and creatine phosphate (CP). CP is produced in the body and stored in the muscle fibers. It is broken down by enzymes to regenerate ATP, which is also stored in the muscle fibers. When the ATP is in turn broken down, the result is a spark of energy that triggers a muscle contraction.

For medium-term energy for repeated near-maximum exertion, the muscles turn to the glycolytic energy systems. In these systems, which are also nonoxidative, glycogen is used to produce energy. Glycogen is the storage form of glucose. It is stored in the liver and muscles, and is readily converted back to glucose when it is needed for energy.

For long-term energy for endurance activities, the muscles use the oxidative energy systems. In these systems, oxygen is used to oxidize long-chain fatty acids, protein, and glucose, which generates energy. For athletes, getting enough oxygen can mean a winning performance rather than a second-place showing.

Every sport involves a variety of skills, and each skill utilizes a unique combination of these three energy sources. The following table lists a number of major skiing events and shows how much your body relies on each of the energy sources when you compete in them. Percentages are also given for two similar sports.

WHERE YOUR ENERGY COMES FROM

For Skiers

	Energy Systems		
	IMMEDIATE	GLYCOLYTIC	OXIDATIVE
Alpine (men's and women's)			
Combined	60%	30%	10%
Downhill	70%	20%	10%
Giant slalom	60%	30%	10%
Slalom	70%	20%	10%
Super-G	60%	30%	10%
Biathlon			
Men's 10k	20%	40%	40%

	Energy Systems		
	IMMEDIATE	GLYCOLYTIC	OXIDATIVE
Men's 20k	10%	20%	70%
Men's 30k relay	20%	40%	40%
Women's 7.5k	20%	40%	40%
Women's 15k	10%	30%	60%
Women's 30k relay	20%	40%	40%
Cross-country			
Men's 10k	15%	35%	50%
Men's 15k pursuit	10%	30%	60%
Men's 30k	5%	15%	80%
Men's 40k relay	15%	35%	50%
Men's 50k	5%	10%	85%
Women's 5k	20%	40%	40%
Women's 10k	15%	35%	50%
Women's 15k	10%	30%	60%
Women's 20k relay	20%	40%	40%
Women's 30k	5%	15%	80%
Freestyle (men's and women's)			
Aerials	80%	15%	5%
Moguls	80%	15%	5%
Nordic combined			
Individual	10%	20%	70%
Team	10%	20%	70%
Ski jumping (men's and women's)	90%	5%	5%
For Similar Sports			
Bobsledding (2- or 4-man)	90%	10%	0%
Grass skiing	90%	5%	5%
Luge (men's and women's singles, and men's doubles)	90%	10%	0%
Snowboarding	80%	15%	5%
Tobogganing	90%	10%	0%

When considering the type of nutritional support to give your training program, keep the following factors in mind:

☐ All athletes need to consume high-quality protein several times a day for effective recovery and adequate repair of damaged muscle tissue.

☐ Athletes whose muscles rely substantially on the immediate or glycolytic energy systems should keep their fat intake to a minimum because fat is not an efficient energy source for their intensive training, which is almost exclusively anaerobic in nature. Since the fat calories consumed by these athletes are not generally used for energy, they are stored as body fat.

☐ Athletes whose muscles rely substantially on the oxidative energy systems can eat more fat because their energy is manufactured through the oxidation of fatty acids. But even these athletes should watch their fat calories if they train aerobically (with oxygen) for less than half an hour at a time.

☐ All athletes should consume a carefully measured amount of high-quality carbohydrates several times a day to ensure an adequate supply of energy.

☐ The carbohydrates in all preworkout meals should consist of foods with low glycemic indexes to ensure that training intensity does not wane and that muscle tissue is not cannibalized for energy. (For the glycemic indexes of some common foods, see page 29.)

The aim of your nutrition program is to make your body healthy enough to accomplish recovery and tissue repair speedily and efficiently—without adding body fat. Your further aim is to do this while maintaining a high strength-to-weight ratio. These aims alone make diet very important for skiers. You must eat just the right amount of food. Eat the wrong foods or the wrong amounts just a few times too often and you will sabotage your fitness efforts.

NUTRITION FOR SKIERS

Skiers are either power, middle-distance, or endurance athletes. Their primary source of energy is determined by the specific type of skiing they specialize in. Some types of skiing require bursts of power, which are supported by energy from the immediate energy systems. Some types of skiing require stamina, which is supported by energy from the glycolytic energy systems. Still other types of skiing require endurance, which is supported by energy from the oxidative energy systems. Therefore, as a skier, you need to plan your nutritional intake, from both food and supplement sources, to support the appropriate systems. In addition, if you are a power or middle-distance skier, your energy expenditure changes in the preseason and/or off-season, and you need to adjust your caloric intake and macronutrient ratio to match. Following are dietary and supplementation guidelines for power skiers to help you in planning your nutrition program. Dietary and supplementation guidelines for middle-distance skiers can be found on page 291, and guidelines for endurance skiers can be found on page 293.

POWER SKIERS

Skiers who compete in events that last for just seconds to minutes are power athletes. Among the typical events they participate in are the downhill, the mogul, and ski jumping.

Dietary Guidelines

The following pie charts illustrate how you should divide up your caloric intake to match the energy demands of power skiing during the preseason, season, and off-season. They show the target percentages of fat, protein, and carbohydrates that your five to six meals should supply each day.

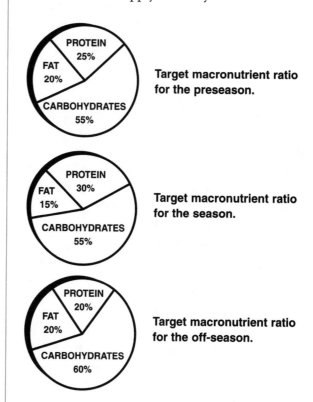

Target macronutrient ratio for the preseason.

Target macronutrient ratio for the season.

Target macronutrient ratio for the off-season.

Note that fat has about 9 calories per gram, while protein and carbohydrates have only 4 calories per gram. Therefore, during the season, if you needed to consume a total of 2,500 calories per day, you would aim for 375 calories (15 percent of your total daily calories) from fat, 750 calories (30 percent of your total daily calories) from protein, and the remaining 1,375 calories (55 percent of your total daily calories) from carbohydrates.

Some other important considerations for power skiers are:

☐ Carbohydrates are the major source of energy for

short-term activities. Complex carbohydrates are the best source because they most effectively refill the glycogen stores in the muscles and liver. In addition, they elevate the blood sugar to a level sufficient for long sessions of intensive training.

☐ As a power athlete, you must make sure that you consume adequate amounts of both carbohydrates and protein. If your energy stores become drastically depleted or you experience lactic-acid buildup, you may suffer temporary muscle fatigue. If you do not refill your glycogen stores before your next workout or competition, your body may begin breaking down muscle tissue for the protein it needs for energy.

☐ Directly before workouts, consume carbohydrate drinks with high glycemic indexes to keep your blood sugar sustained at an appropriate level. This will allow you to train intensively without having your explosiveness hindered by fatigue.

☐ As a power athlete, you need to stimulate the storage of glycogen in your muscles while promoting repair and growth of your muscle tissue and inhibiting buildup of body fat. To do this:

• Train anaerobically on a regular basis. Intensive training stimulates increased storage of glycogen in the muscles and liver, which provides additional energy for greater exercise capacity.

• Consume five to six meals a day. Eating several smaller meals rather than three larger ones will keep your blood-sugar level stable throughout the day and will ensure that a supply of protein is always available for your muscles.

• Keep your fat intake to a minimum. Large amounts of fat in your diet will add to your body fat and will cause you to lose minerals through frequent urination.

• Consume low-glycemic-index foods about two to three hours before workouts and competitions. These foods help sustain the blood-sugar level.

• Drink plenty of water. Not only will this practice reduce your chances of becoming dehydrated, but every ounce of glycogen that is stored within the muscles needs 3 ounces of water stored along with it. Therefore, remaining properly hydrated will also help prevent weakened muscle contractions.

• Do not eat a new food just before a competition. Different people often react differently to the same food. Before a competition, eat just those foods that you know your body will handle well.

As a power skier, you should turn to Appendix C

on page 345 for full discussions of the 20:25:55, 15:30:55, and 20:20:60 dietary plans. Also presented are sample daily diets that use common, healthy foods to meet an athlete's energy and caloric needs. Use the directions on page 150 to estimate your average daily caloric requirement. Then use the directions in Chapter 13 or 14 to adjust your diet for off-season fat loss or muscle building, respectively.

Supplementation Guidelines

In addition to eating a proper diet, you should also take dietary supplements to make sure that any nutrients you lose due to sweating or training are replenished. The following tables will help guide you in selecting the supplements appropriate for you. The first table lists the nutrients recommended for power skiers, as well as the range of intake for each nutrient. (For discussions of these nutrients, see Part One.) Note that within the ranges of intake, the lower amounts are for smaller individuals and lower-activity days, while the higher amounts are for larger individuals and higher-activity days.

RECOMMENDED NUTRIENTS AND RANGES OF INTAKE

For Power Skiers	
NUTRIENT	**RANGE OF INTAKE**
VITAMINS	
Vitamin A	8,000–16,000 IU
Beta-carotene	20,000–35,000 IU
Vitamin B_1 (thiamine)	30–120 mg
Vitamin B_2 (riboflavin)	30–120 mg
Vitamin B_3 (niacin)	40–80 mg
Vitamin B_5 (pantothenic acid)	20–100 mg
Vitamin B_6 (pyridoxine)	20–80 mg
Vitamin B_{12} (cobalamin)	12–120 mcg
Biotin	125–175 mcg
Folate	400–800 mcg
Vitamin C	800–2,000 mg
Vitamin D	400–800 IU
Vitamin E	400–1,000 IU
Vitamin K	60–160 mcg
MINERALS	
Boron	2–8 mg
Calcium	800–1,500 mg
Chromium	200–500 mcg
Copper	1–4 mg

NUTRIENT	RANGE OF INTAKE
Iodine	100–200 mcg
Iron	15–50 mg
Magnesium	250–650 mg
Manganese	12–35 mg
Molybdenum	100–200 mcg
Phosphorus	150–800 mg
Potassium	50–1,000 mg
Selenium	100–200 mcg
Zinc	15–50 mg
AMINO ACIDS	
L-glutamine	1,000–2,000 mg
FATTY ACIDS	
Alpha-linolenic acid	1,500–3,000 mg
Docosahexaenoic acid (DHA)	250–750 mg
Eiocosapentaenoic acid (EPA)	250–750 mg
Gamma linolenic acid (GLA)	100–400 mg
Linoleic acid	3,000–6,000 mg
METABOLITES	
Bioflavonoids	200–800 mg
Choline	100–600 mg
Creatine monohydrate	6,000–20,000 mg
Ferulic acid	25–75 mg
Inosine	500–1,000 mg
Inositol	100–600 mg
L-carnitine	1,000–2,000 mg
Octacosanol	4,000–8,000 mcg

IU = international units, mcg = micrograms, mg = milligrams.

The second table lists the different types of sports supplements available and indicates if their use by power skiers is recommended in the preseason, during the season, or directly before a competition.

RECOMMENDED SPORTS SUPPLEMENTS AND NUTRITIONAL PRACTICES

For Power Skiers

	Intake Recommendation		
	PRESEASON	SEASON	PRE-COMPETITION
SUPPLEMENTS			
Multivitamins	Yes	Yes	No
Multiminerals	Yes	Yes	No
Antioxidants	Yes	Yes	No
Fatty acids	Yes	Yes	No
Metabolites	Optional	Yes	Yes

	Intake Recommendation		
	PRESEASON	SEASON	PRE-COMPETITION
Branched-chain amino acids	Yes	Yes	Yes
Herbs	Yes	Yes	No
Low-calorie protein drink (200–300 calories)	Yes	Yes	Yes
Carbohydrate drink	Yes	Yes	Yes
Fat-burning supplement	Yes	Optional	No
PRACTICES			
Bicarbonate loading	No	Optional	Yes
Carbohydrate loading	No	No	No
Creatine and/or inosine loading	Optional	Yes	Yes
Water loading	No	No	No

The list above also includes a number of popular nutritional practices—bicarbonate loading, carbohydrate loading, creatine and/or inosine loading, and water loading. (For a discussion of any of these supplements or practices, see the appropriate section in Part One or Part Three.)

MIDDLE-DISTANCE SKIERS

Skiers who compete in events that last for up to about a half hour are middle-distance athletes. Among the typical events they participate in are the super-G and 5k.

Dietary Guidelines

The following pie charts illustrate how you should divide up your caloric intake to match the energy demands of middle-distance skiing during the preseason, season, and off-season. They show the target percentages of fat, protein, and carbohydrates that your five to six meals should supply each day.

Note that fat has about 9 calories per gram, while protein and carbohydrates have only 4 calories per gram. Therefore, during the season, if you needed to consume a total of 2,500 calories per day, you would aim for 500 calories (20 percent of your total daily calories) from fat, 625 calories (25 percent of your total daily calories) from protein, and the remaining 1,375 calories (55 percent of your total daily calories) from carbohydrates.

291

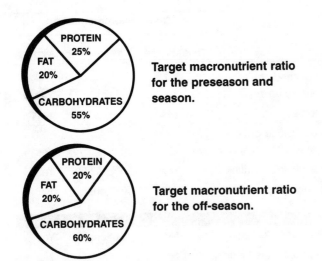

Target macronutrient ratio for the preseason and season.

Target macronutrient ratio for the off-season.

Some other important considerations for middle-distance skiers are:

☐ Carbohydrates are the major source of energy for short-term activities. Complex carbohydrates are the best source because they most effectively refill the glycogen stores in the muscles and liver. In addition, they elevate the blood sugar to a level sufficient for long sessions of intensive training.

☐ As a middle-distance athlete, you must make sure that you consume adequate amounts of both carbohydrates and protein. If your energy stores become drastically depleted or you experience lactic-acid buildup, you may suffer temporary muscle fatigue. If you do not refill your glycogen stores before your next workout or competition, your body may begin breaking down muscle tissue for the protein it needs for energy.

☐ Directly before workouts consume carbohydrate drinks with high glycemic indexes to keep your blood sugar sustained at an appropriate level. This will allow you to train intensively for longer periods of time.

☐ As a middle-distance athlete, you need to stimulate the storage of glycogen in your muscles while promoting repair and growth of your muscle tissue and inhibiting buildup of body fat. To do this:

• Train against your anaerobic threshold (to exhaustion) on a regular basis. Intensive, exhaustive training stimulates increased storage of glycogen in the muscles and liver, which provides additional energy for greater exercise capacity.

• Consume five to six meals a day. Eating several smaller meals rather than three larger ones will keep your blood-sugar level stable throughout the day and will ensure that a supply of protein is always available for your muscles.

• Keep your fat intake to a minimum. Large amounts of fat in your diet will add to your body fat and will cause mineral loss through frequent urination.

• Consume low-glycemic-index foods about two to three hours before workouts. These foods help sustain the blood-sugar level.

• Drink plenty of water. Not only will this practice reduce your chances of becoming dehydrated, but every ounce of glycogen that is stored within the muscles needs 3 ounces of water stored along with it. Therefore, remaining properly hydrated will also help prevent weakened muscle contractions and early onset of fatigue.

• Do not eat a new food just before a competition. Different people often react differently to the same food. Before a competition, eat just those foods that you know your body will handle well.

As a middle-distance skier, you should turn to Appendix C on page 345 for full discussions of the 20:25:55 and 20:20:60 dietary plans. Also presented are sample daily diets that use common, healthy foods to meet an athlete's energy and caloric needs. Use the directions on page 150 to estimate your average daily caloric requirement. Then use the directions in Chapter 13 or 14 to adjust your diet for off-season fat loss or muscle building, respectively.

Supplementation Guidelines

In addition to eating a proper diet, you should also take dietary supplements to make sure that any nutrients you lose due to sweating or training are replenished. The following tables will help guide you in selecting the supplements appropriate for you. The first table lists the nutrients recommended for middle-distance skiers, as well as the range of intake for each nutrient. (For discussions of these nutrients, see Part One.) Note that within the ranges of intake, the lower amounts are for smaller individuals and lower-activity days, while the higher amounts are for larger individuals and higher-activity days.

RECOMMENDED NUTRIENTS AND RANGES OF INTAKE

For Middle-Distance Skiers

NUTRIENT	RANGE OF INTAKE
VITAMINS	
Vitamin A	8,000–16,000 IU
Beta-carotene	20,000–35,000 IU
Vitamin B$_1$ (thiamine)	40–120 mg
Vitamin B$_2$ (riboflavin)	40–120 mg
Vitamin B$_3$ (niacin)	20–40 mg
Vitamin B$_5$ (pantothenic acid)	20–100 mg
Vitamin B$_6$ (pyridoxine)	20–80 mg
Vitamin B$_{12}$ (cobalamin)	12–120 mcg
Biotin	125–175 mcg
Folate	400–800 mcg
Vitamin C	800–2,000 mg
Vitamin D	400–800 IU
Vitamin E	400–1,000 IU
Vitamin K	60–160 mcg
MINERALS	
Boron	2–8 mg
Calcium	800–1,500 mg
Chromium	200–500 mcg
Copper	1–4 mg
Iodine	100–200 mcg
Iron	15–50 mg
Magnesium	250–650 mg
Manganese	12–35 mg
Molybdenum	100–200 mcg
Phosphorus	150–800 mg
Potassium	50–1,000 mg
Selenium	100–200 mcg
Zinc	15–50 mg
AMINO ACIDS	
L-glutamic acid	500–1,000 mg
L-glutamine	1,000–2,000 mg
FATTY ACIDS	
Alpha-linolenic acid	500–1,000 mg
Docosahexaenoic acid (DHA)	250–750 mg
Eiocosapentaenoic acid (EPA)	250–750 mg
Gamma linolenic acid (GLA)	100–400 mg
Linoleic acid	2,000–3,000 mg
METABOLITES	
Bioflavonoids	300–800 mg
Choline	200–600 mg
Inositol	200–600 mg
L-carnitine	500–1,500 mg

NUTRIENT	RANGE OF INTAKE
Octacosanol	4,000–8,000 mcg

IU = international units, mcg = micrograms, mg = milligrams.

The second table lists the different types of sports supplements available and indicates if their use by middle-distance skiers is recommended in the preseason, during the season, or directly before a competition. The list also includes a number of popular nutritional practices—bicarbonate loading, carbohydrate loading, creatine and/or inosine loading, and water loading. (For a discussion of any of these supplements or practices, see the appropriate section in Part One or Part Three.)

RECOMMENDED SPORTS SUPPLEMENTS AND NUTRITIONAL PRACTICES

For Middle-Distance Skiers

	Intake Recommendation		
	PRESEASON	SEASON	PRE-COMPETITION
SUPPLEMENTS			
Multivitamins	Yes	Yes	No
Multiminerals	Yes	Yes	No
Antioxidants	Yes	Yes	No
Fatty acids	Yes	Yes	No
Metabolites	Optional	Yes	Yes
Branched-chain amino acids	Yes	Yes	Yes
Herbs	Yes	Yes	No
Medium-calorie protein drink (300–500 calories)	Yes	Yes	Yes
Carbohydrate drink	Yes	Yes	Yes
Fat-burning supplement	Yes	Optional	No
PRACTICES			
Bicarbonate loading	No	No	No
Carbohydrate loading	No	No	Optional
Creatine and/or inosine loading	No	No	No
Water loading	No	Optional	Optional

ENDURANCE SKIERS

Skiers who compete in events that last longer than about a half hour are endurance athletes. Among the typical events they participate in are cross-country and Nordic skiing.

Dietary Guidelines

The following pie chart illustrates how you should divide up your caloric intake to match the energy demands of endurance skiing during the preseason, season, and off-season. They show the target percentages of fat, protein, and carbohydrates that your five to six meals should supply each day.

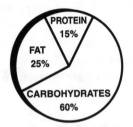

Target macronutrient ratio for the preseason, season, and off-season.

Note that fat has about 9 calories per gram, while protein and carbohydrates have only 4 calories per gram. Therefore, if you needed to consume a total of 2,500 calories per day, you would aim for 625 calories (25 percent of your total daily calories) from fat, 375 calories (15 percent of your total daily calories) from protein, and the remaining 1,500 calories (60 percent of your total daily calories) from carbohydrates.

Some other important considerations for endurance skiers are:

☐ The energy source that is used during an aerobic activity depends upon the duration and intensity of the activity. During the first one and a half to two hours, both glycogen and body fat are the primary sources of energy. After one and a half to two hours, body fat alone becomes the primary source.

☐ While body fat is the primary source of energy during prolonged aerobic activities, it cannot be used efficiently unless some glycogen remains in the muscles and liver. Therefore, even ultra-endurance athletes must make sure to always keep their glycogen stores filled.

☐ As an endurance athlete, you need to encourage glycogen sparing in your body while stimulating the use of fat as your primary energy source. To do this:

• Train for endurance on a regular basis. Regular endurance training stimulates increased storage of both glycogen and fatty acids.

• Consume five to six meals a day. Eating several smaller meals rather than three larger ones will keep your blood-sugar level stable throughout the day.

• Do not load up on dietary fat. Consuming large amounts of fat was originally thought to benefit endurance athletes, whose primary source of energy is fat. However, fat loading can lead to frequent urination, which increases the loss of minerals essential to healthy heart action.

• Consume low-glycemic-index foods about two to three hours before workouts and competitions. These foods help sustain the blood-sugar level.

• Do not consume food or caloric beverages from two hours before an endurance activity to fifteen minutes before. Food and caloric beverages cause the insulin level to rise, which in turn can provoke transient hypoglycemia. Transient hypoglycemia interferes with the energy dynamics during exercise and can induce early onset of fatigue.

• Consume carbohydrates directly before and during endurance activities. Because exercise slows the release of insulin into the bloodstream, the ingestion of carbohydrates spares glycogen and allows the use of fat for energy. Carbohydrate drinks with high glycemic indexes help sustain the blood-sugar level, thereby preserving glycogen stores.

• During endurance activities, drink plenty of water. Endurance activities cause profuse sweating, which results in loss of valuable fluids and minerals. Dehydration not only reduces performance but can seriously affect health.

• Drink electrolyte-containing beverages during endurance activities. These drinks help replace minerals that are lost through sweating.

• During endurance activities, drink 4 to 6 ounces of fluid every fifteen to thirty minutes. For every pound of body weight lost through sweating, 1 pint of fluid should be consumed. Chilled fluids are absorbed the quickest.

• Do not eat a new food just before a competition. Different people often react differently to the same food. Before a competition, eat just those foods that you know your body will handle well.

As an endurance skier, you should turn to Appendix C on page 345 for a full discussion of the 25:15:60 dietary plan. Also presented are sample daily diets that use common, healthy foods to meet an athlete's energy and caloric needs. Use the directions on page 150 to estimate your average daily caloric requirement. Then use the directions in Chapter 13 or 14 to adjust your diet for off-season fat loss or muscle building, respectively.

Supplementation Guidelines

In addition to eating a proper diet, you should also take dietary supplements to make sure that any nutrients you lose due to sweating or training are replenished. The following tables will help guide you in selecting the supplements appropriate for you. The first table lists the nutrients recommended for endurance skiers, as well as the range of intake for each nutrient. (For discussions of these nutrients, see Part One.) Note that within the ranges of intake, the lower amounts are for smaller individuals and lower-activity days, while the higher amounts are for larger individuals and higher-activity days.

RECOMMENDED NUTRIENTS AND RANGES OF INTAKE

For Endurance Skiers

NUTRIENT	RANGE OF INTAKE
VITAMINS	
Vitamin A	8,000–16,000 IU
Beta-carotene	25,000–60,000 IU
Vitamin B$_1$ (thiamine)	100–250 mg
Vitamin B$_2$ (riboflavin)	100–200 mg
Vitamin B$_3$ (niacin)	10–20 mg
Vitamin B$_5$ (pantothenic acid)	100–200 mg
Vitamin B$_6$ (pyridoxine)	20–80 mg
Vitamin B$_{12}$ (cobalamin)	12–120 mcg
Biotin	125–200 mcg
Folate	400–800 mcg
Vitamin C	1,000–2,000 mg
Vitamin D	400–800 IU
Vitamin E	400–1,000 IU
Vitamin K	60–160 mcg
MINERALS	
Boron	2–8 mg
Calcium	800–1,500 mg
Chromium	200–500 mcg
Copper	1–4 mg
Iodine	100–200 mcg
Iron	15–50 mg
Magnesium	250–650 mg
Manganese	12–35 mg
Molybdenum	100–200 mcg

NUTRIENT	RANGE OF INTAKE
Phosphorus	150–800 mg
Potassium	50–1,000 mg
Selenium	100–200 mcg
Zinc	15–50 mg
AMINO ACIDS	
L-glutamic acid	1,000–1,500 mg
L-glutamine	1,000–2,000 mg
FATTY ACIDS	
Alpha-linolenic acid	500–1,000 mg
Docosahexaenoic acid (DHA)	400–1,000 mg
Eiocosapentaenoic acid (EPA)	400–1,000 mg
Gamma linolenic acid (GLA)	200–500 mg
Linoleic acid	500–1,000 mg
METABOLITES	
Bioflavonoids	500–1,000 mg
Choline	500–1,000 mg
Coenzyme Q$_{10}$	60–120 mg
Inositol	500–1,000 mg
L-carnitine	1,000–3,000 mg
Octacosanol	1,000–2,000 mcg
OTHER	
Caffeine*	200–400 mg

IU = international units, mcg = micrograms, mg = milligrams.

*Verify with your sports governing organization that caffeine consumption is permitted during competition.

The second table lists the different types of sports supplements available and indicates if their use by endurance skiers is recommended in the preseason, during the season, or directly before a competition. The list also includes a number of popular nutritional practices—bicarbonate loading, carbohydrate loading, creatine and/or inosine loading, and water loading. (For a discussion of any of these supplements or practices, see the appropriate section in Part One or Part Three.)

RECOMMENDED SPORTS SUPPLEMENTS AND NUTRITIONAL PRACTICES

For Endurance Skiers

	Intake Recommendation		
	PRESEASON	SEASON	PRE-COMPETITION
SUPPLEMENTS			
Multivitamins	Yes	Yes	Yes
Multiminerals	Yes	Yes	Yes
Antioxidants	Yes	Yes	Yes

Intake Recommendation			
	PRESEASON	**SEASON**	**PRE-COMPETITION**
Fatty acids	Yes	Yes	Yes
Metabolites	Optional	Yes	Yes
Branched-chain amino acids	Yes	Yes	Yes
Herbs	Yes	Yes	No
High-calorie protein drink (over 500 calories)	Yes	Yes	Yes
Carbohydrate drink with glycerol and electrolytes	Yes	Yes	Yes
Fat-burning supplement	Yes	No	No
PRACTICES			
Bicarbonate loading	No	No	No
Carbohydrate loading	No	No	Yes
Creatine and/or inosine loading	No	No	No
Water loading	No	Optional	Yes

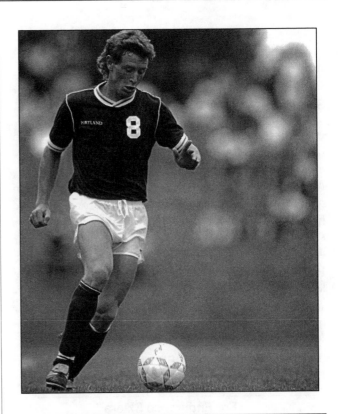

SOCCER

Easily one of the most demanding sports in the world and certainly the most popular, soccer (called football outside of North America) is a game in which conditioning plays as big a role as skill. When you play soccer, you are almost constantly on the run, making many sudden starts, stops, turns, jumps, pivots, and sprints. Therefore, it is essential that you have a solid nutritional foundation, an energy and recovery base to support your training and competition efforts.

Soccer requires a variety of skills. A soccer player must be a combination sprinter, leaper, and even dancer to execute the fundamental movements of the game. Soccer conditioning, therefore, must take each of these areas into account.

Only the most rigorous nutrition and training program can prepare an athlete for the rigors of a soccer season. Increased strength can make you a better soccer player. Through the careful application of scientific training techniques, you can multiply your on-field effectiveness in all areas of the game. You can improve your jumping ability, sprinting ability, endurance, agility, body control, and ball control, playing better even when you are fatigued. Furthermore, the incredible diversity of skills and energy demands of soccer require the support of a carefully constructed nutrition program.

ENERGY SOURCES OF SOCCER PLAYERS

The muscles rely on three major systems to supply the energy they need—the immediate, glycolytic, and oxidative energy systems. For short-term energy for explosive-strength output, the muscles depend on the immediate energy systems. The immediate energy systems are nonoxidative—that is, they do not use oxygen. Instead, these systems generate energy through the use of adenosine triphosphate (ATP) and creatine phosphate (CP). CP is produced in the body and stored in the muscle fibers. It is broken down by enzymes to regenerate ATP, which is also stored in the muscle fibers. When the ATP is in turn broken down, the result is a spark of energy that triggers a muscle contraction.

For medium-term energy for repeated near-maximum exertion, the muscles turn to the glycolytic energy systems. In these systems, which are also nonoxidative, glycogen is used to produce energy. Glycogen is the storage form of glucose. It is stored in the liver and muscles, and is readily converted back to glucose when it is needed for energy.

For long-term energy for endurance activities, the muscles use the oxidative energy systems. In these systems, oxygen is used to oxidize long-chain fatty acids, protein, and glucose, which generates energy. For athletes, getting enough oxygen can mean a winning performance rather than a second-place showing.

Every sport involves a variety of skills, and each skill utilizes a unique combination of these three energy sources. The following table lists the major soccer positions and shows how much your body relies on each of the energy sources when you play them.

WHERE YOUR ENERGY COMES FROM

For Soccer Players			
	Energy Systems		
	IMMEDIATE	GLYCOLYTIC	OXIDATIVE
Forward	50%	30%	20%
Fullback	90%	10%	0%
Goalie	100%	0%	0%
Halfback	60%	20%	20%
Wing	50%	30%	20%

When considering the type of nutritional support to give your training program, keep the following factors in mind:

☐ All athletes need to consume high-quality protein several times a day for effective recovery and adequate repair of damaged muscle tissue.

☐ Athletes whose muscles rely substantially on the immediate or glycolytic energy systems should keep their fat intake to a minimum because fat is not an efficient energy source for their intensive training, which is almost exclusively anaerobic in nature. Since the fat calories consumed by these athletes are not generally used for energy, they are stored as body fat.

☐ Athletes whose muscles rely substantially on the oxidative energy systems can eat more fat because their energy is manufactured through the oxidation of fatty acids. But even these athletes should watch their fat calories if they train aerobically (with oxygen) for less than half an hour at a time.

☐ All athletes should consume a carefully measured amount of high-quality carbohydrates several times a day to ensure an adequate supply of energy.

☐ The carbohydrates in all preworkout meals should consist of foods with low glycemic indexes to ensure that training intensity does not wane and that muscle tissue is not cannibalized for energy. (For the glycemic indexes of some common foods, see page 29.)

The aim of your nutrition program is to make your body healthy enough to accomplish recovery and tissue repair speedily and efficiently—without adding body fat. Your further aim is to do this while maintaining a high strength-to-weight ratio. These aims alone make diet very important for soccer players. You must eat just the right amount of food. Eat the wrong foods or the wrong amounts just a few times too often and you will sabotage your fitness efforts. Even more important, do not be in a hurry. It take *years* to become a great soccer player. Rush the nutrition and training processes and you will become fat, your recovery rate will decline, and your injury rate will rise.

NUTRITION FOR SOCCER PLAYERS

Soccer players are either power or middle-distance athletes. Depending on the position they play, they need bursts of power, which are supported by energy from the immediate energy systems, or stamina, which is supported by energy from the glycolytic energy systems. Therefore, as a soccer player, you need to plan your nutritional intake, from both food and supplement sources, to support the appropriate systems. In addition, if you are a power soccer player, your energy expenditure changes in the off-season, and you need to adjust your caloric intake and macronutrient ratio to match. Following are dietary and supplementation guidelines for power soccer players (fullbacks and goalies) to help you in planning your nutrition program. Dietary and supplementation guidelines for middle-distance soccer players (forwards, halfbacks, and wings) can be found on page 300.

POWER SOCCER PLAYERS

The soccer players who usually play in spurts are power athletes. These players include the fullbacks and goalie.

Dietary Guidelines

The following pie charts illustrate how you should divide up your caloric intake to match the energy demands of your power soccer position during the preseason, season, and off-season. They show the target percentages of fat, protein, and carbohydrates that your five to six meals should supply each day.

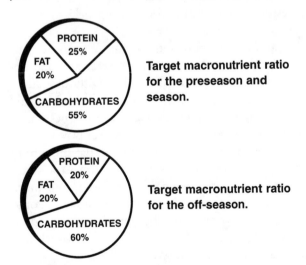

PROTEIN 25%
FAT 20%
CARBOHYDRATES 55%

Target macronutrient ratio for the preseason and season.

PROTEIN 20%
FAT 20%
CARBOHYDRATES 60%

Target macronutrient ratio for the off-season.

Note that fat has about 9 calories per gram, while protein and carbohydrates have only 4 calories per gram. Therefore, during the season, if you needed to consume a total of 2,500 calories per day, you would aim for 500 calories (20 percent of your total daily calories) from fat, 625 calories (25 percent of your total daily calories) from protein, and the remaining

1,375 calories (55 percent of your total daily calories) from carbohydrates.

Some other important considerations for power soccer players are:

☐ Carbohydrates are the major source of energy for short-term activities. Complex carbohydrates are the best source because they most effectively refill the glycogen stores in the muscles and liver. In addition, they elevate the blood sugar to a level sufficient for long sessions of intensive training.

☐ As a power athlete, you must make sure that you consume adequate amounts of both carbohydrates and protein. If your energy stores become drastically depleted or you experience lactic-acid buildup, you may suffer temporary muscle fatigue. If you do not refill your glycogen stores before your next workout or game, your body may begin breaking down muscle tissue for the protein it needs for energy.

☐ Directly before workouts and games, consume carbohydrate drinks with high glycemic indexes to keep your blood sugar sustained at an appropriate level. This will allow you to train or play intensively without having your explosiveness hindered by fatigue.

☐ As a power athlete, you need to stimulate the storage of glycogen in your muscles while promoting repair and growth of your muscle tissue and inhibiting buildup of body fat. To do this:

• Train anaerobically on a regular basis. Intensive training stimulates increased storage of glycogen in the muscles and liver, which provides additional energy for greater exercise capacity.

• Consume five to six meals a day. Eating several smaller meals rather than three larger ones will keep your blood-sugar level stable throughout the day and will ensure that a supply of protein is always available for your muscles.

• Keep your fat intake to a minimum. Large amounts of fat in your diet will add to your body fat and will cause you to lose minerals through frequent urination.

• Consume low-glycemic-index foods about two to three hours before workouts and games. These foods help sustain the blood-sugar level.

• Drink plenty of water. Not only will this practice reduce your chances of becoming dehydrated, but every ounce of glycogen that is stored within the muscles needs 3 ounces of water stored along with it.

Therefore, remaining properly hydrated will also help prevent weakened muscle contractions.

As a power soccer player, you should turn to Appendix C on page 345 for full discussions of the 20:25:55 and 20:20:60 dietary plans. Also presented are sample daily diets that use common, healthy foods to meet an athlete's energy and caloric needs. Use the directions on page 150 to estimate your average daily caloric requirement. Then use the directions in Chapter 13 or 14 to adjust your diet for off-season fat loss or muscle building, respectively.

Supplementation Guidelines

In addition to eating a proper diet, you should also take dietary supplements to make sure that any nutrients you lose due to sweating or training are replenished. The following tables will help guide you in selecting the supplements appropriate for you. The first table lists the nutrients recommended for power soccer players, as well as the range of intake for each nutrient. (For discussions of these nutrients, see Part One.) Note that within the ranges of intake, the lower amounts are for smaller individuals and lower-activity days, while the higher amounts are for larger individuals and higher-activity days.

RECOMMENDED NUTRIENTS AND RANGES OF INTAKE

For Power Soccer Players

NUTRIENT	RANGE OF INTAKE
VITAMINS	
Vitamin A	8,000–16,000 IU
Beta-carotene	15,000–25,000 IU
Vitamin B$_1$ (thiamine)	40–120 mg
Vitamin B2 (riboflavin)	40–120 mg
Vitamin B$_3$ (niacin)	20–40 mg
Vitamin B$_5$ (pantothenic acid)	20–100 mg
Vitamin B$_6$ (pyridoxine)	20–80 mg
Vitamin B$_{12}$ (cobalamin)	12–120 mcg
Biotin	125–175 mcg
Folate	400–800 mcg
Vitamin C	800–2,000 mg
Vitamin D	400–800 IU
Vitamin E	200–800 IU
Vitamin K	60–160 mcg

NUTRIENT	RANGE OF INTAKE
MINERALS	
Boron	2–8 mg
Calcium	800–1,500 mg
Chromium	200–500 mcg
Copper	1–4 mg
Iodine	100–200 mcg
Iron	15–50 mg
Magnesium	250–650 mg
Manganese	12–35 mg
Molybdenum	100–200 mcg
Phosphorus	150–800 mg
Potassium	50–1,000 mg
Selenium	100–200 mcg
Zinc	15–50 mg
AMINO ACIDS	
L-glutamic acid	500–1,000 mg
L-glutamine	1,000–2,000 mg
FATTY ACIDS	
Alpha-linolenic acid	500–1,000 mg
Docosahexaenoic acid (DHA)	250–750 mg
Eiocosapentaenoic acid (EPA)	250–750 mg
Gamma linolenic acid (GLA)	100–400 mg
Linoleic acid	2,000–3,000 mg
METABOLITES	
Bioflavonoids	300–800 mg
Choline	200–600 mg
Creatine monohydrate	6,000–12,000 mg
Inosine	500–1,500 mg
Inositol	200–600 mg
L-carnitine	500–1,500 mg
Octacosanol	1,000–2,000 mcg

IU = international units, mcg = micrograms, mg = milligrams.

The second table lists the different types of sports supplements available and indicates if their use by power soccer players is recommended in the preseason, during the season, or directly before a game. The list also includes a number of popular nutritional practices—bicarbonate loading, carbohydrate loading, creatine and/or inosine loading, and water loading. (For a discussion of any of these supplements or practices, see the appropriate section in Part One or Part Three.)

RECOMMENDED SPORTS SUPPLEMENTS AND NUTRITIONAL PRACTICES

For Power Soccer Players

	Intake Recommendation		
	PRESEASON	SEASON	PREGAME
SUPPLEMENTS			
Multivitamins	Yes	Yes	No
Multiminerals	Yes	Yes	No
Antioxidants	Yes	Yes	No
Fatty acids	Yes	Yes	No
Metabolites	Optional	Yes	Yes
Branched-chain amino acids	Yes	Yes	Yes
Herbs	Yes	Yes	No
Low-calorie protein drink (200–300 calories)	Yes	Yes	Yes
Carbohydrate drink	Yes	Yes	Yes
Fat-burning supplement	Yes	Optional	No
PRACTICES			
Bicarbonate loading	No	No	No
Carbohydrate loading	No	No	Optional
Creatine and/or inosine loading	No	Yes	Yes
Water loading	No	No	Optional

MIDDLE-DISTANCE SOCCER PLAYERS

The soccer players who are in motion for longer periods of time are middle-distance athletes. These players include the forwards, halfbacks, and wings.

Dietary Guidelines

The following pie chart illustrates how you should divide up your caloric intake to match the energy demands of your middle-distance soccer position during the preseason, season, and off-season. It shows the target percentages of fat, protein, and carbohydrates that your five to six meals should supply each day.

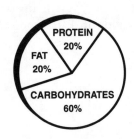

Target macronutrient ratio for the preseason, season and off-season.

Note that fat has about 9 calories per gram, while protein and carbohydrates have only 4 calories per gram. Therefore, if you needed to consume a total of 2,500 calories per day, you would aim for 500 calories (20 percent of your total daily calories) from fat, 500 calories (20 percent of your total daily calories) from protein, and the remaining 1,500 calories (60 percent of your total daily calories) from carbohydrates.

Some other important considerations for middle-distance soccer players are:

☐ Carbohydrates are the major source of energy for short-term activities. Complex carbohydrates are the best source because they most effectively refill the glycogen stores in the muscles and liver. In addition, they elevate the blood sugar to a level sufficient for long sessions of intensive training.

☐ As a middle-distance athlete, you must make sure that you consume adequate amounts of both carbohydrates and protein. If your energy stores become drastically depleted or you experience lactic-acid buildup, you may suffer temporary muscle fatigue. If you do not refill your glycogen stores before your next workout or game, your body may begin breaking down muscle tissue for the protein it needs for energy.

☐ Directly before workouts and games, consume carbohydrate drinks with high glycemic indexes to keep your blood sugar sustained at an appropriate level. This will allow you to train or play intensively for longer periods of time.

☐ As a middle-distance athlete, you need to stimulate the storage of glycogen in your muscles while promoting repair and growth of your muscle tissue and inhibiting buildup of body fat. To do this:

• Train against your anaerobic threshold (to exhaustion) on a regular basis. Intensive, exhaustive training stimulates increased storage of glycogen in the muscles and liver, which provides additional energy for greater exercise capacity.

• Consume five to six meals a day. Eating several smaller meals rather than three larger ones will keep your blood-sugar level stable throughout the day and will ensure that a supply of protein is always available for your muscles.

• Keep your fat intake to a minimum. Large amounts of fat in your diet will add to your body fat and will cause mineral loss through frequent urination.

- Consume low-glycemic-index foods two to three hours before workouts and games. These foods help sustain the blood-sugar level.

- Drink plenty of water. Not only will this practice reduce your chances of becoming dehydrated, but every ounce of glycogen that is stored within the muscles needs 3 ounces of water stored along with it. Therefore, remaining properly hydrated will also help prevent weakened muscle contractions and early onset of fatigue.

- Do not eat a new food just before a game. Different people often react differently to the same food. Before a game, eat just those foods that you know your body will handle well.

As a middle-distance soccer player, you should turn to Appendix C on page 345 for a full discussion of the 20:20:60 dietary plan. Also presented are sample daily diets that use common, healthy foods to meet an athlete's energy and caloric needs. Use the directions on page 150 to estimate your average daily caloric requirement. Then use the directions in Chapter 13 or 14 to adjust your diet for off-season fat loss or muscle building, respectively.

Supplementation Guidelines

In addition to eating a proper diet, you should also take dietary supplements to make sure that any nutrients you lose due to sweating or training are replenished. The following tables will help guide you in selecting the supplements appropriate for you. The first table lists the nutrients recommended for middle-distance soccer players, as well as the range of intake for each nutrient. (For discussions of these nutrients, see Part One.) Note that within the ranges of intake, the lower amounts are for smaller individuals and lower-activity days, while the higher amounts are for larger individuals and higher-activity days.

RECOMMENDED NUTRIENTS AND RANGES OF INTAKE

For Middle-Distance Soccer Players

NUTRIENT	RANGE OF INTAKE
VITAMINS	
Vitamin A	8,000–16,000 IU
Beta-carotene	20,000–30,000 IU
Vitamin B$_1$ (thiamine)	80–160 mg

NUTRIENT	RANGE OF INTAKE
Vitamin B$_2$ (riboflavin)	80–160 mg
Vitamin B$_3$ (niacin)	10–20 mg
Vitamin B$_5$ (pantothenic acid)	60–120 mg
Vitamin B$_6$ (pyridoxine)	20–80 mg
Vitamin B$_{12}$ (cobalamin)	12–120 mcg
Biotin	125–175 mcg
Folate	400–800 mcg
Vitamin C	1,000–2,000 mg
Vitamin D	400–800 IU
Vitamin E	300–800 IU
Vitamin K	60–160 mcg
MINERALS	
Boron	2–8 mg
Calcium	800–1,500 mg
Chromium	200–500 mcg
Copper	1–4 mg
Iodine	100–200 mcg
Iron	15–50 mg
Magnesium	250–650 mg
Manganese	12–35 mg
Molybdenum	100–200 mcg
Phosphorus	150–800 mg
Potassium	50–1,000 mg
Selenium	100–200 mcg
Zinc	15–50 mg
AMINO ACIDS	
L-glutamic acid	500–1,000 mg
L-glutamine	1,000–2,000 mg
FATTY ACIDS	
Alpha-linolenic acid	500–1,000 mg
Docosahexaenoic acid (DHA)	350–750 mg
Eiocosapentaenoic acid (EPA)	350–750 mg
Gamma linolenic acid (GLA)	200–400 mg
Linoleic acid	1,000–2,000 mg
METABOLITES	
Bioflavonoids	400–900 mg
Choline	400–800 mg
Coenzyme Q$_{10}$	60–100 mg
Inositol	400–800 mg
L-carnitine	1,000–2,000 mg
Octacosanol	1,000–2,000 mcg

IU = international units, mcg = micrograms, mg = milligrams.

The second table lists the different types of sports supplements available and indicates if their use by middle-distance soccer players is recommended in the preseason, during the season, or directly before a game. The list also includes a number of popular nutritional practices—bicarbonate loading, carbohydrate loading, creatine and/or inosine loading, and water loading. (For a discussion of any of these supplements or practices, see the appropriate section in Part One or Part Three.)

RECOMMENDED SPORTS SUPPLEMENTS AND NUTRITIONAL PRACTICES

For Middle-Distance Soccer Players

	Intake Recommendation		
	PRESEASON	SEASON	PREGAME
SUPPLEMENTS			
Multivitamins	Yes	Yes	No
Multiminerals	Yes	Yes	No
Antioxidants	Yes	Yes	No
Fatty acids	Yes	Yes	No
Metabolites	Optional	Yes	Yes
Branched-chain amino acids	Yes	Yes	Yes
Herbs	Yes	Yes	No
Medium-calorie protein drink (300–500 calories)	Yes	Yes	Yes
Carbohydrate drink with glycerol	Yes	Yes	Yes
Fat-burning supplement	Yes	Optional	No
PRACTICES			
Bicarbonate loading	No	No	No
Carbohydrate loading	No	No	Optional
Creatine and/or inosine loading	No	No	No
Water loading	No	No	Yes

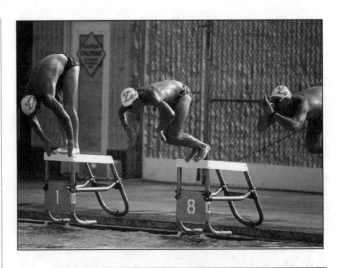

SWIMMING

Also for Skin Diving, Snorkeling, Synchronized Swimming, and Water Polo

What kind of swimmer are you? If you are a relay swimmer, your energy comes primarily from the immediate energy systems and you must eat and train accordingly. If you are a freestyle swimmer, you need to focus the bulk of your nutrition and training efforts on building up your glycolytic energy reserves. If you are a long-distance specialist whose goal is to swim from Florida to Cuba, you need to concentrate on your oxidative energy systems. However, if you enjoy two or all three kinds of swimming, you should combine your nutrition and training programs, stressing one only as a competition nears.

No matter what type of swimmer you are, you cannot completely ignore any facet of the sport. You must address each skill to some extent, whether you use it on a regular basis or not. Therefore, your training, both in and out of the water, should develop strength, anaerobic or aerobic endurance, and speed-strength equally. This calls for specialized training. Furthermore, the unique energy output called for by each swimming event requires the support of a carefully constructed nutrition program.

ENERGY SOURCES OF SWIMMERS

The muscles rely on three major systems to supply the energy they need—the immediate, glycolytic, and oxidative energy systems. For short-term energy for explosive-strength output, the muscles depend on the immediate energy systems. The immediate energy systems are nonoxidative—that is, they do not use oxygen. Instead, these systems generate energy through the use of adenosine triphosphate (ATP) and creatine phosphate (CP). CP is produced in the body and stored in the muscle fibers. It is broken down by enzymes to regenerate ATP, which is also stored in the muscle fibers. When the ATP is in turn broken down, the result is a spark of energy that triggers a muscle contraction.

For medium-term energy for repeated near-maximum exertion, the muscles turn to the glycolytic energy systems. In these systems, which are also nonoxidative, glycogen is used to produce energy. Glycogen is the storage form of glucose. It is stored in the liver and muscles, and is readily converted back to glucose when it is needed for energy.

For long-term energy for endurance activities, the muscles use the oxidative energy systems. In these systems, oxygen is used to oxidize long-chain fatty acids, protein, and glucose, which generates energy. For athletes, getting enough oxygen can mean a winning performance rather than a second-place showing.

Every sport involves a variety of skills, and each skill utilizes a unique combination of these three energy sources. The following table lists a number of major swimming events and shows how much your body relies on each of the energy sources when you compete in them. Percentages are also given for two similar sports.

WHERE YOUR ENERGY COMES FROM

For Swimmers

	Energy Systems		
	IMMEDIATE	GLYCOLYTIC	OXIDATIVE
Average events			
Backstroke, breaststroke, butterfly, and freestyle, 100 yards	90%	10%	0%
Backstroke, breaststroke, butterfly, and freestyle, 200 yards	70%	20%	10%
Freestyle, 400 yards	50%	30%	20%
Freestyle, men's, 1,500 yards	10%	50%	40%
Freestyle, women's, 800 yards	30%	40%	30%
Medley, individual, 400 yards	50%	30%	20%

	Energy Systems		
	IMMEDIATE	GLYCOLYTIC	OXIDATIVE
Medley, individual, women's, 200 yards	70%	20%	10%
Relay, freestyle, 4 X 100 yards	90%	10%	0%
Relay, freestyle, men's, 4 X 200 yards	70%	20%	10%
Relay, medley, 4 X 100 yards	90%	10%	0%
Long distance (over 1 hour)	0%	10%	90%

For Similar Sports

Synchronized swimming, solo, duet, and teams of 8	20%	30%	50%
Water polo	10%	20%	70%

When considering the type of nutritional support to give your training program, keep the following factors in mind:

☐ All athletes need to consume high-quality protein several times a day for effective recovery and adequate repair of damaged muscle tissue.

☐ Athletes whose muscles rely substantially on the immediate and glycolytic energy systems should keep their fat intake to a minimum because fat is not an efficient energy source for their intensive training, which is almost exclusively anaerobic in nature. Since the fat calories consumed by these athletes are not generally used for energy, they are stored as body fat.

☐ Athletes whose muscles rely substantially on the oxidative energy systems can eat more fat because their energy is manufactured through the oxidation of fatty acids. But even these athletes should watch their fat calories if they train aerobically (with oxygen) for less than half an hour at a time.

☐ All athletes should consume a carefully measured amount of high-quality carbohydrates several times a day to ensure an adequate supply of energy.

☐ The carbohydrates in all preworkout meals should consist of foods with low glycemic indexes to ensure that training intensity does not wane and that muscle tissue is not cannibalized for energy. (For the glycemic indexes of some common foods, see page 29.)

The aim of your nutrition program is to make your body healthy enough to accomplish recovery and tissue repair speedily and efficiently—without adding body fat. Your further aim is to do this while maintaining a high strength-to-weight ratio. These aims alone make diet very important for swimmers. You must eat just the right amount of food. Eat the wrong foods or the wrong amounts just a few times too often and you will sabotage your fitness efforts.

NUTRITION FOR SWIMMERS

Swimmers are either power, middle-distance, or endurance athletes. Their primary source of energy is determined by the specific type of swimming they specialize in. Some types of swimming require bursts of power, which are supported by energy from the immediate energy systems. Some types of swimming require stamina, which is supported by energy from the glycolytic energy systems. Still other types of swimming require endurance, which is supported by energy from the oxidative energy systems. Therefore, as a swimmer, you need to plan your nutritional intake, from both food and supplement sources, to support the appropriate systems. In addition, if you are a power or middle-distance swimmer, your energy expenditure changes in the preseason and/or off-season, and you need to adjust your caloric intake and macronutrient ratio to match. Following are dietary and supplementation guidelines for power swimmers to help you in planning your nutrition program. Dietary and supplementation guidelines for middle-distance swimmers can be found on page 306, and guidelines for endurance swimmers can be found on page 308.

POWER SWIMMERS

Swimmers who compete in events that last for just minutes are power athletes. Among the typical events they participate in are the 100-yard backstroke, 200-yard women's individual medley, and 4 X 100 yards freestyle relay.

Dietary Guidelines

The following pie charts illustrate how you should divide up your caloric intake to match the energy demands of power swimming during the preseason, season, and off-season. They show the target percentages of fat, protein, and carbohydrates that your five to six meals should supply each day.

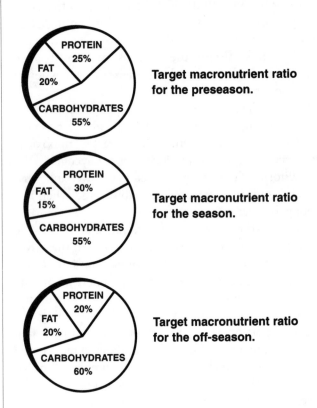

Target macronutrient ratio for the preseason.

Target macronutrient ratio for the season.

Target macronutrient ratio for the off-season.

Note that fat has about 9 calories per gram, while protein and carbohydrates have only 4 calories per gram. Therefore, during the season, if you needed to consume a total of 2,500 calories per day, you would aim for 375 calories (15 percent of your total daily calories) from fat, 750 calories (30 percent of your total daily calories) from protein, and the remaining 1,375 calories (55 percent of your total daily calories) from carbohydrates.

Some other important considerations for power swimmers are:

☐ Carbohydrates are the major source of energy for short-term activities. Complex carbohydrates are the best source because they most effectively refill the glycogen stores in the muscles and liver. In addition, they elevate the blood sugar to a level sufficient for long sessions of intensive training.

☐ As a power athlete, you must make sure that you consume adequate amounts of both carbohydrates and protein. If your energy stores become drastically depleted or you experience lactic-acid buildup, you may suffer temporary muscle fatigue. If you do not refill your glycogen stores before your next workout or competition, your body may begin breaking down muscle tissue for the protein it needs for energy.

☐ Directly before workouts, consume carbohydrate drinks with high glycemic indexes to keep your blood sugar sustained at an appropriate level. This will allow you to train intensively without having your explosiveness hindered by fatigue.

☐ As a power athlete, you need to stimulate the storage of glycogen in your muscles while promoting repair and growth of your muscle tissue and inhibiting buildup of body fat. To do this:

• Train anaerobically on a regular basis. Intensive training stimulates increased storage of glycogen in the muscles and liver, which provides additional energy for greater exercise capacity.

• Consume five to six meals a day. Eating several smaller meals rather than three larger ones will keep your blood-sugar level stable throughout the day and will ensure that a supply of protein is always available for your muscles.

• Keep your fat intake to a minimum. Large amounts of fat in your diet will add to your body fat and will cause you to lose minerals through frequent urination.

• Consume low-glycemic-index foods about two to three hours before workouts and competitions. These foods help sustain the blood-sugar level.

• Drink plenty of water. Not only will this practice reduce your chances of becoming dehydrated, but every ounce of glycogen that is stored within the muscles needs 3 ounces of water stored along with it. Therefore, remaining properly hydrated will also help prevent weakened muscle contractions.

• Do not eat a new food just before a competition. Different people often react differently to the same food. Before a competition, eat just those foods that you know your body will handle well.

As a power swimmer, you should turn to Appendix C on page 345 for full discussions of the 20:25:55, 15:30:55, and 20:20:60 dietary plans. Also presented are sample daily diets that use common, healthy foods to meet an athlete's energy and caloric needs. Use the directions on page 150 to estimate your average daily caloric requirement. Then use the directions in Chapter 13 or 14 to adjust your diet for off-season fat loss or muscle building, respectively.

Supplementation Guidelines

In addition to eating a proper diet, you should also take dietary supplements to make sure that any nutrients you lose due to sweating or training are replenished. The following tables will help guide you in selecting the supplements appropriate for you. The first table lists the nutrients recommended for power swimmers, as well as the range of intake for each nutrient. (For discussions of these nutrients, see Part One.) Note that within the ranges of intake, the lower amounts are for smaller individuals and lower-activity days, while the higher amounts are for larger individuals and higher-activity days.

RECOMMENDED NUTRIENTS AND RANGES OF INTAKE

For Power Swimmers	
NUTRIENT	RANGE OF INTAKE
VITAMINS	
Vitamin A	8,000–16,000 IU
Beta-carotene	15,000–30,000 IU
Vitamin B_1 (thiamine)	30–120 mg
Vitamin B_2 (riboflavin)	30–120 mg
Vitamin B_3 (niacin)	40–80 mg
Vitamin B_5 (pantothenic acid)	20–100 mg
Vitamin B_6 (pyridoxine)	20–80 mg
Vitamin B_{12} (cobalamin)	12–120 mcg
Biotin	125–175 mcg
Folate	400–800 mcg
Vitamin C	800–2,000 mg
Vitamin D	400–800 IU
Vitamin E	200–600 IU
Vitamin K	60–160 mcg
MINERALS	
Boron	2–8 mg
Calcium	800–1,500 mg
Chromium	200–500 mcg
Copper	1–4 mg
Iodine	100–200 mcg
Iron	15–50 mg
Magnesium	250–650 mg
Manganese	12–35 mg
Molybdenum	100–200 mcg
Phosphorus	150–800 mg
Potassium	50–1,000 mg
Selenium	100–200 mcg
Zinc	15–50 mg

NUTRIENT	RANGE OF INTAKE
AMINO ACIDS	
L-glutamine	1,000–2,000 mg
FATTY ACIDS	
Alpha-linolenic acid	1,500–3,000 mg
Docosahexaenoic acid (DHA)	250–750 mg
Eiocosapentaenoic acid (EPA)	250–750 mg
Gamma linolenic acid (GLA)	100–400 mg
Linoleic acid	3,000–6,000 mg
METABOLITES	
Bioflavonoids	200–800 mg
Choline	100–600 mg
Creatine monohydrate	8,000–22,000 mg
Ferulic acid	50–100 mg
Inosine	500–1,000 mg
Inositol	100–600 mg
L-carnitine	750–2,000 mg
Octacosanol	1,000–3,000 mcg

IU = international units, mcg = micrograms, mg = milligrams.

The second table lists the different types of sports supplements available and indicates if their use by power swimmers is recommended in the preseason, during the season, or directly before a competition. The list also includes a number of popular nutritional practices—bicarbonate loading, carbohydrate loading, creatine and/or inosine loading, and water loading. (For a discussion of any of these supplements or practices, see the appropriate section in Part One or Part Three.)

RECOMMENDED SPORTS SUPPLEMENTS AND NUTRITIONAL PRACTICES

For Power Swimmers

	Intake Recommendation		
	PRESEASON	SEASON	PRE-COMPETITION
SUPPLEMENTS			
Multivitamins	Yes	Yes	No
Multiminerals	Yes	Yes	No
Antioxidants	Yes	Yes	No
Fatty acids	Yes	Yes	No
Metabolites	Optional	Yes	Yes
Branched-chain amino acids	Yes	Yes	Yes
Herbs	Yes	Yes	No

	Intake Recommendation		
	PRESEASON	SEASON	PRE-COMPETITION
Low-calorie protein drink (200–300 calories)	Yes	Yes	Yes
Carbohydrate drink	Yes	Yes	Yes
Fat-burning supplement	Yes	Optional	No
PRACTICES			
Bicarbonate loading	No	Optional	Yes
Carbohydrate loading	No	No	No
Creatine and/or inosine loading	Optional	Yes	Yes
Water loading	No	No	No

MIDDLE-DISTANCE SWIMMERS

Swimmers who compete in events that last for up to about twenty minutes are middle-distance athletes. Among the typical events they participate in are the 400-yard, 800-yard women's, and 1,500-yard men's freestyle.

Dietary Guidelines

The following pie charts illustrate how you should divide up your caloric intake to match the energy demands of middle-distance swimming during the preseason, season, and off-season. They show the target percentages of fat, protein, and carbohydrates that your five to six meals should supply each day.

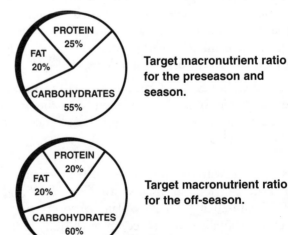

PROTEIN 25%
FAT 20%
CARBOHYDRATES 55%

Target macronutrient ratio for the preseason and season.

PROTEIN 20%
FAT 20%
CARBOHYDRATES 60%

Target macronutrient ratio for the off-season.

Note that fat has about 9 calories per gram, while protein and carbohydrates have only 4 calories per gram. Therefore, during the season, if you needed to consume a total of 2,500 calories per day, you would aim for 500 calories (20 percent of your total daily calories) from fat, 625 calories (25 percent of your total daily calories) from protein, and the remaining 1,375 calories (55 percent of your total daily calories) from carbohydrates.

Some other important considerations for middle-distance swimmers are:

☐ Carbohydrates are the major source of energy for short-term activities. Complex carbohydrates are the best source because they most effectively refill the glycogen stores in the muscles and liver. In addition, they elevate the blood sugar to a level sufficient for long sessions of intensive training.

☐ As a middle-distance athlete, you must make sure that you consume adequate amounts of both carbohydrates and protein. If your energy stores become drastically depleted or you experience lactic-acid buildup, you may suffer temporary muscle fatigue. If you do not refill your glycogen stores before your next workout or competition, your body may begin breaking down muscle tissue for the protein it needs for energy.

☐ Directly before workouts, consume carbohydrate drinks with high glycemic indexes to keep your blood sugar sustained at an appropriate level. This will allow you to train intensively for longer periods of time.

☐ As a middle-distance athlete, you need to stimulate the storage of glycogen in your muscles while promoting repair and growth of your muscle tissue and inhibiting buildup of body fat. To do this:

• Train against your anaerobic threshold (to exhaustion) on a regular basis. Intensive, exhaustive training stimulates increased storage of glycogen in the muscles and liver, which provides additional energy for greater exercise capacity.

• Consume five to six meals a day. Eating several smaller meals rather than three larger ones will keep your blood-sugar level stable throughout the day and will ensure that a supply of protein is always available for your muscles.

• Keep your fat intake to a minimum. Large amounts of fat in your diet will add to your body fat and will cause mineral loss through frequent urination.

• Consume low-glycemic-index foods about two to three hours before workouts and competitions. These foods help sustain the blood-sugar level.

• Drink plenty of water. Not only will this practice reduce your chances of becoming dehydrated, but every ounce of glycogen that is stored within the muscles needs 3 ounces of water stored along with it. Therefore, remaining properly hydrated will also help prevent weakened muscle contractions and early onset of fatigue.

• Do not eat a new food just before a competition. Different people often react differently to the same food. Before a competition, eat just those foods that you know your body will handle well.

As a middle-distance swimmer, you should turn to Appendix C on page 345 for full discussions of the 20:25:55 and 20:20:60 dietary plans. Also presented are sample daily diets that use common, healthy foods to meet an athlete's energy and caloric needs. Use the directions on page 150 to estimate your average daily caloric requirement. Then use the directions in Chapter 13 or 14 to adjust your diet for off-season fat loss or muscle building, respectively.

Supplementation Guidelines

In addition to eating a proper diet, you should also take dietary supplements to make sure that any nutrients you lose due to sweating or training are replenished. The following tables will help guide you in selecting the supplements appropriate for you. The first table lists the nutrients recommended for middle-distance swimmers, as well as the range of intake for each nutrient. (For discussions of these nutrients, see Part One.) Note that within the ranges of intake, the lower amounts are for smaller individuals and lower-activity days, while the higher amounts are for larger individuals and higher-activity days.

RECOMMENDED NUTRIENTS AND RANGES OF INTAKE

For Middle-Distance Swimmers

NUTRIENT	RANGE OF INTAKE
VITAMINS	
Vitamin A	8,000–16,000 IU
Beta-carotene	30,000–45,000 IU
Vitamin B$_1$ (thiamine)	40–120 mg
Vitamin B$_2$ (riboflavin)	40–120 mg
Vitamin B$_3$ (niacin)	20–40 mg
Vitamin B$_5$ (pantothenic acid)	20–100 mg

NUTRIENT	RANGE OF INTAKE
Vitamin B$_6$ (pyridoxine)	20–80 mg
Vitamin B$_{12}$ (cobalamin)	12–120 mcg
Biotin	125–175 mcg
Folate	400–800 mcg
Vitamin C	800–2,000 mg
Vitamin D	400–800 IU
Vitamin E	200–800 IU
Vitamin K	60–160 mcg
MINERALS	
Boron	2–8 mg
Calcium	800–1,500 mg
Chromium	200–500 mcg
Copper	1–4 mg
Iodine	100–200 mcg
Iron	15–50 mg
Magnesium	250–650 mg
Manganese	12–35 mg
Molybdenum	100–200 mcg
Phosphorus	150–800 mg
Potassium	50–1,000 mg
Selenium	100–200 mcg
Zinc	15–50 mg
AMINO ACIDS	
L-glutamic acid	500–1,000 mg
L-glutamine	1,000–2,000 mg
FATTY ACIDS	
Alpha-linolenic acid	500–1,000 mg
Docosahexaenoic acid (DHA)	250–750 mg
Eiocosapentaenoic acid (EPA)	250–750 mg
Gamma linolenic acid (GLA)	100–400 mg
Linoleic acid	2,000–3,000 mg
METABOLITES	
Bioflavonoids	300–800 mg
Choline	200–600 mg
Inositol	200–600 mg
L-carnitine	500–1,500 mg
Octacosanol	1,000–2,000 mcg

IU = international units, mcg = micrograms, mg = milligrams.

The second table lists the different types of sports supplements available and indicates if their use by middle-distance swimmers is recommended in the preseason, during the season, or directly before a competition. The list also includes a number of popular nutritional practices—bicarbonate loading, carbohydrate loading, creatine and/or inosine loading,

and water loading. (For a discussion of any of these supplements or practices, see the appropriate section in Part One or Part Three.)

RECOMMENDED SPORTS SUPPLEMENTS AND NUTRITIONAL PRACTICES

For Middle-Distance Swimmers

	Intake Recommendation		
	PRESEASON	SEASON	PRE-COMPETITION
SUPPLEMENTS			
Multivitamins	Yes	Yes	No
Multiminerals	Yes	Yes	No
Antioxidants	Yes	Yes	No
Fatty acids	Yes	Yes	No
Metabolites	Optional	Yes	Yes
Branched-chain amino acids	Yes	Yes	Yes
Herbs	Yes	Yes	No
Medium-calorie protein drink (300–500 calories)	Yes	Yes	Yes
Carbohydrate drink	Yes	Yes	Yes
Fat-burning supplement	Yes	Optional	No
PRACTICES			
Bicarbonate loading	No	No	Optional
Carbohydrate loading	No	No	No
Creatine and/or inosine loading	No	No	Optional
Water loading	No	No	No

ENDURANCE SWIMMERS

Swimmers who compete in events that last longer than about twenty minutes are endurance athletes. Among the typical events they participate in are long-distance swims such as crossing the English Channel and swimming from Florida to Cuba.

Dietary Guidelines

The following pie chart illustrates how you should divide up your caloric intake to match the energy demands of endurance swimming during the preseason, season, and off-season. It shows the target percentages of fat, protein, and carbohydrates that your five to six meals should supply each day.

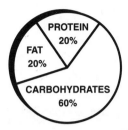

Target macronutrient ratio for the preseason, season and off-season.

Note that fat has about 9 calories per gram, while protein and carbohydrates have only 4 calories per gram. Therefore, if you needed to consume a total of 2,500 calories per day, you would aim for 500 calories (20 percent of your total daily calories) from fat, 500 calories (20 percent of your total daily calories) from protein, and the remaining 1,500 calories (60 percent of your total daily calories) from carbohydrates.

Some other important considerations for endurance swimmers are:

☐ The energy source that is used during an aerobic activity depends upon the duration and intensity of the activity. During the first one and a half to two hours, both glycogen and body fat are the primary sources of energy. After one and a half to two hours, body fat alone becomes the primary source.

☐ While body fat is the primary source of energy during prolonged aerobic activities, it cannot be used efficiently unless some glycogen remains in the muscles and liver. Therefore, even ultra-endurance athletes must make sure to always keep their glycogen stores filled.

☐ As an endurance athlete, you need to encourage glycogen sparing in your body while stimulating the use of fat as your primary energy source. To do this:

• Train for endurance on a regular basis. Regular endurance training stimulates increased storage of both glycogen and fatty acids.

• Consume five to six meals a day. Eating several smaller meals rather than three larger ones will keep your blood-sugar level stable throughout the day.

• Do not load up on dietary fat. Consuming large amounts of fat was originally thought to benefit endurance athletes, whose primary source of energy is fat. However, fat loading can lead to frequent urination, which increases the loss of minerals essential to healthy heart action.

• Consume low-glycemic-index foods about two to three hours before workouts and competitions. These foods help sustain the blood-sugar level.

• Do not consume food or caloric beverages from two hours before an endurance activity to fifteen minutes before. Food and caloric beverages cause the insulin level to rise, which in turn can provoke transient hypoglycemia. Transient hypoglycemia interferes with the energy dynamics during exercise and can induce early onset of fatigue.

• Consume carbohydrates directly before and during endurance activities. Because exercise slows the release of insulin into the bloodstream, the ingestion of carbohydrates spares glycogen and allows the use of fat for energy. Carbohydrate drinks with high glycemic indexes help sustain the blood-sugar level, thereby preserving glycogen stores.

• During endurance activities, drink plenty of water. Endurance activities cause profuse sweating, which results in loss of valuable fluids and minerals. Dehydration not only reduces performance but can seriously affect health.

• Drink electrolyte-containing beverages during endurance activities. These drinks help replace minerals that are lost through sweating.

• During endurance activities, drink 4 to 6 ounces of fluid every fifteen to thirty minutes. For every pound of body weight lost through sweating, 1 pint of fluid should be consumed. Chilled fluids are absorbed the quickest.

• Do not eat a new food just before a competition. Different people often react differently to the same food. Before a competition, eat just those foods that you know your body will handle well.

As an endurance swimmer, you should turn to Appendix C on page 345 for a full discussion of the 20:20:60 dietary plan. Also presented are sample daily diets that use common, healthy foods to meet an athlete's energy and caloric needs. Use the directions on page 150 to estimate your average daily caloric requirement. Then use the directions in Chapter 13 or 14 to adjust your diet for off-season fat loss or muscle building, respectively.

Supplementation Guidelines

In addition to eating a proper diet, you should also take dietary supplements to make sure that any nutrients you lose due to sweating or training are replenished. The following tables will help guide you in selecting the supplements appropriate for you. The first table lists the nutrients recommended for endurance swimmers, as well as the range of intake for each nutrient. (For discussions of these nutrients, see Part One.) Note that within the ranges of intake, the lower amounts are for smaller individuals and lower-activity days, while the higher amounts are for larger individuals and higher-activity days.

RECOMMENDED NUTRIENTS AND RANGES OF INTAKE

For Endurance Swimmers

NUTRIENT	RANGE OF INTAKE
VITAMINS	
Vitamin A	8,000–16,000 IU
Beta-carotene	30,000–50,000 IU
Vitamin B_1 (thiamine)	80–160 mg
Vitamin B_2 (riboflavin)	80–160 mg
Vitamin B_3 (niacin)	10–20 mg
Vitamin B_5 (pantothenic acid)	60–120 mg
Vitamin B_6 (pyridoxine)	20–80 mg
Vitamin B_{12} (cobalamin)	12–120 mcg
Biotin	120–175 mcg
Folate	400–800 mcg
Vitamin C	1,000–2,000 mg
Vitamin D	400–800 IU
Vitamin E	300–800 IU
Vitamin K	60–160 mcg
MINERALS	
Boron	2–8 mg
Calcium	800–1,500 mg
Chromium	200–500 mcg
Copper	1–4 mg
Iodine	100–200 mcg
Iron	15–50 mg
Magnesium	250–650 mg
Manganese	12–35 mg
Molybdenum	100–200 mcg
Phosphorus	150–800 mg
Potassium	50–1,000 mg
Selenium	100–200 mcg
Zinc	15–50 mg
AMINO ACIDS	
L-glutamic acid	500–1,000 mg
L-glutamine	1,000–2,000 mg
FATTY ACIDS	
Alpha-linolenic acid	500–1,000 mg

NUTRIENT	RANGE OF INTAKE
Docosahexaenoic acid (DHA)	350–750 mg
Eiocosapentaenoic acid (EPA)	350–750 mg
Gamma linolenic acid (GLA)	200–400 mg
Linoleic acid	1,000–2,000 mg
METABOLITES	
Bioflavonoids	400–900 mg
Choline	400–800 mg
Coenzyme Q_{10}	60–100 mg
Inositol	400–800 mg
L-carnitine	1,000–2,000 mg
Octacosanol	1,000–2,000 mcg

IU = international units, mcg = micrograms, mg = milligrams.

The second table lists the different types of sports supplements available and indicates if their use by endurance swimmers is recommended in the preseason, during the season, or directly before a competition. The list also includes a number of popular nutritional practices—bicarbonate loading, carbohydrate loading, creatine and/or inosine loading, and water loading. (For a discussion of any of these supplements or practices, see the appropriate section in Part One or Part Three.)

RECOMMENDED SPORTS SUPPLEMENTS AND NUTRITIONAL PRACTICES

For Endurance Swimmers

	Intake Recommendation		
	PRESEASON	SEASON	PRE-COMPETITION
SUPPLEMENTS			
Multivitamins	Yes	Yes	Yes
Multiminerals	Yes	Yes	Yes
Antioxidants	Yes	Yes	Yes
Fatty acids	Yes	Yes	Yes
Metabolites	Optional	Yes	Yes
Branched-chain amino acids	Yes	Yes	Yes
Herbs	Yes	Yes	No
Medium-calorie protein drink (300–500 calories)	Yes	Yes	Yes
Carbohydrate drink with glycerol	Yes	Yes	Yes
Fat-burning supplement	Yes	Optional	No

Intake Recommendation			
	PRESEASON	SEASON	PRE-COMPETITION
PRACTICES			
Bicarbonate loading	No	No	No
Carbohydrate loading	No	Yes	Yes
Creatine and/or inosine loading	No	No	No
Water loading	No	No	Optional

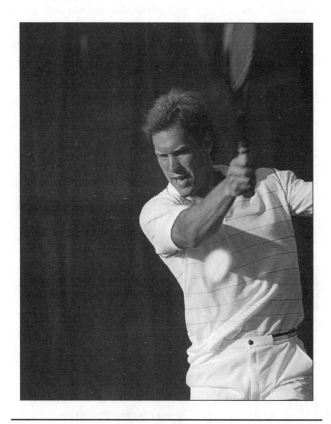

TENNIS

Tennis is a game that involves a wide range of skills and movements. It requires not only speed and strength in short, explosive bursts, but also a high level of anaerobic-strength endurance, as well as flexibility and agility.

Every bit of your training and diet must reflect these elements. These elements are what make tennis explosive in nature. In fact, most of the racket sports, including tennis, are very explosive, so improved recovery and tissue repair plus increased speed and strength are your year-round training and dietary goals. Nutritionally, this means emphasizing short-term energy needs and maximizing the muscles' recovery and tissue-repair processes.

In tennis, the energy output is primarily anaerobic (without oxygen). This does not mean that training for or playing tennis is easy, however. Serving, returning, and volleying the ball all require not only "touch" and finesse but also lightning-quick reflexes and a high tolerance to pain and fatigue from lactic-acid buildup in the muscles. The training for tennis is extremely intensive and grueling. At the highest levels, speed training for successful court play forces you to operate at your anaerobic threshold (the point at which you must receive oxygen).

Muscles grow when they are stressed. In tennis, the aim is to make the muscles grow as strong and as quick as possible. This calls for specialized training. Furthermore, the incredible energy output of tennis, especially coupled with the fast, often explosive aspects of the game, requires the support of a carefully constructed nutrition program.

ENERGY SOURCES OF TENNIS PLAYERS

The muscles rely on three major systems to supply the energy they need—the immediate, glycolytic, and oxidative energy systems. For short-term energy for explosive-strength output, the muscles depend on the immediate energy systems. The immediate energy systems are nonoxidative—that is, they do not use oxygen. Instead, these systems generate energy through the use of adenosine triphosphate (ATP) and creatine phosphate (CP). CP is produced in the body and stored in the muscle fibers. It is broken down by enzymes to regenerate ATP, which is also stored in the muscle fibers. When the ATP is in turn broken down, the result is a spark of energy that triggers a muscle contraction.

For medium-term energy for repeated near-maximum exertion, the muscles turn to the glycolytic energy systems. In these systems, which are also nonoxidative, glycogen is used to produce energy. Glycogen is the storage form of glucose. It is stored in the liver and muscles, and is readily converted back to glucose when it is needed for energy.

For long-term energy for endurance activities, the muscles use the oxidative energy systems. In these systems, oxygen is used to oxidize long-chain fatty acids, protein, and glucose, which generates energy. For athletes, getting enough oxygen can mean a winning performance rather than a second-place showing.

Every sport involves a variety of skills, and each skill utilizes a unique combination of these three energy sources. The following table shows how much your body relies on each of the energy sources during an average singles match and an average doubles match.

WHERE YOUR ENERGY COMES FROM

For Tennis Players			
Energy Systems			
	IMMEDIATE	GLYCOLYTIC	OXIDATIVE
Doubles match	80%	20%	0%
Singles match	70%	20%	10%

When considering the type of nutritional support to give your training program, keep the following factors in mind:

☐ All athletes need to consume high-quality protein several times a day for effective recovery and adequate repair of damaged muscle tissue.

☐ Athletes whose muscles rely substantially on the immediate or glycolytic energy systems should keep their fat intake to a minimum because fat is not an efficient energy source for their intensive training, which is almost exclusively anaerobic in nature. Since the fat calories consumed by these athletes are not generally used for energy, they are stored as body fat.

☐ All athletes should consume a carefully measured amount of high-quality carbohydrates several times a day to ensure an adequate supply of energy.

☐ The carbohydrates in all preworkout meals should consist of foods with low glycemic indexes to ensure that training intensity does not wane and that muscle tissue is not cannibalized for energy. (For the glycemic indexes of some common foods, see page 29.)

The aim of your nutrition program is to make your body healthy enough to accomplish recovery and tissue repair speedily and efficiently—without adding body fat. Your further aim is to do this while maintaining a high strength-to-weight ratio. These aims alone make diet as critical as training for tennis players. You must eat just the right amount of food. Eat the wrong foods or the wrong amounts just a few times too often and you will sabotage your fitness efforts.

NUTRITION FOR TENNIS PLAYERS

Tennis players are power athletes. They obtain most of their energy from the immediate energy systems. Therefore, as a tennis player, you need to plan your nutritional intake, from both food and supplement sources, to support the immediate systems. In addition, since your energy expenditure changes in the preseason and off-season, you need to adjust your caloric intake and macronutrient ratio to match. Following are dietary guidelines for tennis players to help you in planning your nutrition program. Supplementation guidelines for tennis players can be found on page 313.

Dietary Guidelines

The following pie charts illustrate how you should divide up your caloric intake to match the energy demands of tennis during the preseason, season, and off-season. They show the target percentages of fat, protein, and carbohydrates that your five to six meals should supply each day.

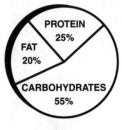

Target macronutrient ratio for the preseason and season.

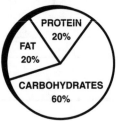

Target macronutrient ratio for the off-season.

Note that fat has about 9 calories per gram, while protein and carbohydrates have only 4 calories per gram. Therefore, during the season, if you needed to consume a total of 2,500 calories per day, you would aim for 500 calories (20 percent of your total daily calories) from fat, 625 calories (25 percent of your total daily calories) from protein, and the remaining 1,375 calories (55 percent of your total daily calories) from carbohydrates.

Some other important considerations for tennis players are:

☐ Carbohydrates are the major source of energy for short-term activities. Complex carbohydrates are the best source because they most effectively refill the glycogen stores in the muscles and liver. In addition, they elevate the blood sugar to a level sufficient for long sessions of intensive training.

☐ As a power athlete, you must make sure that you consume adequate amounts of both carbohydrates and protein. If your energy stores become drastically depleted or you experience lactic-acid buildup, you may suffer temporary muscle fatigue. If you do not refill your glycogen stores before your next workout or match, your body may begin breaking down muscle tissue for the protein it needs for energy.

☐ Directly before workouts and matches, consume carbohydrate drinks with high glycemic indexes to keep your blood sugar sustained at an appropriate level. This will allow you to train or play intensively without having your explosiveness hindered by fatigue.

☐ As a power athlete, you need to stimulate the storage of glycogen in your muscles while promoting repair and growth of your muscle tissue and inhibiting buildup of body fat. To do this:

• Train anaerobically on a regular basis. Intensive training stimulates increased storage of glycogen in the muscles and liver, which provides additional energy for greater exercise capacity.

• Consume five to six meals a day. Eating several smaller meals rather than three larger ones will keep your blood-sugar level stable throughout the day and will ensure that a supply of protein is always available for your muscles.

• Keep your fat intake to a minimum. Large amounts of fat in your diet will add to your body fat and will cause you to lose minerals through frequent urination.

• Consume low-glycemic-index foods about two to three hours before workouts and matches. These foods help sustain the blood-sugar level.

• Drink plenty of water. Not only will this practice reduce your chances of becoming dehydrated, but every ounce of glycogen that is stored within the muscles needs 3 ounces of water stored along with it. Therefore, remaining properly hydrated will also help prevent weakened muscle contractions.

• Do not eat a new food just before a match. Different people often react differently to the same food.

Before a match, eat just those foods that you know your body will handle well.

As a tennis player, you should turn to Appendix C on page 345 for full discussions of the 20:25:55 and 20:20:60 dietary plans. Also presented are sample daily diets that use common, healthy foods to meet an athlete's energy and caloric needs. Use the directions on page 150 to estimate your average daily caloric requirement. Then use the directions in Chapter 13 or 14 to adjust your diet for off-season fat loss or muscle building, respectively.

Supplementation Guidelines

In addition to eating a proper diet, you should also take dietary supplements to make sure that any nutrients you lose due to sweating or training are replenished. The following tables will help guide you in selecting the supplements appropriate for you. The first table lists the nutrients recommended for tennis players, as well as the range of intake for each nutrient. (For discussions of these nutrients, see Part One.) Note that within the ranges of intake, the lower amounts are for smaller individuals and lower-activity days, while the higher amounts are for larger individuals and higher-activity days.

RECOMMENDED NUTRIENTS AND RANGES OF INTAKE

For Tennis Players

NUTRIENT	RANGE OF INTAKE
VITAMINS	
Vitamin A	8,000–16,000 IU
Beta-carotene	30,000–45,000 IU
Vitamin B_1 (thiamine)	40–120 mg
Vitamin B_2 (riboflavin)	40–120 mg
Vitamin B_3 (niacin)	20–40 mg
Vitamin B_5 (pantothenic acid)	20–100 mg
Vitamin B_6 (pyridoxine)	20–80 mg
Vitamin B_{12} (cobalamin)	12–120 mcg
Biotin	125–175 mcg
Folate	400–800 mcg
Vitamin C	800–2,000 mg
Vitamin D	400–800 IU
Vitamin E	200–800 IU
Vitamin K	60–160 mcg

NUTRIENT	RANGE OF INTAKE
MINERALS	
Boron	2–8 mg
Calcium	800–1,500 mg
Chromium	200–500 mcg
Copper	1–4 mg
Iodine	100–200 mcg
Iron	15–50 mg
Magnesium	250–650 mg
Manganese	12–35 mg
Molybdenum	100–200 mcg
Phosphorus	150–800 mg
Potassium	50–1,000 mg
Selenium	100–200 mcg
Zinc	15–50 mg
AMINO ACIDS	
L-glutamic acid	500–1,000 mg
L-glutamine	1,000–2,000 mg
FATTY ACIDS	
Alpha-linolenic acid	500–1,000 mg
Docosahexaenoic acid (DHA)	250–750 mg
Eiocosapentaenoic acid (EPA)	250–750 mg
Gamma linolenic acid (GLA)	100–400 mg
Linoleic acid	1,000–2,000 mg
METABOLITES	
Bioflavonoids	300–800 mg
Choline	200–600 mg
Creatine monohydrate	8,000–20,000 mg
Inositol	200–600 mg
L-carnitine	500–1,500 mg
Octacosanol	8,000–12,000 mcg

IU = international units, mcg = micrograms, mg = milligrams.

RECOMMENDED SPORTS SUPPLEMENTS AND NUTRITIONAL PRACTICES

For Tennis Players

	Intake Recommendation		
	PRESEASON	SEASON	PREMATCH
SUPPLEMENTS			
Multivitamins	Yes	Yes	Yes
Multiminerals	Yes	Yes	Yes
Antioxidants	Yes	Yes	Yes
Fatty acids	Yes	Yes	Yes
Metabolites	Optional	Yes	Yes
Branched-chain amino acids	Yes	Yes	Yes
Herbs	Yes	Yes	No
Medium-calorie protein drink (300–500 calories)	Yes	Yes	Yes
Carbohydrate drink	Yes	Yes	Yes
Fat-burning supplement	Yes	Optional	No
PRACTICES			
Bicarbonate loading	No	No	No
Carbohydrate loading	No	No	Optional
Creatine and/or inosine loading	No	No	Optional
Water loading	No	No	Optional

The second table lists the different types of sports supplements available and indicates if their use by tennis players is recommended in the preseason, during the season, or directly before a match. The list also includes a number of popular nutritional practices—bicarbonate loading, carbohydrate loading, creatine and/or inosine loading, and water loading. (For a discussion of any of these supplements or practices, see the appropriate section in Part One or Part Three.)

314

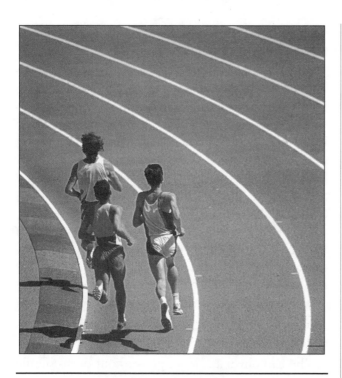

TRACK AND FIELD (ATHLETICS)

Includes Ball Throwing, Cross-Country Running, Decathlon, Discus, Hammer Throwing, Heptathlon, High Jumping, Hurdles, Javelin, Long Jumping, Marathon Running, Pentathlon, Pole Vaulting, Relay, Road Racing, Running, Shot-Putting, Steeplechase, Track, Triple Jumping, Walking, and Weight Throwing

If a champion shot-putter and a champion marathon runner held a contest to see who could run twenty-six miles the fastest, who would win? The marathon runner, of course. But if they raced to see who could run five meters the fastest, the shot-putter would win—every time.

While both shot-putters and marathon runners possess enormous strength, that strength is tempered by the metabolic demands of the particular contest. In a twenty-six-mile race, a marathon runner is able to exert greater force into the ground footfall-per-footfall during the final mile of the race than a shot-putter can—assuming that the shot-putter can even run that far in the first place! In an explosive dash, on the other hand, a shot-putter's legs have such a huge capacity for force output that they can hurl him over the five meters as though he were fired from a cannon.

Track-and-field athletes (called just athletes, since in most of the world, track and field is known simply as athletics) require not only tremendous amounts of aerobic endurance but also high levels of speed, strength, flexibility, and agility. In addition, both track athletes and field athletes need high energy levels to maintain their concentration while competing under often-difficult conditions, such as high temperatures. This calls for specialized training. Futhermore, the physical and mental demands of the sport also require the support of a carefully constructed nutrition program.

ENERGY SOURCES OF TRACK-AND-FIELD ATHLETES

The muscles rely on three major systems to supply the energy they need—the immediate, glycolytic, and oxidative energy systems. For short-term energy for explosive-strength output, the muscles depend on the immediate energy systems. The immediate energy systems are nonoxidative—that is, they do not use oxygen. Instead, these systems generate energy through the use of adenosine triphosphate (ATP) and creatine phosphate (CP). CP is produced in the body and stored in the muscle fibers. It is broken down by enzymes to regenerate ATP, which is also stored in the muscle fibers. When the ATP is in turn broken down, the result is a spark of energy that triggers a muscle contraction.

For medium-term energy for repeated near-maximum exertion, the muscles turn to the glycolytic energy systems. In these systems, which are also nonoxidative, glycogen is used to produce energy. Glycogen is the storage form of glucose. It is stored in the liver and muscles, and is readily converted back to glucose when it is needed for energy.

For long-term energy for endurance activities, the muscles use the oxidative energy systems. In these systems, oxygen is used to oxidize long-chain fatty acids, protein, and glucose, which generates energy. For athletes, getting enough oxygen can mean a winning performance rather than a second-place showing.

Every sport involves a variety of skills, and each skill utilizes a unique combination of these three energy sources. The following table lists a number of major track-and-field events and shows how much your body relies on each of the energy sources when you compete in them. Percentages are also given for an average men's decathlon and women's heptathlon.

WHERE YOUR ENERGY COMES FROM

For Track-and-Field Athletes

	Energy Systems		
	IMMEDIATE	GLYCOLYTIC	OXIDATIVE
Average track events			
100 yards	95%	5%	0%
200 yards	70%	30%	0%
400 yards	45%	50%	5%
800 yards	10%	80%	10%
1,500 yards	5%	50%	45%
5,000 yards	0%	10%	90%
10,000 yards	0%	5%	95%
*Cross-country**	5%	15%	80%
Hurdles, 110 yards	90%	10%	0%
Hurdles, 400 yards	20%	75%	5%
Marathon	0%	0%	100%
Relay, 4 X 100 yards	95%	5%	0%
Relay, 4 X 400 yards	35%	60%	5%
Steeplechase, 3,000 yards (28 hurdles and 7 water jumps)	5%	25%	70%
Walk, 20 kilometers	0%	15%	85%
Walk, 50 kilometers	0%	0%	100%
Average field events			
Discus	100%	0%	0%
Hammer throw	100%	0%	0%
High jump	100%	0%	0%
Javelin	100%	0%	0%
Long jump	100%	0%	0%
Pole vault	100%	0%	0%
Shot put	100%	0%	0%
Triple jump	100%	0%	0%
Weight throw	100%	0%	0%
Average decathlon, men's	60%	30%	10%
Average heptathlon, women's	60%	30%	10%

*Not a sanctioned track-and-field event.

When considering the type of nutritional support to give your training program, keep the following factors in mind:

☐ All athletes need to consume high-quality protein several times a day for effective recovery and adequate repair of damaged muscle tissue.

☐ Athletes whose muscles rely substantially on the immediate or glycolytic energy systems should keep their fat intake to a minimum because fat is not an efficient energy source for their intensive training, which is almost exclusively anaerobic in nature. Since the fat calories consumed by these athletes are not generally used for energy, they are stored as body fat.

☐ Athletes whose muscles rely substantially on the oxidative energy systems can eat more fat because their energy is manufactured through the oxidation of fatty acids. But even these athletes should watch their fat calories if they train aerobically (with oxygen) for less than half an hour at a time.

☐ All athletes should consume a carefully measured amount of high-quality carbohydrates several times a day to ensure an adequate supply of energy.

☐ The carbohydrates in all preworkout meals should consist of foods with low glycemic indexes to ensure that training intensity does not wane and that muscle tissue is not cannibalized for energy. (For the glycemic indexes of some common foods, see page 29.)

The aim of your nutrition program is to make your body healthy enough to accomplish recovery and tissue repair speedily and efficiently—without adding body fat. This aim alone makes diet very important for athletes. You must eat just the right amount of food. Eat the wrong foods or the wrong amounts just a few times too often and you will sabotage your fitness efforts.

NUTRITION FOR TRACK-AND-FIELD ATHLETES

Track-and-field athletes are either power, middle-distance, or endurance athletes. Their primary source of energy is determined by the specific events they specialize in. Some track-and-field events require bursts of power, which are supported by energy from the immediate energy systems. Some track-and-field events require stamina, which is supported by energy from the glycolytic energy systems. Still other track-and-field events require endurance, which is supported by energy from the oxidative energy systems. Therefore, as a track-and-field athlete, you need to plan your nutritional intake, from both food and supplement sources, to support the appropriate systems. In addition, if you are a power or middle-distance track-and-field athlete, your energy expenditure changes in the preseason and/or off-season, and you need to adjust your caloric intake and macronutrient ratio to match. Following are dietary and supplementation guidelines for power track-and-field athletes to help you in planning your nutrition program. Dietary and supplementation guidelines for middle-distance track-and-field athletes can be found on page 319, and guidelines for endurance track-and-field athletes can be found on page 321.

POWER TRACK-AND-FIELD ATHLETES

Track-and-field athletes who compete in events that require bursts of energy are power athletes. Among the typical events they participate in are the 100-yard dash, discus, and triple jump.

Dietary Guidelines

The following pie charts illustrate how you should divide up your caloric intake to match the energy demands of your power track-and-field events during the preseason, season, and off-season. They show the target percentages of fat, protein, and carbohydrates that your five to six meals should supply each day.

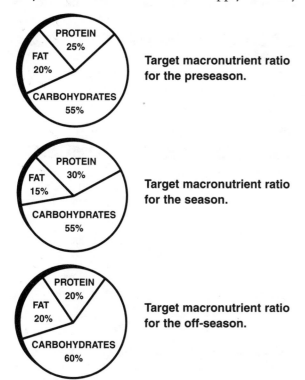

Target macronutrient ratio for the preseason.

Target macronutrient ratio for the season.

Target macronutrient ratio for the off-season.

Note that fat has about 9 calories per gram, while protein and carbohydrates have only 4 calories per

gram. Therefore, during the season, if you needed to consume a total of 2,500 calories per day, you would aim for 375 calories (15 percent of your total daily calories) from fat, 750 calories (30 percent of your total daily calories) from protein, and the remaining 1,375 calories (55 percent of your total daily calories) from carbohydrates.

Some other important considerations for power track-and-field athletes are:

☐ Carbohydrates are the major source of energy for short-term activities. Complex carbohydrates are the best source because they most effectively refill the glycogen stores in the muscles and liver. In addition, they elevate the blood sugar to a level sufficient for long sessions of intensive training.

☐ As a power athlete, you must make sure that you consume adequate amounts of both carbohydrates and protein. If your energy stores become drastically depleted or you experience lactic-acid buildup, you may suffer temporary muscle fatigue. If you do not refill your glycogen stores before your next workout or competition, your body may begin breaking down muscle tissue for the protein it needs for energy.

☐ Directly before workouts, consume carbohydrate drinks with high glycemic indexes to keep your blood sugar sustained at an appropriate level. This will allow you to train intensively without having your explosiveness hindered by fatigue.

☐ As a power athlete, you need to stimulate the storage of glycogen in your muscles while promoting repair and growth of your muscle tissue and inhibiting buildup of body fat. To do this:

• Train anaerobically on a regular basis. Intensive training stimulates increased storage of glycogen in the muscles and liver, which provides additional energy for greater exercise capacity.

• Consume five to six meals a day. Eating several smaller meals rather than three larger ones will keep your blood-sugar level stable throughout the day and will ensure that a supply of protein is always available for your muscles.

• Keep your fat intake to a minimum. Large amounts of fat in your diet will add to your body fat and will cause you to lose minerals through frequent urination.

• Consume low-glycemic-index foods about two to three hours before workouts and competitions. These foods help sustain the blood-sugar level.

• Drink plenty of water. Not only will this practice reduce your chances of becoming dehydrated, but every ounce of glycogen that is stored within the muscles needs 3 ounces of water stored along with it. Therefore, remaining properly hydrated will also help prevent weakened muscle contractions.

• Do not eat a new food just before a competition. Different people often react differently to the same food. Before a competition, eat just those foods that you know your body will handle well.

As a power track-and-field athlete, you should turn to Appendix C on page 345 for full discussions of the 20:25:55, 15:30:55, and 20:20:60 dietary plans. Also presented are sample daily diets that use common, healthy foods to meet an athlete's energy and caloric needs. Use the directions on page 150 to estimate your average daily caloric requirement. Then use the directions in Chapter 13 or 14 to adjust your diet for off-season fat loss or muscle building, respectively.

Supplementation Guidelines

In addition to eating a proper diet, you should also take dietary supplements to make sure that any nutrients you lose due to sweating or training are replenished. The following tables will help guide you in selecting the supplements appropriate for you. The first table lists the nutrients recommended for power track-and-field athletes, as well as the range of intake for each nutrient. (For discussions of these nutrients, see Part One.) Note that within the ranges of intake, the lower amounts are for smaller individuals and lower-activity days, while the higher amounts are for larger individuals and higher-activity days.

RECOMMENDED NUTRIENTS AND RANGES OF INTAKE

For Power Track-and-Field Athletes

NUTRIENT	RANGE OF INTAKE
VITAMINS	
Vitamin A	8,000–16,000 IU
Beta-carotene	20,000–35,000 IU
Vitamin B$_1$ (thiamine)	30–120 mg
Vitamin B$_2$ (riboflavin)	30–120 mg
Vitamin B$_3$ (niacin)	40–80 mg
Vitamin B$_5$ (pantothenic acid)	20–100 mg

NUTRIENT	RANGE OF INTAKE
Vitamin B$_6$ (pyridoxine)	20–80 mg
Vitamin B$_{12}$ (cobalamin)	12–120 mcg
Biotin	125–175 mcg
Folate	400–800 mcg
Vitamin C	800–2,000 mg
Vitamin D	400–800 IU
Vitamin E	200–600 IU
Vitamin K	60–160 mcg
MINERALS	
Boron	2–8 mg
Calcium	800–1,500 mg
Chromium	200–500 mcg
Copper	1–4 mg
Iodine	100–200 mcg
Iron	15–50 mg
Magnesium	250–650 mg
Manganese	12–35 mg
Molybdenum	100–200 mcg
Phosphorus	150–800 mg
Potassium	50–1,000 mg
Selenium	100–200 mcg
Zinc	15–50 mg
AMINO ACIDS	
L-glutamine	1,000–2,000 mg
FATTY ACIDS	
Alpha-linolenic acid	1,500–3,000 mg
Docosahexaenoic acid (DHA)	250–750 mg
Eiocosapentaenoic acid (EPA)	250–750 mg
Gamma linolenic acid (GLA)	100–400 mg
Linoleic acid	3,000–6,000 mg
METABOLITES	
Bioflavonoids	200–800 mg
Choline	100–600 mg
Creatine monohydrate	6,000–22,000 mg
Ferulic acid	30–90 mg
Inosine	1,000–2,000 mg
Inositol	100–600 mg
L-carnitine	750–2,000 mg
Octacosanol	3,000–6,000 mcg

IU = international units, mcg = micrograms, mg = milligrams.

The second table lists the different types of sports supplements available and indicates if their use by power track-and-field athletes is recommended in the preseason, during the season, or directly before a competition. The list also includes a number of popular nutritional practices—bicarbonate loading, carbohydrate loading, creatine and/or inosine loading, and water loading. (For a discussion of any of these supplements or practices, see the appropriate section in Part One or Part Three.)

RECOMMENDED SPORTS SUPPLEMENTS AND NUTRITIONAL PRACTICES

For Power Track-and-Field Athletes

	Intake Recommendation		
	PRESEASON	SEASON	PRE-COMPETITION
SUPPLEMENTS			
Multivitamins	Yes	Yes	No
Multiminerals	Yes	Yes	No
Antioxidants	Yes	Yes	No
Fatty acids	Yes	Yes	No
Metabolites	Optional	Yes	Yes
Branched-chain amino acids	Yes	Yes	Yes
Herbs	Yes	Yes	No
Low-calorie protein drink (200–300 calories)	Yes	Yes	Yes
Carbohydrate drink	Yes	Yes	Yes
Fat-burning supplement	Yes	Optional	No
PRACTICES			
Bicarbonate loading	No	Optional	Yes
Carbohydrate loading	No	No	No
Creatine and/or inosine loading	Optional	Yes	Yes
Water loading	No	No	No

MIDDLE-DISTANCE TRACK-AND-FIELD ATHLETES

Track-and-field athletes who participate in events that require a steady supply of energy for up to about twenty minutes are middle-distance athletes. Among the typical events they participate in are the 800-yard dash, 400-yard hurdles, and 4 x 400 yards relay.

Dietary Guidelines

The following pie charts illustrate how you should divide up your caloric intake to match the energy demands of your middle-distance track-and-field events during the preseason, season, and off-season. They show the target percentages of fat, protein, and

carbohydrates that your five to six meals should supply each day.

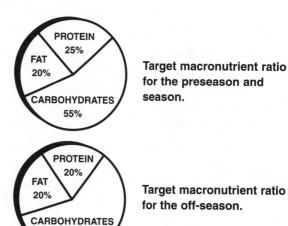

Target macronutrient ratio for the preseason and season.

Target macronutrient ratio for the off-season.

Note that fat has about 9 calories per gram, while protein and carbohydrates have only 4 calories per gram. Therefore, during the season, if you needed to consume a total of 2,500 calories per day, you would aim for 500 calories (20 percent of your total daily calories) from fat, 625 calories (25 percent of your total daily calories) from protein, and the remaining 1,375 calories (55 percent of your total daily calories) from carbohydrates.

Some other important considerations for middle-distance track-and-field athletes are:

☐ Carbohydrates are the major source of energy for short-term activities. Complex carbohydrates are the best source because they most effectively refill the glycogen stores in the muscles and liver. In addition, they elevate the blood sugar to a level sufficient for long sessions of intensive training.

☐ As a middle-distance athlete, you must make sure that you consume adequate amounts of both carbohydrates and protein. If your energy stores become drastically depleted or you experience lactic-acid buildup, you may suffer temporary muscle fatigue. If you do not refill your glycogen stores before your next workout or competition, your body may begin breaking down muscle tissue for the protein it needs for energy.

☐ Directly before workouts, consume carbohydrate drinks with high glycemic indexes to keep your blood sugar sustained at an appropriate level. This will allow you to train intensively for longer periods of time.

☐ As a middle-distance athlete, you need to stimulate the storage of glycogen in your muscles while promoting repair and growth of your muscle tissue and inhibiting buildup of body fat. To do this:

• Train against your anaerobic threshold (to exhaustion) on a regular basis. Intensive, exhaustive training stimulates increased storage of glycogen in the muscles and liver, which provides additional energy for greater exercise capacity.

• Consume five to six meals a day. Eating several smaller meals rather than three larger ones will keep your blood-sugar level stable throughout the day and will ensure that a supply of protein is always available for your muscles.

• Keep your fat intake to a minimum. Large amounts of fat in your diet will add to your body fat and will cause mineral loss through frequent urination.

• Consume low-glycemic-index foods about two to three hours before workouts and competitions. These foods help sustain the blood-sugar level.

• Drink plenty of water. Not only will this practice reduce your chances of becoming dehydrated, but every ounce of glycogen that is stored within the muscles needs 3 ounces of water stored along with it. Therefore, remaining properly hydrated will also help prevent weakened muscle contractions and early onset of fatigue.

• Do not eat a new food just before a competition. Different people often react differently to the same food. Before a competition, eat just those foods that you know your body will handle well.

As a middle-distance track-and-field athlete, you should turn to Appendix C on page 345 for full discussions of the 20:25:55 and 20:20:60 dietary plans. Also presented are sample daily diets that use common, healthy foods to meet an athlete's energy and caloric needs. Use the directions on page 150 to estimate your average daily caloric requirement. Then use the directions in Chapter 13 or 14 to adjust your diet for off-season fat loss or muscle building, respectively.

Supplementation Guidelines

In addition to eating a proper diet, you should also take dietary supplements to make sure that any nutrients you lose due to sweating or training are replen-

ished. The following tables will help guide you in selecting the supplements appropriate for you. The first table lists the nutrients recommended for middle-distance track-and-field athletes, as well as the range of intake for each nutrient. (For discussions of these nutrients, see Part One.) Note that within the ranges of intake, the lower amounts are for smaller individuals and lower-activity days, while the higher amounts are for larger individuals and higher-activity days.

RECOMMENDED NUTRIENTS AND RANGES OF INTAKE

For Middle-Distance Track-and-Field Athletes

NUTRIENT	RANGE OF INTAKE
VITAMINS	
Vitamin A	8,000–16,000 IU
Beta-carotene	25,000–40,000 IU
Vitamin B_1 (thiamine)	40–120 mg
Vitamin B_2 (riboflavin)	40–120 mg
Vitamin B_3 (niacin)	20–40 mg
Vitamin B_5 (pantothenic acid)	20–100 mg
Vitamin B_6 (pyridoxine)	20–80 mg
Vitamin B_{12} (cobalamin)	12–120 mcg
Biotin	125–175 mcg
Folate	400–800 mcg
Vitamin C	800–2,000 mg
Vitamin D	400–800 IU
Vitamin E	200–800 IU
Vitamin K	60–160 mcg
MINERALS	
Boron	2–8 mg
Calcium	800–1,500 mg
Chromium	200–500 mcg
Copper	1–4 mg
Iodine	100–200 mcg
Iron	15–50 mg
Magnesium	250–650 mg
Manganese	12–35 mg
Molybdenum	100–200 mcg
Phosphorus	150–800 mg
Potassium	50–1,000 mg
Selenium	100–200 mcg
Zinc	15–50 mg
AMINO ACIDS	
L-glutamic acid	500–1,000 mg
L-glutamine	1,000–2,000 mg

NUTRIENT	RANGE OF INTAKE
FATTY ACIDS	
Alpha-linolenic acid	500–1,000 mg
Docosahexaenoic acid (DHA)	250–750 mg
Eiocosapentaenoic acid (EPA)	250–750 mg
Gamma linolenic acid (GLA)	100–400 mg
Linoleic acid	1,000–2,000 mg
METABOLITES	
Bioflavonoids	300–800 mg
Choline	200–600 mg
Inositol	200–600 mg
L-carnitine	1,000–2,000 mg
Octacosanol	3,000–6,000 mcg

IU = international units, mcg = micrograms, mg = milligrams.

The second table lists the different types of sports supplements available and indicates if their use by middle-distance track-and-field athletes is recommended in the preseason, during the season, or directly before a competition. The list also includes a number of popular nutritional practices—bicarbonate loading, carbohydrate loading, creatine and/or inosine loading, and water loading. (For a discussion of any of these supplements or practices, see the appropriate section in Part One or Part Three.)

RECOMMENDED SPORTS SUPPLEMENTS AND NUTRITIONAL PRACTICES

For Middle-Distance Track-and-Field Athletes

	Intake Recommendation		
	PRESEASON	SEASON	PRE-COMPETITION
SUPPLEMENTS			
Multivitamins	Yes	Yes	No
Multiminerals	Yes	Yes	No
Antioxidants	Yes	Yes	No
Fatty acids	Yes	Yes	No
Metabolites	Optional	Yes	Yes
Branched-chain amino acids	Yes	Yes	Yes
Herbs	Yes	Yes	No
Medium-calorie protein drink (300–500 calories)	Yes	Yes	Yes
Carbohydrate drink	Yes	Yes	Yes
Fat-burning supplement	Yes	Optional	No

	Intake Recommendation		
	PRESEASON	SEASON	PRE-COMPETITION
PRACTICES			
Bicarbonate loading	No	No	No
Carbohydrate loading	No	No	Optional
Creatine and/or inosine loading	No	No	No
Water loading	No	No	Optional

ENDURANCE TRACK-AND-FIELD ATHLETES

Track-and-field athletes who participate in events that require a steady supply of energy for more than about twenty minutes are endurance athletes. Among the typical events they participate in are the 5,000-yard dash, 50-kilometer walk, and marathon running.

Dietary Guidelines

The following pie chart illustrates how you should divide up your caloric intake to match the energy demands of your endurance track-and-field events during the preseason, season, and off-season. They show the target percentages of fat, protein, and carbohydrates that your five to six meals should supply each day.

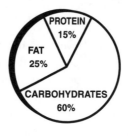

Target macronutrient ratio for the preseason, season, and off-season.

Note that fat has about 9 calories per gram, while protein and carbohydrates have only 4 calories per gram. Therefore, if you needed to consume a total of 2,500 calories per day, you would aim for 625 calories (25 percent of your total daily calories) from fat, 375 calories (15 percent of your total daily calories) from protein, and the remaining 1,500 calories (60 percent of your total daily calories) from carbohydrates.

Some other important considerations for endurance track-and-field athletes are:

☐ The energy source that is used during an aerobic activity depends upon the duration and intensity of the activity. During the first one and a half to two hours, both glycogen and body fat are the primary sources of energy. After one and a half to two hours, body fat alone becomes the primary source.

☐ While body fat is the primary source of energy during prolonged aerobic activities, it cannot be used efficiently unless some glycogen remains in the muscles and liver. Therefore, even ultra-endurance athletes must make sure to always keep their glycogen stores filled.

☐ As an endurance athlete, you need to encourage glycogen sparing in your body while stimulating the use of fat as your primary energy source. To do this:

• Train for endurance on a regular basis. Regular endurance training stimulates increased storage of both glycogen and fatty acids.

• Consume five to six meals a day. Eating several smaller meals rather than three larger ones will keep your blood-sugar level stable throughout the day.

• Do not load up on dietary fat. Consuming large amounts of fat was originally thought to benefit endurance athletes, whose primary source of energy is fat. However, fat loading can lead to frequent urination, which increases the loss of minerals essential to healthy heart action.

• Consume low-glycemic-index foods about two to three hours before workouts and competitions. These foods help sustain the blood-sugar level.

• Do not consume food or caloric beverages from two hours before an endurance activity to fifteen minutes before. Food and caloric beverages cause the insulin level to rise, which in turn can provoke transient hypoglycemia. Transient hypoglycemia interferes with the energy dynamics during exercise and can induce early onset of fatigue.

• Consume carbohydrates directly before and during endurance activities. Because exercise slows the release of insulin into the bloodstream, the ingestion of carbohydrates spares glycogen and allows the use of fat for energy. Carbohydrate drinks with high glycemic indexes help sustain the blood-sugar level, thereby preserving glycogen stores.

• During endurance activities, drink plenty of water. Endurance activities cause profuse sweating, which results in loss of valuable fluids and minerals. Dehydration not only reduces performance but can seriously affect health.

• Drink electrolyte-containing beverages during en-

durance activities. These drinks help replace minerals that are lost through sweating.

• During endurance activities, drink 4 to 6 ounces of fluid every fifteen to thirty minutes. For every pound of body weight lost through sweating, 1 pint of fluid should be consumed. Chilled fluids are absorbed the quickest.

• Do not eat a new food just before a competition. Different people often react differently to the same food. Before a competition, eat just those foods that you know your body will handle well.

As an endurance track-and-field athlete, you should turn to Appendix C on page 345 for a full discussion of the 25:15:60 dietary plan. Also presented are sample daily diets that use common, healthy foods to meet an athlete's energy and caloric needs. Use the directions on page 150 to estimate your average daily caloric requirement. Then use the directions in Chapter 13 or 14 to adjust your diet for off-season fat loss or muscle building, respectively.

Supplementation Guidelines

In addition to eating a proper diet, you should also take dietary supplements to make sure that any nutrients you lose due to sweating or training are replenished. The following tables will help guide you in selecting the supplements appropriate for you. The first table lists the nutrients recommended for endurance track-and-field athletes, as well as the range of intake for each nutrient. (For discussions of these nutrients, see Part One.) Note that within the ranges of intake, the lower amounts are for smaller individuals and lower-activity days, while the higher amounts are for larger individuals and higher-activity days.

RECOMMENDED NUTRIENTS AND RANGES OF INTAKE

For Endurance Track-and-Field Athletes

NUTRIENT	RANGE OF INTAKE
VITAMINS	
Vitamin A	8,000–16,000 IU
Beta-carotene	35,000–60,000 IU
Vitamin B_1 (thiamine)	100–250 mg
Vitamin B_2 (riboflavin)	100–200 mg
Vitamin B_3 (niacin)	10–20 mg

NUTRIENT	RANGE OF INTAKE
Vitamin B_5 (pantothenic acid)	100–200 mg
Vitamin B_6 (pyridoxine)	20–80 mg
Vitamin B_{12} (cobalamin)	12–120 mcg
Biotin	125–200 mcg
Folate	400–800 mcg
Vitamin C	1,000–2,000 mg
Vitamin D	400–800 IU
Vitamin E	400–1,000 IU
Vitamin K	60–160 mcg

MINERALS

Boron	2–8 mg
Calcium	800–1,500 mg
Chromium	200–500 mcg
Copper	1–4 mg
Iodine	100–200 mcg
Iron	15–50 mg
Magnesium	250–650 mg
Manganese	12–35 mg
Molybdenum	100–200 mcg
Phosphorus	150–800 mg
Potassium	50–1,000 mg
Selenium	100–200 mcg
Zinc	15–50 mg

AMINO ACIDS

L-glutamic acid	1,000–1,500 mg
L-glutamine	1,000–2,000 mg

FATTY ACIDS

Alpha-linolenic acid	500–1,000 mg
Docosahexaenoic acid (DHA)	400–1,000 mg
Eiocosapentaenoic acid (EPA)	400–1,000 mg
Gamma linolenic acid (GLA)	200–500 mg
Linoleic acid	500–1,000 mg

METABOLITES

Bioflavonoids	500–1,000 mg
Choline	500–1,000 mg
Coenzyme Q_{10}	60–120 mg
Inositol	500–1,000 mg
L-carnitine	1,000–3,000 mg
Octacosanol	3,000–6,000 mcg

OTHER

Caffeine*	200–400 mg

IU = international units, mcg = micrograms, mg = milligrams.
*Verify with your sports governing organization that caffeine consumption is permitted during competition.

The second table lists the different types of sports supplements available and indicates if their use by endurance track-and-field athletes is recommended in the preseason, during the season, or directly before a competition. The list also includes a number of popular nutritional practices—bicarbonate loading, carbohydrate loading, creatine and/or inosine loading, and water loading. (For a discussion of any of these supplements or practices, see the appropriate section in Part One or Part Three.)

RECOMMENDED SPORTS SUPPLEMENTS AND NUTRITIONAL PRACTICES

For Endurance Track-and-Field Athletes

	Intake Recommendation		
	PRESEASON	SEASON	PRE-COMPETITION
SUPPLEMENTS			
Multivitamins	Yes	Yes	Yes
Multiminerals	Yes	Yes	Yes
Antioxidants	Yes	Yes	Yes
Fatty acids	Yes	Yes	Yes
Metabolites	Optional	Yes	Yes
Branched-chain amino acids	Yes	Yes	Yes
Herbs	Yes	Yes	No
High-calorie protein drink (over 500 calories)	Yes	Yes	Yes
Carbohydrate drink with glycerol and electrolytes	Yes	Yes	Yes
Fat-burning supplement	Yes	No	No
PRACTICES			
Bicarbonate loading	No	No	No
Carbohydrate loading	No	Optional	Yes
Creatine and/or inosine loading	No	No	No
Water loading	No	Optional	Yes

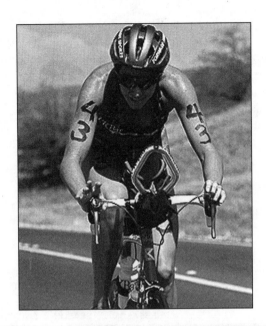

TRIATHLON

Includes Cycling, Running, and Swimming

Also for Road Racing

If a champion triathlete and a champion sprinter held a contest to see who could run five meters the fastest, who would win? The sprinter, of course. But if they raced to see who could run twenty-six miles the fastest, the triathlete would win—every time.

While both triathletes and sprinters possess enormous strength, that strength is tempered by the metabolic demands of the particular contest. In a twenty-six-mile race, a triathlete is able to exert greater force into the ground footfall-per-footfall during the final mile of the race than a sprinter can—assuming that the sprinter can even run that far in the first place! In an explosive dash, on the other hand, a sprinter's legs have such a huge capacity for force output that they can hurl him over the five meters as though he were fired from a cannon.

Triathletes require not only tremendous amounts of aerobic endurance but also high levels of speed, strength, flexibility, and agility. In addition, they need high energy levels to maintain their concentration while competing under often-difficult conditions, such as high temperatures, rough terrain, and choppy water. This calls for specialized training. Futhermore, the physical and mental demands of the sport also require the support of a carefully constructed nutrition program.

ENERGY SOURCES OF TRIATHLETES

The muscles rely on three major systems to supply the energy they need—the immediate, glycolytic, and oxidative energy systems. For short-term energy for explosive-strength output, the muscles depend on the immediate energy systems. The immediate energy systems are nonoxidative—that is, they do not use oxygen. Instead, these systems generate energy through the use of adenosine triphosphate (ATP) and creatine phosphate (CP). CP is produced in the body and stored in the muscle fibers. It is broken down by enzymes to regenerate ATP, which is also stored in the muscle fibers. When the ATP is in turn broken down, the result is a spark of energy that triggers a muscle contraction.

For medium-term energy for repeated near-maximum exertion, the muscles turn to the glycolytic energy systems. In these systems, which are also nonoxidative, glycogen is used to produce energy. Glycogen is the storage form of glucose. It is stored in the liver and muscles, and is readily converted back to glucose when it is needed for energy.

For long-term energy for endurance activities, the muscles use the oxidative energy systems. In these systems, oxygen is used to oxidize long-chain fatty acids, protein, and glucose, which generates energy. For athletes, getting enough oxygen can mean a winning performance rather than a second-place showing.

Every sport involves a variety of skills, and each skill utilizes a unique combination of these three energy sources. The following table lists the three legs of a triathlon and shows how much your body relies on each of the energy sources when you compete in them. Percentages are also given for an average weight-training workout.

WHERE YOUR ENERGY COMES FROM

For Triathletes		
Energy Systems		
IMMEDIATE	GLYCOLYTIC	OXIDATIVE
Average events		
Cycling　0%	10%	90%
Long-distance		
running　0%	0%	100%
Swimming　10%	20%	70%
Average weight-		
training workout　90%	10%	0%

When considering the type of nutritional support to give your training program, keep the following factors in mind:

☐ All athletes need to consume high-quality protein several times a day for effective recovery and adequate repair of damaged muscle tissue.

☐ Athletes whose muscles rely substantially on the oxidative energy systems can eat more fat because their energy is manufactured through the oxidation of fatty acids. But even these athletes should watch their fat calories if they train aerobically (with oxygen) for less than half an hour at a time.

☐ All athletes should consume a carefully measured amount of high-quality carbohydrates several times a day to ensure an adequate supply of energy.

☐ The carbohydrates in your preworkout meals should consist of foods with low glycemic indexes to ensure that training intensity does not wane and that muscle tissue is not cannibalized for energy. (For the glycemic indexes of some common foods, see page 29.)

The aim of your nutrition program is to adequately fill your body's energy stores in preparation for the next competition or workout, plus to make your body healthy enough to accomplish recovery and tissue repair speedily and efficiently—both without adding body fat. Your further aim is to do this while maintaining a high strength-to-weight ratio. These aims alone make diet as critical as training for triathletes. You must eat just the right amount of food. Eat the wrong foods or the wrong amounts just a few times too often and you will sabotage your fitness efforts.

NUTRITION FOR TRIATHLETES

Triathletes are endurance athletes. They obtain most of their energy from the oxidative energy systems. Therefore, as a triathlete, you need to plan your nutritional intake, from both food and supplement sources, to support the oxidative systems. Following are dietary guidelines for triathletes to help you in planning your nutrition program. Supplementation guidelines for triathletes can be found on page 326.

Dietary Guidelines

The following pie chart illustrates how you should divide up your caloric intake to match the energy demands of triathlons during the preseason, season, and off-season. It shows the target percentages of fat, protein, and carbohydrates that your five to six meals should supply each day.

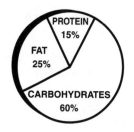

Target macronutrient ratio for the preseason, season, and off-season.

Note that fat has about 9 calories per gram, while protein and carbohydrates have only 4 calories per gram. Therefore, if you needed to consume a total of 2,500 calories per day, you would aim for 625 calories (25 percent of your total daily calories) from fat, 375 calories (15 percent of your total daily calories) from protein, and the remaining 1,500 calories (60 percent of your total daily calories) from carbohydrates.

Some other important considerations for triathletes are:

☐ The energy source that is used during an aerobic activity depends upon the duration and intensity of the activity. During the first one and a half to two hours, both glycogen and body fat are the primary sources of energy. After one and a half to two hours, body fat alone becomes the primary source.

☐ While body fat is the primary source of energy during prolonged aerobic activities, it cannot be used efficiently unless some glycogen remains in the muscles and liver. Therefore, even ultra-endurance athletes must make sure to always keep their glycogen stores filled.

☐ As an endurance athlete, you need to encourage glycogen sparing in your body while stimulating the use of fat as your primary energy source. To do this:

• Train for endurance on a regular basis. Regular endurance training stimulates increased storage of both glycogen and fatty acids.

• Consume five to six meals a day. Eating several smaller meals rather than three larger ones will keep your blood-sugar level stable throughout the day.

• Do not load up on dietary fat. Consuming large amounts of fat was originally thought to benefit endurance athletes, whose primary source of energy is fat. However, fat loading can lead to frequent urination, which increases the loss of minerals essential to healthy heart action.

• Consume low-glycemic-index foods about two to three hours before workouts and competitions. These foods help sustain the blood-sugar level.

• Do not consume food or caloric beverages from two hours before an endurance activity to fifteen minutes before. Food and caloric beverages cause the insulin level to rise, which in turn can provoke transient hypoglycemia. Transient hypoglycemia interferes with the energy dynamics during exercise and can induce early onset of fatigue.

• Consume carbohydrates directly before and during endurance activities. Because exercise slows the release of insulin into the bloodstream, the ingestion of carbohydrates spares glycogen and allows the use of fat for energy. Carbohydrate drinks with high glycemic indexes help sustain the blood-sugar level, thereby preserving glycogen stores.

• During endurance activities, drink plenty of water. Endurance activities cause profuse sweating, which results in loss of valuable fluids and minerals. Dehydration not only reduces performance but can seriously affect health.

• Drink electrolyte-containing beverages during endurance activities. These drinks help replace minerals that are lost through sweating.

• During endurance activities, drink 4 to 6 ounces of fluid every fifteen to thirty minutes. For every pound of body weight lost through sweating, 1 pint of fluid should be consumed. Chilled fluids are absorbed the quickest.

• Do not eat a new food just before a competition. Different people often react differently to the same food. Before a competition, eat just those foods that you know your body will handle well.

As a triathlete, you should turn to Appendix C on page 345 for a full discussion of the 25:15:60 dietary plan. Also presented are sample daily diets that use common, healthy foods to meet an athlete's energy and caloric needs. Use the directions on page 150 to estimate your average daily caloric requirement. Then use the directions in Chapter 13 or 14 to adjust your diet for off-season fat loss or muscle building, respectively.

Supplementation Guidelines

In addition to eating a proper diet, you should also take dietary supplements to make sure that any nutrients you lose due to sweating or training are replenished. The following tables will help guide you in selecting the supplements appropriate for you. The first table lists the nutrients recommended for triathletes, as well as the range of intake for each nutrient. (For discussions of these nutrients, see Part One.) Note that within the ranges of intake, the lower amounts are for smaller individuals and lower-activity days, while the higher amounts are for larger individuals and higher-activity days.

RECOMMENDED NUTRIENTS AND RANGES OF INTAKE

For Triathletes

NUTRIENT	RANGE OF INTAKE
VITAMINS	
Vitamin A	8,000–16,000 IU
Beta-carotene	35,000–60,000 IU
Vitamin B_1 (thiamine)	100–250 mg
Vitamin B_2 (riboflavin)	100–200 mg
Vitamin B_3 (niacin)	10–20 mg
Vitamin B_5 (pantothenic acid)	100–200 mg
Vitamin B_6 (pyridoxine)	20–80 mg
Vitamin B_{12} (cobalamin)	12–120 mcg
Biotin	125–200 mcg
Folate	400–800 mcg
Vitamin C	1,000–2,000 mg
Vitamin D	400–800 IU
Vitamin E	400–1,000 IU
Vitamin K	60–160 mcg
MINERALS	
Boron	2–8 mg
Calcium	800–1,500 mg
Chromium	200–500 mcg
Copper	1–4 mg
Iodine	100–200 mcg
Iron	15–50 mg
Magnesium	250–650 mg
Manganese	12–35 mg
Molybdenum	100–200 mcg
Phosphorus	150–800 mg
Potassium	50–1,000 mg
Selenium	100–200 mcg
Zinc	15–50 mg

NUTRIENT	RANGE OF INTAKE
AMINO ACIDS	
L-glutamic acid	1,000–1,500 mg
L-glutamine	1,000–2,000 mg
FATTY ACIDS	
Alpha-linolenic acid	500–1,000 mg
Docosahexaenoic acid (DHA)	400–1,000 mg
Eiocosapentaenoic acid (EPA)	400–1,000 mg
Gamma linolenic acid (GLA)	200–500 mg
Linoleic acid	500–1,000 mg
METABOLITES	
Bioflavonoids	500–1,000 mg
Choline	500–1,000 mg
Coenzyme Q_{10}	60–120 mg
Inositol	500–1,000 mg
L-carnitine	1,000–3,000 mg
Octacosanol	1,000–2,000 mcg
OTHER	
Caffeine*	200–400 mg

IU = international units, mcg = micrograms, mg = milligrams.

*Verify with your sports governing organization that caffeine consumption is permitted during competition.

The second table lists the different types of sports supplements available and indicates if their use by triathletes is recommended in the preseason, during the season, or directly before a competition. The list also includes a number of popular nutritional practices—bicarbonate loading, carbohydrate loading, creatine and/or inosine loading, and water loading. (For a discussion of any of these supplements or practices, see the appropriate section in Part One or Part Three.)

RECOMMENDED SPORTS SUPPLEMENTS AND NUTRITIONAL PRACTICES

For Triathletes

	Intake Recommendation		
	PRESEASON	SEASON	PRE-COMPETITION
SUPPLEMENTS			
Multivitamins	Yes	Yes	No
Multiminerals	Yes	Yes	No
Antioxidants	Yes	Yes	No
Fatty acids	Yes	Yes	No
Metabolites	Optional	Yes	Yes
Branched-chain amino acids	Yes	Yes	Yes

	Intake Recommendation		
	PRESEASON	SEASON	PRE-COMPETITION
Herbs	Yes	Yes	No
High-calorie protein drink (over 500 calories)	Yes	Yes	Yes
Carbohydrate drink with glycerol and electrolytes	Yes	Yes	Yes
Fat-burning supplement	Yes	No	No
PRACTICES			
Bicarbonate loading	No	No	No
Carbohydrate loading	No	No	Yes
Creatine and/or inosine loading	No	No	No
Water loading	No	Optional	Yes

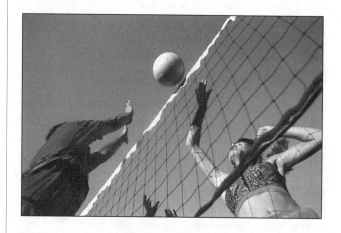

VOLLEYBALL

Includes Beach and Court

Volleyball is one of the most popular sports in the world today. It is a demanding sport that requires excellent physical conditioning. Although most rallies in volleyball last less than thirty seconds, many games last for an hour or two. Therefore, volleyball requires a high level of anaerobic-strength endurance, as well as speed-strength, quickness, and flexibility.

Every bit of your training and diet must reflect these elements. These elements are what make volleyball explosive in nature. In fact, volleyball is very explosive, so improved recovery and tissue repair plus increased speed and strength are your year-round training and dietary goals. Nutritionally, this means emphasizing short-term energy needs and maximizing the muscles' recovery and tissue-repair processes.

In volleyball, the energy output is anaerobic (without oxygen). This does not mean that training for or playing volleyball is easy, however. Especially in beach volleyball, you must explode to the left and right, go for digs, jump, feint, spike the ball, and perform other lightning-quick reflexive movements over and over again, repeatedly testing your tolerance to pain and fatigue, caused by lactic-acid buildup in your muscles. The training for volleyball is extremely intensive and grueling. At the highest levels, training in speed-strength and anaerobic-strength endurance for volleyball forces you to operate at your anaerobic threshold (the point at which you must receive oxygen).

Muscles grow when they are stressed. In volleyball, the aim is to make the muscles grow as strong and as quick as possible. This calls for specialized training. Furthermore, the incredible force output of volleyball, especially coupled with the explosive aspects of the game, requires the support of a carefully constructed nutrition program.

ENERGY SOURCES OF VOLLEYBALL PLAYERS

The muscles rely on three major systems to supply the energy they need—the immediate, glycolytic, and oxidative energy systems. For short-term energy for explosive-strength output, the muscles depend on the immediate energy systems. The immediate energy systems are nonoxidative—that is, they do not use oxygen. Instead, these systems generate energy through the use of adenosine triphosphate (ATP) and creatine phosphate (CP). CP is produced in the body and stored in the muscle fibers. It is broken down by enzymes to regenerate ATP, which is also stored in the muscle fibers. When the ATP is in turn broken down, the result is a spark of energy that triggers a muscle contraction.

For medium-term energy for repeated near-maximum exertion, the muscles turn to the glycolytic energy systems. In these systems, which are also nonoxidative, glycogen is used to produce energy. Glycogen is the storage form of glucose. It is stored in the liver and muscles, and is readily converted back to glucose when it is needed for energy.

For long-term energy for endurance activities, the muscles use the oxidative energy systems. In these systems, oxygen is used to oxidize long-chain fatty acids, protein, and glucose, which generates energy. For athletes, getting enough oxygen can mean a winning performance rather than a second-place showing.

Every sport involves a variety of skills, and each skill utilizes a unique combination of these three energy sources. The following table shows how much your body relies on each of the energy sources during an average game of beach volleyball and an average game of court volleyball.

WHERE YOUR ENERGY COMES FROM

For Volleyball Players			
	Energy Systems		
	IMMEDIATE	GLYCOLYTIC	OXIDATIVE
Beach-volleyball game	65%	30%	5%
Court-volleyball game	75%	20%	5%

When considering the type of nutritional support to give your training program, keep the following factors in mind:

☐ All athletes need to consume high-quality protein several times a day for effective recovery and adequate repair of damaged muscle tissue.

☐ Athletes whose muscles rely substantially on the immediate or glycolytic energy systems should keep their fat intake to a minimum because fat is not an efficient energy source for their intensive training, which is almost exclusively anaerobic in nature. Since the fat calories consumed by these athletes are not generally used for energy, they are stored as body fat.

☐ All athletes should consume a carefully measured amount of high-quality carbohydrates several times a day to ensure an adequate supply of energy.

☐ The carbohydrates in all preworkout meals should consist of foods with low glycemic indexes to ensure that training intensity does not wane and that muscle tissue is not cannibalized for energy. (For the glycemic indexes of some common foods, see page 29.)

The aim of your nutrition program is to make your body healthy enough to accomplish recovery and tissue repair speedily and efficiently—without adding body fat. Your further aim is to do this while maintaining a high strength-to-weight ratio. These aims alone make diet as critical as training for volleyball players. You must eat just the right amount of food. Eat the wrong foods or the wrong amounts just a few times too often and you will sabotage your fitness efforts.

NUTRITION FOR VOLLEYBALL PLAYERS

Volleyball players are power athletes. Whether they play beach or court volleyball, they obtain most of their energy from the immediate energy systems. Therefore, as a volleyball player, you need to plan your nutritional intake, from both food and supplement sources, to support the immediate systems. In addition, since your energy expenditure changes in the off-season, you need to adjust your caloric intake and macronutrient ratio to match. Following are dietary guidelines for volleyball players to help you in planning your nutrition program. Supplementation guidelines for volleyball players can be found on page 330.

Dietary Guidelines

The following pie charts illustrate how you should divide up your caloric intake to match the energy demands of volleyball during the preseason, season, and off-season. They show the target percentages of fat, protein, and carbohydrates that your five to six meals should supply each day.

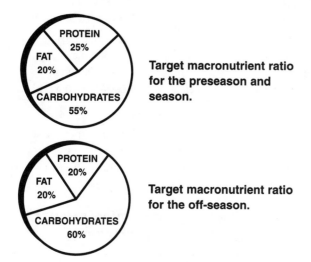

PROTEIN 25%
FAT 20%
CARBOHYDRATES 55%

Target macronutrient ratio for the preseason and season.

PROTEIN 20%
FAT 20%
CARBOHYDRATES 60%

Target macronutrient ratio for the off-season.

Note that fat has about 9 calories per gram, while protein and carbohydrates have only 4 calories per gram. Therefore, during the season, if you needed to consume a total of 2,500 calories per day, you would aim for 500 calories (20 percent of your total daily calories) from fat, 625 calories (25 percent of your total daily calories) from protein, and the remaining 1,375 calories (55 percent of your total daily calories) from carbohydrates.

Some other important considerations for volleyball players are:

☐ Carbohydrates are the major source of energy for short-term activities. Complex carbohydrates are the best source because they most effectively refill the glycogen stores in the muscles and liver. In addition, they elevate the blood sugar to a level sufficient for long sessions of intensive training.

☐ As a power athlete, you must make sure that you consume adequate amounts of both carbohydrates and protein. If your energy stores become drastically depleted or you experience lactic-acid buildup, you may suffer temporary muscle fatigue. If you do not refill your glycogen stores before your next workout or game, your body may begin breaking down muscle tissue for the protein it needs for energy.

☐ Directly before workouts and games, consume carbohydrate drinks with high glycemic indexes to keep your blood sugar sustained at an appropriate level. This will allow you to train or play intensively without having your explosiveness hindered by fatigue.

☐ As a power athlete, you need to stimulate the storage of glycogen in your muscles while promoting repair and growth of your muscle tissue and inhibiting buildup of body fat. To do this:

• Train anaerobically on a regular basis. Intensive training stimulates increased storage of glycogen in the muscles and liver, which provides additional energy for greater exercise capacity.

• Consume five to six meals a day. Eating several smaller meals rather than three larger ones will keep your blood-sugar level stable throughout the day and will ensure that a supply of protein is always available for your muscles.

• Keep your fat intake to a minimum. Large amounts of fat in your diet will add to your body fat and will cause you to lose minerals through frequent urination.

• Consume low-glycemic-index foods about two to three hours before workouts and games. These foods help sustain the blood-sugar level.

• Drink plenty of water. Not only will this practice reduce your chances of becoming dehydrated, but every ounce of glycogen that is stored within the muscles needs 3 ounces of water stored along with it. Therefore, remaining properly hydrated will also help prevent weakened muscle contractions.

• Do not eat a new food just before a game. Different people often react differently to the same food. Before a game, eat just those foods that you know your body will handle well.

As a volleyball player, you should turn to Appendix C on page 345 for full discussions of the 20:25:55 and 20:20:60 dietary plans. Also presented are sample daily diets that use common, healthy foods to meet an athlete's energy and caloric needs. Use the directions on page 150 to estimate your average daily caloric requirement. Then use the directions in Chapter 13 or 14 to adjust your diet for off-season fat loss or muscle building, respectively.

Supplementation Guidelines

In addition to eating a proper diet, you should also take dietary supplements to make sure that any nutrients you lose due to sweating or training are replenished. The following tables will help guide you in selecting the supplements appropriate for you. The first table lists the nutrients recommended for volleyball players, as well as the range of intake for each nutrient. (For discussions of these nutrients, see Part One.) Note that within the ranges of intake, the lower amounts are for smaller individuals and lower-activity days, while the higher amounts are for larger individuals and higher-activity days.

RECOMMENDED NUTRIENTS AND RANGES OF INTAKE

For Volleyball Players

NUTRIENT	RANGE OF INTAKE
VITAMINS	
Vitamin A	8,000–16,000 IU
Beta-carotene	15,000–30,000 IU
Vitamin B_1 (thiamine)	40–120 mg
Vitamin B_2 (riboflavin)	40–120 mg
Vitamin B3 (niacin)	20–40 mg
Vitamin B_5 (pantothenic acid)	20–100 mg
Vitamin B_6 (pyridoxine)	20–80 mg
Vitamin B_{12} (cobalamin)	12–120 mcg
Biotin	125–175 mcg
Folate	400–800 mcg
Vitamin C	800–2,000 mg
Vitamin D	400–800 IU
Vitamin E	200–800 IU
Vitamin K	60–160 mcg
MINERALS	
Boron	2–8 mg
Calcium	800–1,500 mg
Chromium	200–500 mcg
Copper	1–4 mg

NUTRIENT	RANGE OF INTAKE
Iodine	100–200 mcg
Iron	15–50 mg
Magnesium	250–650 mg
Manganese	12–35 mg
Molybdenum	100–200 mcg
Phosphorus	150–800 mg
Potassium	50–1,000 mg
Selenium	100–200 mcg
Zinc	15–50 mg
AMINO ACIDS	
L-glutamic acid	500–1,000 mg
L-glutamine	1,000–2,000 mg
FATTY ACIDS	
Alpha-linolenic acid	1,500–3,000 mg
Docosahexaenoic acid (DHA)	250–750 mg
Eicosapentaenoic acid (EPA)	250–750 mg
Gamma linolenic acid (GLA)	100–400 mg
Linoleic acid	3,000–6,000 mg
VITAMINS	
Bioflavonoids	300–800 mg
Choline	200–600 mg
Creatine monohydrate	8,000–18,000 mg
Inosine	500–1,500 mg
Inositol	200–600 mg
L-carnitine	500–1,500 mg
Octacosanol	6,000–12,000 mcg

IU = international units, mcg = micrograms, mg = milligrams.

The second table lists the different types of sports supplements available and indicates if their use by volleyball players is recommended in the preseason, during the season, or directly before a game.

RECOMMENDED SPORTS SUPPLEMENTS AND NUTRITIONAL PRACTICES

For Volleyball Players

	Intake Recommendation		
	PRESEASON	SEASON	PREGAME
SUPPLEMENTS			
Multivitamins	Yes	Yes	No
Multiminerals	Yes	Yes	No
Antioxidants	Yes	Yes	No
Fatty acids	Yes	Yes	No
Metabolites	Optional	Yes	Yes
Branched-chain amino acids	Yes	Yes	Yes

Intake Recommendation			
	PRESEASON	SEASON	PREGAME
Herbs	Yes	Yes	No
Medium-calorie protein drink (300–500 calories)	Yes	Yes	Yes
Carbohydrate drink	Yes	Yes	Yes
Fat-burning supplement	Yes	Optional	No
PRACTICES			
Bicarbonate loading	No	No	Optional
Carbohydrate loading	No	No	No
Creatine and/or inosine loading	No	Optional	Optional
Water loading	No	No	Optional

The list above also includes a number of popular nutritional practices—bicarbonate loading, carbohydrate loading, creatine and/or inosine loading, and water loading. (For a discussion of any of these supplements or practices, see the appropriate section in Part One or Part Three.)

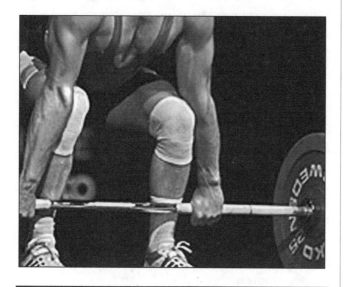

WEIGHTLIFTING

Pound for pound, Olympic weight lifters have more speed-strength than any other type of athlete does. In a study using the athletes at the Mexico City Olympics in 1964, sports scientists found that Olympic lifters were able to both vertical jump higher than any other athletes (including high jumpers) and run the 25-yard dash faster than any other athletes (including sprinters).

While some of a weight lifter's tremendous speed-strength comes from genetics, a good portion also comes from the specialized training. Weightlifting training includes many different kinds of lifts, but it revolves around two in particular—the snatch and the clean and jerk. These are two movements that are completed very quickly. If you ever want to become great at weightlifting, you need to not only lift the greatest load that you can, but you need to lift it as quickly as you can.

In weightlifting, the energy output is primarily anaerobic (without oxygen). This does not mean that training for or competing in weightlifting is easy, however. Weightlifting contests generally require the performance of six limit lifts (the lifting of maximum weight), with perhaps four times as many near-limit lifts done to warm up. On top of this, most contests last four hours or more. Training as a weight lifter is also intensive and grueling. At the highest levels, training for weightlifting forces you to operate at your anaerobic threshold (the point at which you must receive oxygen) for up to an hour and a half.

In weightlifting, the aim is to make the muscles as strong and as quick as possible. This calls for specialized training. Furthermore, the unique energy output of weightlifting requires the support of a carefully constructed nutrition program.

ENERGY SOURCES OF WEIGHT LIFTERS

The muscles rely on three major systems to supply the energy they need—the immediate, glycolytic, and oxidative energy systems. For short-term energy for explosive-strength output, the muscles depend on the immediate energy systems. The immediate energy systems are nonoxidative—they do not use oxygen. Instead, these systems generate energy through the use of adenosine triphosphate (ATP) and creatine phosphate (CP). CP is produced in the body and stored in the muscle fibers. It is broken down by enzymes to regenerate ATP, which is also stored in the muscle fibers. When the ATP is in turn broken down, the result is a spark of energy that triggers a muscle contraction.

For medium-term energy for repeated near-maximum exertion, the muscles turn to the glycolytic energy systems. In these systems, which are also nonoxidative, glycogen is used to produce energy. Glycogen is the storage form of glucose. It is stored in the liver and muscles, and is readily converted back to glucose when it is needed for energy.

For long-term energy for endurance activities, the muscles use the oxidative energy systems. In these systems, oxygen is used to oxidize long-chain fatty acids, protein, and glucose, which generates energy. For athletes, getting enough oxygen can mean a winning performance rather than a second-place showing.

Every sport involves a variety of skills, and each skill utilizes a unique combination of these three energy sources. The following table shows how much your body relies on each of the energy sources during an average weightlifting contest. Percentages are also given for an average warm-up and an average workout.

WHERE YOUR ENERGY COMES FROM

For Weight Lifters			
	Energy Systems		
	IMMEDIATE	**GLYCOLYTIC**	**OXIDATIVE**
Average contest	100%	0%	0%
Average precontest warm-up (1–3 reps per set)	100%	0%	0%
Average off-season workout (5–8 reps per set)	80%	20%	0%

When considering the type of nutritional support to give your training program, keep the following factors in mind:

☐ All athletes need to consume high-quality protein several times a day for effective recovery and adequate repair of damaged muscle tissue.

☐ Athletes whose muscles rely substantially on the immediate energy systems should keep their fat intake to a minimum because fat is not an efficient energy source for their intensive training, which is almost exclusively anaerobic in nature. Since the fat calories consumed by these athletes are not generally used for energy, they are stored as body fat.

☐ All athletes should consume a carefully measured amount of high-quality carbohydrates several times a day to ensure an adequate supply of energy.

☐ The carbohydrates in all preworkout meals should consist of foods with low glycemic indexes to ensure that training intensity does not wane and that muscle tissue is not cannibalized for energy. (For the glycemic indexes of some common foods, see page 29.)

The aim of your nutrition program is to make your body healthy enough to accomplish recovery and tissue repair speedily and efficiently—without adding body fat. Your further aims are to do this while maintaining a high strength-to-weight ratio plus remaining within 3 to 4 percent of your competition body weight. These aims alone make diet as critical as training for weight lifters. You must eat just the right amount of food. Eat the wrong foods or the wrong amounts just a few times too often and you will sabotage your fitness efforts. Even more important, do not be in a hurry. It takes *years* to become a great weight lifter. Rush the nutrition and training processes and you will become injured, not strong.

NUTRITION FOR WEIGHT LIFTERS

Weight lifters are power athletes. Their primary energy sources are the immediate energy systems. Therefore, as a weight lifter, you need to plan your nutritional intake, from both food and supplement sources, to support the immediate systems. In addition, since your energy expenditure changes in the off-season, you need to adjust your caloric intake and macronutrient ratio to match. Following are dietary guidelines for weight lifters to help you in planning your nutrition program. Supplementation guidelines for weight lifters can be found on page 333.

Dietary Guidelines

The following pie charts illustrate how you should divide up your caloric intake to match the energy demands of weightlifting during the preseason, season, and off-season. They show the target percentages of fat, protein, and carbohydrates that your five to six meals should supply each day.

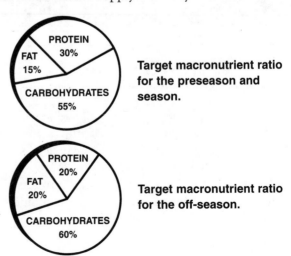

Target macronutrient ratio for the preseason and season.

Target macronutrient ratio for the off-season.

Note that fat has about 9 calories per gram, while protein and carbohydrates have only 4 calories per gram. Therefore, during the season, if you needed to consume a total of 2,500 calories per day, you would aim for 375 calories (15 percent of your total daily calories) from fat, 750 calories (30 percent of your total daily calories) from protein, and the remaining 1,375 calories (55 percent of your total daily calories) from carbohydrates.

Some other important considerations for weight lifters are:

☐ Carbohydrates are the major source of energy for short-term activities. Complex carbohydrates are the best source because they most effectively refill the glycogen stores in the muscles and liver. In addition, they elevate the blood sugar to a level sufficient for long sessions of intensive training.

☐ As a power athlete, you must make sure that you consume adequate amounts of both carbohydrates and protein. If your energy stores become drastically depleted or you experience lactic-acid buildup, you may suffer temporary muscle fatigue. If you do not refill your glycogen stores before your next workout or contest, your body may begin breaking down muscle tissue for the protein it needs for energy.

☐ Directly before workouts, consume carbohydrate drinks with high glycemic indexes to keep your blood sugar sustained at an appropriate level. This will allow you to train intensively without having your explosiveness hindered by fatigue.

☐ As a power athlete, you need to stimulate the storage of glycogen in your muscles while promoting repair and growth of your muscle tissue and inhibiting buildup of body fat. To do this:

• Train anaerobically on a regular basis. Intensive training stimulates increased storage of glycogen in the muscles and liver, which provides additional energy for greater exercise capacity.

• Consume five to six meals a day. Eating several smaller meals rather than three larger ones will keep your blood-sugar level stable throughout the day and will ensure that a supply of protein is always available for your muscles.

• Keep your fat intake to a minimum. Large amounts of fat in your diet will add to your body fat and will cause you to lose minerals through frequent urination.

• Consume low-glycemic-index foods about two to

three hours before workouts and contests. These foods help sustain the blood-sugar level.

• Drink plenty of water. Not only will this practice reduce your chances of becoming dehydrated, but every ounce of glycogen that is stored within the muscles needs 3 ounces of water stored along with it. Therefore, remaining properly hydrated will also help prevent weakened muscle contractions.

• Do not eat a new food just before a contest. Different people often react differently to the same food. Before a contest, eat just those foods that you know your body will handle well.

As a weight lifter, you should turn to Appendix C on page 345 for full discussions of the 15:30:55 and 20:20:60 dietary plans. Also presented are sample daily diets that use common, healthy foods to meet an athlete's energy and caloric needs. Use the directions on page 150 to estimate your average daily caloric requirement. Then use the directions in Chapter 13 or 14 to adjust your diet for off-season fat loss or muscle building, respectively.

Supplementation Guidelines

In addition to eating a proper diet, you should also take dietary supplements to make sure that any nutrients you lose due to sweating or training are replenished. The following tables will help guide you in selecting the supplements appropriate for you. The first table lists the nutrients recommended for weight lifters, as well as the range of intake for each nutrient. (For discussions of these nutrients, see Part One.) Note that within the ranges of intake, the lower amounts are for smaller individuals and lower-activity days, while the higher amounts are for larger individuals and higher-activity days.

RECOMMENDED NUTRIENTS AND RANGES OF INTAKE

For Weight Lifters

NUTRIENT	RANGE OF INTAKE
VITAMINS	
Vitamin A	8,000–16,000 IU
Beta-carotene	15,000–25,000 IU
Vitamin B_1 (thiamine)	30–120 mg
Vitamin B_2 (riboflavin)	30–120 mg
Vitamin B_3 (niacin)	40–80 mg
Vitamin B_5 (pantothenic acid)	20–100 mg

NUTRIENT	RANGE OF INTAKE
Vitamin B$_6$ (pyridoxine)	20–80 mg
Vitamin B$_{12}$ (cobalamin)	12–120 mcg
Biotin	125–175 mcg
Folate	400–800 mcg
Vitamin C	800–2,000 mg
Vitamin D	400–800 IU
Vitamin E	200–600 IU
Vitamin K	60–160 mcg
MINERALS	
Boron	2–8 mg
Calcium	800–1,500 mg
Chromium	200–500 mcg
Copper	1–4 mg
Iodine	100–200 mcg
Iron	15–50 mg
Magnesium	250–650 mg
Manganese	12–35 mg
Molybdenum	100–200 mcg
Phosphorus	150–800 mg
Potassium	50–1,000 mg
Selenium	100–200 mcg
Zinc	15–50 mg
AMINO ACIDS	
L-arginine	1,000–3,000 mg
L-glutamine	1,000–2,000 mg
L-ornithine	1,000–3,000 mg
FATTY ACIDS	
Alpha-linolenic acid	1,500–3,000 mg
Docosahexaenoic acid (DHA)	250–750 mg
Eiocosapentaenoic acid (EPA)	250–750 mg
Gamma linolenic acid (GLA)	100–400 mg
Linoleic acid	3,000–6,000 mg
METABOLITES	
Bioflavonoids	200–800 mg
Choline	100–600 mg
Creatine monohydrate	8,000–22,000 mg
Ferulic acid	50–100 mg
Inosine	1,000–2,000 mg
Inositol	100–600 mg
L-carnitine	1,000–2,000 mg
Octacosanol	1,000–3,000 mcg

IU = international units, mcg = micrograms, mg = milligrams.

The second table lists the different types of sports supplements available and indicates if their use by weight lifters is recommended in the preseason, during the season, or directly before a contest. The list also includes a number of popular nutritional practices—bicarbonate loading, carbohydrate loading, creatine and/or inosine loading, and water loading. (For a discussion of any of these supplements or practices, see the appropriate section in Part One or Part Three.)

RECOMMENDED SPORTS SUPPLEMENTS AND NUTRITIONAL PRACTICES

For Weight Lifters			
	Intake Recommendation		
	PRESEASON	SEASON	PRECONTEST
SUPPLEMENTS			
Multivitamins	Yes	Yes	No
Multiminerals	Yes	Yes	No
Antioxidants	Yes	Yes	No
Fatty acids	Yes	Yes	No
Metabolites	Optional	Yes	Yes
Branched-chain amino acids	Yes	Yes	Yes
Herbs	Yes	Yes	No
Low-calorie protein drink (200–300 calories)	Yes	Yes	Yes
Carbohydrate drink	Yes	Yes	Yes
Fat-burning supplement	Yes	Optional	No
PRACTICES			
Bicarbonate loading	No	Optional	Yes
Carbohydrate loading	No	No	No
Creatine and/or inosine loading	Optional	Yes	Yes
Water loading	No	No	No

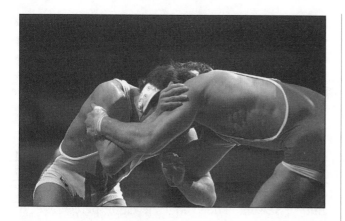

WRESTLING

Wrestling is a multifaceted sport that involves a wide range of skills and movements. There are several different styles of wrestling—such as collegiate, freestyle, and Greco-Roman—and they each require not only speed and strength in short, explosive bursts, but also a high level of anaerobic-strength endurance, as well as flexibility and agility.

Every bit of your training and diet must reflect these elements. These elements are what make wrestling explosive in nature. In fact, wrestling is very explosive, so improved recovery and tissue repair plus increased speed and strength are your year-round training and dietary goals. Nutritionally, this means emphasizing short-term energy needs and maximizing the muscles' recovery and tissue-repair processes.

In wrestling, the energy output is primarily anaerobic (without oxygen). This does not mean that training for or competing in wrestling is easy, however. You must push, pull, grapple, throw, and perform other lightning-quick reflexive movements over and over again, repeatedly testing your tolerance to pain and fatigue, caused by lactic-acid buildup in your muscles. The training for wrestling is extremely intensive and grueling. At the highest levels, it forces you to operate at your anaerobic threshold (the point at which you must receive oxygen).

Muscles grow when they are stressed. In wrestling, the aim is to make the muscles grow as strong and as quick as possible. This calls for specialized training. Furthermore, the incredible force output of wrestling requires the support of a carefully contructed nutrition program.

ENERGY SOURCES OF WRESTLERS

The muscles rely on three major systems to supply the energy they need—the immediate, glycolytic, and oxidative energy systems. For short-term energy for explosive-strength output, the muscles depend on the immediate energy systems. The immediate energy systems are nonoxidative—that is, they do not use oxygen. Instead, these systems generate energy through the use of adenosine triphosphate (ATP) and creatine phosphate (CP). CP is produced in the body and stored in the muscle fibers. It is broken down by enzymes to regenerate ATP, which is also stored in the muscle fibers. When the ATP is in turn broken down, the result is a spark of energy that triggers a muscle contraction.

For medium-term energy for repeated near-maximum exertion, the muscles turn to the glycolytic energy systems. In these systems, which are also nonxidative, glycogen is used to produce energy. Glycogen is the storage form of glucose. It is stored in the liver and muscles, and is readily converted back to glucose when it is needed for energy.

For long-term energy for endurance activities, the muscles use the oxidative energy systems. In these systems, oxygen is used to oxidize long-chain fatty acids, protein, and glucose, which generates energy. For athletes, getting enough oxygen can mean a winning performance rather than a second-place showing.

Every sport involves a variety of skills, and each skill utilizes a unique combination of these three energy sources. The following table shows how much your body relies on each of the energy sources during an average wrestling match. Percentages are also given for two kinds of average workouts.

WHERE YOUR ENERGY COMES FROM

For Wrestlers		
Energy Systems		
IMMEDIATE	GLYCOLYTIC	OXIDATIVE
Average match		
(any style) 40%	50%	10%
Average workouts		
Off-season 60%	30%	10%
Prematch 50%	40%	10%

When considering the type of nutritional support to

give your training program, keep the following factors in mind:

☐ All athletes need to consume high-quality protein several times a day for effective recovery and adequate repair of damaged muscle tissue.

☐ Athletes whose muscles rely substantially on the immediate or glycolytic energy systems should keep their fat intake to a minimum because fat is not an efficient energy source for their intensive training, which is almost exclusively anaerobic in nature. Since the fat calories consumed by these athletes are not generally used for energy, they are stored as body fat.

☐ All athletes should consume a carefully measured amount of high-quality carbohydrates several times a day to ensure an adequate supply of energy.

☐ The carbohydrates in all preworkout meals should consist of foods with low glycemic indexes to ensure that training intensity does not wane and that muscle tissue is not cannibalized for energy. (For the glycemic indexes of some common foods, see page 29.)

The aim of your nutrition program is to make your body healthy enough to accomplish recovery and tissue repair speedily and efficiently—without adding body fat. Your further aims are to do this while maintaining a high strength-to-weight ratio plus remaining within 3 to 4 percent of your competition body weight. These aims alone make diet as critical as training for wrestlers. You must eat just the right amount of food. Eat the wrong foods or the wrong amounts just a few times too often and you will sabotage your fitness efforts. Even more important, do not be in a hurry. It takes *years* to become a great wrestler. Rush the training and nutritional processes and you will become fat, your recovery rate will decline, and your injury rate will rise.

NUTRITION FOR WRESTLERS

Wrestlers are combination power–middle-distance athletes. They obtain most of their energy from a combination of the immediate and glycolytic energy systems. Therefore, as a wrestler, you need to plan your nutritional intake, from both food and supplement sources, to support these nonoxidative systems. In addition, since your energy expenditure changes in the preseason and off-season, you need

to adjust your caloric intake and macronutrient ratio to match. Following are dietary guidelines for wrestlers to help you in planning your nutrition program. Supplementation guidelines for wrestlers can be found on page 337.

Dietary Guidelines

The following pie charts illustrate how you should divide up your caloric intake to match the energy demands of wrestling during the preseason, season, and off-season. They show the target percentages of fat, protein, and carbohydrates that your five to six meals should supply each day.

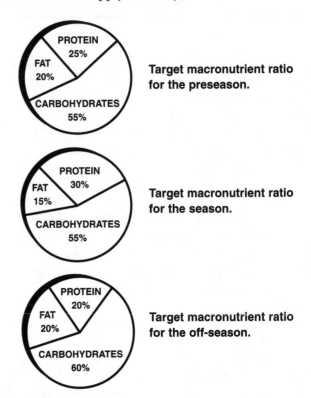

Target macronutrient ratio for the preseason.

Target macronutrient ratio for the season.

Target macronutrient ratio for the off-season.

Note that fat has about 9 calories per gram, while protein and carbohydrates have only 4 calories per gram. Therefore, during the season, if you needed to consume a total of 2,500 calories per day, you would aim for 375 calories (15 percent of your total daily calories) from fat, 750 calories (30 percent of your total daily calories) from protein, and the remaining 1,375 calories (55 percent of your total daily calories) from carbohydrates.

Some other important considerations for wrestlers are:

☐ Carbohydrates are the major source of energy for

short-term activities. Complex carbohydrates are the best source because they most effectively refill the glycogen stores in the muscles and liver. In addition, they elevate the blood sugar to a level sufficient for long sessions of intensive training.

☐ As a combination power–middle-distance athlete, you must make sure that you consume adequate amounts of both carbohydrates and protein. If your energy stores become drastically depleted or you experience lactic-acid buildup, you may suffer temporary muscle fatigue. If you do not refill your glycogen stores before your next workout or match, your body may begin breaking down muscle tissue for the protein it needs for energy.

☐ Directly before workouts, consume carbohydrate drinks with high glycemic indexes to keep your blood sugar sustained at an appropriate level. This will allow you to train intensively for longer periods of time.

☐ As a combination power-middle-distance athlete, you need to stimulate the storage of glycogen in your muscles while promoting repair and growth of your muscle tissue and inhibiting buildup of body fat. To do this:

• Train against your anaerobic threshold (to exhaustion) on a regular basis. Intensive, exhaustive training stimulates increased storage of glycogen in the muscles and liver, which provides additional energy for greater exercise capacity.

• Consume five to six meals a day. Eating several smaller meals rather than three larger ones will keep your blood-sugar level stable throughout the day and will ensure that a supply of protein is always available for your muscles.

• Keep your fat intake to a minimum. Large amounts of fat in your diet will add to your body fat and will cause mineral loss through frequent urination.

• Consume low-glycemic-index foods about two to three hours before workouts and matches. These foods help sustain the blood-sugar level.

• Drink plenty of water. Not only will this practice reduce your chances of becoming dehydrated, but every ounce of glycogen that is stored within the muscles needs 3 ounces of water stored along with it. Therefore, remaining properly hydrated will also help prevent weakened muscle contractions and early onset of fatigue.

• Do not eat a new food just before a match. Different people often react differently to the same food. Before a match, eat just those foods that you know your body will handle well.

As a wrestler, you should turn to Appendix C on page 345 for full discussions of the 20:25:55, 15:30:55, and 20:20:60 dietary plans. Also presented are sample daily diets that use common, healthy foods to meet an athlete's energy and caloric needs. Use the directions on page 150 to estimate your average daily caloric requirement. Then use the directions in Chapter 13 or 14 to adjust your diet for off-season fat loss or muscle building, respectively.

Supplementation Guidelines

In addition to eating a proper diet, you should also take dietary supplements to make sure that any nutrients you lose due to sweating or training are replenished. The following tables will help guide you in selecting the supplements appropriate for you. The first table lists the nutrients recommended for wrestlers, as well as the range of intake for each nutrient. (For discussions of these nutrients, see Part One.) Note that within the ranges of intake, the lower amounts are for smaller individuals and lower-activity days, while the higher amounts are for larger individuals and higher-activity days.

RECOMMENDED NUTRIENTS AND RANGES OF INTAKE

For Wrestlers	
NUTRIENT	RANGE OF INTAKE
VITAMINS	
Vitamin A	8,000–16,000 IU
Beta-carotene	15,000–25,000 IU
Vitamin B$_1$ (thiamine)	30–120 mg
Vitamin B$_2$ (riboflavin)	30–120 mg
Vitamin B$_3$ (niacin)	40–80 mg
Vitamin B$_5$ (pantothenic acid)	20–100 mg
Vitamin B$_6$ (pyridoxine)	20–80 mg
Vitamin B$_{12}$ (cobalamin)	12–120 mcg
Biotin	125–175 mcg
Folate	400–800 mcg
Vitamin C	800–2,000 mg
Vitamin D	400–800 IU
Vitamin E	200–600 IU
Vitamin K	60–160 mcg

NUTRIENT	RANGE OF INTAKE
MINERALS	
Boron	2–8 mg
Calcium	800–1,500 mg
Chromium	200–500 mcg
Copper	1–4 mg
Iodine	100–200 mcg
Iron	15–50 mg
Magnesium	250–650 mg
Manganese	12–35 mg
Molybdenum	100–200 mcg
Phosphorus	150–800 mg
Potassium	50–1,000 mg
Selenium	100–200 mcg
Zinc	15–50 mg
AMINO ACIDS	
L-glutamine	1,000–2,000 mg
FATTY ACIDS	
Alpha-linolenic acid	1,500–3,000 mg
Docosahexaenoic acid (DHA)	250–750 mg
Eiocosapentaenoic acid (EPA)	250–750 mg
Gamma linolenic acid (GLA)	100–400 mg
Linoleic acid	3,000–6,000 mg
METABOLITES	
Bioflavonoids	200–800 mg
Choline	100–600 mg
Creatine monohydrate	8,000–22,000 mg
Ferulic acid	30–60 mg
Inosine	500–1,000 mg
Inositol	100–600 mg
L-carnitine	750–2,000 mg
Octacosanol	6,000–12,000 mcg

IU = international units, mcg = micrograms, mg = milligrams.

The second table lists the different types of sports supplements available and indicates if their use by wrestlers is recommended in the preseason, during the season, or directly before a match. The list also includes a number of popular nutritional practices—bicarbonate loading, carbohydrate loading, creatine and/or inosine loading, and water loading. (For a discussion of any of these supplements or practices, see the appropriate section in Part One or Part Three.)

RECOMMENDED SPORTS SUPPLEMENTS AND NUTRITIONAL PRACTICES

For Wrestlers

	Intake Recommendation		
	PRESEASON	SEASON	PREMATCH
SUPPLEMENTS			
Multivitamins	Yes	Yes	No
Multiminerals	Yes	Yes	No
Antioxidants	Yes	Yes	No
Fatty acids	Yes	Yes	No
Metabolites	Optional	Yes	Yes
Branched-chain amino acids	Yes	Yes	Yes
Herbs	Yes	Yes	No
Low-calorie protein drink (200–300 calories)	Yes	Yes	Yes
Carbohydrate drink	Yes	Yes	Yes
Fat-burning supplement	Yes	Optional	No
PRACTICES			
Bicarbonate loading	No	Optional	Yes
Carbohydrate loading	No	No	No
Creatine and/or inosine loading	Optional	Yes	Yes
Water loading	No	No	No

APPENDIX

A. PERSONAL INVENTORY

Use this inventory sheet to record your weight, lean factor, body composition, basal metabolic rate, and caloric and protein requirements. Keeping these parameters up-to-date and handy will allow you to continually fine-tune your diet to meet your individual needs. You will also need the information if you decide to custom-design a diet for fat loss or muscle gain, as described in Chapters 13 and 14, respectively.

If desired, make photocopies of this blank inventory sheet and fill in a clean copy whenever you make new calculations. Keep all the copies—blank and completed—in a looseleaf binder, along with your Hourly Caloric Breakdown Chart sheets (see page 343), Daily Nutrition Log sheets (see page 373), training and competition records, and anything else that helps you in your performance-improvement efforts.

Name_____ Date_____

Total body weight .... _____

Lean body mass (from page 143) .... _____

Body fat (from page 143) .... _____

Body-fat percentage (from page 143) .... _____

Lean-body-mass percentage (from page 143) .... _____

Basal metabolic rate (from page 149) .... _____

Lean factor (from page 152) .... _____

Lean-factor multiplier (from page 152) .... _____

Average daily caloric requirement, Hour-by-Hour Method (from page 150) .. _____

Average daily caloric requirement, Daily Caloric Requirement Guide (from page 153):

When your activity level is 130 percent...................................... _____

When your activity level is 155 percent...................................... _____

When your activity level is 165 percent .... _____

When your activity level is 200 percent...................................... _____

When your activity level is 230 percent...................................... _____

Daily protein requirement (from page 46) .... _____

B. HOURLY CALORIC BREAKDOWN CHART

Use this chart to estimate your daily caloric expenditure, as explained on page 150. You need to know your daily caloric expenditure to determine your daily caloric intake.

If desired, make photocopies of this blank chart and fill in a clean copy whenever you need to make new calcu-lations. Keep all the copies—blank and completed—in a looseleaf binder, along with your Personal Inventory sheets (see page 341), Daily Nutrition Log sheets (see page 373), training and competition records, and anything else that helps you in your performance-improvement efforts.

Hour	Activity	Percent of BMR	Calories Used
Midnight–1 A.M.			
1–2 A.M.			
2–3 A.M.			
3–4 A.M.			
4–5 A.M.			
5–6 A.M.			
6–7 A.M.			
7–8 A.M.			
8–9 A.M.			
9–10 A.M.			
10–11 A.M.			
11 A.M.–Noon			
Noon–1 P.M.			
1–2 P.M.			
2–3 P.M.			
3–4 P.M.			
4–5 P.M.			
5–6 P.M.			
6–7 P.M.			
7–8 P.M.			
8–9 P.M.			
9–10 P.M.			
10–11 P.M.			
11 P.M.–Midnight			
		Daily total	

C. MEETING YOUR MACRONUTRIENT RATIO

No matter what sport or fitness activity you participate in, your sport-specific plan in Part Four recommends that you consume a diet composed of a certain macronutrient ratio to help maximize your athletic performance. Some of the plans recommend consuming just one diet all year round, while others suggest following two or three different diets during the year. The diets are recommended according to the sport or activity, the energy systems the body primarily uses when participating in the sport or activity, and the season of the athletic year.

Altogether, four different diets are recommended in the twenty-eight sport-specific plans. The diets, as well as the rationales behind them, are as follows:

☐ *The 15:30:55 diet plan.* This diet is for individuals who participate in sports or fitness activities that require explosive strength and power. When training or playing, these individuals rely primarily on the immediate and glycolytic energy systems. They use their large muscles, which are composed mainly of fast-twitch muscle fibers. Because of this, these athletes need to consume large amounts of protein to maintain a positive nitrogen balance and to repair their fragile fast-twitch muscle fibers. A low fat intake and high carbohydrate intake are also recommended, since muscle glycogen is the primary source for replenishing the ATP and CP stores.

☐ *The 20:25:55 diet plan.* This diet is for individuals who participate in sports or fitness activities that require explosive strength and power on a sustained or highly repetitive basis. When training or playing, these individuals rely primarily on the glycolytic energy systems. Muscle glycogen is their primary source of energy. These athletes need to consume large amounts of protein to maintain a positive nitrogen balance and to repair their fragile fast-twitch muscle fibers.

☐ *The 20:20:60 diet plan.* The same as the 20:25:55 diet plan, this diet is for individuals who participate in sports or fitness activities that require explosive strength and power on a sustained or highly repetitive basis. However, while these individuals rely to some extent on the glycolytic energy systems while training or playing, they depend primarily on the oxidative systems. Fatty acids as well as muscle glycogen are their primary sources of energy. Therefore, these athletes need to consume just moderate amounts of protein to maintain a positive nitrogen balance and to repair their fragile fast-twitch muscle fibers.

☐ *The 25:15:60 diet plan.* This diet is for individuals who participate in aerobic sports or fitness activities. When training or playing, these individuals rely primarily on the oxidative energy systems. Their muscles are composed mainly of slow-twitch muscle fibers. Because of this, these athletes need to consume large amounts of carbohydrates to maintain their glycogen stores. Fatty acids are their primary source of energy, so they should consume a moderate amount of fat. The amount of protein that this group consumes is the lowest of the four plans, but it is still about two times more than nonathletes eat.

Meeting these ratios does not require superior intelligence or cunning. However, it does take a little bit of work, and to make that work easier for you, we have done some of it for you. To achieve your recommended macronutrient ratio, as well as your recommended daily caloric and protein totals, you need to plan your diet. For most people, this means sitting down with a piece of paper and a pencil and figuring out their menus. Some people do this in the morning for the coming day; some do it at night for the next day. Some people plan a whole week's menus in advance, and some check labels and reference books for food counts as they stand in front of the open refrigerator looking for the components of a meal or snack. No matter what method you use, however, you must keep track of your calories and your grams of fat, protein, and carbohydrates. Furthermore, at the end of the day, you need to calculate what percentages of the macronutrients you consumed. To help, we have put together lists of the most common foods in the major food categories. (For the lists, see Tables C.1 through C.8 on pages 347 to 356.) We have also provided space at the end of each list to allow you to add items and personalize the lists according to your special dietary needs and preferences. The basic lists are intended to help you get started. The foods, for the most part, are wholesome and readily available in grocery stores. To make the lists functional for you, add your favorite foods to them, including appropriate serving sizes and calorie, protein, carbohydrate, and fat counts. Many packaged foods have all the nutritional information you need right on the label, in the Nutrition Facts box. For the foods that do not have such labels, use a nutritional reference guide such as *The NutriBase Complete Book of Food Counts*, by Dr. Art Ulene. All diets can be accommodated using this method. If you are vegetarian or hypoglycemic, if you have a food allergy, or if you should restrict the intake of a substance such as sodium, just remove the offending foods from the lists and substitute your own. (If you have a medical condition, we strongly recommend that you discuss your proposed diet with your health-care practitioner and get his or her approval of your completed food lists.)

To show you how to turn your food lists into a day's worth of delicious meals that meet your caloric and macronutrient goals, we have also put together sample daily diets for each target macronutrient ratio. (For the diets, see Tables C.9 through C.16 on pages 357 to 372.) The sample daily diets demonstrate how to spread out your calories. Each meal does not need to equal the exact macronutrient ratio. For example, if you are following the 15:30:55 diet, you do not need to consume 15-percent fat, 30-percent protein, and 55-percent carbohydrates at each meal. This ratio is your goal for the *day*. Rather, your main concern at each meal is your carbohydrate intake. On training days, you should plan your diet to supply more carbohydrates around your training sessions. A good approach is to first determine how many calories are supplied by your carbohydrate drink, which you should ingest before, during, and/or after training. Next, determine your morning and afternoon (pretraining) snacks and their macronutrient contents. Finally, figure out your breakfast, lunch, and dinner. Note

that diets of two caloric totals—2,500 calories per day and 3,500 calories per day—are included for each target macronutrient ratio. We chose these two caloric totals because most people who participate in sports or fitness activities should consume diets of this caloric range. If your recommended daily caloric intake should total more or less than this range, you can easily add or subtract foods from the sample diets. (For instructions, see "The Targeted Fat Loss Program" on page 164.) Individuals with enormous caloric requirements, such as 5,000 or 7,000 calories per day, can simply double the portions in the sample diets.

At the same time that you strive to meet your target caloric total and macronutrient ratio, you should not become overly concerned if you have trouble finding foods to exactly meet your goals. It is okay to be flexible. In fact, when scientists calculate the energy and macronutrient contents of foods, they by necessity must make a lot of assumptions, which means that the nutritional-content information of foods is never exact. In fact, a margin of error of up to 10 percent is typical, with up to 20 percent not unheard of.

When following a diet plan, do not torment yourself if you occasionally deviate from it. Just return to the plan with your next meal. To keep the deviations to a minimum, though, you will need to prepare. Make sure that your refrigerator and pantry are well stocked with the foods you should eat. Throw out the foods that you should avoid. Buy a lunch box or a package of paper bags, since meeting your daily nutrition goals may require brown bagging lunch to work or snacks to the gym.

If desired, make photocopies of the basic food lists and sample daily diets, and keep them in a looseleaf binder along with your Personal Inventory sheets (see page 341), Hourly Caloric Breakdown Chart sheets (see page 343), Daily Nutrition Log sheets (see page 373), training and competition records, and anything else that helps you in your performance-improvement efforts. When you run out of the blank lines for adding your favorite foods, use looseleaf paper. When eating out or dining at a friend's house, take the notebook—or just the lists—with you to consult before ordering or deciding which foods to eat. With a little planning and preparation, success can be yours—in the kitchen and on the playing field.

Table C.1. High-Protein Foods (Beef, Pork, Poultry, and Fish)

FOOD	SERVING SIZE	CALORIES	PROTEIN (GRAMS)	CARBS (GRAMS)	FAT (GRAMS)
ABALONE, MIXED SPECIES, raw	3 oz.	89	14.5	5.1	0.7
BACON, ALTERNATIVE, turkey (Louis Rich) heated	1 slice	32	2.4	0.3	2.4
BACON, CANADIAN-STYLE, cured, grilled	2 slices	86	11.3	0.6	3.9
BACON BITS (Hormel)	1 oz.	117	12.0	1.0	7.0
BASS, FRESHWATER, MIXED SPECIES, raw	1 oz.	32	5.3	0.0	1.0
BASS, SEA, MIXED SPECIES, raw	1 oz.	27	5.2	0.0	0.6
BEEF					
bottom round, prime, trimmed, ½-in. fat, raw	1 oz.	45	6.2	0.0	2.1
bottom round, prime, untrimmed, ½-in. fat, raw	1 oz.	64	5.7	0.0	4.4
flank, choice, untrimmed, 0-in. fat, raw	1 oz.	51	5.6	0.0	3.0
tenderloin, choice, untrimmed, ¼-in. fat, raw	1 oz.	82	5.0	0.0	6.7
top sirloin, prime, trimmed, ½-in. fat, raw	1 oz.	44	6.0	0.0	2.0
BEEF, CORNED (Hillshire Farm)	1 oz.	31	6.0	<1.0	0.4
BLUEFISH, raw	1 oz.	35	5.7	0.0	1.2
BUFFALO, AMERICAN, raw	1 oz.	31	6.1	0.0	0.5
BURGER, VEGETARIAN (Green Giant)					
frozen "Harvest Burger" original flavor	1 burger	140	18.0	8.0	4.0
CHICKEN, BROILER-FRYER					
breast meat and skin, raw	1 oz.	49	5.9	0.0	2.6
breast meat only, raw	1 oz.	31	6.5	0.0	0.4
COD, ATLANTIC, raw	1 oz.	23	5.0	0.0	0.2
DEER, raw	1 oz.	34	6.4	0.0	0.7
EGG, ALTERNATIVE (Fleischmann's)					
"Egg Beaters" vegetable omelet	½ cup	50	7.0	5.0	0.0
EGG, CHICKEN, raw, fresh or frozen	1 large	75	6.3	0.6	5.0
EGG WHITE, CHICKEN, raw, fresh or frozen	1 large	17	3.5	0.3	0.0
FLOUNDER, raw	3 oz.	77	16.0	0.0	1.0
FRANKFURTER (Healthy Choice) turkey,					
pork, or beef "Jumbo" lowfat	1 frank	70	8.0	5.0	2.0
HALIBUT, Atlantic, raw	1 oz.	31	5.9	0.0	0.6
HAM, FRESH, leg, rump half, trimmed, raw	1 oz.	39	6.0	0.0	1.5
LUNCHEON MEAT					
chicken, breast (Tyson) hickory smoked	1 slice	25	4.0	0.8	1.0
ham (Kahn's)	1 slice	30	5.0	1.0	1.0
roast beef (Healthy Deli)	1 oz.	30	6.4	0.2	0.4
turkey (Tyson)	1 slice	20	4.0	0.3	0.4
PORK					
chop (Master Choice)	1 chop	120	22.0	0.0	4.0
tenderloin, trimmed, raw	1 oz.	34	5.9	0.0	1.0
TOFU, raw	1 oz.	22	2.3	0.5	1.4
TUNA, BLUEFIN, raw	1 oz.	41	6.6	0.0	1.4
TUNA, CANNED					
light, in soybean oil, solid, drained (Star-Kist)	2 oz.	150	13.0	<1.0	13.0
white, in water, chunk, diet, drained (Star-Kist)	2 oz.	70	15.0	<1.0	1.0
TURKEY, ALL CLASSES					
dark meat only, raw	1 oz.	35	5.7	0.0	1.2
light meat only, raw	1 oz.	33	6.7	0.0	0.4

Use the chart below to fill in the foods you most commonly eat. This will help provide you with nutritional guidelines for your own personalized training diet.

FOOD	SERVING SIZE	CALORIES	PROTEIN (GRAMS)	CARBS (GRAMS)	FAT (GRAMS)

Table C.2. High-Complex-Carbohydrate Foods (Breads, Crackers, Cereals, Grains, Starchy Vegetables, and Starchy Fruits)

FOOD	SERVING SIZE	CALORIES	PROTEIN (GRAMS)	CARBS (GRAMS)	FAT (GRAMS)
BAGEL					
onion, 3½-in. diam.	1 bagel	195	7.5	37.9	1.1
plain, 3½-in. diam.	1 bagel	195	7.5	37.9	1.1
BAGEL, FROZEN, plain (*Lender's*) 2 oz.	1 bagel	150	6.0	30.0	1.0
BAGEL CHIP (*Burns & Ricker*) "Original Bagel Crisps"	1 oz.	130	4.0	20.0	4.0
BISCUIT, plain or buttermilk, commercially baked	1 oz.	103	1.8	13.8	4.7
BREAD					
bran (*Oroweat*) "Bran'nola" original, natural	1 slice	100	4.0	19.0	1.0
French, enriched	1 oz.	78	2.5	14.7	0.9
grain (*Arnold*) "Bran'nola"	1 slice	85	3.9	17.4	1.6
rye (*Pepperidge Farm*) "Family" seeded or seedless	1 slice	80	3.0	16.0	1.0
white (*Wonder*) plain	1 slice	70	3.0	13.0	1.0
whole wheat (*Oroweat*) stoneground, 100%	1 slice	60	3.0	11.0	1.0
BUN, FRANKFURTER, plain	1 bun	123	3.7	21.6	2.2
BUN, HAMBURGER, plain	1 bun	123	3.7	21.6	2.2
CAKE					
chocolate (*Sara Lee*) frozen "Free & Light"	⅛ cake	110	2.0	26.0	0.0
pound (*Sara Lee*) frozen "Free & Light"	¹⁄₁₀ cake	70	1.0	17.0	0.0
CEREAL					
(*General Mills*) "Basic 4"	¾ cup	130	3.0	28.0	2.0
(*General Mills*) "Multi Grain Cheerios"	1 oz.	100	2.0	23.0	1.0
(*Kellogg's*) "All Bran" extra fiber	1 oz.	50	4.0	22.0	0.0
(*Kellogg's*) "Corn Flakes"	1 oz.	110	2.3	24.4	0.1
(*Post*) "Grape-Nuts" wheat and barley	1 oz.	101	3.3	23.3	0.1
CRACKER, saltine (*Premium*) "Fat-Free" ½ oz.	4 crackers	50	1.0	12.0	0.0
ENGLISH MUFFIN (*Thomas'*) plain	1 muffin	130	4.3	25.4	1.3
GRITS, white (*Arrowhead Mills*) dry	2 oz.	200	5.0	43.0	1.0
OATMEAL, instant (*Arrowhead Mills*)	1 oz.	100	5.8	18.0	2.0
PANCAKE MIX					
buttermilk (*Hungry Jack*) prepared w/skim milk/oil/egg whites, 4-in. diam.	3 pancakes	200	6.0	28.0	7.0
extra light (*Hungry Jack*) prepared w/skim milk/oil/egg whites, 4-in. diam.	3 pancakes	170	6.0	28.0	4.0
PASTA, linguine or spaghetti, Jerusalem artichoke (*DeBoles*) dry	2 oz.	210	9.0	41.0	1.0
POPCORN, MICROWAVE					
butter flavor, light (*Jolly Time*) popped	3 cups	60	2.0	12.0	2.0
natural (*Jiffy Pop*) popped	4 cups	140	3.0	17.0	7.0
POTATO					
baked in skin	4 oz.	124	2.6	28.6	0.1
boiled in skin, pulp only	4 oz.	99	2.1	22.8	0.1
PRETZELS (*Featherweight*) "Low Salt"	20 pretzels	110	3.0	23.0	1.0
RICE, BROWN, long grain, dry	1 oz.	105	2.3	21.9	0.8
RICE, WHITE, long grain, unenriched, dry	1 oz.	103	2.0	22.7	0.2

FOOD	SERVING SIZE	CALORIES	PROTEIN (GRAMS)	CARBS (GRAMS)	FAT (GRAMS)
ROLL					
hoagie *(Pepperidge Farm)* soft "Deli Classic"	1 roll	210	8.0	34.0	5.0
kaiser *(Arnold)* "Francisco"	1 roll	184	7.0	35.4	2.9
sandwich *(Arnold)* egg "Dutch"	1 roll	123	4.5	21.6	3.3
SWEET POTATO, baked in skin, pulp only	4 oz.	117	2.0	27.5	0.1

Use the chart below to fill in the foods you most commonly eat. This will help provide you with nutritional guidelines for your own personalized training diet.

FOOD	SERVING SIZE	CALORIES	PROTEIN (GRAMS)	CARBS (GRAMS)	FAT (GRAMS)

Table C.3. Combination High-Protein and High-Carbohydrate Foods

FOOD	SERVING SIZE	CALORIES	PROTEIN (GRAMS)	CARBS (GRAMS)	FAT (GRAMS)
BEEF, CORNED, HASH, canned *(Libby's)* "24 oz. can"	8 oz.	420	19.0	21.0	28.0
CHILI, CANNED					
chicken, w/beans *(Stagg)*	7½ oz.	200	14.0	21.0	6.0
vegetarian *(Health Valley)* 3-bean, mild, fat-free	5 oz.	90	10.0	12.0	0.0
PIZZA, FRENCH BREAD, FROZEN					
(Lean Cuisine) three cheese	5½ oz.	330	23.0	38.0	10.0
POWER BAR	1 bar	230	10.0	45.0	2.5
PROTEIN NUTRITION BAR					
low calorie	1 bar	225	30.0	15.0	5.0
medium calorie	1 bar	470	40.0	64.0	6.0
high calorie	1 bar	548	30.0	80.0	12.0
SNACK/FOOD BAR					
(Bear Valley) "Pemmician" carob-cocoa, 3¾ oz.	1 bar	440	16.0	68.0	12.0
(Earth Grains) "Bagel Power Bar"					
banana apple walnut	1 bar	270	12.0	45.0	6.0
(Health Valley) raspberry, fat-free	1 bar	140	3.0	33.0	0.0

Use the chart below to fill in the foods you most commonly eat. This will help provide you with nutritional guidelines for your own personalized training diet.

FOOD	SERVING SIZE	CALORIES	PROTEIN (GRAMS)	CARBS (GRAMS)	FAT (GRAMS)

Table C.4. Vegetables and Beans

FOOD	SERVING SIZE	CALORIES	PROTEIN (GRAMS)	CARBS (GRAMS)	FAT (GRAMS)
ADZUKI BEAN, raw	1 oz.	93	5.6	17.8	0.2
ARUGULA, raw	1 leaf	1	0.1	0.1	0.0
ASPARAGUS, FROZEN, cuts or spears (Birds Eye)	3.3 oz.	25	3.0	4.0	0.0
BAKED BEANS, CANNED					
barbecue (B&M)	8 oz.	260	15.0	48.0	6.0
in tomato sauce (Campbell's)	8 oz.	200	10.0	43.0	3.0
pea, small (Friends)	8 oz.	360	17.0	62.0	4.0
pork and beans (Bush's Best) "Showboat"	8 oz.	160	12.0	38.0	<1.0
vegetarian (B&M)	8 oz.	230	14.0	50.0	3.0
BLACK BEAN, raw	1 oz.	97	6.1	17.7	0.4
BROCCOLI, raw, trimmed	1 oz.	8	0.8	1.5	0.1
BROCCOLI, FROZEN, spears, whole					
(Birds Eye) "Farm Fresh"	4 oz.	30	4.0	6.0	0.0
CABBAGE, raw, trimmed	1 oz.	7	0.3	1.5	0.1
CARROT, raw, trimmed	1 oz.	12	0.3	2.9	0.1
CAULIFLOWER, raw, trimmed	1 oz.	7	0.6	1.4	0.1
CELERY, raw, trimmed	1 oz.	5	0.2	1.0	<.1
CORN, FROZEN (Health Valley)	½ cup	76	2.0	17.0	0.0
GARBANZO BEAN, raw	1 oz.	103	5.5	17.2	1.7
LETTUCE					
iceberg, trimmed	1 oz.	4	0.3	0.6	0.1
romaine, trimmed	1 oz.	5	0.5	0.7	0.1
LIMA BEAN, raw, trimmed	1 oz.	32	1.9	5.7	0.2
LIMA BEAN, FROZEN (Green Giant) "Harvest Fresh"	½ cup	80	6.0	18.0	0.0
ONION, raw, trimmed	1 oz.	11	0.3	2.4	<.1
SPINACH, raw, chopped	1 oz.	6	0.8	1.0	0.1
TOMATO, raw, 2⅝ in. diam., 4¾ oz.	1 med.	26	1.0	5.7	0.4

Use the chart below to fill in the foods you most commonly eat. This will help provide you with nutritional guidelines for your own personalized training diet.

FOOD	SERVING SIZE	CALORIES	PROTEIN (GRAMS)	CARBS (GRAMS)	FAT (GRAMS)

Table C.5. Fruits

FOOD	SERVING SIZE	CALORIES	PROTEIN (GRAMS)	CARBS (GRAMS)	FAT (GRAMS)
APRICOT, pitted	1 oz.	14	0.4	3.2	0.1
APRICOT, DRIED (Del Monte)	2 oz.	140	2.0	35.0	0.0
BANANA, w/o skin and seeds	1 fruit	105	1.2	26.7	0.6
BLUEBERRY, trimmed	1 oz.	16	0.2	4.0	0.1
FRUIT COCKTAIL, CANNED in light syrup	4 oz.	65	0.5	16.9	0.1
GRAPEFRUIT, pink or red, Florida, fresh (Ocean Spray)	½ med.	50	1.0	13.0	0.0
ORANGE, all commercial varieties, approx. 2⅝ in. diam.	1 med.	62	1.2	15.4	0.2

Use the chart below to fill in the foods you most commonly eat. This will help provide you with nutritional guidelines for your own personalized training diet.

FOOD	SERVING SIZE	CALORIES	PROTEIN (GRAMS)	CARBS (GRAMS)	FAT (GRAMS)

Table C.6. Dairy Products

FOOD	SERVING SIZE	CALORIES	PROTEIN (GRAMS)	CARBS (GRAMS)	FAT (GRAMS)
BUTTER, REGULAR, salted	1 tbsp.	100	0.1	0.0	11.4
CHEESE					
American *(Kraft)* "Deluxe Slices"	1 oz.	110	6.0	1.0	9.0
Cheddar, American domestic	1 oz.	113	7.0	0.4	9.3
cottage cheese, creamed, large curd	4 oz.	117	14.1	3.0	5.1
cottage cheese, creamed, lowfat 2%	1 oz.	25	3.9	1.0	0.5
cottage cheese, creamed, lowfat 1%	1 oz.	20	3.5	0.8	0.3
cream cheese *(Healthy Choice)* fat-free	1 oz.	30	6.0	2.0	0.0
cream cheese, natural	1 oz.	98	2.1	0.7	9.8
Parmesan, grated, natural	1 oz.	128	11.6	1.0	8.4
Swiss, domestic	1 oz.	105	8.0	1.0	7.7
MILK, COW'S, FLUID					
whole *(Borden)*	8 oz.	150	8.0	11.0	8.0
2% fat	8 oz.	121	8.1	11.7	4.7
1% fat	8 oz.	102	8.0	11.7	2.6
skim	8 oz.	86	8.4	11.9	0.4
YOGURT					
mixed berries *(Breyers)* "Lowfat"	8 oz.	250	9.0	48.0	2.0
plain *(Dannon)* "Lowfat"	8 oz.	140	10.0	16.0	4.0
plain *(Dannon)* "Nonfat"	8 oz.	110	11.0	16.0	0.0

Use the chart below to fill in the foods you most commonly eat. This will help provide you with nutritional guidelines for your own personalized training diet.

FOOD	SERVING SIZE	CALORIES	PROTEIN (GRAMS)	CARBS (GRAMS)	FAT (GRAMS)

Table C.7. Condiments, Spreads, and Sauces

FOOD	SERVING SIZE	CALORIES	PROTEIN (GRAMS)	CARBS (GRAMS)	FAT (GRAMS)
APPLESAUCE *(Mott's)* "Natural"	6 oz.	80	0.0	20.0	0.0
CATSUP	1 tbsp.	16	0.2	4.1	0.1
MARGARINE *(Land O'Lakes)*	1 tsp.	35	0.0	0.0	4.0
MAYONNAISE *(Hellmann's)*	1 tbsp.	100	0.0	0.0	11.0
MUSTARD, yellow *(French's)*	1 tbsp.	10	1.0	1.0	1.0
OLIVE OIL *(Hain)*	1 tbsp.	120	0.0	0.0	14.0
PANCAKE SYRUP					
(Hungry Jack) "Lite"	2 tbsp.	50	0.0	14.0	0.0
(Hungry Jack) regular	2 tbsp.	100	0.0	26.0	0.0
SAFFLOWER OIL *(Hain)* "Hi-Oleic"	1 tbsp.	120	0.0	0.0	14.0
SALAD DRESSING					
blue cheese *(Kraft)* "Free"	1 tbsp.	16	0.0	4.0	0.0
blue cheese *(Wish-Bone)* chunky	1 tbsp.	75	0.4	0.7	7.9
French *(Kraft)* "Reduced Calorie"	1 tbsp.	20	0.0	3.0	1.0
Italian *(Wish-Bone)*	1 tbsp.	46	0.0	1.5	4.5
oil and vinegar *(Seven Seas)* "Viva Red Wine!"	1 tbsp.	45	0.0	1.0	4.0
SAUCE					
pasta sauce *(Hunt's)* "Homestyle"	4 oz.	60	2.0	10.0	2.0
pasta sauce, mushroom *(Ragu)* "Thick & Hearty"	4 oz.	100	2.0	15.0	3.0
steak sauce *(A.1)*	1 tbsp.	18	0.0	4.0	0.0

Use the chart below to fill in the foods you most commonly eat. This will help provide you with nutritional guidelines for your own personalized training diet.

FOOD	SERVING SIZE	CALORIES	PROTEIN (GRAMS)	CARBS (GRAMS)	FAT (GRAMS)

Table C.8. Beverages

FOOD	SERVING SIZE	CALORIES	PROTEIN (GRAMS)	CARBS (GRAMS)	FAT (GRAMS)
APPLE GRAPE JUICE *(Red Cheek)*	6 oz.	109	0.3	27.0	0.0
APPLE JUICE					
(Knudsen & Sons) "Natural"	8 oz.	85	<1.0	21.0	0.0
(Ocean Spray)	6 oz.	90	0.0	23.0	0.0
CARBOHYDRATE SPORTS DRINK					
low calorie	8 oz.	50	0.0	13.0	0.0
medium calorie	8 oz.	100	0.0	25.0	0.0
high calorie	8 oz.	200	0.0	50.0	0.0
CRANBERRY JUICE *(Knudsen & Sons)* "Yankee"	8 oz.	125	<1.0	31.0	0.0
GRAPE JUICE *(Welch's)* purple, red, sparkling white,					
or white	6 oz.	120	0.0	30.0	0.0
GRAPEFRUIT JUICE *(Ocean Spray)* "Pink Premium"	6 oz.	60	1.0	15.0	0.0
ORANGE JUICE *(Veryfine)* blend "100%"	8 oz.	120	<1.0	30.0	0.0
PROTEIN DRINK					
low calorie	2 oz.	225	30.0	15.0	5.0
medium calorie	4 oz.	470	40.0	64.0	6.0
high calorie	5 oz.	548	30.0	80.0	12.0
VEGETABLE JUICE *(V•8)*	6 oz.	35	1.0	8.0	0.0

Use the chart below to fill in the foods you most commonly eat. This will help provide you with nutritional guidelines for your own personalized training diet.

FOOD	SERVING SIZE	CALORIES	PROTEIN (GRAMS)	CARBS (GRAMS)	FAT (GRAMS)

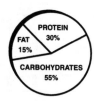

15:30:55 Macronutrient-Ratio Diet
2,500 Calories Per Day

Table C.9. Sample 15:30:55 Diet Supplying Approximately 2,500 Calories Per Day

Daily goals—2,500 calories, 188.0 grams (750 calories) protein, 344.0 grams (1,375 calories) carbohydrates, and 42.0 grams (375 calories) fat

BREAKFAST

Meal goals—500 calories, 40.0 grams protein, 63.0 grams carbohydrates, and 10.0 grams fat
Supplements to take with or after meal—recommended vitamins, minerals, amino acids, fatty acids, metabolites, and/or herbs

FOOD AND PORTION	CALORIES	PROTEIN (GRAMS)	CARBS (GRAMS)	FAT (GRAMS)
2 cups Fleischmann's Vegetable Omelet				
Egg Beaters egg alternative	200	28.0	20.0	0.0
2 slices Canadian-style bacon	86	11.3	0.6	3.9
4 ounces boiled potato, pulp only	99	2.1	22.8	0.1
½ tablespoon salted butter	50	0.1	0.0	5.7
6 ounces Ocean Spray Pink Premium grapefruit juice	60	1.0	15.0	0.0
Meal subtotals	495	42.5	58.4	9.7

MORNING SNACK

Meal goals—225 calories, 30.0 grams protein, 15.0 grams carbohydrates, and 5.0 grams fat
Supplements to take with or after meal—none

1 low-calorie protein nutrition bar	225	30.0	15.0	5.0
Meal subtotals	225	30.0	15.0	5.0

LUNCH

Meal goals—500 calories, 40.0 grams protein, 63.0 grams carbohydrates, and 10.0 grams fat
Supplements to take with or after meal—recommended vitamins, minerals, amino acids, fatty acids, metabolites, and/or herbs

4 ounces skinless chicken breast	124	26.0	0.0	1.6
4 ounces Birds Eye Farm Fresh broccoli spears	30	4.0	6.0	0.0
2 ounces trimmed iceberg lettuce	8	0.6	1.2	0.2
2 ounces raw carrot	24	0.6	5.8	0.2
1 tablespoon Seven Seas Viva Red Wine!				
oil and vinegar salad dressing	45	0.0	1.0	4.0
2 slices Arnold Bran'nola grain bread	170	7.8	34.8	3.2
1 medium orange	62	1.2	15.4	0.2
Meal subtotals	463	40.2	64.2	9.4

AFTERNOON SNACKS

Meal goals—625 calories, 30.0 grams protein, 115.0 grams carbohydrates, and 5.0 grams fat
Supplements to take with or after meal—BCAAs thirty minutes before workout

FOOD AND PORTION	CALORIES	PROTEIN (GRAMS)	CARBS (GRAMS)	FAT (GRAMS)
Two and a half hours before workout:				
2 ounces low-calorie protein drink	225	30.0	15.0	5.0
During workout:				
16 ounces high-calorie carbohydrate sports drink	400	0.0	100.0	0.0
Meal subtotals	625	30.0	115.0	5.0

DINNER

Meal goals—650 calories, 48.0 grams protein, 88.0 grams carbohydrates, and 12.0 grams fat
Supplements to take with or after meal—recommended vitamins, minerals, amino acids, fatty acids, metabolites, and/or herbs

FOOD AND PORTION	CALORIES	PROTEIN (GRAMS)	CARBS (GRAMS)	FAT (GRAMS)
1 Master Choice pork chop	120	22.0	0.0	4.0
8 ounces B&M barbecue baked beans	260	15.0	48.0	6.0
6 ounces raw chopped spinach	36	4.8	6.0	0.6
1 raw medium tomato	26	1.0	5.7	0.4
8 ounces skim milk	86	8.4	11.9	0.4
4 ounces fruit cocktail in light syrup	65	0.5	16.9	0.1
Meal subtotals	593	51.7	88.5	11.5
GRAND TOTALS	2,401	194.4	341.1	40.6

15:30:55 Macronutrient-Ratio Diet
3,500 Calories Per Day

Table C.10. Sample 15:30:55 Diet Supplying Approximately 3,500 Calories Per Day

Daily goals—3,500 calories, 263.0 grams (1,050 calories) protein, 481.0 grams (1,925 calories) carbohydrates, and 58.0 grams (525 calories) fat

BREAKFAST

Meal goals—573 calories, 51.0 grams protein, 64.0 grams carbohydrates, and 13.0 grams fat
Supplements to take with or after meal—recommended vitamins, minerals, amino acids, fatty acids, metabolites, and/or herbs

FOOD AND PORTION	CALORIES	PROTEIN (GRAMS)	CARBS (GRAMS)	FAT (GRAMS)
2½ cups Fleischmann's Vegetable Omelet Egg Beaters egg alternative	250	35.0	25.0	0.0
2 slices Canadian-style bacon	86	11.3	0.6	3.9
4 ounces boiled potato, pulp only	99	2.1	22.8	0.1
⅔ tablespoon salted butter	67	0.1	0.0	7.6
12 ounces Ocean Spray Pink Premium grapefruit juice	120	2.0	30.0	0.0
Meal subtotals	622	50.5	78.4	11.6

MORNING SNACK

Meal goals—470 calories, 40.0 grams protein, 64.0 grams carbohydrates, and 6.0 grams fat
Supplements to take with or after meal—none

1 medium-calorie protein nutrition bar	470	40.0	64.0	6.0
Meal subtotals	470	40.0	64.0	6.0

LUNCH

Meal goals—573 calories, 51.0 grams protein, 64.0 grams carbohydrates, and 13.0 grams fat
Supplements to take with or after meal—recommended vitamins, minerals, amino acids, fatty acids, metabolites, and/or herbs

6 ounces skinless chicken breast	186	39.0	0.0	2.4
4 ounces Birds Eye Farm Fresh broccoli spears	30	4.0	6.0	0.0
2 ounces trimmed iceberg lettuce	8	0.6	1.2	0.2
2 ounces trimmed raw carrot	24	0.6	5.8	0.2
1½ tablespoons Seven Seas Viva Red Wine! oil and vinegar salad dressing	68	0.0	1.5	6.0
2 slices Arnold Bran'nola grain bread	170	7.8	34.8	3.2
1 medium orange	62	1.2	15.4	0.2
Meal subtotals	548	53.2	64.7	12.2

Meal goals—970 calories, 40.0 grams protein, 189.0 grams carbohydrates, and 6.0 grams fat
Supplements to take with or after meal—BCAAs thirty minutes before workout

FOOD AND PORTION	CALORIES	PROTEIN (GRAMS)	CARBS (GRAMS)	FAT (GRAMS)
Two and a half hours before workout:				
4 ounces medium-calorie protein drink	470	40.0	64.0	6.0
During workout:				
20 ounces high-calorie carbohydrate sports drink	500	0.0	125.0	0.0
Meal subtotals	970	40.0	189.0	6.0

DINNER

Meal goals—914 calories, 81.0 grams protein, 100.0 grams carbohydrates, and 20.0 grams fat
Supplements to take with or after meal—recommended vitamins, minerals, amino acids, fatty acids, metabolites, and/or herbs

FOOD AND PORTION	CALORIES	PROTEIN	CARBS	FAT
2½ Master Choice pork chops	300	55.0	0.0	10.0
8 ounces B&M barbecue baked beans	260	15.0	48.0	6.0
6 ounces raw chopped spinach	36	4.8	6.0	0.6
1 raw medium tomato	26	1.0	5.7	0.4
8 ounces skim milk	86	8.4	11.9	0.4
4 ounces fruit cocktail in light syrup	65	0.5	16.9	0.1
Meal subtotals	773	84.7	88.5	17.5
GRAND TOTALS	3,383	268.4	484.6	53.3

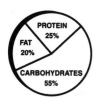

20:25:55 Macronutrient-Ratio Diet
2,500 Calories Per Day

Table C.11. Sample 20:25:55 Diet Supplying Approximately 2,500 Calories Per Day

Daily goals—2,500 calories, 156.0 grams (625 calories) protein, 344.0 grams (1,375 calories) carbohydrates, and 56.0 grams (500 calories) fat

BREAKFAST

Meal goals—465 calories, 27.0 grams protein, 60.0 grams carbohydrates, and 13.0 grams fat
Supplements to take with or after meal—recommended vitamins, minerals, amino acids, fatty acids, metabolites, and/or herbs

FOOD AND PORTION	CALORIES	PROTEIN (GRAMS)	CARBS (GRAMS)	FAT (GRAMS)
1 cup Fleischmann's Vegetable Omelet				
Egg Beaters egg alternative	100	14.0	10.0	0.0
2 slices Canadian-style bacon	86	11.3	0.6	3.9
4 ounces boiled potato, pulp only	99	2.1	22.8	0.1
⅔ tablespoon salted butter	67	0.1	0.0	7.6
9 ounces Ocean Spray Pink Premium grapefruit juice	90	1.5	22.5	0.0
Meal subtotals	442	29.0	55.9	11.6

MORNING SNACK

Meal goals—225 calories, 30.0 grams protein, 15.0 grams carbohydrates, and 5.0 grams fat
Supplements to take with or after meal—none

	CALORIES	PROTEIN	CARBS	FAT
1 low-calorie protein nutrition bar	225	30.0	15.0	5.0
Meal subtotals	225	30.0	15.0	5.0

LUNCH

Meal goals—465 calories, 27.0 grams protein, 60.0 grams carbohydrates, and 13.0 grams fat
Supplements to take with or after meal—recommended vitamins, minerals, amino acids, fatty acids, metabolites, and/or herbs

	CALORIES	PROTEIN	CARBS	FAT
2 ounces skinless chicken breast	62	13.0	0.0	0.8
4 ounces Birds Eye Farm Fresh broccoli spears	30	4.0	6.0	0.0
2 ounces trimmed iceberg lettuce	8	0.6	1.2	0.2
1 raw medium tomato	26	1.0	5.7	0.4
2 ounces trimmed raw carrot	24	0.6	5.8	0.2
2 tablespoons Seven Seas Viva Red Wine!				
oil and vinegar salad dressing	90	0.0	2.0	8.0
2 slices Arnold Bran'nola grain bread	170	7.8	34.8	3.2
1 medium orange	62	1.2	15.4	0.2
Meal subtotals	472	28.2	70.9	13.0

Meal goals—625 calories, 30.0 grams protein, 115.0 grams carbohydrates, and 5.0 grams fat
Supplements to take with or after meal—BCAAs thirty minutes before workout

FOOD AND PORTION	CALORIES	PROTEIN (GRAMS)	CARBS (GRAMS)	FAT (GRAMS)
Two and a half hours before workout:				
2 ounces low-calorie protein drink	225	30.0	15.0	5.0
During workout:				
16 ounces high-calorie carbohydrate sports drink	400	0.0	100.0	0.0
Meal subtotals	625	30.0	115.0	5.0

Meal goals—720 calories, 42.0 grams protein, 94.0 grams carbohydrates, and 20.0 grams fat
Supplements to take with or after meal—recommended vitamins, minerals, amino acids, fatty acids, metabolites, and/or herbs

FOOD AND PORTION	CALORIES	PROTEIN (GRAMS)	CARBS (GRAMS)	FAT (GRAMS)
3 ounces untrimmed prime bottom-round beef	192	17.1	0.0	13.2
2 ounces DeBoles Jerusalem artichoke spaghetti	210	9.0	41.0	1.0
4 ounces Ragu Thick & Hearty mushroom pasta sauce	100	2.0	15.0	3.0
12 ounces raw chopped spinach	72	9.6	12.0	1.2
8 ounces skim milk	86	8.4	11.9	0.4
4 ounces fruit cocktail in light syrup	65	0.5	16.9	0.1
Meal subtotals	725	46.6	96.8	18.9
GRAND TOTALS	2,489	163.8	353.6	53.5

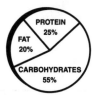

20:25:55 Macronutrient-Ratio Diet
3,500 Calories Per Day

Table C.12. Sample 20:25:55 Diet Supplying Approximately 3,500 Calories Per Day

Daily goals—3,500 calories, 219.0 grams (875 calories) protein, 481.0 grams (1,925 calories) carbohydrates, and 78.0 grams (700 calories) fat

BREAKFAST

Meal goals—579 calories, 38.5 grams protein, 61.0 grams carbohydrates, and 18.5 grams fat

Supplements to take with or after meal—recommended vitamins, minerals, amino acids, fatty acids, metabolites, and/or herbs

FOOD AND PORTION	CALORIES	PROTEIN (GRAMS)	CARBS (GRAMS)	FAT (GRAMS)
1½ cups Fleischmann's Vegetable Omelet				
Egg Beaters egg alternative	150	21.0	15.0	0.0
2 slices Canadian-style bacon	86	11.3	0.6	3.9
4 ounces boiled potato, pulp only	99	2.1	22.8	0.1
1 tablespoon salted butter	100	0.2	0.0	11.4
6 ounces Ocean Spray Pink Premium grapefruit juice	60	1.0	15.0	0.0
4 ounces 2% milk	61	4.1	5.9	2.4
Meal subtotals	556	39.7	59.3	17.8

MORNING SNACK

Meal goals—470 calories, 40.0 grams protein, 64.0 grams carbohydrates, and 6.0 grams fat
Supplements to take with or after meal—none

FOOD AND PORTION	CALORIES	PROTEIN (GRAMS)	CARBS (GRAMS)	FAT (GRAMS)
1 medium-calorie protein nutrition bar	470	40.0	64.0	6.0
Meal subtotals	470	40.0	64.0	6.0

LUNCH

Meal goals—579 calories, 38.5 grams protein, 61.0 grams carbohydrates, and 18.5 grams fat
Supplements to take with or after meal—recommended vitamins, minerals, amino acids, fatty acids, metabolites, and/or herbs

FOOD AND PORTION	CALORIES	PROTEIN (GRAMS)	CARBS (GRAMS)	FAT (GRAMS)
4 ounces skinless chicken breast	124	26.0	0.0	1.6
4 ounces Birds Eye Farm Fresh broccoli spears	30	4.0	6.0	0.0
2 ounces trimmed iceberg lettuce	8	0.6	1.2	0.2
2 ounces trimmed raw carrot	24	0.6	5.8	0.2
3 tablespoons Seven Seas Viva Red Wine!				
oil and vinegar salad dressing	135	0.0	3.0	12.0
1 Pepperidge Farm soft Deli Classic hoagie roll	210	8.0	34.0	5.0
1 medium orange	62	1.2	15.4	0.2
Meal subtotals	593	40.4	65.4	19.2

AFTERNOON SNACKS

Meal goals—970 calories, 40.0 grams protein, 189.0 grams carbohydrates, and 6.0 grams fat
Supplements to take with or after meal—BCAAs thirty minutes before workout

FOOD AND PORTION	CALORIES	PROTEIN (GRAMS)	CARBS (GRAMS)	FAT (GRAMS)
Two and a half hours before workout:				
4 ounces medium-calorie protein drink	470	40.0	64.0	6.0
During workout:				
20 ounces high-calorie carbohydrate sports drink	500	0.0	125.0	0.0
Meal subtotals	970	40.0	189.0	6.0

DINNER

Meal goals—902 calories, 62.0 grams protein, 106.0 grams carbohydrates, and 29.0 grams fat
Supplements to take with or after meal—recommended vitamins, minerals, amino acids, fatty acids, metabolites, and/or herbs

FOOD AND PORTION	CALORIES	PROTEIN	CARBS	FAT
5 ounces trimmed prime bottom-round beef	225	31.0	0.0	10.5
2 ounces DeBoles Jerusalem artichoke spaghetti	210	9.0	41.0	1.0
½ tablespoon Hain olive oil	60	0.0	0.0	7.0
4 ounces Ragu Thick & Hearty mushroom pasta sauce	100	2.0	15.0	3.0
12 ounces raw chopped spinach	72	9.6	12.0	1.2
8 ounces Borden whole milk	150	8.0	11.0	8.0
4 ounces fruit cocktail in light syrup	65	0.5	16.9	0.1
Meal subtotals	882	60.1	95.9	30.8
GRAND TOTALS	3,471	220.2	473.6	79.8

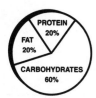

20:20:60 Macronutrient-Ratio Diet
2,500 Calories Per Day

Table C.13. Sample 20:20:60 Diet Supplying Approximately 2,500 Calories Per Day

Daily goals—2,500 calories, 125.0 grams (500 calories) protein, 375.0 grams (1,500 calories) carbohydrates, and 56.0 grams (500 calories) fat

BREAKFAST

Meal goals—425 calories, 23.5 grams protein, 67.0 grams carbohydrates, and 12.5 grams fat

Supplements to take with or after meal—recommended vitamins, minerals, amino acids, fatty acids, metabolites, and/or herbs

FOOD AND PORTION	CALORIES	PROTEIN (GRAMS)	CARBS (GRAMS)	FAT (GRAMS)
3 (4-inch diameter) Hungry Jack buttermilk pancakes prepared with skim milk, oil, and egg whites	200	6.0	28.0	7.0
3½ tablespoons Hungry Jack Lite pancake syrup	88	0.0	24.5	0.0
3 ounces trimmed fresh ham, rump half of leg	117	18.0	0.0	4.5
8 ounces V•8 vegetable juice	47	1.3	10.7	0.0
Meal subtotals	452	25.3	63.2	11.5

MORNING SNACK

Meal goals—270 calories, 12.0 grams protein, 45.0 grams carbohydrates, and 6.0 grams fat
Supplements to take with or after meal—none

	CALORIES	PROTEIN	CARBS	FAT
1 Earth Grains banana apple walnut Bagel Power Bar	270	12.0	45.0	6.0
Meal subtotals	270	12.0	45.0	6.0

LUNCH

Meal goals—425 calories, 23.5 grams protein, 67.0 grams carbohydrates, and 12.5 grams fat
Supplements to take with or after meal—recommended vitamins, minerals, amino acids, fatty acids, metabolites, and/or herbs

	CALORIES	PROTEIN	CARBS	FAT
1 Arnold Dutch egg sandwich roll	123	4.5	21.6	3.3
3 slices Tyson turkey luncheon meat	60	12.0	0.9	1.2
½ ounce Kraft Deluxe Slices American cheese	55	3.0	0.5	4.5
2 ounces trimmed iceberg lettuce	8	0.6	1.2	0.2
3 tablespoons French's yellow mustard	30	3.0	3.0	3.0
2 ounces Del Monte dried apricots	140	2.0	35.0	0.0
Meal subtotals	416	25.1	62.2	12.2

Meal goals—625 calories, 30.0 grams protein, 115.0 grams carbohydrates, and 5.0 grams fat
Supplements to take with or after meal—BCAAs thirty minutes before workout

FOOD AND PORTION	CALORIES	PROTEIN (GRAMS)	CARBS (GRAMS)	FAT (GRAMS)
Two and a half hours before workout:				
2 ounces low-calorie protein drink	225	30.0	15.0	5.0
During workout:				
16 ounces high-calorie carbohydrate sports drink	400	0.0	100.0	0.0
Meal subtotals	625	30.0	115.0	5.0

DINNER

Meal goals—755 calories, 36.0 grams protein, 81.0 grams carbohydrates, and 20.0 grams fat
Supplements to take with or after meal—recommended vitamins, minerals, amino acids, fatty acids, metabolites, and/or herbs

4 ounces bluefin tuna	164	26.4	0.0	5.6
3 ounces dry long-grain brown rice	315	6.9	65.7	2.4
6 ounces trimmed raw cauliflower	42	3.6	8.4	0.6
8 ounces trimmed iceberg lettuce	32	2.4	4.8	0.8
1 raw medium tomato	26	1.0	5.7	0.4
2 ounces trimmed raw onion	22	0.6	4.8	0.2
2 tablespoons Seven Seas Viva Red Wine! oil and vinegar salad dressing	90	0.0	2.0	8.0
3 ounces Welch's grape juice	60	0.0	15.0	0.0
Meal subtotals	751	40.9	106.4	18.0
GRAND TOTALS	2,514	133.3	391.8	52.7

20:20:60 Macronutrient-Ratio Diet
3,500 Calories Per Day

Table C.14. Sample 20:20:60 Diet Supplying Approximately 3,500 Calories Per Day

Daily goals—3,500 calories, 175.0 grams (700 calories) protein, 525.0 grams (2,100 calories) carbohydrates, and 78.0 grams (700 calories) fat

BREAKFAST

Meal goals—489 calories, 36.0 grams protein, 52.5 grams carbohydrates, and 15.0 grams fat
Supplements to take with or after meal—recommended vitamins, minerals, amino acids, fatty acids, metabolites, and/or herbs

FOOD AND PORTION	CALORIES	PROTEIN (GRAMS)	CARBS (GRAMS)	FAT (GRAMS)
3 (4-inch diameter) Hungry Jack buttermilk pancakes prepared with skim milk, oil, and egg whites	200	6.0	28.0	7.0
2 tablespoons Hungry Jack Lite pancake syrup	50	0.0	14.0	0.0
4 ounces trimmed fresh ham, rump half of leg	156	24.0	0.0	6.0
8 ounces skim milk	86	8.4	11.9	0.4
Meal subtotals	492	38.4	53.9	13.4

MORNING SNACK

Meal goals—440 calories, 16.0 grams protein, 68.0 grams carbohydrates, and 12.0 grams fat
Supplements to take with or after meal—none

FOOD AND PORTION	CALORIES	PROTEIN	CARBS	FAT
1 Bear Valley carob-cocoa Pemmician snack/food bar	440	16.0	68.0	12.0
Meal subtotals	440	16.0	68.0	12.0

LUNCH

Meal goals—489 calories, 36.0 grams protein, 52.5 grams carbohydrates, and 15.0 grams fat
Supplements to take with or after meal—recommended vitamins, minerals, amino acids, fatty acids, metabolites, and/or herbs

FOOD AND PORTION	CALORIES	PROTEIN	CARBS	FAT
1 Arnold Dutch egg sandwich roll	123	4.5	21.6	3.3
6 slices Tyson turkey luncheon meat	120	24.0	1.8	2.4
½ ounce Kraft Deluxe Slices American cheese	55	3.0	0.5	4.5
2 ounces trimmed iceberg lettuce	8	0.6	1.2	0.2
3 tablespoons French's yellow mustard	30	3.0	3.0	3.0
1 peeled banana	105	1.2	26.7	0.6
Meal subtotals	441	36.3	54.8	14.0

AFTERNOON SNACKS

Meal goals—1,048 calories, 30.0 grams protein, 205.0 grams carbohydrates, and 12.0 grams fat
Supplements to take with or after meal—BCAAs thirty minutes before workout

FOOD AND PORTION	CALORIES	PROTEIN (GRAMS)	CARBS (GRAMS)	FAT (GRAMS)
Two and a half hours before workout:				
5 ounces high-calorie protein drink	548	30.0	80.0	12.0
During workout:				
20 ounces high-calorie carbohydrate sports drink	500	0.0	125.0	0.0
Meal subtotals	1,048	30.0	205.0	12.0

DINNER

Meal goals—1,034 calories, 57.0 grams protein, 147.0 grams carbohydrates, and 24.0 grams fat
Supplements to take with or after meal—recommended vitamins, minerals, amino acids, fatty acids, metabolites, and/or herbs

FOOD AND PORTION	CALORIES	PROTEIN (GRAMS)	CARBS (GRAMS)	FAT (GRAMS)
6 ounces bluefin tuna	246	39.6	0.0	8.4
3 ounces dry long-grain brown rice	315	6.9	65.7	2.4
6 ounces trimmed raw cauliflower	42	3.6	8.4	0.6
1 ounce garbanzo beans	103	5.5	17.2	1.7
8 ounces trimmed iceberg lettuce	32	2.4	4.8	0.8
1 raw medium tomato	26	1.0	5.7	0.4
2 ounces trimmed raw onion	22	0.6	4.8	0.2
2 tablespoons Seven Seas Viva Red Wine!				
oil and vinegar salad dressing	90	0.0	2.0	8.0
3 ounces Welch's grape juice	60	0.0	15.0	0.0
Meal subtotals	936	59.6	123.6	22.5
GRAND TOTALS	3,357	180.3	505.3	73.9

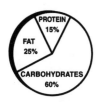

25:15:60 Macronutrient-Ratio Diet
2,500 Calories Per Day

Table C.15. Sample 25:15:60 Diet Supplying Approximately 2,500 Calories Per Day

Daily goals—2,500 calories, 94.0 grams (375 calories) protein, 375.0 grams (1,500 calories) carbohydrates, and 69.0 grams (625 calories) fat

BREAKFAST

Meal goals—440 calories, 20.0 grams protein, 50.0 grams carbohydrates, and 16.5 grams fat
Supplements to take with or after meal—recommended vitamins, minerals, amino acids, fatty acids, metabolites, and/or herbs

FOOD AND PORTION	CALORIES	PROTEIN (GRAMS)	CARBS (GRAMS)	FAT (GRAMS)
3 (4-inch diameter) Hungry Jack buttermilk pancakes prepared with skim milk, oil, and egg whites	200	6.0	28.0	7.0
½ tablespoon salted butter	50	0.1	0.0	5.7
2 tablespoons Hungry Jack Lite pancake syrup	50	0.0	14.0	0.0
2 ounces trimmed fresh ham, rump half of leg	78	12.0	0.0	3.0
12 ounces V•8 vegetable juice	70	2.0	16.0	0.0
Meal subtotals	448	20.1	58.0	15.7

MORNING SNACK

Meal goals—230 calories, 10.0 grams of protein, 45.0 grams of carbohydrates, and 2.5 grams of fat
Supplements to take with or after meal—none

1 power bar	230	10.0	45.0	2.5
Meal subtotals	230	10.0	45.0	2.5

LUNCH

Meal goals—440 calories, 20.0 grams protein, 50.0 grams carbohydrates, and 16.5 grams fat
Supplements to take with or after meal—recommended vitamins, minerals, amino acids, fatty acids, metabolites, and/or herbs

1 Arnold Dutch egg sandwich roll	123	4.5	21.6	3.3
2 slices Tyson turkey luncheon meat	40	8.0	0.6	0.8
1 ounce Kraft Deluxe Slices American cheese	110	6.0	1.0	9.0
2 ounces trimmed iceberg lettuce	8	0.6	1.2	0.2
2 tablespoons French's yellow mustard	20	2.0	2.0	2.0
2 ounces Del Monte dried apricots	140	2.0	35.0	0.0
Meal subtotals	441	23.1	61.4	15.3

AFTERNOON SNACKS

Meal goals—670 calories, 12.0 grams protein, 145.0 grams carbohydrates, and 6.0 grams fat
Supplements to take with or after meal—BCAAs thirty minutes before workout

FOOD AND PORTION	CALORIES	PROTEIN (GRAMS)	CARBS (GRAMS)	FAT (GRAMS)
Two and a half hours before workout:				
1 Earth Grains banana apple walnut Bagel Power Bar	270	12.0	45.0	6.0
During workout:				
16 ounces high-calorie carbohydrate sports drink	400	0.0	100.0	0.0
Meal subtotals	670	12.0	145.0	6.0

DINNER

Meal goals—720 calories, 32.0 grams protein, 85.0 grams carbohydrates, and 27.5 grams fat
Supplements to take with or after meal—recommended vitamins, minerals, amino acids, fatty acids, metabolites, and/or herbs

3 ounces bluefin tuna	123	19.8	0.0	4.2
3 ounces dry long-grain brown rice	315	6.9	65.7	2.4
6 ounces trimmed raw cauliflower	42	3.6	8.4	0.6
4 ounces trimmed iceberg lettuce	16	1.2	2.4	0.4
1 raw medium tomato	26	1.0	5.7	0.4
2 ounces trimmed raw onion	22	0.6	4.8	0.2
4 tablespoons Seven Seas Viva Red Wine! oil and vinegar salad dressing	180	0.0	4.0	16.0
Meal subtotals	724	33.1	91.0	24.2
GRAND TOTALS	2,513	98.3	400.4	63.7

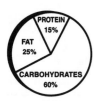

25:15:60 Macronutrient-Ratio Diet
3,500 Calories Per Day

Table C.16. Sample 25:15:60 Diet Supplying Approximately 3,500 Calories Per Day

Daily goals—3,500 calories, 131.0 grams (525 calories) protein, 525.0 grams (2,100 calories) carbohydrates, and 97.0 grams (875 calories) fat

BREAKFAST

Meal goals—560 calories, 24.0 grams protein, 70.0 grams carbohydrates, and 20.5 grams fat
Supplements to take with or after meal—recommended vitamins, minerals, amino acids, fatty acids, metabolites, and/or herbs

FOOD AND PORTION	CALORIES	PROTEIN (GRAMS)	CARBS (GRAMS)	FAT (GRAMS)
3 (4-inch diameter) Hungry Jack buttermilk pancakes prepared with skim milk, oil, and egg whites	200	6.0	28.0	7.0
⅔ tablespoon salted butter	67	0.1	0.0	7.6
4 tablespoons Hungry Jack Lite pancake syrup	100	0.0	28.0	0.0
3 ounces trimmed fresh ham, rump half of leg	117	18.0	0.0	4.5
12 ounces V•8 vegetable juice	70	2.0	16.0	0.0
Meal subtotals	554	26.1	72.0	19.1

MORNING SNACK

Meal goals—440 calories, 16.0 grams protein, 68.0 grams carbohydrates, and 12.0 grams fat
Supplements to take with or after meal—none

FOOD AND PORTION	CALORIES	PROTEIN	CARBS	FAT
1 Bear Valley carob-cocoa Pemmician snack/food bar	440	16.0	68.0	12.0
Meal subtotals	440	16.0	68.0	12.0

LUNCH

Meal goals—560 calories, 24.0 grams protein, 70.0 grams carbohydrates, and 20.5 grams fat
Supplements to take with or after meal—recommended vitamins, minerals, amino acids, fatty acids, metabolites, and/or herbs

FOOD AND PORTION	CALORIES	PROTEIN	CARBS	FAT
1 Arnold Dutch egg sandwich roll	123	4.5	21.6	3.3
3 slices Tyson turkey luncheon meat	60	12.0	0.9	1.2
1 ounce Kraft Deluxe Slices American cheese	110	6.0	1.0	9.0
2 ounces trimmed iceberg lettuce	8	0.6	1.2	0.2
2 tablespoons French's yellow mustard	20	2.0	2.0	2.0
⅓ tablespoon Hain Hi-Oleic safflower oil	40	0.0	0.0	4.7
2 ounces Del Monte dried apricots	140	2.0	35.0	0.0
6 ounces Ocean Spray Pink Premium grapefruit juice	60	1.0	15.0	0.0
Meal subtotals	561	28.1	76.7	20.4

AFTERNOON SNACKS

Meal goals—1,048 calories, 30.0 grams protein, 205.0 grams carbohydrates, and 12.0 grams fat
Supplements to take with or after meal—BCAAs thirty minutes before workout

FOOD AND PORTION	CALORIES	PROTEIN (GRAMS)	CARBS (GRAMS)	FAT (GRAMS)
Two and a half hours before workout:				
5 ounces high-calorie protein drink	548	30.0	80.0	12.0
During workout:				
20 ounces high-calorie carbohydrate sports drink	500	0.0	125.0	0.0
Meal subtotals	1,048	30.0	205.0	12.0

DINNER

Meal goals—892 calories, 37.0 grams protein, 112.0 grams carbohydrates, and 32.0 grams fat
Supplements to take with or after meal—recommended vitamins, minerals, amino acids, fatty acids, metabolites, and/or herbs

FOOD AND PORTION	CALORIES	PROTEIN (GRAMS)	CARBS (GRAMS)	FAT (GRAMS)
3 ounces bluefin tuna	123	19.8	0.0	4.2
4 ounces dry long-grain brown rice	420	9.2	87.6	4.0
6 ounces trimmed raw cauliflower	42	3.6	8.4	0.6
4 ounces trimmed iceberg lettuce	16	1.2	2.4	0.4
1 raw medium tomato	26	1.0	5.7	0.4
2 ounces trimmed raw onion	22	0.6	4.8	0.2
5 tablespoons Seven Seas Viva Red Wine! oil and vinegar salad dressing	225	0.0	5.0	20.0
Meal subtotals	874	35.4	113.9	29.8
GRAND TOTALS	3,477	135.6	535.6	93.3

D. DAILY NUTRITION LOG

Use this log sheet to record your daily caloric, protein, carbohydrate, and fat intakes. Knowing exactly what and how much you eat will help you maintain the macronutrient ratio recommended for you in your sport-specific plan in Part Four. To determine your macronutrient goals, first figure out how many calories you should consume. Next, determine how many calories of protein, carbohydrates, and fat you should eat according to your day's target macronutrient ratio. Finally, convert those caloric totals to grams. To figure out how many calories you should consume, see page 150, as well as Chapter 13 or 14 if you wish to lose fat or build muscle, respectively. For your target macronutrient ratio, see your sport-specific plan in Part Four. To determine your macronutrient intake goals in grams, use the following formulas:

1. To determine the total number of protein grams you should consume, multiply your total daily calories by your target protein percentage. This yields your protein goal in calories. To get your protein goal in grams, divide your total protein calories by 4, which is the number of protein calories per gram.

Total daily calories × target protein percentage
= total protein calories

Total protein calories ÷ 4 calories per gram
= total protein grams

2. To determine the total number of carbohydrate grams you should consume, multiply your total daily calories by your target carbohydrate percentage. This yields your carbohydrate goal in calories. To get your carbohydrate goal in grams, divide your total carbohydrate calories by 4, which is the number of carbohydrate calories per gram.

Total daily calories × target carbohydrate percentage
= total carbohydrate calories

Total carbohydrate calories ÷ 4 calories per gram
= total carbohydrate grams

3. To determine the total number of fat grams you should consume, multiply your total daily calories by your target fat percentage. This yields your fat goal in calories. To get your fat goal in grams, divide your total fat calories by 9, which is the number of fat calories per gram.

Total daily calories × target fat percentage = total fat calories

Total fat calories ÷ 9 calories per gram = total fat grams

For example, if your target macronutrient ratio was 15:30:55 and your total daily caloric requirement was 2,500 calories, you would complete the following calculations:

1. To determine your total grams of protein, you would multiply 2,500 calories (your total daily calories) by 30 percent (your target protein percentage) to get 750 calories (your total protein calories). Then, you would divide 750 (your total protein calories) by 4 (the number of protein calories per gram) to get 187.5 grams (your total protein grams). If desired, round out the total to the nearest whole number, in this case 188 grams.

2,500	Total daily calories
× .30	Target protein percentage
750	Total protein calories
750	Total protein calories
÷ 4	Protein calories per gram
187.5	Total protein grams

2. To determine your total grams of carbohydrates, you would multiply 2,500 calories (your total daily calories) by 55 percent (your target carbohydrate percentage) to get 1,375 calories (your total carbohydrate calories). Then, you would divide 1,375 (your total carbohydrate calories) by 4 (the number of carbohydrate calories per gram) to get 343.75 grams (your total carbohydrate grams). If desired, round out the total to the nearest whole number, in this case 344 grams.

2,500	Total daily calories
× .55	Target carbohydrate percentage
1,375	Total carbohydrate calories

1,375	Total carbohydrate calories
÷ 4	Carbohydrate calories per gram
343.75	Total carbohydrate grams

2,500	Total daily calories
× .15	Target fat percentage
375	Total fat calories

375	Total fat calories
÷ 9	Fat calories per gram
41.67	Total fat grams

3. To determine your total grams of fat, you would multiply 2,500 calories (your total daily calories) by 15 percent (your target fat percentage) to get 375 calories (your total fat calories). Then, you would divide 375 (your total fat calories) by 9 (the number of fat calories per gram) to get 41.67 grams (your total fat grams). If desired, round out the total to the nearest whole number, in this case 42 grams.

Every day, record your target protein, carbohydrate, and fat grams on your nutrition log sheet in the correct spaces. In addition, note the date, whether it is a training or nontraining day, and what your target macronutrient ratio is. If desired, keep all your Daily Nutrition Log sheets in a looseleaf binder, along with your Personal Inventory sheets (see page 341), Hourly Caloric Breakdown Chart sheets (see page 343), food lists and sample daily diets (see page 345), training and competition records, and anything else that helps you in your performance-improvement efforts.

Table D.1. Daily Nutrition Log Sheet

Date _____   Type of day: training ____ or nontraining ____

Macronutrient ratio to follow: 15:30:55 ____ 20:25:55 ____ 20:20:60 ____ or 25:15:60 ____

Daily goals: _____ calories, _____ grams protein, _____ grams carbohydrates, and _____ grams fat

BREAKFAST

Meal goals: _____ calories, _____ grams protein, _____ grams carbohydrates, and _____ grams fat

FOOD AND PORTION	CALORIES	PROTEIN (GRAMS)	CARBS (GRAMS)	FAT (GRAMS)

Meal subtotals: _____

Supplements taken with or after meal: _____

MORNING SNACK

Meal goals: _____ calories, _____ grams protein, _____ grams carbohydrates, and _____ grams fat

_____

_____

Meal subtotals: _____

Supplements taken with or after meal: _____

LUNCH

Meal goals: _____ calories, _____ grams protein, _____ grams carbohydrates, and _____ grams fat

_____

_____

_____

_____

_____

Meal subtotals: _____

Supplements taken with or after meal: _____

AFTERNOON SNACKS

Meal goals: _____ *calories,* _____ *grams protein,* _____ *grams carbohydrates, and* _____ *grams fat*

FOOD AND PORTION	CALORIES	PROTEIN (GRAMS)	CARBS (GRAMS)	FAT (GRAMS)

Meal subtotals: _____

Supplements taken with or after meal: _____

DINNER

Meal goals: _____ *calories,* _____ *grams protein,* _____ *grams carbohydrates, and* _____ *grams fat*

Meal subtotals: _____

Supplements taken with or after meal: _____

GRAND TOTALS: _____

E. REFERENCE DAILY INTAKES AND DAILY REFERENCE VALUES

Table E.1 provides the currently established Reference Daily Intakes (RDIs) of the vitamins and minerals. Note that RDIs have not yet been set for all the known vitamins and minerals. For a full discussion of the RDIs, see page 3.

Table E.2 provides the currently established Daily Reference Values (DRVs) of the macronutrients, potassium, and sodium. For a full discussion of the DRVs, see page 3.

Table E.1. Reference Daily Intakes for Vitamins and Minerals

VITAMIN OR MINERAL	ADULTS AND CHILDREN OVER 4 YEARS OF AGE	PREGNANT WOMEN	LACTATING WOMEN
Vitamin A	5,000 IU	8,000 IU	8,000 IU
Vitamin B_1 (thiamine)	1.5 mg	1.7 mg	1.7 mg
Vitamin B_2 (riboflavin)	1.7 mg	2.0 mg	2.0 mg
Vitamin B_3 (niacin)	20 mg	20 mg	20 mg
Vitamin B_5 (pantothenic acid)	10 mg	10 mg	10 mg
Vitamin B_6 (pyridoxine)	2.0 mg	2.5 mg	2.5 mg
Vitamin B_{12} (cobalamin)	6 mcg	8 mcg	8 mcg
Biotin	300 mcg	300 mcg	300 mcg
Folate	400 mcg	800 mcg	800 mcg
Vitamin C	60 mg	60 mg	60 mg
Vitamin D	400 IU	400 IU	400 IU
Vitamin E	30 IU	30 IU	30 IU
Vitamin K	80 mcg	*	*
Calcium	1,000 mg	1,300 mg	1,300 mg
Chloride	3,400 mg	*	*
Chromium	120 mcg	*	*
Copper	2.0 mg	2.0 mg	2.0 mg
Iodine	150 mcg	150 mcg	150 mcg
Iron	18 mg	18 mg	18 mg
Magnesium	400 mg	450 mg	450 mg
Manganese	2.0 mg	*	*
Molybdenum	75 mcg	*	*
Phosphorus	1,000 mg	1,300 mg	1,300 mg
Selenium	70 mcg	*	*
Zinc	15 mg	15 mg	15 mg

IU = international units, mg = milligrams, mcg = micrograms.
*RDI for this nutrient has not been established for this group.

Table E.2. Daily Reference Values for Macronutrients, Potassium, and Sodium*

NUTRIENT	ADULTS AND CHILDREN OVER 4 YEARS OF AGE	PREGNANT WOMEN	LACTATING WOMEN
Total carbohydrate	300 g	†	†
Fiber	25 g	†	†
Protein	50 g	60 g	65 g
Fat	65 g	†	†
Saturated fat	20 g	†	†
Cholesterol	300 mg	†	†
Potassium	3,500 mg	†	†
Sodium	2,400 mg	†	†

G = grams, mg = milligrams.
*Based on reference daily diet of 2,000 calories.
†DRV for this nutrient has not been established for this group.

F. MUSCLES OF THE HUMAN BODY

Front—Complete Musculature

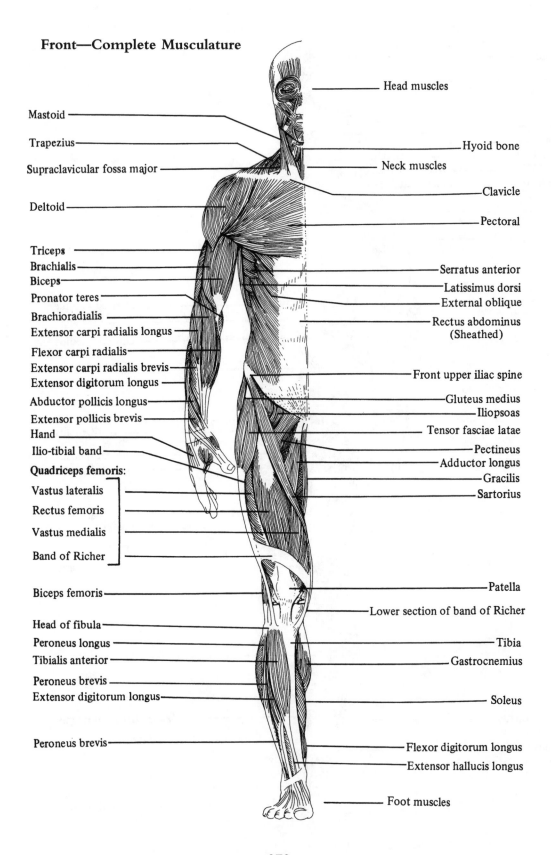

Head muscles

Mastoid

Trapezius

Supraclavicular fossa major

Hyoid bone

Neck muscles

Clavicle

Deltoid

Pectoral

Triceps

Brachialis

Biceps

Serratus anterior

Latissimus dorsi

External oblique

Rectus abdominus
(Sheathed)

Pronator teres

Brachioradialis

Extensor carpi radialis longus

Flexor carpi radialis

Extensor carpi radialis brevis

Extensor digitorum longus

Front upper iliac spine

Abductor pollicis longus

Gluteus medius

Iliopsoas

Extensor pollicis brevis

Tensor fasciae latae

Hand

Ilio-tibial band

Pectineus

Adductor longus

Quadriceps femoris:

Gracilis

Sartorius

Vastus lateralis

Rectus femoris

Vastus medialis

Band of Richer

Biceps femoris

Patella

Lower section of band of Richer

Head of fibula

Peroneus longus

Tibia

Tibialis anterior

Gastrocnemius

Peroneus brevis

Extensor digitorum longus

Soleus

Peroneus brevis

Flexor digitorum longus

Extensor hallucis longus

Foot muscles

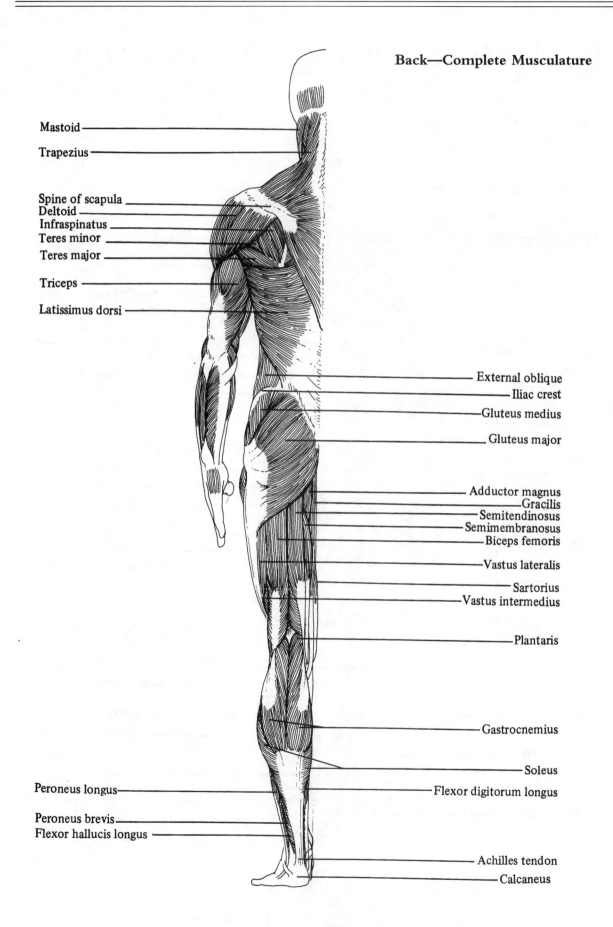

Back—Complete Musculature

Mastoid

Trapezius

Spine of scapula
Deltoid
Infraspinatus
Teres minor
Teres major

Triceps

Latissimus dorsi

External oblique
Iliac crest
Gluteus medius

Gluteus major

Adductor magnus
Gracilis
Semitendinosus
Semimembranosus
Biceps femoris

Vastus lateralis

Sartorius
Vastus intermedius

Plantaris

Gastrocnemius

Soleus

Peroneus longus

Flexor digitorum longus

Peroneus brevis
Flexor hallucis longus

Achilles tendon
Calcaneus

Side—Complete Musculature

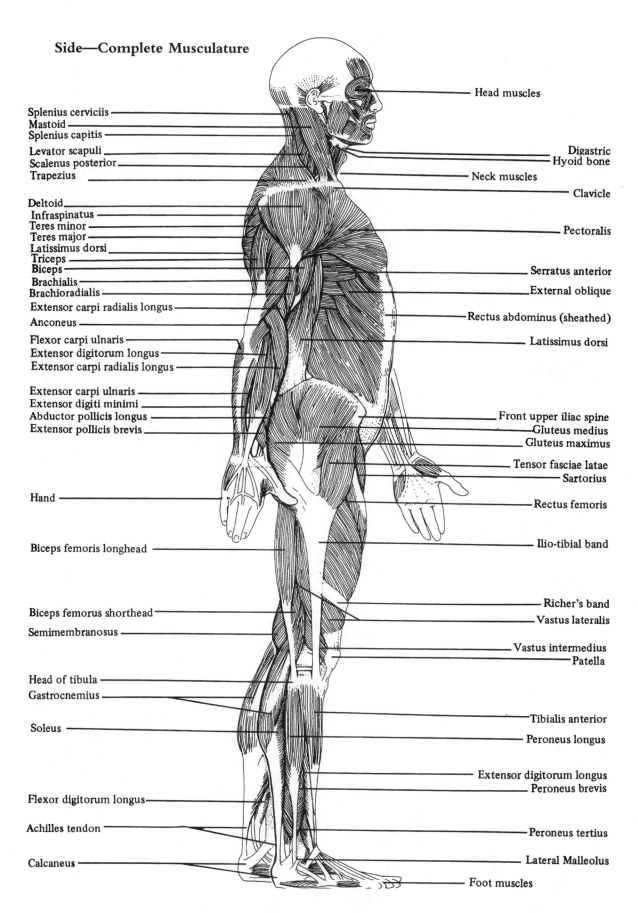

Splenius cerviciis
Mastoid
Splenius capitis
Levator scapuli
Scalenus posterior
Trapezius

Deltoid
Infraspinatus
Teres minor
Teres major
Latissimus dorsi
Triceps
Biceps
Brachialis
Brachioradialis
Extensor carpi radialis longus
Anconeus

Flexor carpi ulnaris
Extensor digitorum longus
Extensor carpi radialis longus

Extensor carpi ulnaris
Extensor digiti minimi
Abductor pollicis longus
Extensor pollicis brevis

Hand

Biceps femoris longhead

Biceps femorus shorthead
Semimembranosus

Head of tibula
Gastrocnemius

Soleus

Flexor digitorum longus

Achilles tendon

Calcaneus

Head muscles

Digastric
Hyoid bone
Neck muscles
Clavicle

Pectoralis

Serratus anterior
External oblique

Rectus abdominus (sheathed)

Latissimus dorsi

Front upper iliac spine
Gluteus medius
Gluteus maximus
Tensor fasciae latae
Sartorius

Rectus femoris

Ilio-tibial band

Richer's band
Vastus lateralis

Vastus intermedius
Patella

Tibialis anterior
Peroneus longus

Extensor digitorum longus
Peroneus brevis

Peroneus tertius

Lateral Malleolus

Foot muscles

GLOSSARY

acetylcholine. A neurotransmitter that is critical for optimum nervous-system functioning.

acid-base balance. The condition in which the pH of the blood is at a constant level of 7.35 to 7.45.

adaptive overload stress. A training method in which the body must adjust to increasingly greater amounts of resistance.

adenosine triphosphate (ATP). A compound that, when broken down, produces the energy that enables the muscles and other organs to function.

adipose tissue. The anatomical fat found in between the skin and muscle.

aerobic. With oxygen.

aerobic activity. A low-intensity, high-endurance activity that requires oxygen for endurance.

aerobic endurance. The ability to maintain aerobic muscle output over long periods of time.

alpha-linolenic acid. An essential fatty acid.

amine. A nitrogen-containing compound in which at least one hydrogen atom has been replaced with a hydrocarbon radical.

ammonia. A toxic metabolic waste product.

anabolism. The biochemical process in which different molecules combine to form larger, more complex molecules.

anaerobic. Without oxygen.

anaerobic activity. A high-intensity, low-endurance activity that requires bursts of energy for power or speed.

anaerobic power-endurance. The ability to exert maximum muscular effort time after time with no appreciable decline in force output.

anemia. A condition in which the oxygen-carrying capacity of the blood is reduced. It is the most common symptom of iron deficiency.

anticatabolic. Describing a substance the prevents catabolism.

antioxidant. A nutrient that has been found to seek out and neutralize free radicals in the body and to stimulate the body to recover more quickly from free-radical damage.

arachidonic acid. A fatty acid that becomes essential when a linoleic-acid deficiency exists.

arteriosclerosis. Hardening of the arteries.

assimilation. Conversion into living tissue.

atherosclerosis. A degenerative illness that causes hardening of the arteries.

beta oxidation. The metabolic process in which fatty acids are used to regenerate adenosine-triphosphate molecules; an oxidative energy system.

betaine. An alkaloid used to treat muscular degeneration.

bile. A substance secreted by the liver that is essential for the digestion and absorption of fats and for the assimilation of calcium.

bioavailability. The ability of an ingested nutrient to cross from the digestive tract into the bloodstream and then from the bloodstream into the cells in which it will be utilized.

biological value (BV). Both the biological efficiency of a protein and any of a number of methods used to measure a protein's biological efficiency.

blood buffer. A substance that helps maintain the pH balance in the blood.

blood plasma. The liquid part of the blood; the substance in the blood that carries the red blood cells.

blood pressure. The pressure of the blood against the walls of the arteries.

blood-brain barrier. A semipermeable membrane that keeps the blood that is circulating in the brain away from the tissue fluids surrounding the brain cells.

calorie. A unit of measurement used to express the energy value of food.

cannibalization. The breakdown of muscle tissue by the body for the purpose of obtaining amino acids for other metabolic purposes.

capillary. A tiny blood vessel through which nutrients and waste products travel between the bloodstream and the body's cells.

carbohydrate drink. A sports beverage designed to replenish the glycogen (energy) stores.

carbon dioxide. A metabolic waste product.

carcinogen. A substance that is either proven or suspected to cause cancer in humans or laboratory animals.

catabolism. The biochemical process in which complex

molecules are broken down for energy production, recycling of their components, or excretion.

catalyze. To initiate.

catecholamine. One of the substances that function, primarily as neurotransmitters, in the sympathetic and central nervous systems. The substances include dopamine, epinephrine, and norepinephrine.

cell membrane. The outer boundary of a cell. Also called the *plasma membrane*.

cellular replication. The process in which a cell is duplicated for the purpose of creating a new cell.

cellular uptake. Absorption by the cells.

chromosome. A unit, located within the cell nucleus, that contains all of a person's genetic information, in the form of genes.

coenzyme. An enzyme cofactor.

cofactor. A substance that must be present for another substance to be able to perform a certain function.

collagen. A simple protein that is the chief component of connective tissue.

complete protein. A protein that contains the essential amino acids in amounts that are sufficient for the maintenance of normal growth rate and body weight.

connective tissue. Tissue that either supports other tissue or joins tissue to tissue, muscle to bone, or bone to bone. It includes cartilage, bone, tendons, ligaments, reticular tissue, areolar tissue, adipose tissue, blood, bone marrow, and lymph.

contraction. The development of tension within a muscle. The two kinds are isotonic, in which the muscle shortens as it becomes tense, and isometric, in which the muscle does not shorten as it becomes tense.

cortisol. A hormone secreted by the adrenal glands that stimulates catabolism.

creatine phosphate. A compound produced in the body, stored in the muscle fibers, and broken down by enzymes to quickly replenish the adenosine-triphosphate stores.

creatinine. A waste product of creatine metabolism.

cross-link. An undesirable bond between molecules that is induced by free radicals and results in deformed molecules that cannot function properly.

cytoplasm. The liquid between the cell membrane and nuclear membrane of a cell. Also called the *cytosol*.

degenerative illness. An illness that causes the body to deteriorate. Examples are cancer and arthritis.

deoxyribonucleic acid (DNA). The substance in the cell nucleus that contains the cell's genetic blueprint and determines the type of life form into which the cell will develop.

depletion. Draining.

dermatitis. A skin condition.

detoxifying agent. A substance that helps rid the body of carcinogens and dangerous chemicals.

diabetes. Diabetes mellitus. A condition in which the body does not properly metabolize carbohydrates due to a lack of or resistance against insulin.

digestive enzyme. An enzyme that acts as catalysts for the breakdown of food components.

di-peptide. Two amino acids linked together.

disaccharide. A simple carbohydrate composed of two sugar molecules.

diuretic. A substance that increases urination.

docosahexaenoic acid (DHA). An omega-3 fatty acid.

dopamine. A catecholamine that often functions as a neurotransmitter.

ectomorph. The slim, linear body type.

eicosanoid. One of a group of substances that help regulate a wide diversity of physiological processes.

eicosapentaenoic acid (EPA). An omega-3 fatty acid.

electrolyte balance. The ratio of chloride, potassium, sodium, and the other electrolytes in the body.

electron transport system. The metabolic process in which electrons are passed between certain protein molecules, releasing energy that is used to regenerate adenosine-triphosphate molecules.

emulsifier. A substance that, during digestion, helps disperse fats in water mediums.

endomorph. The fat, round body type.

endurance. The ability to continue performing without undue discomfort.

endurance sport. A sport that requires the ability to perform for long periods of time at low intensities, such as marathon running and cross-country skiing.

energy metabolism. A series of chemical reactions that break down foodstuffs and thereby produce energy.

energy supplement. A supplement designed to enhance the mental or physical energy levels.

energy system. A sequence of metabolic reactions that produces energy.

enteric coating. A coating on tablets that delays digestion of the tablets until they pass from the stomach into the intestines.

enzyme. One of a group of protein catalysts that initiate or speed chemical reactions in the body without being consumed.

ephedra. A plant that contains ephedrine and pseudoephedrine and is therefore banned by a number of sports governing organizations.

ephedrine. A drug that constricts the blood vessels and widens the bronchial passages.

epinephrine. A hormone secreted by the adrenal gland that prepares the body for the fight-or-flight reaction.

ergogenic. A catchall term that describes anything that can be used to enhance athletic performance. Ergogenic aids can be dietary or nondietary and include dietary supplements, special training techniques, and mental strategies.

essential nutrient. A nutrient that the body cannot produce itself or that it cannot produce in sufficient amounts to maintain good health.

excitatory neurotransmitter. A neurotransmitter that acts as a stimulant to the brain.

extracellular. Outside the cell.

fast-twitch muscle fibers. Muscle fibers that contract quickly, providing short bursts of energy, and therefore are used when strength and power are needed.

fat cell. A cell that stores fatty acids for energy.

fat metabolism. The process by which fat is changed to make new tissue.

fat soluble. Capable of being dissolved in lipid and organic solvents.

free radical. One of the highly reactive molecules that are known to injure cell membranes, cause defects in the deoxyribonucleic acid (DNA), and contribute to the aging process and a number of degenerative illnesses. Free radicals are byproducts of normal chemical reactions in the body that involve oxygen.

free-form amino acids. Amino acids that are in their free state, or single.

fructose. A simple carbohydrate that is a monosaccharide. It is absorbed and utilized by the body much slower than glucose and has therefore become the preferred form of sugar in health foods. Also called *levulose* or *fruit sugar*.

full profile. Containing all the nonessential as well essential nutrients. For example, a full-profile amino-acid supplement contains all the nonessential amino acids as well as the essential amino acids. Also called *full spectrum*.

gluconeogenesis. The metabolic process in which glucose is synthesized from noncarbohydrate sources.

glucose. A simple carbohydrate that is a monosaccharide. Also called *dextrose* or *grape sugar*.

glucose polymer. A processed form of polysaccharides, or complex carbohydrates.

glucose tolerance factor. A substance that helps lower the blood-sugar level.

glucose-alanine cycle. An important biochemical process that occurs during exercise to produce energy. Glycogen is broken down to glucose and then to pyruvate, some of which is used directly for energy and the remainder of which is converted to alanine. The alanine is returned to the liver and stored as glucose, then once again broken down to glycogen and then to pyruvate.

glycogen. A complex carbohydrate that occurs only in animals; the form in which glucose is stored in the body.

glycogen depletion. The draining of the body's glycogen stores.

glycogen replenishment. The refilling of the body's glycogen stores.

glycogen sparing. The saving of glycogen by the body for other functions.

glycogen-bound water. The water that is stored in the muscles along with glycogen. About 3 ounces of water must be stored with every 1 ounce of glycogen.

glycogenolysis. The metabolic process in which glycogen is broken down.

glycolysis. The metabolic process in which glucose is converted to lactic acid.

glycolytic energy systems. The energy systems that produce energy through glycolysis. They include nonoxidative glycolysis and oxidative glycolysis.

glycoprotein. A conjugated protein found in blood.

glycosaminoglycans (GAGs). Long chains of modified sugars that are the main component of proteoglycan.

gram. A measurement of weight equal to approximately one twenty-eighth of an ounce.

guarana. A plant that contains caffeine and is therefore banned by a number of sports governing organizations.

hard gainer. A person who has trouble gaining weight.

heart rate. The rate at which the heart pumps the blood through the body.

hemoglobin. The oxygen carrier in red blood cells.

hemolytic anemia. A condition in which the hemoglobin becomes separated from the red blood cells.

hemorrhage. Bleed excessively.

herbal bitter. A liquor prepared with bitter herbs and used for various therapeutic purposes.

high-density lipoproteins (HDLs). The good lipoproteins that help prevent cholesterol buildup in the arteries.

hitting the wall. The sensation felt by marathon runners when they deplete their body's glycogen stores and begin running primarily on stored body fat.

homeostasis. The tendency of the body to maintain an internal equilibrium.

hormone. One of the numerous substances produced by the endocrine glands that regulate bodily functions.

hyaluronic acid. The principal glycosaminoglycan in proteoglycan.

hydrochloric acid. A stomach secretion that functions in protein metabolism, helps keep the stomach relatively bacteria-free, and assists in the maintenance of a low pH balance in the stomach.

hydrogenation. The process in which unsaturated fatty acids are saturated with hydrogen atoms to make them more solid.

hydrolysis. The breakdown of a substance throught the use of water.

hydrolyzed protein. A protein that has already been broken down, usually by enzymes, and is a mixture of free-form, di-peptide, and tri-peptide amino acids.

hydrostatic weighing. A method for determining body composition that involves weighing the body under water.

hypertension. High blood pressure.

hypervitaminosis. *See* **Vitamin toxicity**.

hypoglycemia. Low blood sugar.

immediate energy systems. The nonoxidative energy systems that supply immediate energy for bursts of power through the use of adenosine triphosphate and creatine phosphate.

immunoglobulin. A protein that functions as an antibody in the body's immune system.

incomplete protein. A protein that is usually deficient in one or more of the essential amino acids. Most plant proteins are incomplete.

inhibitory neurotransmitter. A neurotransmitter that is calming to the brain.

inorganic. Referring to something that is not biologically produced and that does not contain any living material.

insulin resistance. A condition in which the body is resistant against the effects of insulin.

insulin-like growth factors (IGFs). Substances that promote growth in the muscles. The two kinds are insulin-like growth factor I (IGF-I) and insulin-like growth factor II (IGF-II).

intermediary. A substance that plays a role in the middle of a process.

international unit (IU). A measure of potency based on an accepted international standard. It is usually used with beta-carotene and vitamins A, D, and E. Because it is a measure of potency, not weight or volume, the number of milligrams in an IU varies, depending on the substance being measured.

interstitial spaces. The tiny spaces between tissues or organ parts.

intracellular. Inside the cell.

involuntary muscle. A muscle that acts independently of the will.

ionic form. In the form of ions, which are atoms or groups of atoms that have either a positive or negative charge from having lost or gained one or more electrons.

ketone. An acidic substance produced during the incomplete metabolism of fatty acids. It can upset the physiology.

Krebs cycle. The metabolic process in which energy is released from glucose, fatty-acid, or protein molecules and used to regenerate adenosine-triphosphate molecules.

lactic acid. A byproduct of glycolysis.

lean body mass. All of a body's tissues apart from the body fat—the bones, muscles, organs, blood, and water. Also called *fat-free mass*.

limiting nutrient. A nutrient that has the ability, through its absence or presence, to restrict the utilization of other nutrients or the functioning of the body.

linoleic acid. An essential fatty acid.

lipolysis. The process in which lipids are broken down into their constituent fatty acids.

lipoprotein. A conjugated protein that transports cholesterol and fats in the blood.

lipotropic agent. A substance that prevents fatty buildup in the liver and helps the body metabolize fat more efficiently.

long-chain fatty acid. A fatty acid with a chain of thirteen to nineteen carbon atoms.

lymphatic fluid. A clear fluid derived from blood plasma that circulates throughout the body to nourish tissue cells and to return waste matter to the bloodstream.

lymphatic system. The system of vessels that carries the lymphatic fluid through the body.

macronutrient. One of the nutrients that are required daily in large amounts and that are thought of in quantities of ounces and grams. They include carbohydrates, protein, lipids, and water.

macronutrient modulation. The practice of varying the ratio of the macronutrients in the diet to meet specific metabolic needs to enhance performance. Also called *macronutrient manipulation*.

malabsorption. Incorrect absorption.

meal-replacement drink. A nutrient drink that is low in calories and designed to replace meals for weight-loss purposes.

medium-chain fatty acid. A fatty acid with a chain of six to twelve carbon atoms.

megadose. An extremely large dose.

mesomorph. The muscular body type.

metabolic booster. A substance whose digestion causes the body to produce more than the normal amount of energy. Also called *thermogenic aid*.

metabolic pathway. A sequence of metabolic reactions.

metabolic rate. The body's total daily caloric expenditure.

metabolic water. The water that is produced in the body as a result of energy production.

metalloenzyme. A mineral-containing enzyme.

metaloprotein. A conjugated protein found in blood.

microgram. A measurement of weight equal to one one-thousandth of a milligram.

micronutrient. One of the nutrients present in the diet and the body in small amounts. Micronutrients are measured in milligrams and micrograms. They include the vitamins, minerals, metabolites, and herbs.

microtrauma. Small but widespread tears in the muscle cells from training stress.

milligram. A measurement of weight equal to one one-thousandth of a gram.

mineralization. Hardening.

mitochondrion. The organelle that produces the cellular energy required for metabolism.

monosaccharide. A simple carbohydrate composed of one sugar molecule, such as glucose and fructose.

monounsaturated fatty acid. A fatty acid that has one unsaturated carbon molecule.

muscle fiber. A long muscle cell.

muscle mass. Muscle tissue.

muscle tissue. Tissue that has the ability to contract, either voluntarily or involuntarily. It can be striated or smooth. The three kinds are skeletal muscle tissue, cardiac muscle tissue, and smooth muscle tissue.

neurotransmitter. A chemical substance that helps transmit nerve impulses.

nonessential nutrient. A nutrient that is not considered essential—that is, a nutrient that the body does make in sufficient amounts to maintain good health.

nonoxidative energy systems. The systems that supply energy for high-intensity, low-endurance activities lasting up to several minutes, such as powerlifting and sprinting. They include the immediate energy systems and nonoxidative glycolysis.

nonoxidative glycolysis. The metabolic process in which a glucose molecule is split in half to regenerate adenosine diphosphate back into adenosine triphosphate; a nonoxidative energy system that is the major contributor of energy during near-maximum efforts lasting up to about one and a half minutes.

norepinephrine. A hormone secreted by the adrenal glands for a number of purposes and also released by the sympathetic nerve endings as a neurotransmitter.

nuclear membrane. The membrane surrounding the cell nucleus.

nucleic acid. A conjugated protein found in chromosomes.

nucleoplasm. The liquid within the cell nucleus in which the chromosomes are suspended.

nucleus. The control center of the cell.

organelle. One of the variety of components that make up a cell. The organelles include the cell membrane, nucleus, ribosome, endoplasmic reticulum, Golgi apparatus, lysosome, and mitochondrion.

organic. Biologically produced and containing carbon atoms as part of its structure.

osteoporosis. A condition in which the bones are very porous and can break very easily.

oxidation. A chemical reaction in which an atom or molecule loses electrons or hydrogen atoms.

oxidation-reduction reaction. A chemical reaction in which one substance loses electrons or hydrogen atoms while, at the same time, another substance gains electrons or hydrogen atoms.

oxidative energy systems. The systems that supply energy for low-intensity, high-duration activities lasting more than approximately three or four minutes, such as marathon running and aerobic dance. They include oxidative glycolysis and beta oxidation.

oxidative glycolysis. The metabolic process in which a glucose molecule is split in half to form pyruvate to regenerate adenosine triphosphate; an oxidative energy system that is a major contributor of energy during near-maximum efforts lasting up to about three or four minutes.

peptide-bonded amino acids. Amino acids that are linked together.

peroxidation. The formation of a peroxide compound.

pH. Potential of hydrogen. A measure of the concentration of hydrogen ions in a solution.

phosphoinositide. An inositol-containing phospholipid that has a profound effect on cellular functioning and on metabolism, particularly the metabolism of fats.

phosphoprotein. A conjugated protein found in casein, or milk protein.

polypeptide. Four or more amino acids linked together.

polysaccharide. A complex carbohydrate.

polyunsaturated fatty acid. A fatty acid that has more than one unsaturated carbon molecule. Polyunsaturated fatty acids tend to be liquid at room temperature.

potentiator. A substance that helps another substance perform its function.

power. Strength combined with speed.

power sport. A sport that requires the ability to perform at high intensities for short periods of time, such as powerlifting and golf.

precursor. An intermediate substance in the body's production of another substance.

prostaglandin. A hormone important in metabolism.

prostanoid. A derivative of the prostaglandin.

protected nutrient. A nutrient that the body reserves (protects against being used) for a certain function.

protein supplement. A supplement that supplies extra protein.

pseudoephedrine. A decongestant; a drug that reduces nasal congestion.

pyruvate. A compound that is produced during the glucose-alanine cycle. Some of the pyruvate that is produced is used directly for energy, while the remainder is converted back to alanine, which is eventually converted into glucose and used for energy.

quick-release tablet. A tablet that releases its contents quickly.

red blood cell. The cell that carries the hemoglobin in blood.

renal. Pertaining to the kidneys.

replenishment. Refilling.

ribonucleic acid (RNA). The substance that carries the coded genetic information from the deoxyribonucleic acid (DNA), in the cell nucleus, to the ribosomes, where the instructions are translated into the form of protein molecules.

saturated fatty acid. A fatty acid that has the maximum number of hydrogen atoms that it can hold, with no unsaturated carbon molecules. Saturated fatty acids tend to be solid at room temperature.

series-1 prostaglandins. A group of hormones that regulate many cellular activities.

serotonin. A neurotransmitter that helps control the sleep cycle.

short-chain fatty acid. A fatty acid with a chain of four to five carbon atoms.

skeletal muscle. One of the muscles that work in conjunction with the skeletal system to create motion.

skin-fold calipers. The specialized calipers used to measure the thickness of skin folds.

skin-fold measurement. A method for determining body composition that involves measuring the thickness of selected folds of skin using special calipers.

slow-twitch muscle fibers. Muscle fibers that produce a steady, low-intensity, repetitive contraction and therefore are used when endurance is needed.

sodium bicarbonate. A bicarbonate that boosts performance in power sports.

somatotropin. Growth hormone.

somatotype. Body type.

sports rehydration drink. A drink that replaces water, glucose, and the electrolytes after exercising.

sports supplement. A dietary supplement with ergogenic benefits.

sports-nutrition drink. A beverage formulated to fulfill special athletic needs by providing specific nutrients.

starch. A complex carbohydrate that occurs only in plants.

strength. Force output.

strength-power. *See* **Power.**

striated muscle. A muscle that has a grainy appearance.

sulfur. An acid-forming mineral that is part of the chemical structure of several amino acids. Because of its ability to protect against the harmful effects of radiation and pollution, it slows down the aging process.

superoxide dismutase. An antioxidant.

sustained power. The ability to maintain power output over long periods of time.

sustained-release tablet. A tablet that releases its contents slowly and continuously over an extended period of time.

synthesis. Formation.

thermogenesis. The process by which the body generates heat, or energy, by increasing the metabolic rate above normal.

thermogenic response. The rise in the metabolic rate. Also known as the *thermogenic effect* or *specific dynamic action (SDA).*

timed-release tablet. A tablet that releases its contents in spurts over several hours.

tissue metabolism. The process by which foodstuffs are changed to make new tissues.

transamination reaction. The process in which an amino group is transferred from an amino acid to a molecule, usually to produce another amino acid.

transmethylation. The metabolic process in which an amino acid donates a methyl group to another compound.

triiodothyronine. A thyroid hormone.

tri-peptide. Three amino acids linked together.

ultra-endurance event. An event lasting longer than two hours.

urea cycle. The metabolic process in which ammonia is converted to the waste product urea, which is then excreted from the body.

uric acid. A toxic metabolic waste product.

vascularization. The creation of new blood vessels in the tissues.

vasodilator. A substance that increases blood flow.

very long chain fatty acid. A fatty acid with a chain of twenty or more carbon atoms.

vitamin toxicity. Vitamin poisoning.

VO_2 max. The maximum rate at which oxygen can be consumed.

voluntary muscle. A muscle that responds to an act of the will.

water soluble. Capable of being dissolved in water.

whole food. Food that is in its natural, complete state; unprocessed food.

BIBLIOGRAPHY

Allen, Markku, Matti Reinla, and Reijo Vihko. "Response of Serum Hormones to Androgen Administration in Power Athletes." *Medicine and Science in Sports and Exercise*, Vol. 17 (1985), pp. 354–359.

Anderson, Helen L., Mary Belle Heindel, and Hellen Linkswiler. "Effect on Nitrogen Balance of Adult Man of Varying Source of Nitrogen and Level of Calorie Intake." *Journal of Nutrition* (1969), pp. 82–90.

Anderson, M., et al. "Pre-Exercise Meal Affects Ride Time to Fatigue in Trained Cyclists." *Journal of the American Dietetic Association*, Vol. 94 (1994), pp. 1152–1153.

Apfelbaum, Marian, Jacques Fricker, and Lawrence Igoin-Apfelbaum. "Low and Very Low Calorie Diets." *American Journal of Clinical Nutrition*, Vol. 45 (1987), pp. 1126–1134.

Armstrong, R. B. "Mechanisms of Exercise-Induced Delayed Onset Muscular Soreness: A Brief Review." *Medicine and Science in Sports and Exercise*, Vol. 16 (1984), No. 6, pp. 529–538.

Armstrong, R. B. "Muscle Damage and Endurance Events." *Sports Medicine*, Vol. 3 (1986), pp. 370–381.

Baker, O., et al. "Absorption and Excretion of L-Carnitine During Single or Multiple Dosings in Humans." *International Journal of Vitamin and Nutrition Research*, Vol. 63 (1993), pp. 22–26.

Ball, T., et al. "Periodic Carbohydrate Replacement During 50 Minutes of High-Intensity Cycling Improves Subsequent Sprint Performance." *International Journal of Sport Science* (1995), pp. 151–158.

Bamman, M. M., et al. "Changes in Body Composition, Diet, and Strength of Bodybuilders During the 12 Weeks Prior to Competition." *Journal of Sports Medicine and Physical Fitness*, Vol. 33 (1993), p. 383.

Belanger, A. Y., and A. J. McComas. "A Comparison of Contractile Properties in Human Arm and Leg Muscles." *European Journal of Applied Physiology*, Vol. 54 (1985), pp. 26–33.

Bell, R. D., J. D. MacDougall, R. Billeter, and H. Howald. "Muscle Fiber Types and Morphometric Analysis of Skeletal Muscle in Six-Year-Old Children." *Medicine and Science in Sports and Exercise*, Vol. 12 (1980), No. 1, pp. 28–31.

Bergstrom, Jonas, and Eric Hultman. "Nutrition for Maximal Sports Performance." *Journal of the American Medical Association*, Vol. 221 (1972), No. 9, pp. 999–1004.

Berning, J. R. "The Role of Medium-Chain Triglycerides in Exercise." *International Journal of Sport Nutrition*, Vol. 6 (1996), No. 3, pp. 121–133.

Bier, Dennis M., and Vernon R. Young. "Exercise and Blood Pressure: Nutritional Considerations." *Annals of Internal Medicine*, Part 2 (1983), pp. 864–869.

Bonde-Petersen, Flemming, Howard G. Knuttgen, and Jan Henriksson. "Muscle Metabolism During Exercise With Concentric and Eccentric Contractions." *Journal of Applied Physiology*, Vol. 33 (1972), pp. 792–795.

Bonke, D., and B. Nickel. "Improvement of Fine Motoric Movement Control by Elevated Dosages of Vitamin B_1, B_6 and B_{12} in Target Shooting." *International Journal of Vitamin and Nutrition Research*, Vol. 30 (1989), p. 198.

Borum, Peggy R. "Carnitine." *Annual Reviews of Nutrition*, Vol. 3 (1983), pp. 233–259.

Brilla, L. R., and T. E. Landerholm. "Effect of Fish Oil Supplementation and Exercise on Serum Lipid and Aerobic Fitness." *Journal of Sports Medicine*, Vol. 30 (1990), No. 2, p. 173.

Brodan, V., E. Kuhn, J. Pechar, Z. Placer, and Z. Slabochova. "Effects of Sodium Glutamate Infusion on Ammonia Formation During Intense Physical Exercise in Man." *Nutrition Reports International*, Vol. 9 (1974), No. 3, pp. 223–232.

Brown, C. Harmon, and Jack H. Wilmore. "The Effects of Maximal Resistance Training on the Strength and Body Composition of Women Athletes." *Medicine and Science in Sports*, Vol. 6 (1974), No. 3, pp. 174–177.

Bucci, L. *Nutrients as Ergogenic Aids for Sports and Exercise*. Boca Raton, FL: CRC Press, 1993.

Bucci, L. *Nutrition Applied to Injury Rehabilitation and Sports Medicine*. Boca Raton, FL: CRC Press, 1995.

Buono, Michael J., Thomas R. Clancy, and Jeff R. Cook. "Blood Lactate and Ammonium Ion Accumulation During Graded Exercise in Humans." *The American Physiological Society* (1984), pp. 135–139.

Burke, Edmond R., Frank Cerny, David Costill, and William Fink. "Characteristics of Skeletal Muscle in Competitive Cyclists." *Medicine and Science in Sports*, Vol. 9 (1977), No. 2, pp. 109–112.

Buskirk, Elsworth R., and José Mendez. "Sports Science and Body Composition Analysis: Emphasis on Cell and Muscle

Mass." *Medicine and Science in Sports and Exercise*, Vol. 16 (1984), No. 6, pp. 584–593.

Butterfield, G. "Ergogenic Aids: Evaluating Sport Nutrition Products." *International Journal of Sport Nutrition*, Vol. 6 (1996), No. 3, pp. 191–197.

Butterfield, Gail E., and Doris H. Calloway. "Physical Activity Improves Protein Utilization in Young Men." *British Journal of Nutrition*, Vol. 51 (1984), pp. 171–184.

Calles-Escandon, Jorge, John J. Cunningham, Peter Snyder, Ralph Jacob, Gabor Huszar, Jacob Loke, and Philip Felig. "Influence of Exercise on Urea, Creatinine, and 3-Methylhistidine Excretion in Normal Human Subjects." *The American Physiological Society* (1984), pp. E334–E338.

Campbell, C. J., A. Bonen, R. L. Kirby, and A. N. Belcastro. "Muscle Fiber Composition and Performance Capacities of Women." *Medicine and Science in Sports*, Vol. 11 (1979), pp. 260–265.

Campbell, M. J., A. J. McComas, and F. Petitio. "Physiological Changes in Aging Muscles." *Journal of Neurology, Neurosurgery, and Psychiatry*, Vol. 36 (1973), pp.174–182.

Carlson, Bruce M., and John A. Faulkner. "The Regeneration of Skeletal Muscle Fibers Following Injury: A Review." *Medicine and Science in Sports and Exercise*, Vol. 15 (1983), No. 3, pp. 187–198.

Carter, J. E. Lindsay, and William H. Phillips. "Structural Changes in Exercising Middle-Aged Males During a 2-Year Period." *Journal of Applied Physiology*, Vol. 27 (1969), pp. 787–794.

Casanueva, F. F., L. Villanueva, J. A. Cabranes, J. Cabezas-Cerrato, and A. Fernandez-Cruz. "Cholinergic Mediation of Growth Hormone Secretion Elicited by Arginine, Clonidine, and Physical Exercise in Man." *Journal of Clinical Endocrinology and Metabolism*, Vol. 59 (1984), No. 3, pp. 526–530.

Celejowa, I., and M. Homa. "Food Intake, Nitrogen and Energy Balance in Polish Weight Lifters, During Training Camp." *Nutrition and Metabolism*, Vol. 12 (1970), pp. 259–274.

Chang, Tse Wen, and Alfred L. Goldberg. "The Metabolic Fates of Amino Acids and the Formation of Glutamine in Skeletal Muscle." *Journal of Biological Chemistry*, Vol. 253 (1978), No. 10, pp. 3685–3695.

Christensen, H. "Muscle Activity and Fatigue in the Shoulder Muscles During Repetitive Work." *European Journal of Applied Physiology*, Vol. 54 (1986), pp. 596–601.

Clarkson, P., and E. Haymes. "Trace Mineral Requirements for Athletes." *International Journal of Sports Nutrition*, Vol. 4 (1994), p. 104.

Clarkson, Priscilla M., Walter Kroll, and Thomas C. McBride. "Plantar Flexion Fatigue and Muscle Fiber Type in Power and Endurance Athletes." *Medicine and Science in Sports and Exercise*, Vol. 12 (1980), pp. 262–267.

Conzolazio, C. Frank, Herman L. Johnson, Richard A. Nelson, Joseph G. Dramise, and James H. Skala. "Protein Metabolism During Intensive Physical Training in the Young Adult." *American Journal of Clinical Nutrition*, Vol. 28 (1975), pp. 29–35.

Cook, James D., and Elaine R. Monsen. "Vitamin C, the Common Cold, and Iron Absorption." *American Journal of Clinical Nutrition* (1977), pp. 235–241.

Copinschi, Georges, Laurence C. Wegienka, Satoshi Hane, and Peter H. Forsham. "Effect of Arginine on Serum Levels of Insulin and Growth Hormone in Obese Subjects." *Metabolism*, Vol. 16 (1967), pp. 485–491.

Cossack, Zafrallah T., and Ananda Prasad. "Effect of Protein Source on the Bioavailability of Zinc in Human Subjects." *Nutrition Research*, Vol. 3 (1983), pp. 23–31.

Costill, D. L., A. Barnett, R. Sharp, W. J. Fink, and A. Katz. "Leg Muscle pH Following Sprint Running." *Medicine and Science in Sports and Exercise*, Vol. 15 (1983), pp. 325–329.

Costill, D. L., and M. Hargreaves. "Carbohydrate Nutrition and Fatigue." *Sports Medicine*, Vol. 13 (1992), p. 86.

Costill, David L., Michael G. Flynn, John P. Kirwan, Joseph A. Houmard, Joel B. Mitchell, Robert Thomas, and Sung Han Park. "Effects of Repeated Days of Intensified Training on Muscle Glycogen and Swimming Performance." *Medicine and Science in Sports and Exercise*, Vol. 20 (1987), No. 3, pp. 249–254.

Coyle, Edward F., and Andrew R. Coggan. "Effectiveness of Carbohydrate Feeding in Delaying Fatigue During Prolonged Exercise." *Sports Medicine* (1984), pp. 446–458.

Craig, B. "The Influence of Fructose on Physical Performance." *American Journal of Clinical Nutrition*, Vol. 58 (1993), p. S819.

Davies, Kelvin J. A., Alexandre T. Quintanilha, George A. Brooks, and Lester Packer. "Free Radicals and Tissue Damage Produced by Exercise." *Biochemical and Biophysical Research Communications*, Vol. 107 (1982), No. 4, pp. 1198–1205.

Davis, Teresa A., Irene E. Karl, Elise D. Tegtmeyer, Dale F. Osborne, Saulo Klahr, and Herschel R. Harter. "Muscle and Protein Turnover: Effects of Exercise Training and Renal Insufficiency." *The American Physiological Society* (1985), pp. E337–E345.

Despres, J. P., C. Bouchard, R. Savard, A. Tremblay, M. Marcotte, and G. Theriault. "Level of Physical Fitness and Adipocyte Lipolysis in Humans." *The American Physiological Society* (1984), pp.1157–1161.

Despres, J. P., C. Bouchard, A. Tremblay, R. Savard, and M. Marcotte. "Effects of Aerobic Training on Fat Distribution in Male Subjects." *Medicine and Science in Sports and Exercise*, Vol. 17 (1985), No. 1, pp. 113–118.

DiPasquale, M. G. *The Bodybuilding Supplement Review*. N.P.: Optimum Training Systems, 1995.

DiPrampero, P. Enrico. "Energetics of Muscular Exercise." *Biochemical Pharmacology*, Vol. 89 (1981), pp. 143–209.

Dohm, G. Lynis, George J. Kasperek, Edward B. Tapscott, and Gary R. Beecher. "Effect of Exercise on Synthesis and

Degradation of Muscle Protein." *Biochemical Journal*, Vol. 188 (1980), pp. 255–262.

Ehn, Lars, Bjorn Carlmark, and Sverker Hoglund. "Iron Status in Athletes Involved in Intense Physical Activity." *Medicine and Science in Sports and Exercise*, Vol. 12 (1980), No. 1, pp. 61–64.

Erickson, Mark A., Robert J. Schwarzkopf, and Robert D. McKenzie. "Effects of Caffeine, Fructose, and Glucose Ingestion on Muscle Glycogen Utilization During Exercise." *Medicine and Science in Sports and Exercise*, Vol. 19 (1987), No. 6, pp. 579–583.

Essen, B. E., J. Jansson, J. Henriksson, A. W. Taylor, and B. Saltin. "Metabolic Characteristics of Fibre Types in Human Skeletal Muscle." *Acta Physiolgica Scandinavica*, Vol.19 (1975), pp.153–165.

Fahey, Thomas D., Lahsen Akka, and Richard Rolph. "Body Composition and VO$_2$ Max of Exceptional Weight-Trained Athletes." *Journal of Applied Physiology*, Vol. 19 (1975), No. 4, pp. 559–561.

Food and Nutrition Board. *Recommended Dietary Allowances*, 9th Ed. Washington, DC: National Academy of Sciences, 1980.

Forbes, Gilbert B. "Body Composition as Affected by Physical Activity and Nutrition." *Metabolic and Nutritional Aspects of Physical Exercise: Federation Proceedings*, Vol. 44 (1985), No. 2., pp. 334–352.

Forbes, Gilbert B. "Growth of the Lean Body Mass in Man." *Growth*, Vol. 36 (1972), pp. 325–338.

Forbes, Richard M., and John W. Erdman, Jr. "Bioavailability of Trace Mineral Elements." *Annual Reviews of Nutrition*, Vol. 3 (1983), pp. 213–231.

Fournier, Mario, Joe Ricci, Albert W. Taylor, Ronald J. Ferguson, Richard R. Montpetit, and Bernard R. Chaitman. "Skeletal Muscle Adaptation in Adolescent Boys: Sprint and Endurance Training and Detraining." *Medicine and Science in Sports and Exercise*, Vol. 14 (1982), No. 6, pp. 453–456.

Fox, Edward L., Robert L. Bartels, James Klinzing, and Kerry Ragg. "Metabolic Responses to Interval Training Programs of High and Low Power Output." *Medicine and Science in Sports*, Vol. 9 (1977), No. 3, pp.191–196.

Friedman, J. E., et al. "Regulation of Glycogen Resynthesis Following Exercise." *Sports Medicine*, Vol. 11 (1991), p. 232.

Galton, David J., and George A. Bray. "Studies on Lipolysis in Human Adipose Cells." *Journal of Clinical Investigation*, Vol. 46 (1967), No. 4, pp. 621–629.

Gao, J. P., D. I. Costill, C. A. Horswill, and S. H. Park. "Sodium Bicarbonate Ingestion Improves Performance in Interval Swimming." *European Journal of Applied Physiology*, Vol. 58 (1988), pp. 171–174.

Garza, C., N. S. Scrimshaw, and V. R. Young. "Human Protein Requirements: The Effect of Variations in Energy Intake Within the Maintenance Range." *American Journal of Clinical Nutrition*, Vol. 29 (1976), pp. 280–287.

Gastelu, D. L. "Developing State-of-the-Art Amino Acids." *Muscle Magazine International*, May 1989, pp. 58–64.

Goldberg, Alfred L., Joseph D. Etlinger, David F. Goldspink, and Charles Jablecki. "Mechanism of Work-Induced Hypertrophy of Skeletal Muscle." *Medicine and Science in Sports*, Vol. 7 (1975), No. 3, pp.185–198.

Goldspink, David F. "The Influence of Activity on Muscle Size and Protein Turnover." *Journal of Physiology*, Vol. 264 (1976), pp. 283–296.

Gollnick, P. D., R. B. Armstrong, B. Saltin, C. W. Saubert IV, W. L. Sembrowich, and R. E. Shepherd. "Effect of Training on Enzyme Activity and Fiber Composition of Human Skeletal Muscle." *Journal of Applied Physiology*, Vol. 34 (1973), No. 1, pp. 107–111.

Gollnick, Philip D. "Metabolism of Substrates: Energy Substrate Metabolism During Exercise and as Modified by Training." *Metabolic and Nutritional Aspects of Physical Exercise: Federation Proceedings*, Vol. 44 (1985), No. 2, pp. 353–368.

Gontzea, I., P. Sutzescu, and S. Dumitrache. "The Influence of Muscular Activity on Nitrogen Balance and on the Need of Man for Proteins." *Nutrition Reports International*, Vol.10 (1974), pp. 35–43.

Green, Jerry Franklin, and Alan P. Jackman. "Peripheral Limitations to Exercise." *Medicine and Science in Sports and Exercise*, Vol. 16 (1984), No. 3, pp. 299–305.

Greenhaff, P., et al. "Effect of Oral Creatine Supplementation on Skeletal Muscle Phosphocreatine Resynthesis." *American Journal of Physiology*, Vol. 266 (1994), pp. E725–E730.

Haralambie, G., and A. Berg. "Serum Urea and Amino Nitrogen Changes With Exercise Duration." *European Journal of Applied Physiology* (1976), pp. 39–48.

Hargreaves, M., David L. Costill, A. Katz, and W. J. Fink. "Effect of Fructose Ingestion on Muscle Glycogen Usage During Exercise." *Medicine and Science in Sports and Exercise*, Vol. 17 (1985), pp. 360–363.

Harmsen, Eef, Peter P. DeTombe, Jan Willem DeJong, and Peter W. Achterberg. "Enhanced ATP and GTP Synthesis From Hypoxanthine or Inosine After Myocardial Ischemia." *The American Physiological Society* (1984), pp. H37–H43.

Hartog, M., R. J. Havel, G. Copinschi, J. M. Earll, and B. C. Ritchie. "The Relationship Between Changes in Serum Levels of Growth Hormone and Mobilization of Fat During Exercise in Man." *Quarterly Journal of Experimental Physiology*, Vol. 52 (1967), pp. 86–96.

Hatfield, F. C. *Fitness: The Complete Guide*, 3rd Edition. Santa Barbara, CA: International Sports Sciences Association, 1996.

Hatfield, F. C. *Hardcore Bodybuilding: A Scientific Approach*. Chicago: Contemporary Books, 1993.

Hatfield, F. C., and M. Krotee. *Personalized Weight Training for Fitness and Athletics: From Theory to Practice*. Dubuque, IA: Kendall/Hunt Publishing Co., 1978.

Helie, R., J.-M. Lavoie, and D. Cousineau. "Effects of a 24-Hour Carbohydrate-Poor Diet on Metabolic and Hormonal Responses During Glucose-Infused Leg Exercise." *European Journal of Applied Physiology*, Vol. 54 (1985), pp. 420–426.

Henneman, Dorothy, and Philip H. Henneman. "Effects of Human Growth Hormone on Levels of Blood and Urinary Carbohydrate and Fat Metabolites in Man." *Journal of Clinical Investigation*, Vol. 39 (1960), pp. 1239–1245.

Herbert, Victor, Elizabeth Jacob, and Kit-Tai Judy Wong. "Destruction of Vitamin B_{12} by Vitamin C." *American Journal of Clinical Nutrition*, Vol. 30 (1976), pp. 297–303.

Hermansen, Lars, Eric Hultman, and Bengt Saltin. "Muscle Glycogen During Prolonged Severe Exercise." *Acta Physiolgica Scandinavica*, Vol. 71 (1967), pp. 129–139.

Heymsfield, Steven B., Carlos Arteaga, Clifford McManus, Janet Smith, and Steven Moffitt. "Measurement of Muscle Mass in Humans: Validity of the 24-Hour Urinary Creatinine Method." *American Journal of Clinical Nutrition*, Vol. 37 (1983), pp. 478–494.

Hickson, James F., Jr., and Klaus Hinkelmann. "Exercise and Protein Intake Effects on Urinary 3-Methylhistidine Excretion." *American Journal of Clinical Nutrition*, Vol. 41 (1985), pp. 32–45.

Hickson, Robert C., and Maureen A. Rosenkoetter. "Reduced Training Frequencies and Maintenance of Increased Aerobic Power." *Medicine and Science in Sports and Exercise*, Vol. 13, No. 1 (1981), pp. 13–16.

Hill, J. O., and R. Commerford. "Physical Activity, Fat Balance, and Energy Balance." *International Journal of Sport Nutrition*, Vol. 6 (1996), No. 3, pp. 80–92.

Hofman, Z., et al. "Glucose and Insulin Responses After Commonly Used Sport Feedings Before and After a 1-Hour Training Session." *International Journal of Sport Nutrition*, Vol. 5 (1995), pp. 194–205.

Holloszy, John O. "Adaptation of Skeletal Muscle to Endurance Exercise." *Medicine and Science in Sports*, Vol. 7 (1975), No. 3, pp. 155–164.

Holloszy, John O. "Exercise, Health, and Aging: A Need for More Information." *Medicine and Science in Sports and Exercise*, Vol. 15 (1983), No. 1, pp. 1–5.

Horton, E., and R. Terjung. *Exercise, Nutrition, and Energy Metabolism*. New York: Macmillan Publishing Company, 1988.

Horton, Edward S. "Metabolic Aspects of Exercise and Weight Reduction." *Medicine and Science in Sports and Exercise*, Vol. 18 (1986), p. 10.

Ivy, J. L., R. T. Withers, P. J. Van Handel, D.L.L. Elger, and D. L. Costill. "Muscle Respiratory Capacity and Fiber Type as Determinants of the Lactate Threshold." *American Physiological Society* (1980), pp. 523–527.

Jacobs, Ira, Mona Esbjornsson, Christer Sylven, Ingemar Holm, and Eva Jansson. "Sprint Training Effects on Muscle Myoglobin, Enzymes, Fiber Types, and Blood Lactate." *Medicine and Science in Sports and Exercise*, Vol. 19 (1987), No. 4, pp. 369–374.

Jakeman, P., and S. Maxwell. "Effect of Antioxidant Vitamin Supplementation on Muscle Function After Eccentric Exercise." *European Journal of Applied Physiology*, Vol. 67 (1993), p. 426.

Jezova, D., M. Vigas, P. Tatar, R. Kvetnansky, K. Nazar, H. Kaciuba-Uscilko, and S. Kozlowski. "Plasma Testosterone and Catecholamine Responses to Physical Exercise of Different Intensities in Men." *European Journal of Applied Physiology*, Vol. 54 (1985), pp. 62–66.

Kanter, M. "Free Radicals, Exercise, and Antioxidant Supplementation." *International Journal of Sports Nutrition*, Vol. 4 (1994), p. 205.

Karagiorgos, Athanase, Joseph F. Garcia, and George A. Brooks. "Growth Hormone Response to Continuous and Intermittent Exercise." *Medicine and Science in Sports*, Vol. 11 (1979), No. 3, pp. 302–307.

Karlsson, Jan, Lars-Olof Nordesjo, and Bengt Saltin. "Muscle Glycogen Utilization During Exercise After Physical Training." *Acta Physiolgica Scandinavica*, Vol. 90 (1974), pp. 210–217.

Karlsson, Jan, and Bengt Saltin. "Diet, Muscle Glycogen, and Endurance Performance." *Journal of Applied Physiology*, Vol. 31 (1971), No. 2, pp. 203–206.

Karlsson, Jan, and Bengt Saltin. "Lactate, ATP, and CP in Working Muscles During Exhaustive Exercise in Man." *Journal of Applied Physiology*, Vol. 29 (1970), No. 5, pp. 598–602.

Kasai, Kikuo, Masami Kobayashi, and Shin-Ichi Shimoda. "Stimulatory Effect of Glycine on Human Growth Hormone Secretion." *Metabolism*, Vol. 27 (1978), pp. 201–208.

Kasai, Kikuo, Hitoshi Suzuki, Tsutomu Nakamura, Hiroaki Shiina, and Shin-Ichi Shimoda. "Glycine Stimulates Growth Hormone Release in Man." *Acta Endocronologica*, Vol. 90 (1980), pp. 283–286.

Kasperek, George J., and Rebecca D. Snider. "Increased Protein Degradation After Eccentric Exercise." *European Journal of Applied Physiology*, Vol. 54 (1985), pp. 30–34.

Katch, F. "U.S. Government Raises Serious Questions About Reliability of U.S. Department of Agriculture's Food Composition Database." *International Journal of Sport Nutrition*, Vol. 5 (1995), pp. 62–67

Katch, Victor L., Frank I. Katch, Robert Moffatt, and Michael Gittleson. "Muscular Development and Lean Body Weight in Body Builders and Weight Lifters." *Medicine and Science in Sports and Exercise*, Vol. 12 (1980), No. 5, pp. 340–344.

Kirkendall, D. "Effect of Nutrition on Performance in Soccer." *Medicine and Science in Sports and Exercise*, Vol. 25 (1993), pp. 1370.

Kirwan, John P., David L. Costill, Michael G. Flynn, Joel B. Mitchell, William J. Fink, P. Darrell Neufer, and Joseph A.

Houmard. "Physiological Responses to Successive Days of Intense Training in Competitive Swimmers." *Medicine and Science in Sports and Exercise*, Vol. 20 (1988), No. 3, pp. 255–259.

Klissouras, Vassilis, Freddy Pirnay, and Jean-Marie Petit. "Adaptation to Maximal Effort: Genetics and Age." *Journal of Applied Physiology*, Vol. 35 (1973), No. 2, pp. 288–293.

Knopf, R. F., J. W. Conn, S. S. Fajans, J. C. Floyd, E. M. Guntsche, and J. A. Rull. "Plasma Growth Hormone Response to Intravenous Administration of Amino Acids." *Journal of Clinical Endocrinology*, Vol. 25 (1965), pp. 1140–1144.

Koeslag, J. H. "Post-Exercise Ketosis and the Hormone Response to Exercise: A Review." *Medicine and Science in Sports and Exercise*, Vol. 14 (1982), No. 5, pp. 327–334.

Lander, Jeffrey E., Barry T. Bates, James A. Sawhill, and Joseph Hamill. "A Comparison Between Free-Weight and Isokinetic Bench Pressing." *Medicine and Science in Sports and Exercise*, Vol. 17 (1985), No. 3, p. 344.

Lemon, P.W.R., et al. "Protein Requirements and Muscle Mass/Strength Changes During Intensive Training in Novice Bodybuilders." *Journal of Applied Physiology*, Vol. 73 (1992), pp. 767–775.

Lemon, P.W.R., and J. P. Mullin. "Effect of Initial Muscle Glycogen Levels on Protein Catabolism During Exercise." *The American Physiological Society* (1980), pp. 624–629.

Lemon, P.W.R., and F. J. Nagle. "Effects of Exercise on Protein and Amino Acid Metabolism." *Medicine and Science in Sports and Exercise*, Vol. 13 (1981), No. 3, pp. 141–149.

Lemon, P.W.R., and D. Proctor. "Protein Intake and Athletic Performance." *Sports Medicine*, Vol. 12 (1991), No. 5, p. 313.

Leung, A.Y., and S. Foster. *Encyclopedia of Common Natural Ingredients Used in Food, Drugs, and Cosmetics.* New York: John Wiley & Sons, 1996.

Lewis, Steven M. A., William L. Haskell, Peter D. Wood, Norman M. A. Manoogian, Judith E. Bailey, and MaryBeth B. A. Pereira. "Effects of Physical Activity on Weight Reduction in Obese Middle-Aged Women." *American Journal of Clinical Nutrition*, Vol. 29 (1976), pp. 151–156.

Linderman, J., and T. D. Fahey. "Sodium Bicarbonate Ingestion and Exercise Performance." *Sports Medicine*, Vol. 11, No. 9, p. 71.

Lucke, Christoph, and Seymour Glick. "Experimental Modification of the Sleep-Induced Peak of Growth Hormone Secretion." *Journal of Clinical Endocrinology and Metabolism*, Vol. 32 (1971), pp. 729–736.

MacDougall, J. D., D. G. Sale, S. E. Alway, and J. R. Sutton. "Muscle Fiber Number in Biceps Brachii in Bodybuilders and Control Subjects." *The American Physiological Society* (1984), p. 1399.

MacDougall, J. D., D. G. Sale, G.C.B. Elder, and J. R. Sutton. "Muscle Ultrastructural Characteristics of Elite Powerlifters and Bodybuilders." *European Journal of Applied Physiology*, Vol. 48 (1982), pp. 117–126.

MacDougall, J. D., D. G. Sale, J. R. Moroz, G.C.B. Elder, J. R. Sutton, and H. Howald. "Mitochondrial Volume Density in Human Skeletal Muscle Following Heavy Resistance Training." *Medicine and Science in Sports and Exercise*, Vol. 11 (1979), No. 2, pp. 164–166.

Mackova, Eva V., Jan Melichna, Karel Vondra, Toivo Jurimae, Thomas Paul, and Jaroslav Novak. "The Relationship Between Anaerobic Performance and Muscle Metabolic Capacity and Fibre Distribution." *European Journal of Applied Physiology*, Vol. 54 (1985), pp. 413–415.

MacLean, William C., Jr., and George G. Graham. "The Effect of Level of Protein Intake in Isoenergetic Diets on Energy Utilization." *American Journal of Clinical Nutrition* (1979), pp. 1381–1387.

Malina, Robert M., William H. Mueller, Claude Bouchard, Richard F. Shoup, and Georges Lariviere. "Fatness and Fat Patterning Among Athletes at the Montreal Olympic Games, 1976." *Medicine and Science in Sports and Exercise*, Vol. 14 (1982), No. 6, pp. 445–452.

Manore, M. "Vitamin B_6 and Exercise." *International Journal of Sports Nutrition*, Vol. 4 (1994), p. 89.

Marable, N. L., J. F. Hickson Jr., M. K. Korslund, W. G. Herbert, R. F. Desjardins, and F. W. Thye. "Urinary Nitrogen Excretion as Influenced by a Muscle-Building Exercise Program and Protein Intake Variation." *Nutrition Reports International*, Vol. 19 (1979), No. 6, pp. 795–805.

Maresh, C., et al. "Dietary Supplementation and Improved Anaerobic Performance." *International Journal of Sport Nutrition*, Vol. 4 (1994), p. 387.

Marriott, B. *Food Components to Enhance Performance.* Washington, DC: National Academy Press, 1994.

Maughan, Ronald. "Creatine Supplementation and Exercise Performance." *International Journal of Sport Nutrition* (1995), pp. 94–101.

Mayer, Jean, Roy Purnima, and Kamakhya Prasad Mitra. "Relation Between Caloric Intake, Body Weight, and Physical Work: Studies in an Industrial Male Population in West Bengal." *American Journal of Clinical Nutrition*, Vol. 4 (1956), No. 2, pp. 169–175.

Merimee, T. J., D. Rabinowitz, and S. E. Fineberg. "Arginine-Initiated Release of Human Growth Hormone." *New England Journal of Medicine* (1969), pp. 1434–1438.

Merimee, Thomas J., David Rabinowitz, Lamar Riggs, John A. Burgess, David L. Rimoin, and Victor A. McKusick. "Plasma Growth Hormone After Arginine Infusion." *New England Journal of Medicine*, Vol. 23 (1967), pp. 434–438.

Mertz, Walter. "Assessment of the Trace Element Nutritional Status." *Nutrition Research* (1985), pp. 169–174.

Meydani, M., et al. "Protective Effect of Vitamin E on Exercise-Induced Oxidative Damage in Young and Older Adults." *American Journal of Physiology*, Vol. 264 (1993), pp. R992–R998.

Mikesell, Kevin A., and Gary A. Dudley. "Influence of Intense Endurance Training on Aerobic Power of Competitive

Distance Runners." *Medicine and Science in Sports and Exercise,* Vol. 16 (1984), No. 4, pp. 371–375.

Mitchell, J. B., D. L. Costill, J. A. Houmard, M. G. Flynn, W. J. Fink, and J. D. Beltz. "Effects of Carbohydrate Ingestion on Gastric Emptying and Exercise Performance." *Medicine and Science in Sports and Exercise,* Vol. 20 (1988), No. 2, pp. 110–115.

Morgan, William P. "Affective Beneficence of Vigorous Physical Activity." *Medicine and Science in Sports and Exercise,* Vol. 17 (1985), No. 1, pp. 94–100.

Murphy, T., et al. "Performance Enhancing Ration Components Project: U.S. Army." Abstract of the 11th annual symposium of Sports and Cardiovascular Nutritionists, Atlanta, Georgia, 22–24 April 1994.

Murray, Robert; Dennis E. Eddy, Tami W. Murray, John G. Seifert, Gregory L. Paul, and George A. Halaby. "The Effect of Fluid and Carbohydrate Feedings During Intermittent Cycling Exercise." *Medicine and Science in Sports and Exercise,* Vol. 19 (1987), No. 6, pp. 597–604.

Mutch, B.J.C., and E. W. Banister. "Ammonia Metabolism in Exercise and Fatigue: A Review." *Medicine and Science in Sports and Exercise,* Vol. 15 (1983), No. 1, pp 41–50.

Nishizawa, N., M. Shimbo, S. Hareyama, and R. Funabiki. "Fractional Catabolic Rates of Myosin and Actin Estimated by Urinary Excretion of N-Methylhistidine: The Effect of Dietary Protein Level on Catabolic Rates Under Conditions of Restricted Food Intake." *British Journal of Nutrition,* Vol. 37 (1976), pp. 345–421.

Okano, Goroh, Hidekatsu Takeda, Isao Morita, Mitsuru Katoh, Zuien Mu, and Shosuke Miyake. "Effect of Pre-Exercise Fructose Ingestion on Endurance Performance in Fed Men." *Medicine and Science in Sports and Exercise,* Vol. 20 (1987), No. 7, pp. 105–109.

Oscai, Lawrence B., and John O. Holloszy. "Effects of Weight Changes Produced by Exercise, Food Restriction, or Overeating on Body Composition." *Journal of Clinical Investigation,* Vol. 48 (1969), pp. 2124–2128.

Palmer, Warren K. "Introduction to Symposium: Cyclic AMP Regulation of Fuel Metabolism During Exercise." *Medicine and Science in Sports and Exercise,* Vol. 20 (1988), No. 6, pp. 523–524.

Parkhouse, W. S., and D. C. McKenzie. "Possible Contribution of Skeletal Muscle Buffers to Enhanced Anaerobic Performance: A Brief Review." *Medicine and Science in Sports and Exercise,* Vol. 16 (1984), No. 4, 328–338.

Pavlou, Konstantin N., William P. Steffee, Robert H. Lerman, and Belton A. Burrows. "Effects of Dieting and Exercise on Lean Body Mass, Oxygen Uptake, and Strength." *Medicine and Science in Sports and Exercise,* Vol. 17 (1974), No. 4, pp. 466–471.

Piehl, Karin. "Time Course for Refilling of Glycogen Stores in Human Muscle Fibres Following Exercise-Induced Glycogen Depletion." *Acta Physiologica Scandinavica,* Vol. 90 (1974), pp. 297–302.

Pizza, F., et al. "A Carbohydrate Loading Regimen Improves High Intensity, Short Duration Exercise Performance." *International Journal of Sport Science* (1995), pp. 110–116.

Prasad, Ananda S. "Role of Trace Elements in Growth and Development." *Nutrition Research* (1985), pp. 295–299.

Prud'homme, D. C. Bouchard, C. Leblanc, F. Landry, and E. Fontaine. "Sensitivity of Maximal Aerobic Power to Training Is Genotype-Dependent." *Medicine and Science in Sports and Exercise,* Vol. 16 (1984), No. 5, pp. 489–493.

Romieu, Isabelle, Walter C. Willett, Meir J. Stampfer, Graham A. Colditz, Laura Sampson, Bernard Rosner, Charles Hennekens, and Frank E. Speizer. "Energy Intake and Other Determinants of Relative Weight." *American Journal of Clinical Nutrition,* Vol. 47 (1988), pp. 406–412.

Brilla, L. R., and T. E. Landerholm. "Effect of Fish Oil Supplementation and Exercise on Serum Lipids and Aerobic Fitness." *Journal of Sports Medicine and Physical Fitness,* Vol. 30 (1990), No. 2, pp. 173–180.

Saitoh, Shin-ichi, Yutaka Yoshitake, and Masahige Suzuki. "Enhanced Glycogen Repletion in Liver and Skeletal Muscle With Citrate Orally Fed After Exhaustive Treadmill Running and Swimming." *Journal of Nutritional Science and Vitaminology,* Vol. 29 (1983), pp. 45–52.

Salleo, Alberto, Guiseppe Anastasi, Guiseppa LaSpada, Guiseppina Falzea, and Maria G. Denaro. "New Muscle Fiber Production During Compensatory Hypertrophy." *Medicine and Science in Sports and Exercise,* Vol. 12 (1980), No. 4, pp. 268–273.

Satabin, Pascale, Pierre Portero, Gilles Defer, Jacques Bricout, and Charles-Yannick Guezennec. "Metabolic and Hormonal Responses to Lipid and Carbohydrate Diets During Exercise in Man." *Medicine and Science in Sports and Exercise,* Vol. 19 (1987), No. 3, pp. 218–223.

Saudek, Christopher D. "The Metabolic Events of Starvation." *American Journal of Medicine,* Vol. 60 (1976), pp. 117–126.

Schalch, Don S. "The Influence of Physical Stress and Exercise on Growth Hormone and Insulin Secretion in Man." *Journal of Laboratory and Clinical Medicine,* Vol. 69 (1967), No. 2, pp. 256–267.

Sen, C., et al. "Oxidative Stress After Human Exercise: Effect of N-Acetylcysteine Supplementation." *Journal of Applied Physiology,* Vol. 76 (1994), pp. 2570–2577.

Short, S. "Dietary Surveys and Nutrition Knowledge." In Hickson, J. F., and I. W. Wolinsky, Eds., *Nutrition in Exercise and Sport.* Boca Raton, FL: CRC Press, 1989.

Simoneau, J.-A., G. Lortie, M. R. Boulay, M. Marcotte, M.-C. Thibault, and C. Bouchard. "Human Skeletal Muscle Fiber Type Alteration With High-Intensity Intermittent Training." *European Journal of Applied Physiology,* Vol. 54 (1985), pp. 250–253.

Simon-Schnass, I., and H. Pabst. "Influence of Vitamin E on Physical Performance." *International Journal of Vitamin Nutrition Research* (1987), pp. 49–54.

Soares, M. J., et al. "The Effect of Exercise on Riboflavin Status of Adult Men." *British Journal of Nutrition*, Vol. 69 (1993), pp. 541–551.

Thomas, D., et al. "Plasma Glucose Levels After Prolonged Strenuous Exercise Correlate Inversely With Glycemic Response to Food Consumed Before Exercise." *International Journal of Sport Nutrition*, Vol. 4 (1994), p. 361.

Thompson, Deborah A., Larry A. Wolfe, and Roelof Eikelboom. "Acute Effects of Exercise Intensity on Appetite in Young Men." *Medicine and Science in Sports and Exercise*, Vol. 20 (1988), No. 3, pp. 222–227.

Thorland, William G., Glen O. Johnson, Thomas G. Fagot, Gerald D. Tharp, and Richard W. Hammer. "Body Composition and Somatotype Characteristics of Junior Olympic Athletes" *Medicine and Science in Sports and Exercise*, Vol. 13 (1981), No. 5, pp. 332–338.

Todd, Karen S., Gail E. Butterfield, and Doris Howes Calloway. "Nitrogen Balance in Men With Adequate and Deficient Energy Intake at Three Levels of Work." *Journal of Nutrition*, Vol. 114 (1984), pp. 2107–2118.

Torun, B., N. S. Scrimshaw, and V. R. Young. "Effect of Isometric Exercises on Body Potassium and Dietary Protein Requirements of Young Men." *American Journal of Clinical Nutrition*, Vol. 30 (1977), pp. 1983–1993.

Tric, I., and E. Haymes. "Effects of Caffeine Ingestion on Exercise-Induced Changes During High-Intensity, Intermittent Exercise." *International Journal of Sport Nutrition*, Vol. 5 (1995), pp. 37–44.

Valeriani, A. "The Need for Carbohydrate Intake During Endurance Exercise." *Sports Medicine*, Vol. 12 (1991), No. 6, p. 349.

Viru, A. *Adaptation in Sports Training*. Boca Raton, FL: CRC Press, 1995.

Walberg, Janet L., V. Karina Ruiz, Sandra L. Tarlton, Dennis E. Hinkle, and Forrest W. Thye. "Exercise Capacity and Nitrogen Loss During a High or Low Carbohydrate Diet." *Medicine and Science in Sports and Exercise*, Vol. 20 (1986), pp. 34–43.

Ward, P. S., and D.C.L. Savage. "Growth Hormone Responses to Sleep, Insulin Hypoglycemia and Arginine Infusion." *Hormone Research*, Vol. 22 (1985), pp. 7–11.

Weir, Jane, Timothy D. Noakes, Kathryn Myburgh, and Brett Adams. "A High Carbohydrate Diet Negates the Metabolic Effects of Caffeine During Exercise." *Medicine and Science in Sports and Exercise*, Vol. 19 (1986), pp. 100–105.

Weltman, Arthur, Sharleen Matter, and Bryant A. Stamford. "Caloric Restriction and/or Mild Exercise: Effects on Serum Lipids and Body Composition." *American Journal of Clinical Nutrition*, Vol. 33 (1980), pp. 1002–1009.

Wilcox, Anthony R. "The Effects of Caffeine and Exercise on Body Weight, Fat-Pad Weight, and Fat-Cell Size." *Medicine and Science in Sports and Exercise*, Vol. 14 (1981), pp. 317–321.

Williams, M. H. "Vitamin Supplementation and Athletic Performance." *International Journal of Vitamin and Nutrition Research*, Vol. 30 (1989), p. 163.

Wolinsky, I., and J. Hickson. *Nutrition in Exercise and Sport*, Second Edition. Boca Raton, FL: CRC Press, 1994.

Young, K., and C.T.M. Davies. "Effect of Diet on Human Muscle Weakness Following Prolonged Exercise." *European Journal of Applied Physiology*, Vol. 53 (1984), pp. 81–85.

Young, Vernon R., and Peter L. Pellett. "Protein Intake and Requirements With Reference to Diet and Health." *American Journal of Clinical Nutrition*, Vol. 45 (1987), pp. 1323–1343.

ABOUT THE AUTHORS

Daniel Gastelu, M.S., M.F.S., is a pioneer in performance nutrition. He is a graduate of Rutgers University, where he has also taught undergraduate biological science and graduate level computer programming and biostatistical analysis. During the past fifteen years, Mr. Gastelu has developed personal-care products and dietary supplements designed to boost athletic performance, aid fat loss, and improve health. He has also authored numerous manuals, articles, books, and infomercials on fitness and nutrition, and is a certified master of fitness science, certified fitness trainer, and certified specialist in performance nutrition. In addition, he is currently serving as a professor for the International Sports Sciences Association, as well as the director of its Nutritional Sciences Department. *Dynamic Nutrition for Maximum Performance* is based on his Specialist in Performance Nutrition course, which is used to certify doctors, trainers, strength coaches, therapists, and fitness trainers worldwide. Mr. Gastelu and his family live in northern New Jersey.

Fred Hatfield, Ph.D, is a graduate of Temple University. He has specialized in sports nutrition and fitness for over thirty years, and is co-founder and president of the International Sports Sciences Association. He is a world-champion power lifter, and has trained hundreds of professional and elite athletes and their trainers. Outside the gym, Dr. Hatfield has taught sports psychology, strength physiology, and physical education at the University of Wisconsin, Newark State College, Bowie State College, the University of Illinois, and Temple University. He has acted as a consultant to the U.S. Olympic Committee, West German Body Building Federation, Australian Powerlifting Federation, and CBS Sports; coached the U.S. National Powerlifting team; and served on the executive committees of the U.S. Olympic Weightlifting Federation and U.S. Powerlifting Federation. He is the founding editor of *Sports Fitness* and *BodyCraft* magazines, and has written over sixty books and hunerds of articles on fitness and nutrition. He has also helped develop a number of athletic-performance products. Because of his frequent world-record–breaking performances in the squat, Dr. Hatfield has come to be known as "Dr. Squat" in powerlifting circles. Dr. Hatfield and his family currently reside in Clearwater, Florida.

INDEX

Index